Developing Practical Nursing Skills

Developing Practical Nursing Skills

Fourth edition

Edited by

Lesley Baillie PhD, MSc, BA (Hons), RNT, RGN

Florence Nightingale Foundation Chair of Clinical Nursing Practice
London South Bank University, University College London Hospitals,
Florence Nightingale Foundation

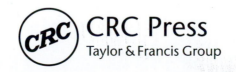

CRC Press
Taylor & Francis Group

CRC Press
Taylor & Francis Group
6000 Broken Sound Parkway NW, Suite 300
Boca Raton, FL 33487-2742

© 2014 by Taylor & Francis Group, LLC
CRC Press is an imprint of Taylor & Francis Group, an Informa business

No claim to original U.S. Government works
Printed and bound in India by Replika Press Pvt. Ltd.
Printed on acid-free paper
Version Date: 20130808

International Standard Book Number-13: 978-1-4441-7595-0 (Paperback)

This book contains information obtained from authentic and highly regarded sources. While all reasonable efforts have been made to publish reliable data and information, neither the author[s] nor the publisher can accept any legal responsibility or liability for any errors or omissions that may be made. The publishers wish to make clear that any views or opinions expressed in this book by individual editors, authors or contributors are personal to them and do not necessarily reflect the views/opinions of the publishers. The information or guidance contained in this book is intended for use by medical, scientific or health-care professionals and is provided strictly as a supplement to the medical or other professional's own judgement, their knowledge of the patient's medical history, relevant manufacturer's instructions and the appropriate best practice guidelines. Because of the rapid advances in medical science, any information or advice on dosages, procedures or diagnoses should be independently verified. The reader is strongly urged to consult the drug companies' printed instructions, and their websites, before administering any of the drugs recommended in this book. This book does not indicate whether a particular treatment is appropriate or suitable for a particular individual. Ultimately it is the sole responsibility of the medical professional to make his or her own professional judgements, so as to advise and treat patients appropriately. The authors and publishers have also attempted to trace the copyright holders of all material reproduced in this publication and apologize to copyright holders if permission to publish in this form has not been obtained. If any copyright material has not been acknowledged please write and let us know so we may rectify in any future reprint.

Library of Congress Cataloging-in-Publication Data

Developing practical nursing skills / edited by Lesley Baillie. -- Fourth edition.
   p. ; cm.
   Preceded by: Developing practical adult nursing skills / edited by Lesley Baillie. 3rd ed. 2009.
   Includes bibliographical references and index.
   ISBN 978-1-4441-7595-0 (hardcover : alk. paper)
   I. Baillie, Lesley, editor of compilation.
   [DNLM: 1. Nursing Care--methods. 2. Clinical Competence. WY 100]

RT62
610.7306'93--dc23
                        2013030985

**Visit the Taylor & Francis Web site at
http://www.taylorandfrancis.com**

**and the CRC Press Web site at
http://www.crcpress.com**

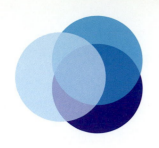

Contents

Contents

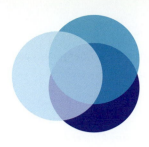

Foreword

Nurses are in a unique and privileged position to deliver skilled and compassionate care that promotes comfort and dignity to people who are most vulnerable. The practical skills that nurses carry out with people of all ages, and in many different care settings, are central to people's experiences of healthcare and for their recovery and well-being. Although we are aware that many people experience excellent nursing care, we also come across patient experiences devoid of skilled and compassionate care with sometimes devastating effects on the individuals concerned. Such examples highlight the importance of ensuring that the nursing workforce consistently provides the highest standards of compassionate and dignified nursing care across all settings.

In December 2012, we launched *Compassion in Practice* in which we presented our shared purpose as nurses, midwives and care staff to deliver high-quality, compassionate care and to achieve excellent health and well-being outcomes. *Compassion in Practice* was launched after a wide consultation with nurses, midwives, care staff, the public, service users and other stakeholders. The vision and strategy is underpinned by six fundamental values and behaviours: care, compassion, competence, communication, courage and commitment; the 6Cs focus on 'putting the person being cared for at the heart of the care given' (p. 13). *Compassion in Practice* also sets out six areas of action to support the delivery of excellent care.

The fourth edition of the popular nursing textbook *Developing Practical Nursing Skills* retains the caring, person-centred and holistic approach to carrying out practical nursing skills, which the earlier editions established. The first two chapters of the book introduce concepts of caring, compassion, communication and dignity, emphasising and explaining how these underpin the practical skills that nurses carry out in everyday practice. The subsequent chapters focus on essential aspects of nursing practice, explaining how to integrate competent, safe and evidence-based actions with excellent communication and a caring and compassionate approach. The book applies nursing skills across healthcare settings to people with physical and/or mental health needs and to people with learning disabilities. The chapters of the book include the practical application of nursing skills when caring for people with dementia, which is both welcome and timely.

This book will be a valuable guide for student nurses, and other care staff, as it will support them in developing their practical skills for nursing care, underpinned by core nursing values. The interactive approach of the book will encourage readers to engage with their own learning and reflect on, and learn from, their practice experiences. I recommend this book to students and care staff and also to nurse educators and nurses who are supervising and guiding students and care staff in delivering skilled, compassionate and dignified nursing care.

Jane Cummings
Chief Nursing Officer for England

Preface

This book, fully updated and expanded from the third edition, aims to assist readers in developing the practical skills necessary to care for adults in varied healthcare settings. Practical nursing skills, when carried out with competence and compassion, are highly valued by those who need care from nurses and their families and will promote health, recovery, dignity and comfort, making an essential contribution to positive healthcare experiences. In 2010, the Nursing and Midwifery Council (NMC) published new standards for preregistration nurse education. These standards included the Essential Skills Clusters for preregistration nursing students, first released in 2007, and this fourth edition covers all of these essential skills as well as other skills which are important in nursing practice. In some environments, nurses are more likely to supervise or support others than directly carry out these practical skills. To supervise others in providing quality fundamental care requires leadership, a sound knowledge and understanding of these skills and a commitment to their importance and value.

This book's practical skills are applied through scenarios to adults with physical health needs, adults with mental health needs and adults with learning disabilities. However, as the NMC's (2010) standards include generic competencies and recognise that all nurses should be able to provide essential care across the life span, each chapter includes boxes with practice points for caring for children, and women who are pregnant, or after childbirth. These boxes highlight key points that all nurses should be aware of with recommended further reading and suggested resources. This fourth edition has increased content about caring for people with dementia. This is in response to reports highlighting the high proportion of people with dementia needing healthcare, along with the need to improve care for people with dementia, particularly in a hospital setting (Alzheimer's Society 2009; Royal College of Psychiatrists 2011).

The first chapter explains the caring context for skills, emphasising the importance of the underpinning knowledge and attitudes of the caregiver, as well as the practical components of skills and safe practice. Chapter 1 also provides guidance to help students maximise learning from their practical experiences. Dignity in care is explored, and subsequent chapters address how to promote the dignity of people when undertaking specific skills in practice. Skills are discussed with application to the scenarios, emphasising problem-solving skills and a reflective and caring approach. The book is interactive, evidence-based and promotes theory—practice links and reflective practice.

Although this fourth edition is particularly applicable to preregistration nursing students following the adult, mental health and learning disability fields of nursing, it is also relevant to people who are studying for qualifications in care, to students on a range of assistant practitioner (foundation degree) healthcare-related programmes and to all those involved in the teaching of practical skills, including university and college lecturers, and practitioners.

Nurses care for people in a wide range of settings in different circumstances, and hence no single term is appropriate to be used in every situation. In this book, the terms 'person' and 'people' are often used, but in some contexts the terms 'patient', 'client', 'individual', 'resident' or 'service user' are referred to in relation to people nurses care for.

I hope that this book will be really helpful to students who are learning skills for nursing adults, and I wish all those using the book a successful and rewarding nursing career.

Lesley Baillie

References

Alzheimer's Society. 2009. *Counting the Cost: Caring for People with Dementia on Acute Hospital Wards*. London: Alzheimer's Society.

Nursing and Midwifery Council (NMC). 2010. *Standards for Pre-Registration Nursing Education*. London: NMC.

Royal College of Psychiatrists (RCP). 2011. *Report of the National Audit of Dementia Care in General Hospitals*. In: Young, J., Hood, C., Woolley, R., Gandesha, A. and Souza, R. (eds.). London: Healthcare Quality Improvement Partnership.

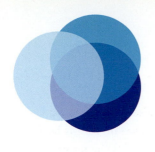

Acknowledgements

Grateful thanks to the following people for their help in preparing the manuscript:

- Friends, family and colleagues for their invaluable support and encouragement during the preparation of this fourth edition
- Alan Baillie, Senior Lecturer, Mental Health, Buckinghamshire New University, for advice on mental health content
- The staff at Taylor & Francis for their support and encouragement throughout the development of this fourth edition, in particular, Naomi Wilkinson.

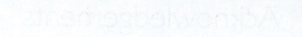

Editor Biography

Lesley Baillie, PhD, MSc, BA (Hons), RNT, RGN, is an experienced acute care nurse, educator and researcher. She is particularly interested in developing and improving clinical practice and promoting integrated care, and she has published widely on patient dignity and clinical practice developments. Lesley edited the first edition of *Developing Practical Nursing Skills*, which was published in 2001, and she has continued to edit subsequent editions. In 2011, she co-edited *Dignity in Healthcare: A Practical Approach for Nurses and Midwives*. From 2006 to 2010, Lesley led clinical skills and simulation developments at London South Bank University. Lesley was Reader in Healthcare at University of Bedfordshire from 2010 to 2012, where she worked on projects to promote dignified and competent healthcare. In 2012, Lesley was appointed Florence Nightingale Foundation Chair of Clinical Nursing Practice, in a joint appointment between London South Bank University, University College London Hospitals and the Florence Nightingale Foundation.

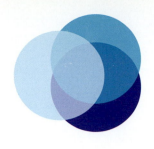

Contributors

Kirsty Andrews
Senior Lecturer, Faculty of Health, Social Care and Education, Anglia Ruskin University, UK

Janine Ashton
Tissue Viability Nurse, Airedale NHS Foundation Trust, UK

Lesley Baillie
Professor of Clinical Nursing Practice, Faculty of Health and Social Care, London South Bank University, UK

Dee Burrows
Independent Consultant Nurse, Chronic Pain; Honorary Lecturer, Cardiff University, UK; Clinical Nurse Specialist, Chronic Pain, South Devon Healthcare NHS Foundation Trust

Rachel Busuttil Leaver
Lecturer Practitioner, Urological Care, Faculty of Health and Social Care, London South Bank University, UK

Patricia Folan
Infection Prevention & Control Matron; Deputy Director of Infection Prevention & Control, Microbiology Department, Whittington NHS Trust, UK

Stephanie Forge
Community Nurse, North East London Foundation Trust, London, UK

Sue Maddex
Senior Lecturer, Adult Nursing, Faculty of Health and Social Care, London South Bank University, UK

Nicola M. Neale
Macmillan Cancer Information and Support Manager, Heatherwood and Wexham Park Hospitals NHS Foundation Trust, UK

Martina O'Brien
Senior Lecturer, Adult Nursing, London South Bank University, UK

Glynis Pellatt
Formerly Senior Lecturer, Adult Nursing, Faculty of Health and Social Sciences, University of Bedfordshire, UK

Joanne Sale
Senior Lecturer, Mental Health, University of Bedfordshire, UK

Tracey Valler-Jones
Senior Lecturer (Pre-registration Nursing), University of Birmingham, Birmingham, UK

Moira Walker
Lecturer (Practice – Adult Acute), University of Bedfordshire, UK

Consultants

Pregnancy and birth: practice points: Melanie Brooke-Read, Senior Lecturer (Midwifery), University of Bedfordshire, UK

Children: practice points: Rebecca Jones, Tutor (Child Health), University of Surrey, UK

Learning disability review: Sherry Forchione, Community Learning Disability Nurse, Southern Health NHS Foundation Trust, UK

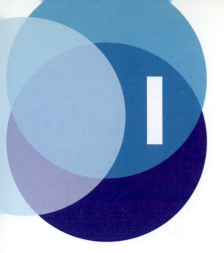

Practical Nursing Skills: A Caring Approach

Lesley Baillie

Nursing care should be delivered compassionately and competently in a way that promotes the dignity of the people being cared for. All student nurses need to learn to perform a range of practical skills safely, with a caring approach (Nursing and Midwifery Council [NMC] 2010). Healthcare support workers and assistant practitioners also need to develop practical skills, as they work within nursing teams. This book aims to assist readers in developing a caring approach to a range of practical nursing skills, for application with people across different healthcare settings. Practical nursing skills comprise not only the hands-on (psychomotor) element but also an underpinning evidence-based knowledge, effective communication skills, an ethical approach, creative and reflective thinking and an appropriate professional, caring attitude. These elements are considered throughout the chapters in this book.

This chapter discusses the nature and context of practical skills in nursing and how this book can help you in developing your nursing skills. There is an emphasis on developing and valuing these practical skills as holistic, caring skills that contribute to people's healthcare experiences in a positive way, promote their dignity and support their comfort and well-being.

This chapter includes the following topics:

- The nature of practical nursing skills
- The context for practical nursing skills
- Practical skills and their application across the life span and in different healthcare settings
- A caring and compassionate approach to practical nursing skills
- Cultural competence and practical nursing skills
- Dignity and practical nursing skills
- Learning practical nursing skills

THE NATURE OF PRACTICAL NURSING SKILLS

Nurses need to develop a range of abilities, including skills in practical nursing, communication and management. These skills are often integrated within the role of nursing because carrying out practical nursing skills effectively also requires skills in communication and teamwork. Practical nursing skills are the hands-on skills that nurses use in their care of people; some of these skills are performed by other professionals in caring roles too. Healthcare support workers and assistant practitioners carry out many of these skills, and hence, this book is relevant for them too.

Practical nursing skills are used to promote comfort and maintain health for people who, due to acute or long-term physical or mental health conditions, cannot care for themselves independently or need help to maintain their health.

ACTIVITY

Reflect on all the activities you carry out to keep yourself comfortable and healthy each day. What would happen if you could not carry out these activities?

You might have reflected that you carry out these activities, often referred to as 'activities of daily living' (Roper et al. 2000) with little thought much of the time: sleeping, eating and drinking, going to the toilet, moving about, and carrying out personal hygiene. You also might take medication for one or more health conditions or if you have pain, take painkilling medicines or manage your pain another way. However, any mental or physical health condition can affect these self-care activities; without help, people would quickly become debilitated and uncomfortable, with their health and well-being at risk. There are more than 6 million unpaid carers in the United Kingdom (UK) who help family, friends or neighbours with care due to health issues (Buckner and Yeandle 2011). Many nurses are involved in supporting people and their carers at home, for example, teaching them to keep their skin healthy when they lack mobility; to manage medication; to cope with mental health issues; or to deal with altered elimination, such as a urinary catheter. When people are admitted to hospital, nursing teams must support people with activities that they cannot manage themselves as part of their holistic care.

Practical nursing skills are also carried out when assessing a person's condition and delivering interventions to improve or maintain their health; these skills are carried out in acute situations, for people with long-term conditions and people with multiple health needs. When we feel unwell, we self-assess; for example, we might measure our body temperature. Some people are unable to self-assess or communicate that they feel unwell, for example, a person with advanced dementia or a person with a severe learning disability. Nurses need to be highly skilled in using a range of assessment skills for people with different health needs, and they must be able to interpret and act on the results appropriately and often speedily. People who are acutely ill or who have long-term health conditions that fluctuate in severity, need careful and skilful monitoring. Nurses must also be able to use a wide range of practical skills to promote comfort, safety and well-being, including administration of medication.

ACTIVITY

Almost everyone has had an injection at some stage, and you may have had recent immunisations before starting to study nursing. You probably took it for granted that the skill would be performed competently. What are the different elements of carrying out this skill?

You probably considered technical aspects such as preparing the correct medicine accurately and safely. You also may have identified that the nurse required underlying knowledge of the drug's actions and potential side effects and that the nurse should use a calm and friendly approach to relax you and relieve anxiety. This example illustrates that effective practical nursing skills require a skilled motor performance (the doing element) and a sound knowledge based on best evidence (the cognitive aspect), with both accompanied by an appropriate attitude (the affective aspect).

Oermann (1990) suggested that the motor (doing) element of a practical (psychomotor) skill is often emphasised to the exclusion of the cognitive and affective components. She highlighted the importance of the cognitive base (the scientific principles underlying the performance of the skill) and the affective domain, which reflects the nurse's values and concern for the person while the skill is being performed. These three aspects are now explored further.

The affective domain

The affective domain is underpinned by values, which can be defined as 'core beliefs that guide and motivate attitudes and actions' (see http://www.ethics.org/resource/definitions-values). Nurses bring their own personal values into nursing; these values are influenced by a range of factors (e.g. family, education) and hopefully include integrity, compassion, dignity and kindness. Nurses must also embrace professional values, directed by the National Health Service (NHS) and the Nursing and Midwifery Council (NMC). Values are important as they influence attitudes and behaviour. For example, Nåden and Eriksson (2004) found that nurses who promoted dignity had a strong moral attitude, underpinned by values such as respect, honesty and responsibility; such nurses had a 'genuine interest and desire to help patients' (p. 90).

Bush and Barr's (1997) study of critical care nurses' experiences of caring identified the affective process as including sensitivity, empathy, concern and interest. One participant was quoted saying, 'instead of just saying, "I'm taking your blood pressure, your temperature", you really care about what the patient is going through – how they must feel'. Bjork (1999a) argued that caring intentions are necessary in practical nursing actions because 'they can transform the acts of handling and helping into tolerable or even meaningful experiences for the patient'. She suggested that nurses can demonstrate respect for and interest in patients while carrying out skills, conveying the message that 'it is not just a body that is being handled'. While carrying out practical skills, such as bathing, nurses can foster confidence and develop trusting relationships with patients.

Bjork (1999a) also suggested being aware of the meaning of the practical skill for the individual and how it fits into the person's overall experience. For example, a wound dressing may exemplify the change in body image after invasive surgery, and bathing someone may highlight their loss of independence due to physical or mental health problems. Box 1.1 details the positive experience of Dee Burrows (one of the authors of Chapter 12) of being assisted with a shower postoperatively. Her story illustrates the significance of the nurse's approach while carrying out her care,

Box 1.1 Illustrative example of the significance of the nurse's approach to a patient while assisting with showering

About 5 days after I had had major abdominal surgery, after which I had been seriously ill, a nurse got me up for the first time and took me in a wheelchair to the bathroom for a shower. I was weak, afraid of being naked in front of her and I felt uncomfortable about my wound being on show. She helped me off with my clothes and helped me have a shower, during which she sensitively used humour to make me relaxed. She washed my body and hair, and at intervals put her hand gently on my shoulder in a comforting way. At one point, she knelt down and gently put her hands either side of my large wound and said 'It looks beautiful — it's going to heal up really well. You'll be back in a bikini within a month'. (I was!) I got this tremendous sense of relief that even though I had this massive scar I would still be me again. She had encouraged me to accept my scar. By the end of the whole episode of care, I felt wonderfully clean from top to toe, relaxed and had begun to recover a sense of self. The fear had just disappeared.

and its impact on her recovery. Each time you carry out a practical skill with a person, you convey a message about your state of being (Paterson and Zderad 1988); for example, are you anxious, in a hurry, distracted or uninterested? Chapter 2 considers the nurse's approach to people during practical nursing skills application.

The cognitive domain

The cognitive domain reflects the thinking element behind the skill, including the application of best evidence in practice and problem solving. Being able to adapt a skill in practice requires a sound underlying knowledge of why it is being performed and the rationale for each stage. For example, understanding the principles behind oxygen therapy administration enables nurses to choose an administration method that is safe and acceptable to people in specific healthcare situations. Practical skills should be based on best available evidence, which may be derived from research, but could be based on experience, and from reflection on practice. Benner (1984) identified that practice is always more complex and presents many more realities than theory ever can, and she highlighted the value of theory derived from practice (see section 'Learning from experience and reflection').

Nurses are accountable for their actions, so they must be able to explain the knowledge base underpinning their practice. Benner (1984) explored how expert nurses develop knowledge from their practice, learning to recognise, for example, subtle changes in people's conditions. Not all nursing skills have a firm evidence base on which to implement practice, but in many areas research-based knowledge is available. Within this book, authors have searched for up-to-date evidence to underpin practical skills, and they refer to evidence-based guidelines where available. These guidelines include the National Institute for Health and

Clinical Excellence (NICE) evidence-based guidelines and quality standards (see www.nice.org.uk) and the Cochrane Library systematic reviews of research. Be aware: these guidelines are regularly reviewed, so check the websites for updates. An excellent source of information is the 'Evidence Search Health and Social Care' website (http://www.evidence.nhs.uk), which includes access to resources for evidence-based practice and a facility to search for evidence. Often, NHS Trusts and other healthcare organisations have their own clinical guidelines, based on best evidence, to assist nurses and other healthcare professionals to implement evidence-based practice in the local context. You should always work with your employer's guidelines, if available.

The motor domain

Learning the motor dimension of a skill is important for an effective outcome as lack of a skilled motor performance jeopardises both safety and comfort. Knowing how to execute a practical skill can be termed know-how type of knowledge – practical expertise and skill that is really acquired through practice and experience (Manley 1997). Nursing skills are performed in a changing clinical environment, with people who respond and react in different ways. Therefore, nurses need to adapt skills accordingly, so practical nursing skills can never be wholly automatic in nature.

The importance of practical nursing skills for quality care

The importance of high-quality nursing care cannot be overstated, and the application of practical nursing skills is central to patients' experiences. The National Nursing Research Unit (2008) identified that from patients' perspectives, the features of high-quality care are as follows:

- A holistic approach to physical, mental and emotional needs, patient-centred and continuous care
- Efficiency and effectiveness combined with humanity and compassion
- Professional, high-quality evidence-based practice
- Safe, effective and prompt nursing interventions
- Patient empowerment, support and advocacy
- Seamless care through effective teamwork with other professions

Nurses valued being able to make a difference to patients' lives, having close contact with patients, delivering excellent care, working in a team and being a role model to others and continually developing through learning and improving.

However, over the past decade or so, there have been increasing concerns about fundamental care being neglected in healthcare settings, with media headlines about poor attention to nutrition and continence, and reports from the Patients Association (2009, 2011), the Health Service Ombudsman (2011) and the inquiry into care standards in Mid Staffordshire (Mid Staffordshire NHS Foundation Trust Inquiry 2013), all revealing a lack of care with poor patient experiences and outcomes. Nurses should deliver high-quality fundamental care, and they have a professional and ethical duty to do so. People who are cared for and their families should be confident that nurses will deliver care in a compassionate and competent way and promote comfort and dignity when people are at their most vulnerable. Technology is integral to the application of many practical nursing skills, but its use should be accompanied by a caring and humanistic approach.

This book emphasises that practical skills should be person-centred and delivered within the context of a caring philosophy, with value attached to fundamental as well as technical care. For example, there is great skill involved in helping an older person regain the ability to wash and dress after a stroke, or in assisting a person with confusion to maintain continence.

THE CONTEXT FOR PRACTICAL NURSING SKILLS

Practical nursing skills must be applied within the context of the individual person and the nurse–patient relationship. The wider context for skills application is also relevant: the legal, professional and health policy context.

Legislation

Nursing practice takes place in the context of legislation; some Acts of Parliament with particular relevance to practical skills are briefly presented here. The Human Rights Act (Great Britain 1998) recognised that all individuals have minimal and fundamental human rights including the right to dignity and privacy; dignity and privacy are important principles during delivery of care and are discussed in relation to practical skills throughout this book. The Mental Capacity Act (Great Britain 2005) is also particularly relevant to practical nursing skills and is considered further in relation to consent in Chapter 2.

The Equality Act (Great Britain 2010) aims to protect all people against discrimination. The act established protected characteristics that cannot be used as a reason to treat people unfairly and include the following: age, disability, gender reassignment, marriage and civil partnership, pregnancy and maternity, race, religion and belief, sex and sexual orientation. Unfortunately, there is evidence that discrimination in healthcare persists and that discriminatory behaviour diminishes the dignity of people being cared for (Baillie and Matiti 2013). For example, a UK Commission to investigate dignified care for older people highlighted that older people continue to experience discrimination despite being the major group of health service users (Commission on Dignity in Care 2012). An independent inquiry into access to healthcare for people with learning disabilities (Sir Jonathan Michael and the Independent Inquiry into Access to Healthcare for People with Learning Disabilities 2008) highlighted inequalities in relation to people with learning disabilities. Mencap (2004, 2007, 2012), a UK charity campaigning for equal rights for children and adults with a learning disability, reports that people with learning disabilities continue to encounter direct discrimination from NHS staff who fail to treat them with dignity and respect. Mencap (2012) highlighted the legal requirement to provide equality in healthcare, so nurses must give the same quality of care and treatment to all patients, including those with a learning disability. Mencap (2012) suggested that discrimination occurs due to the lack of value afforded to the life of a person with a learning disability, indicating that, despite the Equality Act 2010 and professional codes of practice, some healthcare workers do not recognise the human dignity of people with learning disabilities. The 2012 Mencap report revealed cases where nurses failed to provide even basic care to people with learning disabilities, neglecting nutrition, hydration and pain relief.

Professional requirements

The NMC requirements are an important context for the development of practical nursing skills, so you should become familiar with the NMC's guidance and standards. The NMC's (2011) guidance on professional conduct for nursing and midwifery students explains the role of the NMC as the professional regulator with regard to safeguarding the health and well-being of the public, and how this role is carried out. The NMC's (2008a) *Code: Standards of Conduct, Performance and Ethics for Nurses and Midwives* is applicable to every nursing care activity that you take part in as nurses must provide 'a high standard of practice and care at all times'. The code also requires that nurses treat people kindly and considerately, respect their dignity, respond to concerns and preferences, gain consent and involve people in decisions about their care. All these elements should be integral to carrying out practical nursing skills. The NMC's (2010) *Standards for Pre-Registration Nursing Education* include skills that students must develop prior to registration; these are termed the 'Essential Skills Clusters'. This book's chapters address all of these:

- Care, compassion and communication (Chapters 1, 2, 8, 9, 10 and 12)
- Organisational aspects of care (Chapters 4, 6 and 11)
- Infection prevention and control (Chapters 3 and 7)
- Nutrition and fluid balance (Chapter 10)
- Medicines management (Chapter 5)

The Department of Health (DH 2012b) has set out a vision for nursing that has care at its core; for further exploration, see section 'A caring and compassionate approach to practical nursing skills' and Chapter 2, which particularly focuses on communication.

Health policy and guidelines

There are many UK health and social care policy documents that provide context and guidance to nursing practice; on the website of the Royal College of Nursing (RCN), there is a section on clinical governance, which is a useful resource with documents for all four countries in the UK (see http://www.rcn.org.uk/development/practice/clinical_governance). Some key documents that are particularly relevant are discussed next. The NHS Constitution (DH 2012a) sets out core values; these

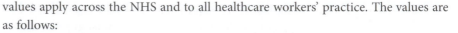

values apply across the NHS and to all healthcare workers' practice. The values are as follows:

- Respect and dignity
- Quality of care
- Compassion
- Improving lives
- Working together for patients
- Everyone counts

The NHS Constitution acknowledges to patients that they have 'the right to be treated with dignity and respect, in accordance with your human rights' (DH 2012a, p. 6), thus firmly embedding dignity as a human right within UK healthcare.

The DH's (2010) *Essence of Care 2010* sets out benchmarking standards for best practice in fundamental care for people of all ages (Box 1.2); these standards are referred to in applicable chapters. The Care Quality Commission for England inspects all health and social care providers on essential standards of safety and quality, and some of these standards are particularly relevant to practical nursing skills, for example, 'Respecting and involving people who use services', 'Meeting nutritional needs' and 'Cleanliness and infection control' (see http://www.cqc.org.uk/content/essential-standards-quality-and-safety).

In 2012, NICE produced a quality standard for patient experience in adult NHS services in England, so these standards apply to all nursing practice with adults, in both inpatient and other healthcare settings. These standards recommend that patients are 'treated with dignity, kindness, compassion, courtesy, respect, understanding and honesty'. The standards also include that patients should have regular assessment of their physical and psychological needs, which include nutrition, hydration, pain relief, personal hygiene and anxiety. The standards

---

Box 1.2 Essence of Care 2010: benchmarks

- Bladder, bowel and continence care
- Care environment
- Communication
- Food and drink
- Prevention and management of pain
- Personal hygiene
- Prevention and management of pressure ulcers
- Promoting health and well-being
- Record keeping
- Respect and dignity
- Safety
- Self-care

Source: Department of Health (DH). 2010. *Essence of Care 2010*. Gateway Ref: 14641. London: The Stationery Office.

highlight the importance of meeting both emotional support and fundamental needs such as pain management and nutrition, and of respecting confidentiality, listening in a sensitive and empathetic way and establishing trusting relationships.

Many health policies aim to set out strategy and guidance for particular areas of healthcare, and many of these approaches are applicable to nursing practice. Some key documents are reviewed next, in relation to care of people with learning disabilities, people with mental health problems and people with dementia.

Healthcare for people with learning disabilities

Many people with a learning disability do not have family and carers to advocate for them (Mencap 2012), increasing their vulnerability when accessing healthcare. Nurses care for people with learning disabilities across healthcare settings when they have health needs and have an important role in ensuring the delivery of high quality, safe care that addresses their individual needs in a dignified manner. In 2001, the DH published *Valuing People: A New Strategy for Learning Disability for the 21st Century*, which stressed that people with learning disabilities are people first and there should be a focus on what they can do rather than what they cannot. This document set out that all people with learning disabilities should have a health facilitator – who may be a keyworker, relative or health or social care professional – appointed to ensure they get the healthcare they need, and a Health Action Plan. An individual's Health Action Plan includes details of health interventions, oral health and dental care, fitness and mobility, continence, vision, hearing, nutrition, emotional needs, medication and records of screening. Any nurse carrying out practical skills with people with learning disabilities, or supporting their carers, should refer to the person's Health Action Plan.

Since 2001, the DH has carried out progress reviews. In *Good Practice in Learning Disability Nursing*, the DH (2007) emphasised that learning disability nurses are essential for making the 'Valuing People' vision happen and that they can help people with learning disabilities to stay healthy as long as possible. The DH (2009a) published *Valuing People Now: A New Three-Year Strategy for Learning Disabilities*, stating the key objective for all people with learning disabilities to get the healthcare and the support they need to live healthy lives. The report again acknowledged that better health for people with learning disabilities is a key priority, as there is clear evidence that most people with learning disabilities have poorer health than the rest of the population. The DH (2009a) further stated that access to the NHS is often poor and characterised by problems that undermine personalisation, dignity and safety. Mencap has launched a 'Getting it right' charter for healthcare providers to sign up to, with helpful resources provided (see http://www.mencap.org.uk/campaigns/take-action/getting-it-right). The website 'Improving Health and Lives Observatory' (http://www.improvinghealthandlives.org.uk/) monitors the health and healthcare of people with learning disabilities and is very informative. The site includes a 'Hospital Traffic Light Assessment' that, when completed, gives hospital staff important information about a person with learning disabilities who is admitted to hospital (see http://www.improvinghealthandlives.org.uk/securefiles/130921_1310//Traffic%20Light%20Assessment%20Notts.pdf).

Other countries in the UK have published documents regarding services for people with learning disabilities; check their websites for current documents and strategy. The RCN (2011) provides helpful guidance for nurses about meeting the health needs of people with learning disabilities.

Healthcare for people with mental health problems

At least one in four people will experience a mental health problem at some point in their life, and one in six adults has a mental health problem at any one time (McManus et al. 2009). The DH (2011) published the strategy *No Health without Mental Health* that highlighted the importance of mental health for all ages. One of the objectives is that 'more people with mental health problems will have good physical health' and that 'fewer people with mental health problems will die prematurely, and more people with physical ill health will have better mental health' (p. 6). The strategy highlights that having a mental health problem increases the risk of physical health problems; all nurses should understand the links between mental and physical health and be able to recognise and address the physical health needs of people who have mental health problems.

The National Collaborating Centre for Mental Health (2011) has produced the guidelines *Service User Experience in Adult Mental Health: Improving the Experience of Care for People Using Adult NHS Mental Health Services*. These guidelines highlight that healthcare professionals who demonstrated support and qualities of empathy and respect could facilitate service users' access to healthcare. The guidelines set out that health and social care professionals should have the knowledge, skills and attitude to assess service users in a sensitive and professional manner and endeavour to build trusting, respectful and empowering therapeutic relationships with service users. The guidelines also highlight that service users want to feel valued and listened to during the process, and for professionals to treat them with dignity, respect and genuine concern. Service users expressed that the most productive relationship with professionals was when it was collaborative, when staff were non-judgemental and caring, and respectful.

Healthcare for people with dementia

Nurses may care for people with dementia in any healthcare setting as they are likely to have both physical and mental healthcare needs. Several different health conditions can lead to dementia; the Alzheimer's Society and the Social Care Institute for Excellence websites are excellent resources for more information. Dementia primarily affects older people, so many people with dementia have other conditions common to old age that precipitate hospital admission. In the UK, one in four of all adult hospital beds are occupied by people older than 65 years with dementia (Alzheimer's Society 2009), so they are key service users for whom nurses should be providing high-quality, dignified and compassionate care. In relation to learning disability, people with Down's syndrome have an increased risk of developing dementia due to Alzheimer's disease in middle age (Stanton and Coetzee 2004).

The DH (2009b) launched a national dementia strategy which included an objective to improve the quality of hospital care for people with dementia. Unfortunately, reports have revealed that care for people with dementia in hospital

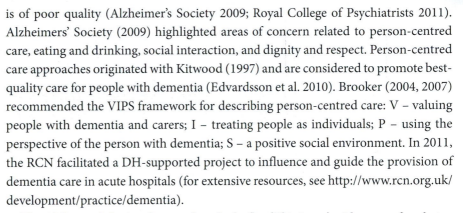

is of poor quality (Alzheimer's Society 2009; Royal College of Psychiatrists 2011). Alzheimers' Society (2009) highlighted areas of concern related to person-centred care, eating and drinking, social interaction, and dignity and respect. Person-centred care approaches originated with Kitwood (1997) and are considered to promote best-quality care for people with dementia (Edvardsson et al. 2010). Brooker (2004, 2007) recommended the VIPS framework for describing person-centred care: V – valuing people with dementia and carers; I – treating people as individuals; P – using the perspective of the person with dementia; S – a positive social environment. In 2011, the RCN facilitated a DH-supported project to influence and guide the provision of dementia care in acute hospitals (for extensive resources, see http://www.rcn.org.uk/development/practice/dementia).

The Alzheimer's Society has produced a leaflet, 'This is me', with spaces for photos and information, to support people with dementia, so that nurses and other healthcare staff can better understand the person's perspectives and take into account their preferences. When caring for people with dementia, be proactive about using 'This is me' (downloadable from the website http://www.alzheimers.org.uk/thisisme) and getting to know the person and their family. Alzheimer's Society has also produced 'Top tips for nurses' on aspects of care that nurses have reported finding challenging and that carers have raised concerns with. These practical guides are referred to throughout this book in the relevant chapters.

PRACTICAL SKILLS AND THEIR APPLICATION ACROSS THE LIFE SPAN AND IN DIFFERENT HEALTHCARE SETTINGS

This book includes a range of practical skills that student nurses need to develop during their preregistration programme. Many of these skills are addressed in courses for healthcare support workers too.

Each chapter begins with scenarios of adults in physical healthcare, learning disability and mental healthcare settings, and the chapter links the skills back to these scenarios, thus encouraging theory–practice links. The book aims to include a selection of scenarios, from a variety of settings, but it is not intended that all possible situations are represented. All scenarios have been developed from experience with similar people with health needs. Any identifying details have been changed or omitted, and pseudonyms were allocated at random.

As the NMC (2010) standards expect nurses to care for people across the life span, with specialist skills in their own field of practice, the book includes 'Practice points' boxes for care of children, and for pregnancy and birth, with reference to further reading and resources. Nurses encountering pregnant women in different settings should remember that they are adapting to a life-changing event that may make them feel vulnerable: physically, emotionally and socially. Pregnant women may access healthcare in many different healthcare settings and should be partners in their care choices. Contemporaneous, evidence-based information should always be provided to women and families to support this partnership.

All healthcare staff should be able to assess a collapsed person and administer basic life support (BLS). These procedures are updated regularly by the Resuscitation Council (UK) and outlined in detail on their website (http://www.resus.org.uk). Therefore, these procedures, although referred to where appropriate, are not reproduced in detail here. The Resuscitation Council's (UK) very informative website includes other useful sections as well as guidelines, for example, information about legal aspects of resuscitation and decisions relating to cardiopulmonary resuscitation. You must undergo supervised BLS practice in the skills laboratory with a trained instructor, and it is mandatory for all healthcare staff to attend these sessions annually. Chapter 6 covers some principles underpinning moving and handling skills. However, these skills are frequently updated, and you must attend the training sessions provided for you, both as a student and as a registered nurse, so that you can practise and update your skills under supervision.

A CARING AND COMPASSIONATE APPROACH TO PRACTICAL NURSING SKILLS

When asked your reasons for wanting to be a nurse, you might well have responded that you wanted to care for people. Many nursing theorists have recognised that caring and nursing are interrelated. For example, Watson (1979) stated that 'the practice of caring is central to nursing' (p. 9), whereas Roach (2002) identified caring both as a natural attribute of being human and as the core of nursing. Benner and Wrubel (1989) asserted that the 'nature of the caring relationship is central to most nursing interventions' (p. 5). They identified that the same act done in a non-caring way, as opposed to a caring way, has very different consequences so that 'nursing can never be reduced to mere technique' (p. 4). Woodward (1997) identified two dimensions of professional caring: *instrumental* caring (the technique comprising skills and knowledge) and *expressive* caring (the emotional element which includes respect for the individual). She suggested that it is expressive caring which transforms nursing actions into caring. Bjork's (1999b) model of practical skill performance included aspects such as sequence and fluency, but it also included a 'caring comportment', explained as being how the nurse creates a respectful, accepting and encouraging atmosphere, which includes concern for the whole person. Roach (2002) made a study of caring in relation to nursing and developed the '6Cs' framework: compassion, competence, confidence, conscience, commitment and comportment.

Halldorsdottir (1991) identified a 'life-sustaining mode of being with a patient' which included 'compassionate competence, genuine concern for the patient as a person, undivided attention when the nurse is with the patient, and cheerfulness' (p. 44). This approach is described as 'professional caring'. Research participants felt relief when they felt cared for, and they believed that their diminished anxiety gave them time to concentrate on getting better. In Thorsteinsson's (2002) study, nurses perceived as giving high-quality care were described as 'joyful, warm,

Box 1.3 An uncaring approach

An older, frail man had been admitted to a surgical ward in the night. He was confused and had a hearing impairment (his hearing aid lay on his bedside locker). The nurse (or healthcare assistant) approached him to find out what he wanted for breakfast but was impatient and clearly irritated by his inability to answer coherently. Two other patients observed the interaction and found it quite upsetting. Mr. A said of the situation: 'This poor chap opposite me who was clearly quite deaf and obviously very confused – didn't know where he was – and she was shouting at him – she was a bully. She shouldn't be in that job'.

Source: Baillie, L. 2007. *A Case Study of Patient Dignity in an Acute Hospital Setting*. Unpublished thesis. London: London South Bank University, p. 155.

tender, smiling, positive, polite and understanding'. All these attributes relate to the nurse's approach; clinical competence was also expected but did not lead to an experience of high-quality care unless accompanied by these other aspects.

Arman and Rehnsfeldt's (2007) study led them to conclude that 'the essence of uncaring was that patients were not seen as whole human beings and their existential suffering was not noticed by caregivers' (p. 373). Box 1.3 provides an example of unkindness to a patient who was clearly vulnerable, and the staff member, instead of being understanding, was impatient and harsh. As mentioned, in the UK media and other reports, concerns have been expressed about some nurses lacking compassion with a negative impact on patients' care experiences (Mid Staffordshire NHS Foundation Trust Public Inquiry 2013).

The aforementioned review highlights the value of a caring and compassionate approach from patients' perspectives. The DH (2012b) released *Compassion in Practice: Nursing, Midwifery and Care Staff: Our Vision and Strategy*, and this guidance promotes a 6Cs framework, with care at the centre and the values of compassion, competence, communication, courage and commitment included (for a summary, see Box 1.4). The vision aims to embed these values in all nursing, midwifery and caregiving settings across the NHS and social care, to improve care for patients.

ACTIVITY

Read through Box 1.4. Now reflect on the 6Cs and how you can apply these values in your everyday nursing practice.

All the values are important for people being cared for by nurses to have positive experiences. Roach (2002) argued that compassion is needed more than ever to humanise the ever-increasing cold and impersonal technology used within healthcare. Box 1.5 illustrates this need with a nurse's act of compassion that occurred in the highly technical environment of the intensive therapy unit. Communication is essential for portraying compassion and building relationships and is discussed in detail in Chapter 2. Hudacek (2008) found that compassion requires nurses to

Box 1.4 6 Cs of caring

Care

Care is our core business and that of our organisations, and the care we deliver helps the individual person and improves the health of the whole community. Caring defines us and our work. People receiving care expect it to be right for them, consistently, throughout every stage of their life.

Compassion

Compassion is how care is given through relationships based on empathy, respect and dignity – it can also be described as intelligent kindness and is central to how people perceive their care.

Competence

Competence means all those in caring roles must have the ability to understand an individual's health and social needs and the expertise, clinical and technical knowledge to deliver effective care and treatments based on research and evidence.

Communication

Communication is central to successful caring relationships and to effective teamworking. Listening is as important as what we say and do and essential for 'no decision about me without me'. Communication is the key to a good workplace with benefits for those in our care and staff alike.

Courage

Courage enables us to do the right thing for the people we care for, to speak up when we have concerns and to have the personal strength and vision to innovate and to embrace new ways of working.

Commitment

A commitment to our patients and populations is a cornerstone of what we do. We need to build on our commitment to improve the care and experience of our patients; to take action to make this vision and strategy a reality for all; and to meet the health, care and support challenges ahead.

Source: Department of Health (DH). 2012. *Compassion in Practice: Nursing, Midwifery and Care Staff: Our Vision and Strategy.* Gateway reference 18479. London: DH, p. 13.

be present for patients both emotionally and physically and to focus on alleviating suffering and pain through empathic concern. In a study of compassion within the relationship between nurses and older people with a chronic disease, van der Cingel (2011) revealed seven dimensions of compassion: attentiveness, listening, confronting, involvement, helping, presence and understanding. Concerning competence, practical skills must be carried out competently to ensure safe, effective care. The NMC (2008a) specifies that nurses must provide a high standard of practice, displaying up-to-date knowledge and skills for safe and effective practice. Roach (2002) stated that 'while competence without compassion can be

> **Box 1.5 Compassion: an illustrative example from an intensive therapy unit**
>
> James was in the final stages of heart and lung failure, and his nurse, about to go home after a 12-hour shift and knowing that she would not see him again, asked him if there was anything she could get him before she left. He replied 'Oh, a port and brandy please!' Phone calls around the hospital were unsuccessful in locating any, and the nurse went off shift. She returned half an hour later with a small glass of port and brandy brought from home. As James was unable to swallow she dipped sponge mouth sticks into the drink and put them in his mouth for him to suck. James grinned and said it was 'wonderful'. This act of compassion brought tenderness to this patient's final hours and made an immeasurable difference to his relatives' feelings about his death.

brutal and inhumane, compassion without competence may be no more than a meaningless, if not harmful, intrusion into the life of a person or persons needing help' (p. 54).

Courage is an important value in caring. Nurses have an important role in safeguarding people who are vulnerable and must raise any concerns about people who may be at risk. Nurses must also speak out if they feel that care is compromised; speaking up for the vulnerable is an NHS Constitution requirement of all NHS staff, including students (DH 2012a). Commitment as part of care requires that nurses will carry out necessary care in a consistent, reliable and timely way, regardless of barriers and constraints. Henderson et al. (2007) found that nurses needed to respond to patients' needs in a timely manner to be perceived as caring; patients were dissatisfied when nurses apparently forgot patients and their needs. In Box 1.5, the nurse's action exemplified compassion and also demonstrated commitment to James, by bringing the drink from home despite just finishing a 12-hour shift.

CULTURAL COMPETENCE AND PRACTICAL NURSING SKILLS

Britain is a multicultural society, and practical nursing skills must be carried out with sensitivity and in a culturally appropriate manner for each individual and family. The American nurse and anthropologist Madeleine Leininger (1981) studied transcultural caring over many years and identified how acts of caring such as comforting and physical care, and the meaning attached to them, can vary between cultures. Leininger suggested that culture and caring cannot be separated within nursing actions and decision making. Papadopoulos (2006a) presents the Papadopoulos–Tilki–Taylor model for transcultural nursing and health, consisting of four linked elements: cultural awareness, cultural knowledge, cultural sensitivity and cultural competence.

- **Cultural awareness** includes examining and questioning one's personal value-base and beliefs. Chapter 2 of this book will help you to develop self-awareness.
- **Cultural knowledge** may be drawn from sources such as sociology, anthropology and research, and from experience of people. Where appropriate to specific practical skills, cultural variations (particularly related to religious beliefs) are considered in this book. However, there are often individual and regional variations, so it is important to avoid stereotyping and making ethnocentric judgements that serve as barriers to cultural sensitivity. In Cioffi's (2005) Australian study, the nurses used experiences of caring for culturally diverse patients to develop their knowledge; sources were bilingual health workers and colleagues, patients, their families and support persons. Some nurses used stereotypical views of the patient's cultural group to give care, but others used the individual patient's perspective: 'You actually have to ask the person. You can't assume they're going to be the traditional Chinese or Arabic lady' (Cioffi 2005).
- **Cultural sensitivity** can be achieved by nurses working with people as partners, offering choices in care. In Cioffi's study, one nurse said that when caring for culturally diverse patients, 'If I am not sure, I just say to the patient "What is the right thing for me to do?", "Can I do this" or "Would you mind if I do this?"'. Another nurse said, 'It's just finding out what they believe and what they don't believe in and then you can work it out from there with them and individualise their care'. Communication skills, respect and empathy are all very important for cultural sensitivity (see Chapter 2).
- **Cultural competence** requires the application of cultural awareness, knowledge and sensitivity to achieve effective healthcare which addresses people's cultural beliefs, behaviour and needs. The culturally competent nurse also challenges prejudice, discrimination and inequality. Leishman (2006) highlighted the importance of mental health nurses developing cultural competence in an increasingly culturally diverse UK society.

In Cortis's (2000) UK study, Pakistani adults provided some examples of good healthcare experiences where staff were sensitive to their rights for privacy, provided for their need to pray and offered opportunities to maintain cultural practices in the hospital environment. However, nurses were generally perceived as seriously lacking cultural knowledge about this community; they lacked awareness of appropriate support systems, hygiene practices, the significance of Halal food and practices associated with caring and spiritual needs. One participant said, 'Nurses are not particularly interested to find out about our way of life. I feel that it is [the] nurses' duty to get to know some things about our customs or at least learn from us. This will be a great help to nurses as well, but they do not ask us anything either' (Cortis 2000, p. 114). This comment indicated the willingness of the participant to share cultural knowledge but their perception that nurses were not interested in learning. In contrast, Leever (2011) reports examples of nurses who took time to listen to patients so that they could understand their perspectives and be able to adjust care delivery so that it was culturally comfortable and acceptable.

Reflect on your own cultural competence at this stage. Jot down a few notes about your personal values and beliefs, your cultural knowledge and your skills that will aid you to demonstrate cultural sensitivity.

Several models have been proposed for assessment with diverse groups (Higginbottom et al. 2011). Narayanasamy and Narayanasamy (2012) suggest using the 'ACCESS model' as a framework for responding to diversity in healthcare: **A**ssessment, **C**ommunication, **C**ultural negotiation and compromise, **E**stablishing respect and rapport, **S**ensitivity and **S**afety. Assessment using the ACCESS model will provide a cultural awareness that is a deliberate, cognitive process in which health providers appreciate and become sensitive to the values, beliefs, practices and problems of each individual person, as the basis for enhancing involvement in decision making.

Papadopoulos' (2006b) textbook *Transcultural Health and Social Care: Development of Culturally Competent Practitioners* provides a comprehensive guide to this important dimension of practice and is recommended further reading.

DIGNITY AND PRACTICAL NURSING SKILLS

It is a professional requirement for nurses to respect people's dignity in care (NMC 2008a). However, dignity can be difficult to define, and people may have different interpretations of its meaning.

ACTIVITY

Spend a few minutes reflecting on the following:
- What is dignity?
- How does it feel to have your dignity?
- How does it feel to lose your dignity?

Now ask someone else for their views and compare these with your own.

The RCN (2008) developed a working definition to guide nursing practice (Box 1.6). How does this definition compare with your ideas?

Whether people are treated with dignity in healthcare affects perceptions of their whole experience and their satisfaction with care (Beach et al. 2005; Valentine et al. 2008). Health policy documents increasingly emphasise the importance of compassionate and dignified care (DH 2012b). There is a 'Dignity in Care' network with a website (http://www.dignityincare.org.uk) that provides many resources for health and social care and where you can sign up to be a dignity champion. Look out for the annual Dignity in Care action day, promoted on this site, and get involved if you can. There is also a 10-point 'dignity challenge', originally produced by the DH (Box 1.7).

Box 1.6 Definition of dignity

Dignity is concerned with how people feel, think and behave in relation to the worth or value of themselves and others. To treat someone with dignity is to treat them as being of worth, in a way that is respectful of them as valued individuals. When dignity is present, people feel in control, valued, confident, comfortable and able to make decisions for themselves. When dignity is absent people feel devalued, lacking control and comfort. They may lack confidence and be unable to make decisions for themselves. They may feel humiliated, embarrassed or ashamed. Dignity applies equally to those who have capacity and to those who lack it. Everyone has equal worth as human beings and must be treated as if they are able to feel, think and behave in relation to their own worth or value. Dignity applies equally to those who have capacity and to those who lack it.

Source: Royal College of Nursing (RCN). 2008. *Defending Dignity: Challenges and Opportunities for Nurses*. London: RCN, p. 8. Reproduced with permission from Royal College of Nursing.

Box 1.7 The dignity challenge

High-quality services that respect people's dignity should
• show zero tolerance towards all forms of abuse;
• treat people with the same respect as you would want for yourself and your family;
• treat each person as an individual;
• ensure people are able to maintain maximum levels of independence, choice and control;
• support people in expressing their needs;
• respect people's rights to privacy;
• ensure people can complain without fear of retribution;
• work with patients' families and their partners in their care;
• help people to maintain confidence and self-esteem; and
• alleviate people's loneliness and isolation.

Source: Reproduced with permission from the Department of Health, www.dh.gov.uk/dignityincare.

ACTIVITY

Look at the dignity challenge in Box 1.7. From your healthcare experiences to date, as either a patient, relative or professional, which of the 10 challenges do you feel are usually achieved? Are there any that you feel are rarely achieved? If so, reflect on what barriers might stop these being achieved in healthcare.

Although government health policies have often focused on dignity of older people, studies have indicated that people across the life span are concerned about their dignity and can be vulnerable to a loss of dignity in healthcare (Matiti and Baillie 2011). A survey of the nursing workforce illuminated how three key areas affected dignity:

- **Place:** the physical environment and organisational culture
- **People:** the attitudes and behaviour of nurses and others
- **Processes:** care activities and how they are carried out (RCN 2008)

The RCN's (2008) survey highlighted many care activities during which patients were vulnerable to a loss of dignity, but nurses described in detail the actions they took to prevent dignity being lost, which related to privacy, communication and physical actions (Table 1.1). When carrying out skills with people in practice, you need to ensure that your behaviour promotes their dignity. Chapter 2 focuses in detail on your communication, and how it can portray care and compassion. Other chapters highlight dignity in relation to specific skills.

Table 1.1: How nurses protect dignity during care activities

Privacy	Communication	Physical care actions
Physical environment • Side rooms • Quiet/private room/area • Bathroom/toilet use • Curtains/blinds • Curtain clips/pegs/signs • Managing smells • Auditory privacy	Interactions that make patients feel comfortable • Sensitivity • Empathy • Developing relationships • Non-verbal communication • Conversation • Reassurance • Professionalism • Family involvement	Preparation • Procedure • Environment • Timeliness • Equipment
Staff behaviour • Discretion • Prevent/manage interruptions • Sensitivity to culture/religion • Respect for personal space	Interactions that make patients feel in control • Explanations and information giving • Choices and negotiation • Gaining consent	Staff management Promoting independence Physical comfort
Managing people in the environment • Staff: number present, gender • Other patients • Family • Ward visitors/public	Interactions that make patients feel valued • Giving time • Concern for patients as individuals • Courteousness	
Bodily privacy • Covering body • Minimising time exposed • Privacy during undressing • Clothing		

Source: Royal College of Nursing (RCN) 2008. *Defending Dignity: Challenges and Opportunities for Nurses.* London: RCN, p. 8. Reproduced with permission from Royal College of Nursing.

In Baillie's (2007) research, one man's description of the nurse who promoted his dignity was that she:

> . . . is sensitive, explains what she's going to do before she does it, she's cheerful, she has a sense of humour, she appears interested in me as an individual, she has a caring approach, appears to enjoy her work – doesn't appear as though it's a chore. (p. 205)

Baillie found that in situations where dignity was threatened, staff behaviour could prevent dignity being lost. One man said that the student nurse who inserted his suppositories (a procedure that he felt could have threatened his dignity) 'did it nicely' so he did not lose his dignity. A woman in her fifties with terminal cancer identified that she could have lost her dignity in the bathroom, but her 'bath had been handled well' as she had been given choices which promoted her dignity. In a study of UK nurses' strategies to promote dignity, Baillie and Gallagher (2011) found that treating people as valued individuals was the core factor. The nurses recognised the vulnerability of people to dignity loss in their specific care settings. The nurses were proactive in promoting dignity through enhancing privacy, improving communication with patients and their families and building relationships, enhancing the care environment and addressing issues that mattered to individuals.

The Social Care Institute for Excellence (SCIE) produced a series of practice guides on Dignity in Care (www.scie.org.uk). For further reading and a detailed exploration of dignity in different care settings across the life span, see Matiti and Baillie (2011).

LEARNING PRACTICAL NURSING SKILLS

To make the most of opportunities to learn practical skills, it is helpful to think about how skills are learned.

ACTIVITY

Reflect back on a practical skill which you have learned, for example, learning to drive. How did you learn this skill?

You may recall that you built up the skill in step-by-step stages, learning each subskill one at a time. You could probably focus only on the skill and found that it was difficult to do anything else (e.g. have a conversation) at the same time. Benner (1984) identified that when learning any new skill, the performance is initially 'halting and rigid' (p. 37) and that one must pay careful attention to the explicit rules relating to the skill.

As a student, you are not expected to be an expert in your practical skills; expertise develops through substantial experience. Benner's research adapted a skill acquisition model by Dreyfus and Dreyfus to describe different levels of performance in nurses.

She conducted paired interviews with beginners and experienced nurses and also used participant observation to study nurses with various levels of experience. The five stages of performance are as follows:

- **Stage 1 – Novice.** Novice nurses have no experience on which to draw; this lack of experience applies not only to new students but also to experienced nurses moving to an unfamiliar area of practice. Benner describes the novice as being 'rule-governed' in behaviour; that is, the novice needs explicit guidelines about what to do and in which sequence. However, these guidelines need to be adapted to the actual situation, and novice nurses need help and guidance to make these adaptions.

- **Stage 2 – Advanced beginner.** Advanced beginners can use previous experience and apply it in practice but continue to need adequate support, particularly with aspects that are situational, such as prioritising. They have difficulty seeing a situation as a whole and focus on the specific skill to be carried out, regardless of additional situational factors.

- **Stage 3 – Competent.** Competent nurses are able to carry out conscious and deliberate planning and prioritise and manage their work. However, they lack the flexibility and speed of proficient nurses.

- **Stage 4 – Proficient.** Proficient nurses perceive situations holistically, recognise important and less important elements and make decisions quickly. Benner found proficiency in nurses who have worked in an area for some time.

- **Stage 5 – Expert.** Expert nurses have a deep understanding and an intuitive grasp of situations, gained from substantial experience in the practice setting. You may observe this level in some practitioners with whom you work. In her book, Benner gives many examples of expert nurses' care for clients. Such nurses may be excellent and inspirational role models, but it is important not to feel inadequate or overawed by such expertise.

Developing the affective, cognitive and motor dimensions of a skill

The affective dimension

This book includes activities that focus on the affective dimension, asking you to think about, for example, how a patient might be feeling in a particular situation. Chapter 2 concentrates on the affective dimension of practical skills and will help you to understand the concept of self-awareness and how your values might affect how you carry out your care.

The cognitive dimension

Learning the cognitive elements of skills involves you acquiring and understanding the underpinning knowledge and rationale. Throughout this book, the evidence base for practical skills is discussed, but there are also activities encouraging you to draw on other sources of knowledge, such as reflecting on your experience. These activities will help you to develop an enquiring and problem-solving approach to your nursing practice.

The motor dimension

Learning the motor dimension of a psychomotor skill requires practice – the opportunity to try out and repeat performance. It is only with practice that movement becomes refined and a smooth, coordinated performance can develop. The amount of practice needed varies according to motivation to learn the skill, previous related skills learning, familiarity with equipment, level of anxiety, the physical resources and the learner's coordination (Oermann 1990). More complex skills need more practice. Motivation affects mastery as many skills are initially difficult, but highly motivated students will persevere. If you have had previous experience of a related skill, some of the skill's component parts will be familiar, so then your practice can focus on parts of the skill not already learned. Familiarity with equipment also eases the learning of a new skill. This book will help by explaining what type of equipment is used for the skills discussed and includes illustrations of equipment. There is also advice about where you can access equipment with which to become familiar.

Support for learning skills

There are key points a facilitator can do to help when you are learning a new skill (Box 1.8). You can be active about promoting these conditions. For example, the best time to ask a nurse to supervise you drawing up an injection for the first time is not in the middle of an emergency situation, as the stress and anxiety in the environment are unlikely to be conducive to learning. Thus, when asking to be supervised carrying out a skill, pick the right moment! Be open about your prior knowledge, saying explicitly that you have, for example, practised injection technique in the skills laboratory, have observed injection administration in practise and now feel ready to be supervised preparing and administering an injection. Supervisors should avoid the temptation to take over, but they will need to do so if safety is compromised. Learning practical skills requires the opportunity to practise and gain feedback (Quinn and Hughes 2007) to reinforce correct behaviour and eliminate error.

Box 1.8 How a facilitator can help a student learn a practical skill

- Provide an atmosphere conducive to learning.
- Carry out a skills analysis.
- Determine the procedure sequence.
- Assess the student's prior knowledge.
- Demonstrate the skill at normal speed.
- Teach the procedure sequence.
- Teach the skill by either whole learning or part learning.
- Allocate sufficient time to practise.
- Provide feedback on performance.
- Prompt student to self-evaluate.
- Encourage transfer of skills.

Source: Adapted from Quinn, F. and Hughes, S.J. 2007. *Quinn's Principles and Practice of Nurse Education*, 5th edn. Cheltenham: Nelson-Thornes.

The importance of obtaining feedback

Gaining feedback when you are developing skills is important for your learning. Staff supervising you can give you feedback; it is more helpful if the comments are specific rather than a general comment such as 'very good' or 'you need to be quicker'. It will help your supervisor if you identify any aspects for which you particularly want feedback. For example, you might state that when performing the skill last time, the supervisor said that you needed to give a clearer explanation to the client, so ask that the supervisor now give you feedback on this specific aspect. Patients and clients also can give you feedback. They may make spontaneous comments, such as that they feel 'much more comfortable now' or thank you for your kindness, but you can also seek feedback specifically, by asking how they feel at different stages. If you are approachable in the way you seek feedback, people are more likely to give honest responses. Your observation of people while you are carrying out practical skills will also give you feedback; for example, you can observe for facial expressions that might indicate fear or discomfort.

The sources of feedback outlined so far will provide *extrinsic* feedback. Combined with *intrinsic* feedback, you get a balanced view of your performance. Intrinsic feedback involves you reflecting on your performance and asking yourself what were the strengths and weaknesses and how you could improve your performance next time.

Learning from experience and reflection

Carrying out practical nursing skills with different individuals in different circumstances provides rich opportunities for learning from practical experience. Developing your reflective skills will help you in learning and developing your practice so that you optimise your learning. Dewey (1929), an educational theorist, argued that we do not 'learn by doing' but by 'doing and realizing what came of what we did' (p. 367). Dewey's theories were developed further by Kolb and Fry (1975) and then more fully by Kolb (1984). The theory of how we learn from experience is often referred to as *experiential learning* and is portrayed as a cycle. The process starts at the point of a concrete experience or event, after which observations and reflections occur, followed by abstract conceptualisation, where new ideas are developed, linked to other knowledge and experience, and then the new knowledge arising from the experience is tested out in a new situation. This new experience then starts the experiential learning cycle once again.

Reflection enables you to consider what you did and why, and it provides opportunities to develop knowledge from experience and link theory and practice. Knowledge gained from reflection on practice has been termed *practical knowledge* (Schön 1987), and reflection can enable the uncovering of knowledge embedded in practice (Lawler 1991). Reflecting on your practice helps you to examine your experience and consider other explanations for what happened and alternative ways of doing things (Howartson-Jones 2010).

Reflection may occur during the experience (reflection-in-action) or following the experience (reflection-on-action) (Schön 1991). There are various models and frameworks to provide a structure for reflection; you will be introduced to these models during your course, and you should pursue further reading from the many texts on reflective practice available.

To help you develop your reflective skills, you could write reflective accounts that may be included in your portfolio, recording significant events that you experience in your nursing practice. This activity can assist you in developing analytical skills and help you in learning from your experience, linking theory and practice. *Remember*: You must not identify patients or clients (either by name or by other identifying material) in your reflective writing, to maintain confidentiality. You may take part in reflective activities within the classroom setting where you will be encouraged to reflect on specific incidents from practice.

Skills laboratories and simulation

As students need opportunities to rehearse skills in a safe environment, most universities have simulation facilities: skills laboratories or centres where you can practise skills. In simulation, students learn in a realistic clinical environment where they practise a range of skills without the risk of harming patients and then apply these skills in the clinical setting (Wilford and Doyle 2006). Learning in the skills laboratory can help in reducing anxiety about clinical placement experience and develop confidence. Skills laboratories provide a more controlled environment for familiarisation with skills than do practice settings. Practice in simulation also provides opportunities for reflection in and on practice. Your skills may be tested in simulation too, through objective structured clinical examination (OSCE). As far as possible, you should behave in an OSCE as you would in the clinical practice setting; take this opportunity to show how you can carry out your skills safely and compassionately, and based on best evidence.

Skills laboratories vary in complexity and resources, but they usually contain clinical equipment for practising technical procedures. Some skills, such as blood pressure measurement, can be practised safely on your peers, and there will be simulation models for practising other skills. Some skills laboratories organise volunteer patients for students' practice. Universities have different systems for learning in skills laboratories, which you should become familiar with. There may be compulsory sessions, optional workshops and formal or informal sessions. There may be a behaviour and dress code; for example, you may be expected to wear uniform and will certainly be expected to behave in a professional and considerate manner, maintaining safety at all times. Activities within the chapters of this book often suggest that you access equipment to practise with, if possible. You will need to find out about your local policies and procedures for use of equipment in the skills laboratory, and there may be a code of behaviour for users to ensure safety. Your placement provider or employing organisation also may have simulation facilities for skills learning.

Learning in the practice setting

Skills laboratory practice does not replace skills practice within clinical placements; practising skills with people in the healthcare environment is essential to develop competent, caring skills. Practical skills development and practice should take place within the context of the nurse–patient relationship, as part of their holistic care. Obviously, you should take every opportunity to develop new skills, but not within a task-orientated framework that is dehumanising and objectifies people. Learning practical skills should thus occur within the total care required for each individual.

When starting a new clinical placement, you may well feel anxious or even fearful, but be reassured that you are not alone in these feelings. Starting a new practice placement has been likened to starting a new job! You will need to familiarise yourself with the environment and staff. Some practice settings send you information before your placement to help you feel welcome and reduce anxiety, and often a preplacement visit is encouraged. Alternatively, this information may be available to you on the Internet; do make sure you access it and make good use of this facility.

In *Standards to Support Learning and Assessment in Practice*, the NMC (2008b) details how students' effective learning and assessment in practice can be facilitated. When students enter a new practice setting, they can sometimes feel overwhelmed by the range of learning opportunities. Placement areas often identify what specific learning opportunities are available, and these opportunities will include learning practical skills. In any practice setting, you will have an assigned mentor, whose remit includes supporting you in the following:

- Identifying your learning needs
- Addressing these learning needs through enabling you to practise, and giving feedback
- Assessing your performance

The NMC (2008b) identifies the mentor's role in detail. Your role should be an active role throughout this learning process.

Identifying your learning needs

When identifying your learning needs, you should take into account the following:

- Learning outcomes for your stage of the course
- Your prior learning, from previous practice placements, and any relevant experience before entering nurse education
- Any learning needs that were identified during your previous practice placements
- Specific learning opportunities identified by this placement

Your mentor will discuss these learning needs with you and can advise of the learning opportunities in the practice area that can assist you, but you must be honest about your strengths and areas needing improvement. Your learning needs are likely to include practical skills, but they will address other needs too.

Addressing your learning needs

The section 'Learning from experience and reflection' provides ideas on how you can benefit the most from your clinical experience. You need to be active in seeking out your learning opportunities. Being aware of how to learn practical skills will help you to make the best use of opportunities available, ensuring that you observe a skill first, and ask for supervised practice until you feel confident to practise the skill independently. Although some skills need minimal practice, others are much more complex and need repeated practice. You should not attempt a skill unsupervised unless you are confident of your ability. You will be given feedback during practice placements to guide your learning. As mentioned, the practical skills you develop should be considered within the holistic care of patients and not as isolated tasks that you have learned to perform.

You can be more proactive about learning in the practice setting if you are aware of different learning methods. There is much you can learn from observing others in the practice setting, but you need to distinguish between good professional role models and poor models. In some practice settings, there may be formal teaching sessions organised. This approach might be particularly appropriate when there are several students in a placement area, and where workload is predictable so that a specific time can be set aside for teaching sessions. Formal teaching sessions enable you to prepare, by pre-reading for example. Informal teaching occurs more spontaneously, that is, on the spot. Such sessions can be particularly meaningful as they are likely to be linked with the clinical practice occurring at that time. Sometimes, a critical incident can be used as a basis for reflection in the practice setting. This incident might be a situation that has occurred which was difficult or challenging, such as where a relative has raised a concern. Critical incident analysis can aid reflection and learning from such situations.

Here is an example of how you might use different learning methods in the practice setting. When taking part in medicine administration, you can actively observe a qualified nurse, either asking questions at the time (if appropriate) or making a note of questions for later or of specific medicines you want to find out about. The nurse you are with might ask you questions to check your understanding and encourage you to think about what is happening. You may be able to take part in practical elements such as dispensing of tablets or preparing a nebuliser. If a difficult situation occurs, for example, a patient declines their tablets, you could use this incident to reflect on afterwards and develop knowledge from this experience. You could consider, for example, whether a different approach to the patient would have made any difference, or whether an adequate explanation about the tablets was given. You could also follow up later by looking up information about medicines that you encountered and were not familiar with.

RECOMMENDED READING

As stated, the remit of this book is to help you to develop a foundation in practical nursing skills. For guidance about reading material and for other aspects, you should refer to the recommended reading list for your course.

Many practical nursing skills require an underlying biological knowledge base. For example, when taking and recording blood pressure, it is necessary to understand what blood pressure is and how it is maintained. However, a foundation in biology is not within the scope of this book, and you should gain your biological knowledge from the biology texts available, many of which are aimed specifically at student nurses. When working through each chapter of this book, it is sensible to have an understanding of the related biology, so each chapter includes biology questions. Use your recommended text to check your biological knowledge by finding out the answers to the questions posed. Studying the relevant biology and then working through the chapter can help to make the biology more comprehensible and memorable, as you can see its immediate relevance and applicability to nursing practice.

Your recommended reading list is likely to include ethics, sociology and psychology texts, all of which also provide underpinning knowledge for nursing skills, assisting you to care for people holistically.

CHAPTER SUMMARY

All nurses must be competent in a range of practical nursing skills and apply these in practice in a compassionate manner. This book addresses skills that are generally applicable to nurses working with adults in a range of settings, and all the Essential Skills Clusters (NMC 2010) are included. Practical nursing skills include motor, affective and cognitive dimensions, and they should be carried out within the context of a caring relationship and within the wider legal, professional and health policy context. Nurses need to develop cultural competence. Nurses applying skills with people in any healthcare setting must ensure that they promote their dignity while carrying out care.

To develop competent, compassionate caring skills, practice and experience are required, which should include gaining feedback and reflection, thus maximising learning from experience. Through classroom preparation in a skills laboratory or equivalent setting, students can develop familiarity with equipment and the sequential steps of a skill, and the cognitive and affective domains can also be introduced. Carrying out practical skills in the dynamic and variable environment of the clinical setting is affected by many factors. Repeated practice in the clinical setting is needed to become competent and confident in practical skills, and students need to be proactive in seeking out opportunities for learning.

REFERENCES

Alzheimer's Society. 2009. *Counting the Cost: Caring for People with Dementia on Acute Hospital Wards*. London: Alzheimer's Society.

Arman, M. and Rehnsfeldt, A. 2007. The 'little extra' that alleviates suffering. *Nursing Ethics* 14: 372–86.

Baillie, L. 2007. *A Case Study of Patient Dignity in an Acute Hospital Setting*. Unpublished thesis. London South Bank University.

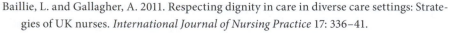

Baillie, L. and Gallagher, A. 2011. Respecting dignity in care in diverse care settings: Strategies of UK nurses. *International Journal of Nursing Practice* 17: 336–41.

Baillie, L. and Matiti, M. 2013. Dignity, equality and diversity: An exploration of how discriminatory behaviour of healthcare workers affects patient dignity. *Diversity and Equality in Health Care* 10: 5–12.

Beach, C., Sugarman, J., Johnson, R., et al. 2005. Do patients treated with dignity report higher satisfaction, adherence and receipt of preventive care. *The Annals of Family Medicine* 3: 331–8.

Benner, P. 1984. *From Novice to Expert.* Boston, MA: Addison-Wesley.

Benner, P. and Wrubel, J. 1989. *The Primacy of Caring.* Boston, MA: Addison-Wesley.

Bjork, I.T. 1999a. What constitutes a nursing practical skill? *Western Journal of Nursing Research* 21: 51–70.

Bjork, I.T. 1999b. Practical skill development in new nurses. *Nursing Inquiry* 6: 34–47.

Brooker, D. 2004. What is person-centred care in dementia? *Reviews in Clinical Gerontology* 13: 215–22.

Brooker, D. 2007. *Person Centred Dementia Care: Making Services Better.* London: Jessica Kingsley.

Buckner, L. and Yeandle, S. 2011. *Valuing Carers 2011: Calculating the Value of Carers' Support.* London: Carers UK. Available from: http://www.carersuk.org (Accessed on 7 February 2013).

Bush, H.A. and Barr, W.J. 1997. Critical care nurses' lived experiences of caring. *Heart and Lung* 26: 387–98.

Cioffi, J. 2005. Nurses' experiences of caring for culturally diverse patients in an acute care setting. *Contemporary Nurse* 20(1): 78–96.

Commission on Dignity in Care. 2012. *Delivering Dignity: Securing Dignity in Care for Older People in Hospitals and Care Homes.* Available from: http://www.nhsconfed.org/Publications/Documents/Delivering_Dignity_final_report150612.pdf (Accessed on 29 October 2012).

Cortis, J.D. 2000. Perceptions and experiences with nursing care: A study of Pakistani (Urdu) Communities in the United Kingdom. *Journal of Transcultural Nursing* 11: 111–18.

Department of Health (DH). 2001. *Valuing People: A New Strategy for Learning Disability for the 21st Century.* London: DH.

Department of Health (DH). 2007. *Good Practice in Learning Disability Nursing.* London: DH.

Department of Health (DH). 2009a. *Valuing People Now: A New Three-Year Strategy for Learning Disabilities.* London: DH.

Department of Health (DH). 2009b. *Living Well with Dementia – A National Dementia Strategy.* Gateway Reference 11198. London: DH.

Department of Health (DH). 2010. *Essence of Care 2010.* Gateway Reference 14641. London: The Stationery Office.

Department of Health (DH). 2011. *No Health without Mental Health: A Cross-Government Mental Health Outcomes Strategy for People of All Ages.* Gateway Reference 14679. London: DH.

Department of Health (DH). 2012a. *The NHS Constitution for England.* Gateway Reference 17278. London: DH.

Department of Health (DH). 2012b. *Compassion in Practice: Nursing, Midwifery and Care Staff: Our Vision and Strategy.* Gateway Reference 18479. London: DH.

Dewey, J. 1929. *Experience and Nature.* New York: Grove Press.

Edvardsson, D., Fetherstonhaugh, D. and Nay, R. 2010. Promoting a continuation of self and normality: Person-centred care as described by people with dementia, their family members and aged care staff *Journal of Clinical Nursing* 19: 2611–2618.

Great Britain. 1998. *Human Rights Act c. 42.* HMSO, London. Available from: http://www.legislation.gov.uk/ukpga/1998/42/contents (Accessed on 12 February 2013).

Great Britain. 2005. *Mental Capacity Act.* Available from: http://www.legislation.gov.uk/ukpga/2005/9/contents (Accessed on 12 February 2013).

Great Britain. 2010. *The Equality Act.* Available from: http://www.legislation.gov.uk/ukpga/2010/15/contents (Accessed on 12 February 2013).

Halldorsdottir, S. 1991. Five basic modes of being with another. In: Gaut, D.A. and Leininger, M.M. (eds.) *Caring: The Compassionate Healer.* New York: National League for Nursing Press, 37–49.

Health Service Ombudsman. 2011. *Care and Compassion? Report of the Health Service Ombudsman on Ten Investigations into NHS Care of Older People.* Available from: http://www.ombudsman.org.uk/care-and-compassion/home (Accessed on 12 February 2013).

Henderson, A., van Eps, M.A., Pearson, K., James, C., Henderson, P. and Osborne, Y. 2007. 'Caring for' behaviours that indicate to patients that nurses 'care about' them. *Journal of Advanced Nursing* 60(2): 146–53.

Higginbottom, G.M.A., Richter, M.S., Mogale, R.S., Ortiz, L., Young, S. and Mollel, O. 2011. Identification of nursing assessment models/tools validated in clinical practice for use with diverse ethno-cultural groups: An integrative review of the literature. *BMC Nursing* 10(16): doi:10.1186/1472-6955-10-16.

Howartson-Jones, L. 2010. *Reflective Practice in Nursing.* Exeter: Learning Matters.

Hudacek, S. 2008. Dimensions of caring: A qualitative analysis of nurses' stories. *Journal of Nursing Education* 47(3): 124–9.

Kitwood, T. 1997. *Dementia Reconsidered: The Person Comes First.* Buckingham: Open University Press.

Kolb, D.A. 1984. *Experiential Learning: Experience as the Source of Learning and Development.* London: Prentice Hall International.

Kolb, D.A. and Fry, R. 1975. Towards an applied theory of experiential learning. In: Cooper, C.L. (ed.) *Theories of Group Processes.* London: John Wiley, 33–57.

Lawler, J. 1991. *Behind the Screens: Nursing Somology and the Problem of the Body.* London: Churchill Livingstone.

Leever, M.G. 2011. Cultural competence: Reflections on patient autonomy and patient good. *Nursing Ethics* 18(4): 560–57.

Leininger, M. 1981. Transcultural nursing: Its progress and its future. *Nursing and Health Care* 2: 365–71.

Leishman, J.L. 2006. Culturally sensitive mental health care: A module for 21st century education and practice. *International Journal of Psychiatric Nursing Research* 11(3): 1310–21.

Manley, K. 1997. Knowledge for nursing practice. In: Perry, A. and Jolley, M. (eds.) *Nursing: A Knowledge Base for Practice,* 2nd edn. London: Arnold, 301–33.

Matiti, M. and Baillie, L. (eds.) 2011. *Dignity in Healthcare: A Practical Approach for Nurses and Midwives.* London: Radcliffe Publishers.

McManus, S., Meltzer, H., Brugha, T., Bebbington, P. and Jenkins, R. 2009. *Adult Psychiatric Morbidity in England, 2007: Results of a Household Survey.* Leeds: NHS Information Centre for Health and Social Care.

Mencap. 2004. *Treat Me Right! Better Healthcare for People with a Learning Disability.* London: Mencap.

Mencap. 2007. *Death by Indifference: Following Up the Treat Me Right! Report.* London: Mencap.

Mencap. 2012. *Death by Indifference: 74 Deaths and Counting: A Progress Report 5 Years On.* London: Mencap.

Mid Staffordshire NHS Foundation Trust Public Inquiry. 2013. *Report of the Mid Staffordshire NHS Foundation Trust Public Inquiry.* Available from: http://www.midstaffspublicinquiry.com/report (Accessed on 12 February 2013).

Nåden, D. and Eriksson, K. 2004. Understanding the importance of values and moral attitudes in nursing care and preserving human dignity. *Nursing Science Quarterly* 17(1): 86–91.

Narayanasamy, A. and Narayanasamy, G. 2012. Diversity in caring. In: McSherry, W., McSherry, R. and Watson, R. (eds.) *Care in Nursing: Principles, Values and Skills.* Oxford: Oxford University Press, 61–77.

National Collaborating Centre for Mental Health. 2011. *Service User Experience in Adult Mental Health: Improving the Experience of Care for People Using Adult NHS Mental Health Services.* Clinical Guidelines 136. London: NICE.

National Institute for Health and Clinical Excellence (NICE). 2012. *Patient Experience in Adult NHS Services: Improving the Experience of Care for People Using Adult NHS Services.* Clinical Guidelines 138. London: NICE.

National Nursing Research Unit. 2008. *What Matters to Patients: The Nursing Contribution.* Policy + Issue 9. London: Kings College London.

Nursing and Midwifery Council (NMC). 2008a. *The Code: Standards of Conduct, Performance and Ethics for Nurses and Midwives.* London: NMC.

Nursing and Midwifery Council (NMC). 2008b. *Standards to Support Learning and Assessment in Practice*, 2nd edn. London: NMC.

Nursing and Midwifery Council (NMC). 2010. *Standards for Pre-Registration Nursing Education.* London: NMC.

Nursing and Midwifery Council (NMC). 2011. *Guidance on Professional Conduct for Nursing and Midwifery Students.* London: NMC.

Oermann, M.H. 1990. Psychomotor skill development. *Journal of Continuing Education in Nursing* 21: 202–4.

Papadopoulos, I. 2006a. The Papadopoulos, Tilki and Taylor model of developing cultural competence. In: Papadopoulos, I. (ed.) *Transcultural Health and Social Care: Development of Culturally Competent Practitioners.* Edinburgh: Churchill Livingstone, 7–24.

Papadopoulos, I. (ed.) 2006b. *Transcultural Health and Social Care: Development of Culturally Competent Practitioners.* Edinburgh: Churchill Livingstone.

Paterson, J. and Zderad, L. 1988. *Humanistic Nursing.* New York: League for Nursing.

Patients Association. 2009. *Patients…Not Numbers, People…Not Statistics.* London: Patients Association.

Patients Association. 2011. *We've Been Listening, Have You Been Learning?* London: Patients Association.

Quinn, F. and Hughes, S.J. 2007. *Quinn's Principles and Practice of Nurse Education,* 5th edn. Cheltenham: Nelson-Thornes.

Roach, M.S. 2002. *Caring, the Human Mode of Being: A Blueprint for the Health Professions,* 2nd rev. edn. Ottawa: Canadian Hospital Association Press.

Roper, N., Logan, W.W. and Tierney, A.J. 2000. *The Roper–Logan–Tierney Model of Nursing: Based on Activities of Living.* Edinburgh: Elsevier Health Sciences.

Royal College of Nursing (RCN). 2008. *Defending Dignity: Challenges and Opportunities for Nurses.* London. Available from: http://www.rcn.org.uk/publications (Accessed on 21 September 2013).

Royal College of Nursing (RCN). 2011. *Meeting the Health Needs of People with Learning Disabilities.* London: RCN.

Royal College of Psychiatrists. 2011. *Report of the National Audit of Dementia Care in General Hospitals.* Young, J., Hood, C., Woolley, R., Gandesha, A. and Souza, R. (eds.) London: Healthcare Quality Improvement Partnership.

Schön, D. 1987. *Educating the Reflective Practitioner.* San Francisco, CA: Jossey-Bass.

Schön, D. 1991. *The Reflective Practitioner.* Aldershot: Ashgate Publishing Ltd.

Sir Jonathan Michael and the Independent Inquiry into Access to Healthcare for People with Learning Disabilities. 2008. *Healthcare for All: Report of the Independent Inquiry into Access to Healthcare for People with Learning Disabilities.* London: Crown.

Stanton, L.R. and Coetzee, R.H. 2004. Down's syndrome and dementia. *Advances in Psychiatric Treatment* 10: 50–8.

Thorsteinsson, L. 2002. The quality of nursing care as perceived by individuals with chronic illnesses: The magic touch of nursing. *Journal of Advanced Nursing* 11: 32–40.

Valentine, N., Darby, C. and Bonsel, G.J. 2008. Which aspects of quality of care are most important? Results from WHO's general population surveys of 'health system responsiveness' in 41 countries. *Social Science & Medicine* 66: 1939–50.

van der Cingel, M. 2011. Compassion in care: A qualitative study of older people with a chronic disease and nurses. *Nursing Ethics* 18(5): 672–85.

Watson, J. 1979. *Nursing: The Philosophy and Science of Caring.* Boston, MA: Little Brown.

Wilford, A. and Doyle, T.J. 2006. Integrating simulation training into the nursing curriculum. *British Journal of Nursing* 15(11): 604–7.

Woodward, V.M. 1997. Professional caring: A contradiction in terms? *Journal of Advanced Nursing* 26: 999–1004.

USEFUL WEBSITES

Alzheimer's Society: http://www.alzheimers.org.uk/

Care Quality Commission: http://www.cqc.org.uk

DepartmentofHealth:https://www.gov.uk/government/organisations/department-of-health

Dignity in Care: http://www.dignityincare.org.uk

Evidence Search: Health and Social Care: http://www.evidence.nhs.uk

Improving Health and Lives Observatory: http://www.improvinghealthandlives.org.uk/

Mencap: http://www.mencap.org.uk

National Institute for Health and Clinical Excellence: www.nice.org.uk

Nursing and Midwifery Council: www.nmc-uk.org

Resuscitation Council (UK): www.resus.org.uk

Royal College of Nursing: http://www.rcn.org.uk

Social Care Institute for Excellence: www.scie.org.uk

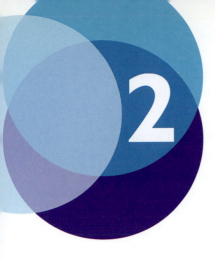

2 The Nurse's Approach and Communication: Foundations for Compassionate Care

Joanne Sale and Nicola M. Neale

> If we want to know ourselves then we need to observe what others are doing. If we want to understand others we need to search within ourselves. (Hamacheck 1992 in Rungapadiachy 2008, p. 17)

When we communicate with others, they are inevitably influenced by our behaviour and responses. Our actions and those of others do not happen in isolation; they are a reflection of the internal and external environment of all involved in the interaction. Any interaction is a two-way process; therefore, nurses must be aware that their approach to clients and patients in any setting affects the outcome. This book focuses on practical nursing skills, and in this chapter, we explore nurse–client interactions while carrying out skills. The chapter addresses the 'Care, compassion and communication' theme in the Nursing and Midwifery Council's (NMC 2010) Essential Skills Clusters (ESCs), which outline expectations of students and newly qualified nurses.

This chapter includes the following topics:

- Understanding what influences the nurse's approach to care
- The communication process
- Developing and maintaining therapeutic relationships
- Communication in challenging situations

PRACTICE SCENARIOS

The following scenarios, taken from later chapters, are referred to in the text. Definitions of medical terms in these scenarios can be found in the chapters in which they appear.

Chapter 4 – Measuring and monitoring vital signs

Natalie Turney is 21 years old. She has been admitted as a voluntary patient to an acute mental health ward with severe depression. After going home for a day, she returns, appearing unsteady on her feet and she has a strong smell of alcohol. Her speech is very slurred, and she is quite uncommunicative. When the staff asks her if she has taken any tablets, she mentions some 'little yellow pills' and paracetamol. However, she won't give details about the quantity or when she took them.

Chapter 8 – Meeting personal hygiene needs

William Newton, who likes to be called 'Bill', is a retired accountant aged 73. He is terminally ill with a history of oesophageal cancer and metastases in his lungs. He is cared for by his wife at home with the support of community nurses and the Macmillan nurse. He is taking regular oral morphine for pain control. He has a very low haemoglobin value and has been admitted for a blood transfusion. He is weak and breathless, and his general condition is poor. He has a body mass index (BMI) of 16. Bill can swallow only very small amounts of liquidised food and drink. He has some of his own teeth but also a partial denture that he likes to wear, although it is now ill fitting. His tongue appears coated and his mouth is dry.

Chapter 12 – Managing pain and promoting comfort and sleep

Maria is a 58-year-old woman with a moderate learning disability who has been living in a group home for the past 5 years. She has long-standing diabetes mellitus treated with insulin and has recently developed painful diabetic neuropathy. She has pain in both legs below the knees, which she finds particularly distressing when she is walking and during the night; her sleep is disturbed. She is in the care of both her general practitioner and the diabetic team at her local hospital. Maria's mother, who is 85 years old and recently widowed, visits weekly and is concerned about Maria's distress. Her community learning disability nurse would like to understand more about how he can support Maria, her mother and the group home staff on how to manage Maria's pain and increase her comfort.

Chapter 12 – Managing pain and promoting comfort and sleep

Violet Davies, aged 76, has moderate Alzheimer's disease. She has been admitted to a care home for respite as her husband is physically and emotionally exhausted and needs a break. He has refused help in the past as he has been determined to look after his wife, but he has now agreed to take a holiday visiting friends. Violet is physically well, but she is also known to have osteoarthritis in her right hip. She looks permanently worried and is agitated; she keeps repeating the same phrase over and over. Mr Davies looks shaky and tearful at the thought of leaving his wife for a week.

UNDERSTANDING WHAT INFLUENCES THE NURSE'S APPROACH TO CARE

LEARNING OUTCOMES

By the end of this section you will be able to:

1 explain the terms *self-concept* and *self-awareness* and apply them in a reflective manner within a caring context;
2 reflect on how personality may be important in nurse–client relationships;
3 discuss attitudes, values and beliefs and their impact in the care environment;
4 explain the terms *stereotyping* and *labelling* and discuss their significance to the care environment.

Learning outcome 1: Explain the terms *self-concept* and *self-awareness* and apply them in a reflective manner within a caring context

Rungapadiachy (2008) suggests that self-awareness includes focusing on self and recognising, knowing and being accepting of self. He also sees self-awareness as a skill that nurses need to develop, comprising three components: *cognitive*, how we think and form an understanding; *affective*, our feelings and emotions; and *behavioural*, the outward expression – verbal or non-verbal. There is a dynamic relationship between these components, and an awareness of self is essential to inform supportive therapeutic relationships. So, for example, you need to be aware of what you think about a client who has an alcohol problem and how this impression may affect your feelings and behaviour towards that client.

One way of developing self-awareness is to use a model such as the Johari window (Luft and Ingram 1955) (Figure 2.1), a model developed to help individuals identify aspects of self. This model suggests that self-disclosure and receiving feedback – that is, telling others about yourself and seeking feedback from them – help increase your awareness of self. Improved self-awareness will mean that the public area increases in relation to the other three areas as your understanding of your own strengths and weaknesses grows (Figure 2.1).

Consider how being self-aware might be important for you when carrying out practical skills. For example, if you have had an argument at home you may understand why you feel impatient with a person who appears to lack motivation to assist with hygiene needs. Acknowledging your emotional state will help you to understand your feelings and the subsequent effects on your caregiving. This increased awareness may highlight a need to adapt your behaviour. Pearce (2011) suggests that it is only through being self-aware that you will realise that you could be making a situation worse through your own behaviour. Healthcare professionals should develop understanding of how and why they behave in certain circumstances because, as Jack and Smith (2007) suggest, having an increased self-awareness helps us to relate to others. Therefore, the crucial point about self-awareness is its impact on our communication with others, and how it can help us to recognise the effects of our behaviour.

In Chapter 1, reflection was identified as being a conscious activity that usually involves a change in behaviour. Reflection, therefore, should help to increase awareness of how psychological, sociological, physical and contextual factors influence relationships with others.

	You know	You do not know
Others know	Public area	Blind area
Others do not know	Hidden area	Unknown area

Figure 2.1: Johari window. (From Luft, J. and Ingram, H. 1955. *The Johari Window: A Graphic Model of Interpersonal Relations*. Los Angeles, CA: University of Los Angeles Press.)

ACTIVITY

Think about a recent situation where your behaviour might have had an impact upon the interaction. Recall your thoughts, feelings and emotions related to this incident and whether these affected your actions, choice of words or your relationship with others.

For example, you may have considered the following:

- If you were angry at the time, did you shout?
- Did you say things that you regretted? Did you storm off?
- If you were sad, did you cry? Were you too emotional to speak?
- Were you able to listen effectively or were you distracted?

Now consider how your behaviour might have influenced the situation, either positively or negatively:

- If you raised your voice, did the other person also raise their voice or did they withdraw and become quiet?
- Did they become angry, aggressive or cry?

It is helpful for nurses to reflect upon their own behaviour because it will *always* affect the response of others to a lesser or greater degree. A lack of self-awareness can lead to serious problems in nurse–client relationships, and Eckroth-Bucher (2001, p. 33) reiterates this stance stating that 'understanding another begins with understanding yourself'. The ESC 'Care, compassion and communication' theme (1.9) states that the newly qualified graduate nurse needs to be self-aware and self-confident and know their own limitations (NMC 2010).

Self-concept can be defined as the information and beliefs that individuals have about their own nature, qualities and behaviour (Rogers 1961). However, Gross and Kinnison (2007, p. 295) suggest that it is a 'hypothetical construct' that each of us develops about ourselves: this construct is dynamic, never complete and helps us to understand not only who we are but also how we fit into society. Our sense of who we are is influenced and affected by how other people act towards us (Pearce 2011), and this supports Schaffer's (2004) suggestion that self-concept is *always* affected by how other people evaluate us.

It is generally accepted that there are three components to self-concept (Gross and Kinnison 2007): self-image, self-esteem and the ideal self.

Self-image

Self-image is the way in which we would describe ourselves, and this description may include social roles, physical characteristics and personality traits.

Self-esteem

Self-esteem is the extent to which we value and approve of ourselves and relates to how much we like ourselves.

Ideal self

The ideal self is the person we would like to be.

ACTIVITY

Describe yourself, including your strengths and weaknesses. Spend 5 minutes writing down the aspects of yourself that you would like a stranger to know. Then ask one of your friends to describe you and compare as follows:
- Does their view match yours?
- Were there things that you did not know about yourself?
- What do any differences tell you about yourself?
- Were there any aspects about yourself that you would choose to keep hidden?

When you have analysed your responses, identify how these responses reflect the three components self-image, self-esteem and ideal self. Now link this information back to the Johari window.

Self-image

Related to self-image, you may have thought about your social roles, physical characteristics and personality traits (Figure 2.2). In relation to your social roles, did you consider the different roles you have in your life: student, friend, nurse, parent, lover, partner, sibling and child? Did you consider your lifestyle and how it might affect choices you make? Did you consider whether your religious or spiritual beliefs and how your sexuality may affect your sense of who you are? For example, looking at the scenarios Mr Davies may now consider one of his roles to be 'a carer' and he may perceive a change in his role as husband, lover or partner. You may also have included your physical characteristics, for example, your height, weight and skin colour. How you view your body is referred to as 'body image'.

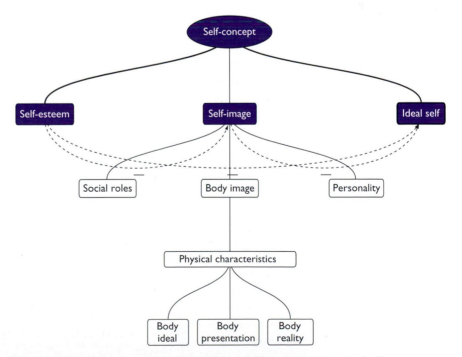

Figure 2.2: Pictorial representation of how self-concept links to other aspects of self.

Body image is the individual's interpretation of their bodily self, and it includes physical characteristics such as being tall, short, fat, thin, brown eyed or blond haired. Price (1990) identifies three aspects of body image:

- **Body ideal** is how we would like to look. This ideal may be guided by society's views and is a dynamic process that is influenced by social norms and cultural variations about what is considered desirable at any specific time.
- **Body presentation** is how we present ourselves, for example, our clothes, hair style and how we sit and walk. Social expectations may influence this presentation; you would probably choose different clothes to wear to a party than for a job interview. The NMC's (2010) ESC 'Care, compassion and communication' (1.10) states that for entry to the register, the newly qualified graduate nurse needs to act as a role model in promoting a professional image. Consider the effect of a nurse having dirty nails when about to give an injection; it is unlikely to demonstrate a professional manner and might affect the client's or a relative's confidence in the nurse.
- **Body reality** is the way we are, which may be very far from our body ideal; this reality might be thinner, taller, stronger or weaker than we really are. For example, Bill, as a result of his cancer, may have a completely different body reality having lost substantial weight in a short space of time.

During the earlier activity, you may also have considered aspects of your personality that you consider to be important in how you view yourself and your strengths and weaknesses. For example, do you see yourself as an outgoing person or a shy person? How might your personality characteristics be important in establishing and maintaining communication with your clients? We return to the concept of personality in more detail later in this chapter.

Self-esteem

Self-esteem is also one of the aspects of self-concept, and it can be viewed as a critical, personal evaluation of our own self-worth. Walker et al. (2012) suggest that self-esteem is an essential part of psychological well-being and believe that childhood and adolescence are especially important periods for the development of self-esteem. This evaluation of ourselves can be general or specific (Gross and Kinnison 2007); for example, we might like ourselves generally but might not like a particular aspect, such as how tall we are, or our short temper. Society appears to value certain characteristics more highly than others. For example, people with healthy physical and psychological attributes are seen positively and as possessing qualities to be attained. However, some health conditions that may be seen in more negative terms include physical disfigurement, physical disability, mental illness and certain physical illnesses such as human immunodeficiency virus (HIV). If a disfigurement or disability is visible to others, there may be a particularly acute effect on body image and self-esteem; for example, an adolescent with acne or a child with a facial port-wine stain.

Some illnesses may be stigmatising as a result of the way society views them. Stigma has been defined as something that is shameful and may set people apart and can lead to discrimination. It is also thought to lead to marginalisation and low self-esteem in children (National CAMHS Support Services 2010). For example, many people such as Natalie, who are labelled with a mental illness, are often treated less favourably than others in society, and this discrimination is not only unlawful and damaging but can potentially have a negative impact upon their view of self. Stigma can affect people at all ages, but for adolescents and young adults, like Natalie, these stages are a particularly important time of their development, and their social skills, identity and psychological well-being are vulnerable to negative attitudes (Department of Health [DH] 2011).

Ideal self

Ideal self relates to our desire to have certain qualities. However, this desire is not just about physical characteristics but also considers wider issues such as personality and relationships. We might want to change some aspects of ourselves, or we might wish we were a different person altogether, perhaps kinder or more intelligent. In relation to your nursing, you may yearn to feel more confident when starting a new placement, wish that you could remember people's names better, or perhaps wish you could perform more confidently when calculating medication for injection. Sometimes, through illness, people undergo changes in their ideal self; these changes may be sudden as in surgery or might progress slowly such as the changes that occur in rheumatoid arthritis. For example, Bill has lost weight and feelings related to this loss may contribute to how he responds and copes with his illness.

ACTIVITY

Consider the scenarios at the beginning of this chapter. How might Maria and Mrs Davies's perceptions of self be influenced by what they are experiencing?

Maria may have difficulty understanding what is happening to her due to her moderate learning disability. Her diagnosis, her increasing lack of mobility and pain could also affect her body image and contribute to a low self-esteem. Mrs Davies's Alzheimer's disease might affect her sense of self from any or all perspectives – physical, psychological and social. It is possible that she might have periods of insight into her loss of intellectual functioning and that she might be aware of other people's reactions and a change in their attitude and approach towards her.

Many people in different care settings have changes to their self-concept due to their illness experiences; therefore, it is vital that nurses are aware that their approach, while carrying out practical skills, can negatively or positively affect clients' self-image, self-esteem and potentially acceptance of their health conditions.

The concept of self is complex, and all of the above aspects are interrelated and dynamic. They are influenced by individual, family and societal experiences and expectations throughout the life span. Self-esteem and self-image are connected, and as Rogers (1961) suggests, the greater the gap between your self-image and your ideal self, the lower your self-esteem, thus reiterating the importance for health professionals to have an awareness and understanding about how an illness may impact upon the sense of self.

Learning outcome 2: Reflect on how personality may be important in nurse–client relationships

Personality is part of what makes people unique but at the same time allows people to be compared with each other. Personality is seen in psychological theories as being either a relatively stable component of the self or as varying depending on an individual's situation. There have been many approaches to the study of personality and how personality may be relevant within healthcare settings. Eysenck (1965) proposed one approach to explaining personality, identifying two principal dimensions: introversion–extroversion and neuroticism–stability. For example, an introverted nurse may find communicating with patients or colleagues in groups more stressful than an extrovert nurse. However, on a one-to-one basis, introvert nurses might be comfortable in this situation and thus may be more effective in their communication.

The behaviour that you observe may give small, but important, insights into a person's personality; however, inappropriate interpretation of personality traits can be unhelpful as it may lead to the perception that the patient is not responsive to change (Walker et al. 2012). For example, Natalie may be quiet and uncommunicative. What conclusions could you draw from this behaviour? You might decide that Natalie is introverted and shy, or that she is thoughtful and polite. These views might indicate to you something about her personality from your viewpoint, but how can you be assured as to the accuracy of these views? Although it is important to be cautious when judging personality traits, Gosling (1995), cited by Gross and Kinnison (2007), suggests that an understanding of personality can help nurses to understand patients and their illnesses and, therefore, may enhance the delivery of individualised patient-centred care.

Nichols (2003, 2005) suggests that patient-centred psychological care, of which communication is a key area, is often unsystematic and arbitrary, leading to unmet needs that can affect recovery, their **concordance** with interventions and their response to illness.

> **Concordance**
>
> A partnership process between patients and healthcare professionals to agree on treatment (Chapter 5 discusses concordance further in relation to medicines).

ACTIVITY

> When you are next on an adult medical or surgical ward, randomly choose one patient on the ward and ask their named nurse 'who is handling this patient's psychological care and how is it going?' (Nichols 2005).

Although Nichols was writing more than 5 years ago, he was still finding that the psychological care for adults in a hospital setting remained hit-and-miss. This was despite 20 years of psychological study, leaving some patients distressed and with unmet needs, as seen in recent examples from both Winterbourne Vale (DH 2012a) and Mid Staffordshire Trust (Mid Staffordshire NHS Foundation Trust Inquiry 2010; Mid Staffordshire NHS Foundation Trust Public Inquiry 2013). Nichols (2005) suggests that unless hospitals and health centres 'develop psychological care as part of the thinking, culture and routines […] then this situation will continue to affect patients' responses and thus their recovery' (p. 26).

Learning outcome 3: Discuss attitudes, values and beliefs and their impact in the care environment

The ESC for 'Care, compassion and communication' (5.10) recommends that the newly qualified graduate nurse has 'insight into their own values and how these may impact on interactions with others' (NMC 2010).

First, some definitions (Gross and Kinnison 2007):

- **Value** – the person's sense of desirability, worth or utility of obtaining some outcome.
- **Belief** – an opinion held about something: the information, knowledge or thoughts about a particular thing.

Our values and beliefs underpin our attitudes and affect how we behave with others. Attitudes have been described as feelings that give order and shape to our lives, but defining attitudes is difficult. For example, what is your opinion about smokers receiving healthcare? You may value life but believe in the right to freedom of choice; therefore, your attitude might be ambivalent.

Similarly to self-awareness (discussed earlier), Rosenberg and Hovland (1960, cited in Gross and Kinnison 2013) suggested that there are three components to attitudes:

- **Affective** – how we feel about a person, object or situation.
- **Cognitive** – our thoughts and perceptions about the person, object or situation.
- **Behavioural** – how we act towards the person, object or situation.

ACTIVITY

Consider the scenario concerning Mrs Davies. Would you feel any differently about her if you found out that her dementia was related to alcohol or drug abuse? Be as honest with yourself as possible.

You might feel less keen to care for Mrs Davies because you believe her condition to be her own fault, or you might even openly criticise her behaviour. Morrison and Burnard (1997) suggest that caregivers constantly make decisions about whether or not people deserve care, citing Rajecki (1982), who suggested that attitudes play a crucial part in influencing caring behaviours. However, the NMC (2008) states that nurses should treat clients as individuals and respect their dignity, be kind and considerate and not discriminate in any way.

ACTIVITY

Are there other illnesses where health professionals may decide that the individual or their lifestyle is responsible for the health problem?

Some examples are as follows:

- A person who is HIV positive as a result of unsafe sex (in contrast to someone infected due to a contaminated blood transfusion).
- A person who has deliberately taken an overdose (in contrast to someone who has mistakenly taken an overdose).
- A cocaine addict who is experiencing hallucinations (in contrast to someone who is experiencing hallucinations either because of their treatment or due to an infection).

These examples are linked to diagnosis. However, in reality, there are many subtle, social factors that influence our judgements in client-centred relationships (Johnson and Webb 1995). It is therefore important to be aware that values, beliefs and attitudes are central to how we behave, and to examine whether these affect the quality of our communication, how we care and our compassion for individuals and their circumstances. Pope (2012), citing McCormack and McCance's (2010) person-centred framework, suggests that amongst the prerequisites of the nurse are clarity of personal beliefs and values, and self-knowledge. These qualities are seen as a necessity for the newly qualified nurse who must 'act professionally to ensure that personal judgements, prejudices, values, attitudes do not compromise care' [ESC 'Care, compassion and communication' in NMC 2010].

Learning outcome 4: Explain the terms *stereotyping* and *labelling* and discuss their significance to the care environment

Stereotyping is the assigning of attributes to an individual based on their membership of a particular group (Walker et al. 2012). **Labelling** is a form of stereotyping where we categorise people by, for example, aspects such as their behaviour or their age.

ACTIVITY

When next in the practice setting, listen carefully to how nurses and other healthcare professionals speak about clients and their families. Are value judgements being made, and if so do these judgements affect caring relationships? Are patients labelled according to diagnosis? If so, how?

What did you notice about the words used to describe clients and their behaviour? Examples that we have heard include 'difficult', 'attention-seeking', 'lovely', 'a pain in the neck', 'demanding' and 'bless him'. You might also have observed body language that reflects attitude: sighing, raising eyes to the ceiling and shrugging shoulders. What kind of labels may be used about the people in the scenarios from any of the chapters? Are you aware of any times where you have used labels that could have influenced other people's views and as a result the care given? Higgins et al. (2007) suggested that handover was an opportunity for nurses to state their subjective beliefs in regard to older people and that these beliefs were then assimilated into other nurses' beliefs about the patient.

The NMC's (2010) ESC for 'Care, compassion and communication' includes the need to be non-judgemental, stating that nurses must deliver care that is warm, sensitive and compassionate and free from discrimination and harassment. Recent high-profile cases such as Winterbourne Vale (DH 2012a) and Mid Staffordshire (Mid Staffordshire NHS Foundation Trust Inquiry 2010) demonstrate the devastating effect upon individual patients and their families when nurses lose sight of the core elements of their role. Although all nurses need knowledge to perform skills within the clinical setting, these skills also must be practised in a manner that continually demonstrates an awareness of the person and their needs at each stage of the care experience. Compassion in Practice (DH 2012b) is a response

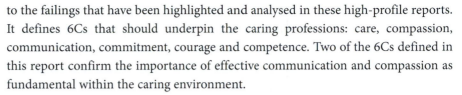

to the failings that have been highlighted and analysed in these high-profile reports. It defines 6Cs that should underpin the caring professions: care, compassion, communication, commitment, courage and competence. Two of the 6Cs defined in this report confirm the importance of effective communication and compassion as fundamental within the caring environment.

As discussed, the judgements we make of others may affect the care that we give. Sometimes, we make these judgements as a result of personal bias, thus failing to see the individual as a unique human being and leading to prejudice in the care provided. The word *prejudice* means 'to prejudge', and it is a constant challenge in our interpersonal relationships to remain as non-judgemental as possible.

There are two manifestations of prejudice – direct and indirect (Pettigrew and Meertens 1995). Direct or open prejudice is blatant and obvious, for example, a patient refusing to be looked after by a nurse who is black. Indirect or closed prejudice is more subtle; for example, a nurse who does not approve of a patient who has acquired HIV through their choice of lifestyle might provide the minimum acceptable level of care and not talk to them or make eye contact.

ACTIVITY

Consider the practice scenarios. How might both direct and indirect prejudice manifest itself?

If Maria is judged as a result of her learning disability, staff may not explain what they are doing or what is happening to her, assuming that she won't understand. However, Valuing People Now (DH 2009) suggests that people with learning difficulties have rights to choice and inclusion. Therefore, Maria should be included, and careful thought should be given to the use of appropriate communication skills to enable her to contribute to any decisions about her care. Mrs Davies may be avoided by staff if she is agitated, as they might consider her difficult, resulting in her physical needs not being met.

We make attempts at ordering the world around us in an effort to understand what is happening, but this ordering can lead to erroneous perceptions that can affect care delivery. Our communication with our patients/clients can reflect our underlying prejudices. At one time, labelling of patients was considered fairly fixed in nature, so that once labelled, this label would remain with the patient/client (Stockwell 1972). However, Johnson and Webb (1995) found that labels were more flexible and transient, changing with time and experience. When approaching patient care, you should be aware of your behaviour and if it is affected by any labels or stereotypical views.

Within an adult care setting, nurses need to be aware that individuals who have a mental illness or learning disability are vulnerable to disadvantage and exclusion (Cabinet Office Social Exclusion Task Force 2007). Nurses in any sector may care for people with learning disabilities or with a history of mental health problems; if nurses hold stereotypical or prejudiced views, such views could affect their approach to care and their interactions. These points relate to the NMC's (2010) ESC for

'Care, compassion and communication', which identified that nurses must act professionally, ensuring that personal judgements, prejudices, values, attitudes and beliefs do not compromise care provision.

Summary
- An understanding of self-concept and related aspects informs and enhances nurse–client relationships.
- Developing self-awareness improves nurses' approach to patients/clients.
- Personality and attitudes are influential in affecting nurse–client relationships.
- Awareness of attitudes, prejudices and labelling – and responding to these appropriately – helps to reduce negative effects.

THE COMMUNICATION PROCESS

LEARNING OUTCOMES

By the end of this section you will be able to:
1 explain appropriate verbal and non-verbal communication skills;
2 identify barriers to communication and reflect on how these barriers can be addressed;
3 discuss elements of effective written communication;
4 outline elements of appropriate telephone communication;
5 appreciate the importance of effective communication between members of the multidisciplinary team.

Communication is the 'successful transfer of a message and meaning from one person or group to another' (McCorry and Mason 2011, p. 6).

Learning outcome 1: Explain appropriate verbal and non-verbal communication skills

In everyday life, we constantly communicate, either verbally, or through the written word, or by our gestures or body language. Communication involves transmitting information and messages from one individual to another, but it is also one of the fundamental ways of demonstrating care and compassion. It is therefore important for nurses to have an understanding of the different aspects of communication to maximise positive effects within the nurse–patient relationship. Communication is essential for initiating, forming and maintaining relationships.

ACTIVITY

Write down as many different ways that you can think of to send a message.

You may have thought of speaking to someone either face to face individually or in a group. You may have considered the telephone, writing a note, sending a text message or an e-mail or participating in an online forum. Did you think of sign language too? In 2003, the United Kingdom (UK) government recognised British Sign Language as a language in its own right (British Deaf Association 2008).

There are two aspects of interpersonal communication: *verbal* and *non-verbal*.

ACTIVITY

List under the headings 'Verbal' and 'Non-verbal' as many aspects of communication you can think of.

The verbal aspects you may have thought of include tone of voice, pitch (or loudness), use of silence and pauses. These verbal components express our emotions and communicate information about our interpersonal attitudes. Sometimes, a person's speed of speech indicates their emotional state – someone who is depressed may speak in a slow, flat, monotone voice. Mrs Davies, who is increasingly agitated, keeps repeating the same phrase over and over again and her speech may become faster and louder. Sometimes, the way we use communication alters the meaning of the words used. For example, consider the different ways 'What do you want?' can be said. Non-verbal aspects include proximity, posture, body movements, touch, eye contact, facial expression and gesture. Both verbal and non-verbal behaviour are culturally determined (Arnold and Bloggs 2011) – which is further discussed in learning outcome 2.

Several authors have developed models or frameworks of the communication process to portray the complexity of interpersonal interactions. Some suggest that communication is something that people do to one another, rather than a process where there is continual receiving, responding and interacting (Rungapadiachy 2008). Many frameworks now incorporate wider aspects in relation to communication. The framework in Figure 2.3 has been developed from reviewing several previous models published in the literature: steps in the communication process (Porritt 1984, adapted from Berlo 1960), a conceptual model of message transmission and reception (Minardi and Riley 1997), and a skill model of interpersonal communication (Hargie et al. 1994).

The framework in Figure 2.3 illustrates that the social context and environment encompass and influence all areas of the interaction process. It also shows that, at any given moment, the sender of a message is also the receiver of messages. Our thoughts, feelings and behaviour (verbal and non-verbal) influence our interpretation and, therefore, our response to the message and its perceived meaning. *Encoding* entails turning our thoughts and feelings into a recognisable message that is in many cases reflected in our responses. *Decoding* is about how we interpret a message we have received, to make sense of it. Therefore, we are continually receiving and sending messages in this dynamic process of interaction.

Listening is an essential part of the communication process, and there are many different definitions of listening emphasising the aural (hearing), oral (spoken) and environmental aspects. Stein-Parbury (2009) underlines the importance of recognising that listening is an active process that requires concentration and effort to enable appropriate skills development.

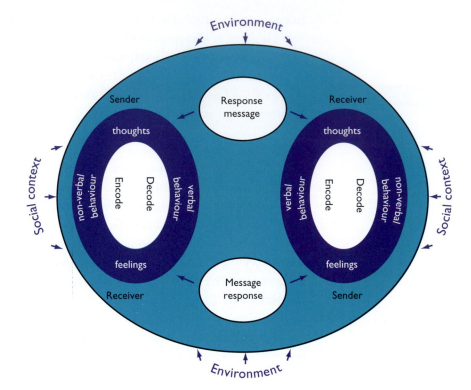

Figure 2.3: A framework for communication.

Reflect on a recent occasion when you were speaking to a friend, a colleague or a client. What can you recall about the following:

- Verbal ways that you showed that you were listening
- Body positions: yours and theirs
- Eye contact
- Facial expressions
- Other non-verbal communication, for example, gestures

What can you remember about the content?

How we select, perceive and retain messages is influenced by our values and beliefs and by our cultural upbringing. How are these aspects relevant to your reflections in the activity above? Was it easier to remember what you discussed with your friend rather than a colleague? This exercise may demonstrate how important attention and memory are within the listening process, as well as context.

Egan (2010) uses the acronym SOLER to help us to remember how to use our body position when listening:

- **Sit** squarely in relation to the client.
- Maintain an **Open** position.
- **Lean** slightly towards the client.
- Maintain reasonable **Eye** contact.
- **Relax**.

Did you identify these aspects of body language? You may also have reflected on use of space, silence, touch and gestures, such as nodding in agreement or using facial expression to show interest or understanding. You or others may have used verbal signals to indicate that you were listening – for example, 'umm', 'aah', 'uh-huh', 'oh' or 'I see'. Sometimes, when we are supposed to be actively listening, we can slip into automatic pilot and are not really fully responsive to the message. Stein-Parbury (2009) suggests that there are many barriers to effective listening, both external and internal, such as our own thoughts, value judgements and feelings.

When we are with patients, we need to demonstrate that we have heard and understood both the emotional and factual content of their message. This acknowledgment can be done by paraphrasing important statements that the patient has said, allowing both patient and carer to seek clarification. We must also be alert to any non-verbal messages, as this information may reflect the patient's feelings and help to achieve a true understanding of their needs. For example, Natalie may say that she is 'OK', but you determine from her non-verbal cues that she is anxious. A recognition of this discrepancy may be important in her therapeutic care.

To recognise incongruence between the verbal and non-verbal message, sensitive observational skills and an empathetic approach are required. Empathy can be described as 'a form of emotional knowing or the experience of another person's feelings' (Rungapadiachy 2008, p. 20). Being empathetic requires the appropriate use of skills mentioned earlier – touch, eye contact and use of voice. Vocal features may encompass not only the words we use but also, just as importantly, the tone and manner. An example would be using a calm and soothing voice. It has been suggested that self-aware nurses are more likely to be empathetic (Wiseman 2007) and may be more effective listeners too (Rungapadiachy 2008).

Learning outcome 2: Identify barriers to communication and reflect on how these barriers can be addressed

The NMC (2010) stressed the importance of nurses acquiring effective communication skills, including verbal and non-verbal aspects and identifying possible barriers.

ACTIVITY

Identify factors that may act as barriers to your communication and relationships with clients.

The NMC (2010) identified that nurses should be able to recognise and overcome barriers affecting the development of therapeutic relationships. Barriers can be physical, psychological or social, although the distinction between these types is not always clear-cut.

- **Physical barriers** could include visual, auditory or speech impairment, pain, or how the surrounding environment is organised (a desk between two participants, one person sitting and the other standing, or background noise).

- **Psychological barriers** may relate to personality (e.g. if someone is very shy), attitudes, beliefs and labelling (either the caregiver's or the client's), the emotional state of either party (e.g. anxiety), and cognition or thought processes, which may affect language, understanding or both. For example, Maria, who has a learning disability, might understand what is said to her, but she may be unable to express herself verbally.

- **Social barriers** may include social status, culture, religious and spiritual beliefs. Social status may affect how we interact with others due to our place in the hierarchy or the context of the relationship. Is there a difference in how you would communicate with a doctor or a healthcare assistant?

The influence of an individual's culture and their religious and spiritual beliefs are important factors that are often overlooked in nurse–client interactions. The NMC (2010) requires that nurses be culturally competent (see Chapter 1 for an explanation of cultural competence). Leininger (1985, cited in Allen and Crouch 2007, p. 450) described 'culture' as the 'learned, shared and transmitted values and beliefs, norms and lifestyle practices of a particular group that guide thinking, decisions and actions in patterned fashions'. Vydelingum's (2000) study, which included Hindu, Sikh and Muslim clients, highlighted how communication difficulties led to patients feeling isolated due to language barriers. For example, nurses did not provide sufficient information in relation to diagnosis or medication. Furthermore, language barriers may disadvantage the patient because it is more difficult to develop a rapport, to obtain relevant clinical information and to emotionally engage. The patient is also less able to convey their concerns and needs (McCorry and Mason 2011). Perceptions about causation of illness are also important because they affect how the person explains to themselves and others what is happening and why it is happening. For example, beliefs about possession by spirits have been demonstrated in some cultures; in Malaysia, 53% of those diagnosed with a mental health problem attributed the problem to supernatural agents such as witchcraft (Razali et al. 1996). Therefore, an understanding of the individual's cultural background will help to ensure that their needs are fully addressed.

There are differences in the use of eye contact, gesture, proximity and touch that may affect communication. For example, looking directly into the other person's eyes can be considered disrespectful or a sign of honesty, depending on the culture. The unspoken conventions that accompany language in different cultures, such as politeness, degrees of directness, pace and the use of silence, may also cause misunderstandings. Fuller (2003) suggests ways to facilitate communication with individuals from different ethnic groups – for example, keeping an even tone, maintaining consistent speed of delivery and avoiding shouting.

Communication can be aided by using pictures, photos and mime, and these strategies may help to ascertain and enhance understanding. Translators and interpreters may be necessary, but where possible professional interpreters should be used rather than untrained personnel or family members. Dein (2006) suggests that using informal interpreters may inadvertently alter the meaning of the message in translation, leading to inadequate information or a lack of understanding. Family members may be reluctant to discuss sensitive and personal subjects with their relatives, particularly if communication is influenced by cultural taboos, for instance about bodily functions.

ACTIVITY

Looking at the section above, reflect on a recent clinical experience and list some of the factors that may have affected your ability to deliver culturally sensitive care and the effect upon the communication process.

You may have included whether
- individuals' food preferences were addressed (e.g. Halal meat or vegetarian);
- provisions were made for particular religious beliefs or practices;
- the number of visitors was limited, making it difficult for extended families to visit;
- eye contact, personal space and touch were adjusted appropriately;
- adjustments were made in the interaction if a patient's English language skills were limited.

The above-mentioned points all highlight the importance of recognising a range of influences within the communication experience and the potential barriers to the supportive nurse–client relationship.

Learning outcome 3: Discuss elements of effective written communication

Written communication is an important but often neglected area in nursing and is increasingly emphasised in relation to documentation and record-keeping. The NMC (2009) states that 'Good record keeping is an integral part of nursing and midwifery practice, and is essential to the provision of safe and effective care' (p. 3). Good record-keeping helps to protect patients' welfare by promoting high standards of continuity and clinical care. It also ensures effective and accurate communication and dissemination of information between healthcare team members.

The NMC (2009, p. 5) outlines principles of good record keeping. Some of these principles are considered below, with application to the scenarios. Patient and client records should:
- *be factual and accurate:* Mrs Davies's behaviour should be documented in an unbiased and non-judgemental way.
- *be written in real time, in chronological order, and as close to the actual time of care as possible.* When Bill, who is terminally ill, is at home, he will be cared for by various community and specialist nurses. Therefore his care must be documented immediately and in sufficient detail.
- *be written clearly and be readable when photocopied or scanned.* If any changes have to be made, you must write your name and job title, and sign and date the original documentation.

- *not include abbreviations, jargon, meaningless phrases, irrelevant speculation or coded expressions of sarcasm.*

Carry out the activity below and see how confusing and potentially dangerous using abbreviations can be.

ACTIVITY

What do the following abbreviations mean: CF, CPA, PID, TPR, BP, OE, RXT, ABC, ETA, TTA, DNA, DOA, GCS? All of these abbreviations can be applicable in healthcare settings. Discuss them with a friend or colleague.

How many of these abbreviations did you know without further investigation? (see definitions at the end of this chapter). Were there any that could have more than one meaning? One example is that PID can mean either 'prolapsed intervertebral disc' or 'pelvic inflammatory disease'. Other examples are that BP could mean 'blood pressure' or 'bedpan' and DOA might mean 'dead on arrival' or 'date of admission'. You might think DNA is to do only with genetics, but it is often used to abbreviate the phrase 'did not attend (an appointment)'.

The context of the clinical environment may influence your interpretation of an abbreviation. Generally, although abbreviations are part of everyday life, there are few that are acceptable in healthcare practice, especially in written records.

When completing nursing records, nurses must have a comprehensive awareness of all the pertinent issues contained in the NMC (2009) guidelines as these guidelines are professional standards for practice. Nurses who have a diagnosis of dyslexia may have particular need for support when completing written records and should be supported appropriately by colleagues and the organisation.

The Internet now plays a vital role in healthcare communications. Nurses should be aware of issues relating to the use of e-mail. Redfern-Jones (2006) advises the following:

- Keep it concise.
- Do not include confidential information.
- Check your spelling and grammar.
- Avoid abbreviations and acronyms.
- Reply quickly.

In relation to the last point, it is also important to remember the immediacy of e-mail messages and the possibility that a hurried, ill-thought-through response may be a source of regret in the future. Therefore, although responding in a timely manner is important, there is also the need to think carefully about any response. It may be more appropriate that some issues are dealt with either by a formal written response or by a telephone conversation.

Most employers will have related policy concerning information governance and data protection, and it is vital that nurses are aware of local as well as national requirements.

Learning outcome 4: Outline elements of appropriate telephone communication

ACTIVITY

Reflect on the last time you telephoned someone to make an appointment or to clarify something. Did you know who you were speaking to? Did they give you the information you wanted? How did it feel if your needs were met or not met; for example, you ended up being directed to a message box or a queue?

Increasingly, telephones are an important mode of communication within healthcare settings (Royal College of Nursing [RCN] 2012). However, there is little guidance about using them appropriately. Organisations provide their own corporate guidance about telephone use; therefore, you must ensure that you are aware of local policy.

- **Answering the telephone.** It is important that you clearly state where you are and who you are.
- **Maintaining confidentiality.** It is essential that you ensure confidentiality. You need to know who you are talking to at the other end of the telephone. If someone asks about a client by name, you must ensure that the client is happy for information to be passed on. If possible, and the client has access to a telephone, they should be encouraged to make contact independently.
- **Acknowledging your level of competence.** For example, if you were asked to take down a message or a set of laboratory results and you did not understand what you were being told, you should explain to the caller that you need to get someone else to take the details.
- **Documenting and disseminating the information.** Make sure that messages are documented accurately and clearly and that they are promptly passed on to the relevant individuals. This dissemination includes passing messages to patients; knowing that others are thinking of them is good for their sense of belonging and self-esteem.

Telephone consultations are becoming more common for nurses to engage in; thus, the RCN (2012) have provided helpful specific guidelines for communicating with patients with long-term conditions.

Learning outcome 5: Appreciate the importance of effective communication between members of the multidisciplinary team

Effective communication within the multidisciplinary team is important in all areas of nursing, both in hospital and community settings, and it is essential for maintaining a high standard of care management. Gibbons (2008) suggests that communication with colleagues is one of the most important areas for ensuring that we are working in the patients' best interests – it is vital that health professionals coordinate and share verbal and written information so that communication with patients about their care is clear and relevant. If you look back at the scenarios at the start of this chapter, you can see that nurses would need to communicate with a wide range of healthcare professionals. Some upcoming chapters explore the multidisciplinary teamwork necessary for the effective care of these patients.

<table>
<tr><td>**ACTIVITY**</td><td>Look at Maria's scenario. Identify members of the multidisciplinary team between whom communication would be necessary to address her ongoing care needs. What form of communication would be used?</td></tr>
</table>

You might have identified that effective communication must occur between Maria, her mother, and the community and specialist health and social care staff including: the pain specialist nurse, group home staff, diabetes team, medical staff, pharmacist, social worker and community learning disability nurse. Other staff might be involved, too, depending on her assessed needs (e.g. dietician, chaplain, physiotherapist, occupational therapist, voluntary organisations). Communication will be verbal (including telephone) and written (including documentation, e-mail, fax).

In relation to skills, nurses must ensure that information is recorded accurately and communicated unambiguously and concisely to other team members, for example, communicating with medical staff about changes to observations that may require medication adjustment, or communicating with the physiotherapist to ensure analgesics are given if needed before exercise. The key principles relating to effective communication discussed in this chapter also apply to communication within the multidisciplinary team.

Children: practice points for communication

Communicating with children in any healthcare setting must take into account their cognitive ability and understanding. Communication is undertaken in partnership with parents/carers to ensure their needs are met and appropriately supported. Parents/carers are in the best position to understand their young child's communication. They may be anxious or frightened when their child is ill or injured, so appropriate communication will reduce this anxiety. Play is often used as a means to communicate effectively with children.

For a review of communication with children and families, see

Glasper, A. 2010. Communicating with children, young people and their families. In: Glasper, A., Aylott, M. and Battrick, C. (eds.) *Developing Practical Skills for Nursing Children and Young People*. London: Hodder Arnold, 40–51.

Macqueen, S., Bruce, E.A. and Gibson, F. 2012. Play as a therapeutic tool. In: *The Great Ormond Street Hospital Manual of Children's Nursing Practices*. Chichester: Wiley-Blackwell, 609–24.

Summary

- Communication can be both verbal and non-verbal.
- Identifying barriers to communication and having an awareness of how these barriers might be overcome are important.
- Effective written communication skills are an essential component of nursing practice.
- Telephone communication is an important method of sharing information and must be conducted in a professional manner.
- Effective communication within the multidisciplinary team is essential for patients'/clients' well-being and safety.

DEVELOPING AND MAINTAINING THERAPEUTIC RELATIONSHIPS

LEARNING OUTCOMES

By the end of this section, you will be able to:

1 appreciate important aspects of initiating successful interactions;
2 identify how to give clear explanations;
3 demonstrate an awareness of a range of questioning styles;
4 explain key features of gaining informed consent;
5 reflect on the features of appropriate professional behaviour.

Learning outcome 1: Appreciate important aspects of initiating successful interactions

Stein-Parbury (2009) suggests that the initial phase of a nurse–patient relationship is full of uncertainty and that there is a need to reduce this uncertainty. Therefore, gaining trust is essential and can be achieved through learning about each other. For nurses, this trust should be within the boundaries of the professional role (NMC 2008).

ACTIVITY

Imagine you are meeting the people from the scenarios (see the beginning of the chapter). Write down how you think you would introduce yourself to each of them.

You might introduce yourself by giving your first name: for example, 'Hello, I'm Jane' or 'I'm Jane Smith', or perhaps 'Hello, I'm student nurse Smith'. If you offer your first name, you may make it difficult for clients not to give you their first name. Some people prefer to be called by their formal titles, for example, Mrs Davies rather than Violet. Usually, if the person wants you to call them by their first name, they will give you permission sometime in the relationship. Using a formal title is a sign of respect, whereas first names imply intimacy or familiarity. In their 'Top tips for care', the Alzheimer's Society (2011) suggests that many patients with dementia may respond more positively if they are addressed in a more formal manner initially. Think back to the first time you met the practitioner in charge of a recent placement – how did you address them? It is likely that you adopted a formal approach until told otherwise.

Here again, cultural aspects should be considered. For example, it would be disrespectful for a nurse to call a Sikh man by his first name or to ask him for his 'Christian' name. As highlighted earlier, cultural norms determine all aspects of the communication process, including the verbal and non-verbal.

ACTIVITY

Imagine that you have been asked to measure Natalie's blood pressure. You are meeting her for the first time. How would you establish rapport?

Opening introductions often involve some small talk. You might, for example, see that Natalie is wearing a scarf of a local football team. You could comment, 'I see you are wearing City's colours, how do you think they're doing this season?' Any introductory conversation should focus on putting the client at ease, thus enabling assessment to be more accurate. Trust can be achieved only if the client experiences the nurse as consistent in approach, be it in attitude, behaviour or communication. Therefore, how we initiate interactions is important for developing therapeutic relationships.

Learning outcome 2: Identify how to give clear explanations

Explanations are only effective if they are given clearly and help individuals to remember what has been said to them.

ACTIVITY

Imagine you are looking after Bill and you need to explain to him about his blood transfusion. What principles should you remember when giving him an explanation?

- Did you think about identifying his *understanding* about his anaemia and the need for a transfusion?
- Did you think about the importance of the *language* you used?
- Did you think about the need to check his *understanding throughout*?
- Did you consider the *order* in which you would give information – for example, important aspects first?
- Did you acknowledge that you need to give *specific rather than general or vague information*?
- Did you consider the need to *emphasise certain information, repeating it* where necessary?

ACTIVITY

Consider the principles highlighted above. How might you explain to any of the people in the scenarios what practical skill you are about to carry out?

You might have thought about how you would ensure Maria understands you when assessing her pain. You should use clear, short questions, and communication methods could include interpreting non-verbal cues, using pictures and signing. The nurse should work closely with Maria and her carers to explain things in an understandable manner. The Department of Health's *Valuing People Now* (DH 2009) emphasised that people with learning disabilities should be able to access healthcare as easily as any other member of the public, and this healthcare includes communication matters. The onus is on staff to adapt and use different approaches to meet individuals' needs. When discussing Bill's pain management, you should check and recheck that he understands what you are saying, as his deteriorating condition may lead to confusion and an inability to concentrate. Having completed an explanation, you should check that patients understand the information accurately (Nichols 2003).

An important part of giving explanations is the *words* that we use. Thompson (2002) suggests language can reinforce social and cultural divisions, emphasising that it is not just the words we use but the way that we use them. Imagine that Bill needed to wear an incontinence pad and the nurse said, 'Let's put your nappy on'. How do you think he would feel? How would you feel if someone spoke to your father or grandfather in this way? Crawford et al. (2006) emphasises the unacceptability of baby talk and the harmful effects it may have on nurse–client relationships.

Stein-Parbury (2009) suggests that acknowledging the client's experience encourages further interaction. Explanations should be high quality and adjusted to meet the individual's needs, and they should receive comprehensive information about all aspects of their care.

Learning outcome 3: Demonstrate an awareness of a range of questioning styles

There are many different types of questions that may be utilised within the therapeutic relationship. It is important for nurses to be aware of how these questions may enhance (or detract from) the quality of information gathered, specifically within the assessment process in relation to ascertaining important and relevant aspects of the person's thoughts, feelings and attitudes to their situation.

Consider the following:

- **Closed questions** (e.g. 'Would you like a cup of tea?', 'Have you got pain?'). Closed questions can gain factual information, but they do not allow further exploration. They frequently require a yes/no answer and are helpful for gaining information from patients who can only respond briefly (e.g. in acute breathlessness). Often, closed questions are used in initial patient assessments and lead to the second major type of question.

- **Open questions** (e.g. 'What symptoms have you experienced in the last week?', 'How would you describe your pain?'). Open questions allow a fuller response, enabling people to reply in their own manner. Sometimes, open questions precipitate a long and not necessarily relevant response, and a closed question can refocus the conversation. Thus, both closed and open questions are valuable when interviewing.
- **Probing questions** (e.g. 'You say that the pain is worse in the mornings. Tell me when else it is particularly bad?'). Probes or prompts can assist people to talk about their thoughts and feelings and express their concerns.
- **Leading questions** (e.g. 'You don't look as if you are in pain. Are you?'). Leading questions are best avoided as they can pressure people to respond in a particular way. However, nurses are often unaware of using them.
- **Affective questions.** Affective questions specifically address people's emotions and indicate concern. For example, if Natalie is quiet and uncommunicative, she could be asked how she feels about being in hospital. We need to have established a good rapport before asking this kind of question and should ensure that we can give time for responses. We should also know our own limitations in terms of helping responses.

Learning outcome 4: Explain key features of gaining informed consent

Nurses must ensure that they gain consent before any care or treatment is given (NMC 2008). The ESC for 'Care, compassion and communication' (8) states that nurses need to gain consent based on sound understanding and informed choice prior to any intervention (NMC 2010). Seeking consent is a common courtesy, but patients also have a legal and ethical right to determine what happens to them within healthcare settings, so consent, as stated above, is needed before any action is taken with patients – for example, administering an injection or helping with personal hygiene. Informed consent is an ongoing agreement by a person to receive treatment, undergo procedures or participate in research, after risks, benefits and alternatives have been adequately explained to them. The RCN (2011) advised that for informed consent to be valid, the patient must:

- be competent to make the particular decision;
- have received sufficient information to make the decision;
- not be acting under duress.

For example, if Mrs Davies were to be asked to consent to having an x-ray of her right hip, informed consent would include ensuring that she understands what an x-ray will show, why she needs it, what would happen when she goes for this x-ray, and the implications of not having the x-ray.

People have different information needs, and these needs should be discussed as early as possible. Some patients would choose to have the minimum amount of information and prefer others to make choices. Other patients will want to be involved throughout any decision-making process. Assessing and meeting individual information needs minimise undue anxiety and distress.

Acts of Parliament, the Mental Capacity Act (MCA) (Great Britain 2005) and the Mental Health Act (Great Britain 2007) have strengthened protection for those who lack the mental capacity to consent to the care or treatment they need. The MCA 2005 Code of Practice (Department of Constitutional Affairs [DCA] 2007) provides a detailed guide to practical implementation of the MCA, including methods of communication, and it is recommended further reading. One of the statutory principles of the MCA is that it is important to take all practical and appropriate steps to enable people to make decisions for themselves before deciding that an individual lacks capacity to make a particular decision (DCA 2007). A person's capacity (or lack of capacity) refers specifically to their capacity to make a particular decision at the time it needs to be made, and individual circumstances and needs must be taken into account. For example, someone with a learning disability, such as Maria, may need a different approach, to a person with dementia, such as Mrs Davies.

The DCA's Code of Practice (2007, pp. 29–30) suggests the following good practice in relation to helping someone to make a decision for themselves:

Providing relevant information
- Does the person have all the relevant information they need to make a particular decision?
- If they have a choice, have they been given information on all the alternatives?

Communicating in an appropriate way
- Could the information be explained or presented in a way that is easier for the person to understand (e.g. by using simple language or visual aids)?
- Have different methods of communication been explored if required, including non-verbal communication?
- Could anyone else help with communication (e.g. a family member, support worker, interpreter, speech and language therapist or advocate)?

Making the person feel at ease
- Are there particular times of day when the person's understanding is better?
- Are there particular locations where they may feel more at ease?
- Could the decision be put off to see whether the person can make the decision at a later time when circumstances are right for them?

Supporting the person
- Can anyone else help or support the person to make choices or express a view?

Care home staff should apply the above-mentioned suggestions in the care of Mrs Davies, enabling her to make her own decisions wherever possible; for example, use of pictures may help her to make choices and Mr Davies may be able to help her to express her views. If decisions are made on her behalf, they must be in her best interests and the least restrictive interventions should be used (Great Britain 2005).

These interventions would need to be discussed within the multidisciplinary team and involve her husband too.

Children: practice points for consent

Children and young people are able to consent for procedures or treatments if they are deemed competent; thus, have a cognitive understanding for the rationale, what is involved, outcome, etc. Informed consent must be achieved with the healthcare professional. Consent is usually undertaken in partnership with parents/carers, and if the child is under 18 years of age, the parent/carer who has parental responsibility may give consent.

For further information regarding consent in children, see

Great Britain (GB) and Department of Health (DH). 2009. *Reference Guide to Consent for Examination and Treatment*, 2nd edn. Available from: http://www.dh.gov.uk/en/Publicationsandstatistics/Publications/PublicationsPolicyAndGuidance/DH_103643

Learning outcome 5: Reflect on the features of appropriate professional behaviour

The code (NMC 2008) assumes that nurses are in positions of trust, and to justify this trust, they must act with integrity to uphold the profession's reputation. The code further highlights two areas of particular concern:

- *The receipt of gifts/money.* This aspect specifically relates to anything that could be considered an attempt to receive preferential treatment or care.
- *The need to establish and maintain clear sexual boundaries with clients, their families and carers.* Thus, any over-familiarity or intimacy is absolutely inappropriate and cannot be sanctioned under any circumstances.

Other relevant aspects to maintaining appropriate professional boundaries within therapeutic relationships include avoidance of

- being over-friendly;
- inappropriate self-disclosure;
- doing too much for a client at the expense of others;
- taking advantage of a client for one's own needs or gain;
- taking too much interest in the client beyond the confines of the supportive relationship.

Most clients and patients are vulnerable to some extent, including those with short episodes of illness and temporary dependence or individuals with severe and ongoing physical, emotional or cognitive impairments. For example, suppose you are the only person Natalie seems to communicate with; therefore, when she asks for your personal mobile number you may be tempted to give her this number. However, this would be an inappropriate response that compromises the professional relationship, potentially making her more dependent in the relationship.

Summary
- Establishing initial rapport is an important stage in developing trusting nurse–patient/client relationships.
- Clear explanations are essential to ensure understanding.
- There are different types of question that should be used appropriately for effective interactions.
- Informed consent must be gained. Where patients or clients lack the mental capacity for consent, care must be conducted in their best interests.
- It is vital to behave in an appropriate professional manner at all times, in accordance with the NMC's (2008) code.

COMMUNICATION IN CHALLENGING SITUATIONS

LEARNING OUTCOMES

By the end of this section, you will be able to:
1 appreciate how anxiety is experienced and managed;
2 discuss how depression is recognised and managed;
3 reflect on how to recognise and manage anger;
4 appreciate ways of communicating with people who are confused;
5 discuss how to communicate with people who are receiving unwelcome news;
6 consider communication in relation to sensitive issues, such as sexuality.

The code (NMC 2008) states that the nurse must 'provide a high standard of care at all times' (p. 1). This standard would include showing sensitivity and compassion at all times, even in difficult and challenging situations.

Learning outcome 1: Appreciate how anxiety is experienced and managed

Anxiety is one of our basic emotions and can range from mild to very severe, serving as a warning and helping us to cope with threatening situations. However, if anxiety is excessive and left untreated, it may be detrimental and interfere with a person's normal day-to-day life and interactions. Excessive anxiety can cause suffering and disability and can be costly at both an individual and societal level. Someone who has unresolved anxiety may have difficulty sustaining relationships, maintaining employment or both. This anxiety could lead to a loss of confidence, loss of role, loss of job/earnings and in the extreme perhaps loss of housing. The National Institute for Health and Clinical Excellence (NICE 2011a) asserts that anxiety disorders are common across all care settings.

If you think about the scenarios, Maria may be anxious because she may not understand what is happening or she may be a naturally anxious person. She may be lonely and have more time to worry about what is happening to her.

- What are the cues that may lead you to think a person is anxious?
- What aspects of Bill's situation may give rise to anxiety?

In answer to the first question, you might have considered facial expression, restlessness, wringing hands and profuse sweating, indicators that an individual is anxious due to a feeling of impending doom. The resulting fear, which can be intense, may also cause some or all of the following: dryness of the mouth, racing heart, butterflies in the stomach, shortness of breath, having to go to the toilet repeatedly, irregular heart beats (palpitations), cognitive impairment including poor concentration, impatience, irritability, painful or missed periods and difficulty in falling or staying asleep (see NHS Choices, http://www.nhs.uk/Conditions/Anxiety/Pages/Symptoms.aspx).

Anxiety about illness and implications for the future are often linked to fearfulness, uncertainty or both. Bill could have fears for the future and uncertainty about his situation, causing anxiety; for example, how he will cope in a hospital setting as opposed to the home environment. He may also be anxious about whether he will continue to be given his pain medication when he needs it, as he may no longer perceive himself to be in control of when he is able to take this medication.

Other factors that may cause healthcare recipients anxiety include:
- awaiting a life-threatening or life-changing diagnosis;
- fear of an operative procedure;
- fear about treatments;
- fear about the short- and long-term effects of treatments;
- fear of the unknown environment, leading to feelings of vulnerability and insecurity;
- fear of being treated in an uncaring manner.

Any or all of the above-mentioned factors may be relevant to individuals, so we should make no assumptions about what may be causing their anxiety. Careful assessment, including observation and information gathering, and the development of trusting relationships can enable nurses to accurately identify causes of anxiety.

Anxiety management techniques include:
- explanation of the process of anxiety and the symptoms experienced;
- breathing control;
- relaxation therapy;

- challenging of cognition (thoughts);
- assertiveness training.

Nichols (2003) suggests that effective communication and information-giving skills can reduce anxiety, fear and uncertainty, enabling clients to work in partnership and follow treatment in a more relaxed manner, while positively contributing to recovery. NICE (2011a) provides a detailed evidence-based approach to anxiety disorders.

Children: practice points – dealing with distress

Much can be done to prepare children for procedures or investigations and help them to cope through, for example, distraction and play. However, sometimes children may become distressed about procedures or investigations that are necessary, and then nurses should work with the child and family and try to calm and de-escalate these situations. Brenner and Noctor (2010) explore communication in situations where children may resist procedures, and they suggest four key questions when assessing the situation:

1. What am I feeling now? The nurse's feelings could affect communication and exacerbate the situation.

2. What does this child feel, want or need – try to understand the motivation behind the child's behaviour.

3. How is this environment affecting this child – could the environment be modified? Hospitalisation is always stressful for children.

4. How can I best respond? Respond to the child's distress in a timely and helpful way.

For further information, see

Brenner, M. and Noctor, C. 2010. Clinical holding of children and young people. In: Glasper, A., Aylott, M. and Battrick, C. (eds.) *Developing Practical Skills for Nursing Children and Young People*. London: Hodder Arnold, 18–25.

Macqueen, S., Bruce, E.A. and Gibson, F. 2012. Moving and handling, therapeutic holding & restraint. In: *The Great Ormond Street Hospital Manual of Children's Nursing Practices*. Chichester: Wiley-Blackwell, 412–5.

For guidance on therapeutic holding of children, for example, for procedures, and legal and ethical aspects, see

Royal College of Nursing (RCN). 2010. *Restrictive Physical Intervention and Therapeutic Holding for Children and Young People: Guidance for Nursing Staff*. London: RCN.

Mental health problems, including depression and anxiety, are common in young people; see

Noctor, C. 2010. Managing children and young people with mental health problems. In: Glasper, A., Aylott, M. and Battrick, C. (eds.) *Developing Practical Skills for Nursing Children and Young People*. London: Hodder Arnold, 518–30.

Learning outcome 2: Discuss how depression is recognised and managed

Depression is a common mental disorder characterised by sadness, loss of interest in activities and decreased energy. It is differentiated from normal mood changes by the extent of its severity, the symptoms and the duration of the disorder. It is estimated that 350 million people worldwide experience depression (WHO 2012). Depression is estimated to be two to three times more common in people with a chronic physical health issue, such as heart disease, diabetes or neurological disorder, occurring in about 20% of these people (NICE 2011b). A depressed mood is common when a patient has a life-threatening illness and is often a stage of adjustment to their illness, and it is estimated that 50% of people who are terminally ill can suffer from some degree of depression (Davis 2007). The impact of this depression may be that having both physical and mental health problems can delay recovery from both (NICE 2009a). In fact, depression increases the risk of mortality by 50% and, for example, doubles the risk of coronary heart disease in adults (NICE 2009a).

Depression is difficult to diagnose and can be unrecognised in acute hospital care settings; therefore, it is important to differentiate between someone who is sad, perhaps due to receiving unwelcome news about their prognosis, and someone who is in need of clinical support for depression. NICE (2009a,b) guidelines for managing depression detail the assessment of depression and recommend a stepped care approach. Nurses need to be able to assess patients accurately to recognise these differences and to ensure appropriate referral for those in need of specialist support (NICE 2009b). Nurses have an important role in identifying depression, and their communication skills can help the effective assessment and screening of vulnerable people. Assessment can highlight those at risk – for example, those who have a past history of brain pathology, those who have not maintained good relationships with healthcare professionals in the past, or clients who have poor social support. It is recognised that many patients with functional illness are at high risk of developing depression (NICE 2009a).

Depression has various physical and psychological symptoms, but they may not be identified in the clinical setting for various reasons, including the knowledge and attitudes of healthcare staff or resource and time issues. People may also not complain of depression, or depression may manifest itself in other symptoms – for example, pain that is difficult to control. Nurses are best placed in recognising the physical and psychological changes that may indicate a client is in need of support.

ACTIVITY

What might indicate to you that a person is depressed? List features that you are aware of. Then, read about symptoms of depression on Mind's website at http://www.mind.org.uk/mental_health_a-z/7980_understanding_depression?gclid=CJuO-7DY97QCFYLHtAodj3oA_A.
Have you seen any assessment tools used in practice to help assess depression?

As detailed on Mind's website, there are many signs and symptoms of depression. People who are depressed may also be anxious, and it is not always clear whether the anxiety leads to the depression or whether depression causes the anxiety. Various assessment tools are used in healthcare settings to assess depression and anxiety – for example, the Hospital Anxiety and Depression Scale (Zigmund and Snaith 1983) and the Beck's Depression Inventory (Beck et al. 1961) – so you may have seen these assessments or similar tools.

NICE (2009a) advises that treatment and care should:

- take into account patient's needs;
- take into account patient's preferences;
- provide the opportunity to make informed decisions;
- include the opportunity to make advance decisions and statements;
- be culturally appropriate;
- be accessible to people with additional needs, such as physical, sensory or learning disabilities;
- be accessible to people who do not speak or read English;
- be supported by evidence-based written information tailored to the patient's needs.

The healthcare team should be fully aware of all the above principles, and good communication skills will be essential throughout the patient's care experience. It is important to recognise 'normal' responses to adverse events/life-threatening illnesses, as opposed to responses which indicate a person needs further psychological assessment and support.

Learning outcome 3: Reflect on how to recognise and manage anger

Anger is a natural response to feeling attacked, injured or violated. It is part of being human; it is energy that is seeking expression (Mind 2012). Nurses are sometimes confronted with people who are displaying strong emotions, such as anger and aggression. It is important to use good interpersonal skills at these times to minimise the psychological impact of the emotions. People who are in hospital can become angry for many reasons, and this anger is often related to a loss of control over their circumstances and may be a reaction to the uncertainty around their situation. Anger from both patients and their relatives is also associated with a lack of effective therapeutic communication. It is important to recognise when a patient is becoming angry and to be able to manage this anger is an effective way.

ACTIVITY

Think back to the last time you were with anyone who was angry. How did you recognise that the person was becoming angry? What can you remember about how you felt and your responses?

Examples that you might remember may include both verbal and non-verbal aspects related to anger. Verbal indications include a raised voice, tense tone, fast speech or using obscenities. Non-verbal indications include changes in body language: the person may display exaggerated movements, clenched fists, pace back and forth or throw or kick objects. There may be changes in facial expression, for example, frowning, and eye contact may be negligible or it might be extended – glaring. These expressions are just some indications that an individual is becoming angry. In terms of your own reaction, did you feel angry, did you feel that you were able to remain calm? Did the way you responded influence the situation positively or negatively?

A nurse who has recognised these signs should act to disperse the anger by the following means:

- Maintaining a calm, respectful demeanour (McCorry and Mason 2011).
- Listening actively to what the person has to say, thus showing a non-judgemental stance. However, eye contact that is held for too long may be seen as threatening (Crawford et al. 2006).
- Maintaining adequate space.
- Keeping an open posture (McCorry and Mason 2011).
- Acknowledging the anger, thereby demonstrating empathy with what the person is feeling (Crawford et al. 2006).
- Encouraging the person to identify the cause of the anger, through use of skilful questioning.
- Where possible, empowering the person to resolve any causes.

The ESC 'Care, compassion and communication' states that nurses need to be able to manage and diffuse situations effectively and to be able to recognise and respond to verbal and non-verbal cues (NMC 2010).

The aim in any situation where a patient may become aggressive is a peaceful resolution. Meeting anger with anger – through direct confrontation, defensiveness or questioning of the person's feelings – may lead to an escalation in anger and maybe to aggression, even violence. Appropriate communication skills and good self-awareness can minimise and de-escalate potential points of conflict.

Learning outcome 4: Appreciate ways of communicating with people who are confused

Acute *confusion* is defined as having a rapid onset and 'is a condition characterised by changeable levels of consciousness [...] with an impaired ability to think and concentrate' (Trenoweth et al. 2011, p. 56). Dementia is 'a serious reduction in cognitive ability that is greater than the normal ageing process' (Trenoweth et al. 2011, p. 182). Dementia involves a progressive, irreversible decline in mental function. There are estimated to be 800,000 people with dementia in the UK in 2012, two-thirds are women, and there are 670,000 carers of people with dementia (Alzheimer's Society 2012).

ACTIVITY   Make a list of the characteristics of someone with dementia.

You may have thought about the following:

- Impairment in memory.
- Difficulty with understanding.
- Difficulty undertaking certain tasks.
- Poor judgement and difficulty reasoning.

A person with dementia can become confused, as a result of cognitive impairment, and it can gradually affect the person's ability to communicate. This confusion can result in patients being excluded from being involved in their care, which can be upsetting and frustrating for the patient and their loved ones.

Confusion is often a relatively permanent feature in the later stages of dementia; however, for someone like Mrs Davies who is in the earlier stage of dementia, confusion may be unpredictable, transient and intermittent. However, the nurse must avoid making assumptions about her confusion as it may be due to other factors, such as the physical factors of malnutrition, dehydration, constipation or an acute infection. She may also be disorientated because she is in an unfamiliar environment, and this disorientation would be compounded if she had a visual or hearing impairment.

Sometimes, despite all attempts to help a patient, their confusion makes it difficult to make needs known and for nurses to identify appropriate interventions. In these situations, the patient's safety and best interests are paramount, as previously discussed, with reference to the Mental Capacity Act (Great Britain 2005). The code (NMC 2008) highlights the nurse's responsibility to ensure that 'people who lack capacity remain at the centre of decision-making and are fully safeguarded' (p. 4). It is important in these situations to remember to continue to provide person-centred care that promotes respect and dignity in line with benchmarks for best practice (DH 2010a) and the standards for preregistration nursing education (NMC 2010).

ACTIVITY

Mrs Davies is looking for her husband, who has just said goodbye and told her he is going home, and she is becoming more agitated. Suggest strategies you could use to help her.

Strategies to consider include:

- orientation to time and place;
- use of appropriate and understandable language;
- a calm, clear voice;
- a calm manner, for example, avoiding sudden or exaggerated movements;
- use of active listening skills.

The Alzheimer's Society (2011) has produced some top tips in relation to communication with someone who has dementia, and these tips include the best way to approach someone with dementia and the importance of minimising distractions. They also give tips about how vital an awareness of non-verbal behaviour is, such as tone of voice, eye contact and body contact. People with dementia often have difficulty processing questions and information; therefore, attention needs to be given to the speed of delivery; careful listening; and not being patronising, arguing and contradicting.

Whether the patient has an acute confusional state or has dementia, as in the case of Mrs Davies, nurses are in a unique position to ensure accurate assessment and to ensure that patients are treated with respect, dignity and compassion at all times. The ESC for 'Care, compassion and communication' requires nurses to act with dignity and respect at all times and to act autonomously to challenge situations or others when someone's dignity may be compromised (NMC 2010).

Learning outcome 5: Discuss how to communicate with people who are receiving unwelcome news

Breaking unwelcome or bad news is often medical staff's role, but increasingly specialist nurses and other healthcare professionals are involved. Nurses should understand how to facilitate the situation to minimise distress for patients and relatives. It is often at times of intimate contact (e.g. bed-bathing) that patients ask searching questions. Bad news can be defined as any news that adversely and seriously affect how an individual views their future (Buckman 2005).

Giving bad news is often cited as the most difficult part of the healthcare professional's role and can engender feelings of guilt, distress and fear for one's own mortality. Healthcare staff may sometimes avoid telling the whole truth either because they fear the reactions of patients and relatives or they fear acknowledging their own feelings. Although it can be distressing for patients and relatives to receive bad news, it is rarely acceptable to withhold the truth from them. Society holds the belief that truth is a fundamental and valued principle and is essential for establishing effective relationships. Furthermore, patients need correct information for making informed choices in decision-making (Ryan and McQuillan 2006). Current government strategy has recognised the importance of patients participating in decisions about their care and treatment, and the phrase 'no decision about me without me' sums up this person-centred approach (DH 2010b).

Patients generally want to be told the truth, and the code (NMC 2008) states that nurses must be open and honest. Arguments relating to deception in healthcare stress the importance of respecting patient autonomy. This respect involves acknowledging aspects such as individual preference and establishing an environment of trust that enables clients to feel accepted, respected and involved in their care (Collis 2006).

Price (2004) emphasises the importance of conducting interviews in a sensitive and structured way to elicit information about clients' beliefs, attitudes and values. A supportive environment helps patients to disclose their concerns, enabling nurses to adapt information according to individuals' emotional needs.

Buckman's (2005) SPIKES strategy centres on addressing and recognising the emotional aspects of the patient experience.
- **Setting** – ensuring privacy, adequate time, set up of room, removing the chance of interruptions, listening mode.
- **Perception** – how the person views the seriousness of their situation and the language and vocabulary they use to describe it.

- **Invitation** – finding out how much the patient would like to know about their situation.
- **Knowledge** – giving a warning that you are going to give bad news, using similar language to the patient, avoiding technical jargon.
- **Empathy** – listening for and identifying emotions and their source and acknowledging these emotions and sources.
- **Strategy and summary** – checking understanding, summarising and allowing time for questions and clarification.

Although SPIKES is directed primarily towards medical staff, it provides valuable insight for nurses dealing with patients at this sensitive time.

ACTIVITY

Think of a situation where a patient has been given bad news. Write down some of the factors you would need to have considered had you been the one breaking the bad news.

You may have considered the following:
- **Setting** – Where would you give the bad news? Was there somewhere private?
- **Perception** – How serious did you think the patient thought their condition was?
- **Invitation** – Was the patient asked about what they wanted to know? How would you do this?
- **Knowledge** – Did you think about the words and language you might use and how you might ascertain the patient's current understanding?
- **Empathy** – What emotions might you expect and how do you think you would respond?
- **Strategy and summary** – How did you check the patient's understanding and did you consider making arrangements for future meetings?

Buckman (2005) suggests that if breaking bad news is perceived to have been handled insensitively, it can have adverse long-term consequences for the patient and family in adjusting to the illness. Therefore, nurses have a role to play in ensuring that breaking difficult news is handled sensitively and that sufficient time is given to the process including any follow-up.

Pregnancy and birth: practice points – pregnancy loss and stillbirth

Nursing staff may be directly involved with pregnant or recently delivered women in a variety of healthcare settings. In gynaecology or surgical wards, women may experience spontaneous abortion (miscarriage), termination of pregnancy (TOP) for foetal anomaly or evacuation of retained products of conception after delivery. Intensive care unit (ITU) staff may provide care for critically ill women after obstetric emergencies or severe illness/accident and on rare occasions, deal with a maternal death. Community nurses may work alongside practice nurses, performing blood tests or baby immunisations.

Whatever the context of care, the approach must be compassionate, considerate and respectful.

Read the following and consider how it makes you feel:

> *It should have been the happiest day*
> *To remember all our life*
> *But joy has turned to heartache*
> *No breath, no beat, no life (Anon)*

For further suggested reading to support women and families through pregnancy loss or stillbirth, see

Pregnancy Loss and the Death of a Baby: Guidelines for Professionals, available from the Child Bereavement Charity at www.childbereavement.org.uk/

Other useful websites:

www.winstonswish.org.uk (Winston's Wish-charity for bereaved children)

www.miscarriageassociation.org.uk (Miscarriage Association)

www.fsid.org.uk (Foundation for Sudden Infant Death) (Foundation for Sudden Infant Death)

www.uk-sands.org.uk (support for bereaved parents) (Support for bereaved parents)

Learning outcome 6: Consider communication in relation to sensitive issues, such as sexuality

There are various sensitive issues that nurses may need to discuss with patients and clients; sexuality is one such area. Sexuality plays an important part in the development of self-concept and who we are as human beings. The way individuals perceive themselves sexually affects self-image, body image and self-esteem (Volman and Landeen 2007). Indeed, the nurse's own sexuality may have an impact on their assessment of situations and behaviour. It is important that nurses are aware of the various ways individuals may identify in relation to their sexuality, for example, heterosexual, gay, lesbian, transgender or bisexual. Explorations of how illness affects an individual's sexuality is often neglected due to nurses' own inhibitions about discussing intimate issues and other institutional and client-related factors (Magnan et al. 2006).

Gregory (2000) outlines the difference between sexuality (concepts of identity) and sexual functioning (bodily function). Major illness such as cancer, stroke and arthritis can affect sexuality either because of the effects of the illness itself or due to hospitalisation, treatments or medication.

ACTIVITY   Reflect upon situations where clients' sexuality needed to be considered.

Did you think of the following examples?
- How the client identifies in relation to their sexuality.
- After a mastectomy or other surgery that alters body image.
- Where appearance has been altered due to medication (e.g. chemotherapy may cause a loss of hair and steroid therapy may cause weight gain).

- Effects of long-term medication use (e.g. some medications used for hypertension and mental illnesses can cause impotence/sexual dysfunction).
- People with long-term urinary catheters.
- People who are paralysed or have had a stroke.
- Patients who have had genital or reproductive surgery.

Assessment can help to discover the physical, psychological and relational aspects of an individual's sexual needs, but a sensitive and skilled approach is vital. Gregory (2000) outlines the importance of a structured approach, suggesting that the benefits of including sexuality in patient assessment include:

- helping patients to understand their situation/condition and possible effects on their sexual functioning;
- helping to relieve fear and anxiety;
- helping towards an understanding of treatment options.

Gregory (2000) suggests that managing sexual problems is primarily about giving information and allowing patients to respond to options in care and treatment. Davis (2006) highlights research that suggests that patients often do not voice concerns about their sexuality as they prefer nurses to raise the subject. However, Krebbs and Marrs (2006) suggest that the nurses' own beliefs may hinder their exploration and communication with clients about sexuality. Nurses might be unsure about when to raise the topic and be concerned that patients themselves might feel uncomfortable. Price (2010) also highlights the fact that nurses often have difficulty with discussions about sexuality and sexual relationships with patients but emphasises that it is important to be able to have sensitive discussions. He suggests that open dialogue will help the patient to make sense of how the illness or treatment may impact on their sexuality and intimate relationships. However, it is important that nurses are able to discuss sensitive issues; as we have seen, illness often affects sexuality.

Summary
- This section highlighted and raised awareness of communication with people who are angry, depressed and confused or who have sensitive issues to address.
- Breaking bad news is one of the most difficult aspects of a healthcare professional's role and demands sensitive, compassionate care.
- Excellent interpersonal communication skills are particularly needed in challenging situations.
- Key aspects of communication in challenging situations are as follows:
  - Be prepared to listen and hear what clients are saying.
  - Give clients permission to raise their concerns.
  - Ask questions sensitively.
  - Give timely information.
  - Respond and refer appropriately.

CHAPTER SUMMARY

Understanding influences such as self-awareness, personality, attitudes and stereotyping are important aspects in the provision of sensitive, compassionate communication – and therefore of care. Communication takes many forms and has verbal and non-verbal components. Nurses need to use a range of interpersonal skills effectively. In relation to practical nursing skills, initiating interactions, listening, non-verbal communication, questioning and giving explanations are all of particular importance. There are many situations where communication is challenging and requires nurses to be skilled and empathetic.

In conclusion, this chapter aimed to provide insight into the importance of nurse–patient relationships. It included a discussion about the impact of self within this relationship, and how it affects communication and thus the care of people. The scenarios highlighted how communication principles are applied in a variety of care settings with different patients and within multidisciplinary teams. This chapter has emphasised the vital role that communication plays throughout the patients' care experiences. The following chapters focus on specific practical nursing skills and demonstrate the importance of effective communication for all nurses, in all care settings at all times.

ANSWER TO ABBREVIATIONS (activity Section 2)

CF: Cystic fibrosis
CPA: Care Programme Approach
PID: Pelvic inflammatory disease or prolapsed intervertebral disc
TPR: Temperature, pulse and respiration
BP: Blood pressure or bedpan
OE: On examination
RXT: Radiotherapy
ETA: Estimated time of arrival
TTA: To take away
DNA: Did not attend or deoxyribonucleic acid
DOA: Dead on arrival or date of admission
GCS: Glasgow Coma Scale

REFERENCES

Allen, S. and Crouch, A. 2007. Cultural and spiritual health assessment. In: Crouch., A. and Meurier, C. (eds.) *Vital Notes for Nurses: Health Assessment*. Oxford: Blackwell, 311–30.

Alzheimer's Society. 2011. Top tips for nurses. London: Alzheimer's Society. Available from: http://www.alzheimers.org.uk/site/scripts/documents_info.php?documentID = 1211 (Accessed on 20 January 2013).

Alzheimer's Society. 2012. Statistics. Available from: http://www.alzheimers.org.uk/site/scripts/documents_info.php?documentID = 341 (Accessed on 20 January 2013).

Arnold, E. and Bloggs, K. 2011. *Interpersonal Relationships: Professional Communication Skills for Nurses*, 6th edn. London: Saunders.

Beck, A.T., Ward, C.H., Mendelssohn, M.J. and Erbaugh, J. 1961. An inventory for measuring depression. *Archives of General Psychiatry* 4: 561–71.

British Deaf Association. 2008. *About British Sign Language (BSL)*. London: BDA. Available from: http://bda.org.uk/British_Sign_Language-i-14.html (Accessed on 20 January 2013).

Buckman, R.A. 2005. Breaking bad news: The S-P-I-K-E-S strategy. *Community Oncology* 2:138–42.

Cabinet Office Social Exclusion Task Force. 2007. *Prioritising the Most Disadvantaged Adults*. Available from: http://webarchive.nationalarchives.gov.uk/+/http://www.cabinetoffice.gov.uk/social_exclusion_task_force/psa.aspx (Accessed on 20 January 2013).

Collis, S.P. 2006. The importance of truth-telling in health care. *Nursing Standard* 20(17): 41–5.

Crawford, P., Brown, B. and Bonham, P. 2006. *Communication in Clinical Settings*. Cheltenham: Nelson Thornes.

Davis, C. 2007. Depression and cancer. *Cancer Nursing Practice* 6(9): 10–11.

Davis, T.B. 2006. Using the extended PLISSIT model to address sexual healthcare needs. *Nursing Standard* 21(11): 35–40.

Dein, S. 2006. *Culture and Cancer Care: Anthropological Insights in Oncology*. Maidenhead: Open University Press.

Department for Constitutional Affairs (DCA). 2007. *Mental Capacity Act 2005 Code of Practice*. Norwich, UK: The Stationery Office. Available from: http://www.justice.gov.uk/downloads/protectingthe-vulnerable/mca/mca-code-practice-0509.pdf (Accessed on 20 January 2013).

Department of Health (DH). 2009. *Valuing People Now: A Three Year Strategy for Learning Disability*. London: DH.

Department of Health (DH). 2010a. *Essence of Care 2010*. London: DH.

Department of Health (DH). 2010b. *Equity and Excellence Liberating the NHS*. London: DH.

Department of Health (DH). 2011. *No Health without Mental Health: A Cross-Government Mental Health Outcomes Strategy for People of All Ages*. London: DH.

Department of Health (DH). 2012a. *Transforming Care: A National Response to Winterbourne View Hospital: Department of Health Review Final Report*. London: DH.

Department of Health (DH). 2012b. *Compassion in Practice: Nursing, Midwifery and Care Staff: Our Vision and Strategy*. London: DH.

Eckroth-Bucher, M. 2001. The philosophical basis and practice of self-awareness in psychiatric nursing. *Journal of Psychosocial Nursing and Mental Health Services* 39(2): 32–9.

Egan, G. 2010. *The Skilled Helper: A Problem-Management and Opportunity-Development Approach to Helping*, 9th edn. California: Brooks/Cole.

Eysenck, H.J. 1965. *Fact and Fiction in Psychology*. Harmondsworth: Penguin Books.

Fuller, J. 2003. Effective cross-cultural communication. In: Kai, J. (ed.) *Ethnicity, Health and Primary Care: A Practical Guide*. Oxford: Oxford University Press.

Gibbons, P. 2008. Ethical dimensions of care. In: Hinchliff, S., Norman, S. and Schoeber, J. (eds.) *Nursing Practice and Health Care*, 5th edn. London: Hodder Arnold, 175–200.

Great Britain. 2005. *Mental Capacity Act*. Available from: http://www.legislation.gov.uk. (Accessed on 7 February 2013).

Great Britain. 2007. *Mental Health Act*. Available from: http://www.legislation.gov.uk. (Accessed on 7 February 2013).

Gregory, P. 2000. Patient assessment and care planning: Sexuality. *Nursing Standard* 15(9): 38–41.

Gross, R. and Kinnison, N. 2013. *Psychology for Nurses and Health Professionals.* 2nd edn. Boca Raton, FL: CRC Press.

Hargie, O., Saunders, C. and Dickson, D. 1994. *Social Skills in Interpersonal Communication*, 3rd edn. London: Routledge.

Higgins, I., Van Der Riet, P., Slater, L., et al. 2007. The negative attitudes of nurses towards older patients in the acute hospital setting: a qualitative descriptive study. *Contemporary Nurse* 26(2): 225–37.

Jack, K. and Smith, A. 2007. Promoting self-awareness in nurses to improve nursing practice. *Nursing Standard* 21(32): 47–52.

Johnson, M. and Webb, C. 1995. Rediscovering unpopular patients: Concept of social judgement. *Journal of Advanced Nursing* 21: 466–75.

Krebbs, L. and Marrs, J.A. 2006. What should I say? Talking with patients about sexuality issues. *Clinical Journal of Oncology Nursing* 10(3): 313–15.

Luft, J. and Ingram, H. 1955. *The Johari Window: A Graphic Model of Interpersonal Relations.* Los Angeles, CA: University of Los Angeles Press.

Magnan, M.A., Reynolds, K.E. and Galvin, E.A. 2006. Barriers to addressing patient sexuality in nursing practice. *Dermatology Nursing* 18(5): 448–54.

McCormack, B. and McCance, T. 2010. *Person-Centred Nursing Theory and Practice.* Oxford: Wiley-Blackwell.

McCorry, L.K. and Mason, J. 2011. *Communication Skills for the Healthcare Professional.* Baltimore, MD: Lippincott.

Mid Staffordshire NHS Foundation Trust Inquiry. 2010. *Independent Inquiry into Care Provided by Mid Staffordshire NHS Foundation Trust.* January 2005–March 2009, Volume I & 2. Available from: http://www.official-documents.gov.uk/document/hc0910/hc03/0375/0375_ii.pdf (Accessed on 20 January 2013).

Mid Staffordshire NHS Foundation Trust Public Inquiry. 2013. *Report of the Mid Staffordshire NHS Foundation Trust Public Inquiry.* Available from: http://www.midstaffspublicinquiry.com/report (Accessed on 12 February 2013).

Minardi, H.A. and Riley, M.J. 1997. *Communication in Health Care: A Skills Based Approach.* Oxford: Butterworth Heinemann.

Mind. 2012. *How to Deal with Anger.* Available from: http://www.mind.org.uk/assets/0002/1357/How_to_deal_with_anger_2012.pdf (Accessed on 20 January 2013).

Morrison, P. and Burnard, P. 1997. *Caring and Communicating: The Interpersonal Relationship in Nursing,* 2nd edn. Basingstoke: Macmillan.

National CAMHS Support Services. 2010. *Tackling Stigma: A Practical Toolkit.* London: National CAMHS Support Services.

National Institute for Health and Clinical Excellence (NICE). 2009a. *Depression with a Chronic Physical Health Problem.* Clinical Guidelines 91. Available from: http://www.nice.org.uk (Accessed on 15 February 2013).

National Institute for Health and Clinical Excellence (NICE). 2009b. *Depression. The Treatment and Management of Depression in Adults.* Clinical Guidelines 90. Available from: http://www.nice.org.uk (Accessed on 15 February 2013).

National Institute for Health and Clinical Excellence (NICE). 2011a. *Generalised Anxiety Disorder and Panic Disorder (with or without Agoraphobia) in Adults. Management in Primary, Secondary and Community Care.* Clinical Guideline 113. London: NICE.

National Institute for Health and Clinical Excellence (NICE). 2011b. *Depression in Adults Quality Standard.* London: NICE.

Nichols, K. 2003. *Psychological Care for Ill and Injured People: A Clinical Guide.* Maidenhead: Open University Press.

Nichols, K. 2005. Why is psychology still failing the average patient? *The Psychologist* 18(1): 26–7.

Nursing and Midwifery Council (NMC). 2008. *The Code: Standards of Conduct, Performance and Ethics for Nurses and Midwives.* London: NMC.

Nursing and Midwifery Council (NMC). 2009. *Record Keeping: Guidance for Nurses and Midwives.* London: NMC.

Nursing and Midwifery Council (NMC). 2010. *Standards for Pre-Registration Nursing Education.* London: NMC.

Pearce, R. 2011. Clarifying your own personal values and beliefs. In: Trenoweth, S., Docherty T., Franks, J. and Pearce, R. (eds.) *Nursing and Mental Health Care: An Introduction for All Fields of Practice.* Exeter: Learning Matters Ltd.

Pettigrew, T. and Meertens, R. 1995. Subtle and blatant prejudice in Western Europe. *European Journal of Social Psychology* 25: 55–75.

Pope, T. 2012. How person centred care can improve nurses' attitudes to hospitalised older patients. *Nursing Older People* 24(1): 32–6.

Porritt, L. 1984. *Communication: Choices for Nurses.* London: Churchill Livingston.

Price, B. 1990. *Body Image: Nursing Concepts and Care.* London: Prentice-Hall.

Price, B. 2004. Conducting sensitive patient interviews. *Nursing Standard* 18(38): 45–52.

Price, B. 2010. Sexuality: Raising the issue with patients. *Cancer Nursing Practice* 9, 5: 29–35.

Rajecki, D.W. (1982) *Attitudes: Themes and Advances.* Sunderland Mass: Sinauer Associates.

Razali, S.M., Kahn, U.A. and Hasanah, C.I. 1996. Belief in super-natural causes of mental health illness among Malay patients: Impact on treatment. *Acta Psychiatrica Scandanavica* 94(4): 229–33.

Redfern-Jones, J. 2006. Sending the right message. *Nursing Standard* 20(41): 72.

Rogers, C.R. 1961. *On Becoming a Person.* Boston, MA: Houghton Mifflin.

Royal College of Nursing (RCN). 2012. *Informed Consent in Health and Social Care Research: RCN Guidance for Nurses,* 2nd edn. London: RCN.

Royal College of Nursing (RCN). 2012. *Using Telephone Advice for Patients with Long-Term Conditions: An RCN Guide to Using Technology to Complement Nursing Practice.* London: RCN.

Rungapadiachy, D.M. 2008. *Self-Awareness in Health Care Engaging in Helping Relationships.* Hampshire: Palgrave Macmillan.

Ryan, K. and McQuillan, R. 2006. Ethical decision-making. In: Read, S. (ed.) *Palliative Care for People with Learning Disabilities.* London: MA Healthcare Ltd, 75–91.

Schaffer, H.R. 2004. *Introducing Child Psychology.* Oxford: Blackwell.

Stein-Parbury, J. 2009. *Patient and Person: Interpersonal Skills in Nursing,* 4th edn. London: Churchill Livingstone.

Stockwell, F. 1972. *The Unpopular Patient.* London: Royal College of Nursing.

Thompson, N. 2002. *People Skills,* 2nd edn. Hampshire: Palgrave Macmillan.

Trenoweth, S., Docherty, T., Franks, J. and Pearce, R. 2011. *Nursing and Mental Health Care; An Introduction for All Fields of Nursing.* Exeter: Learning Matters Ltd.

Volman, L. and Landeen, J. 2007. Uncovering the sexual self in people with schizophrenia. *Journal of Psychiatric and Mental Health Nursing* 14: 411–7.

Vydelingum, V. 2000. South Asian patients' lived experience of acute care in an English hospital. *Journal of Advanced Nursing* 32: 100–7.

Walker, J., Payne, S., Smith, P., Jarrett, N. and Ley, T. 2012. *Psychology for Nurses and the Caring Professions,* 4th edn. Maidenhead: Open University Press.

Wiseman, T. 2007. Toward a holistic conceptualization of empathy for nursing practice. *Advances in Nursing Science* 30(3): E61–72.

World Health Organization (WHO). 2012. Depression. Available from: http://www.who.int/mediacentre/factsheets/fs369/en/index.html (Accessed on 7 February 2013).

Zigmund, A.S. and Snaith, R.P. 1983. The hospital anxiety and depression scale. *Acta Psychiatrica Scandinavica* 67(6): 361–70.

3 Infection Prevention and Control

Patricia Folan and Lesley Baillie

Prevention and management of infection are the responsibilities of all staff working in health and social care and are applicable across all settings in which care is delivered (Royal College of Nursing [RCN] 2012a). However, within hospital and residential situations, where many nurses work, the risk of cross-infection is high. In any healthcare setting, unless adequate care is taken, healthcare workers, including nurses, can unwittingly transmit microorganisms from one person to another. Healthcare-associated infection (HCAI), previously referred to as hospital-acquired infection or nosocomial infection, is defined as 'Infection acquired as a result of the delivery of healthcare either in an acute (hospital) or non-acute setting' (Pratt et al. 2007, S62). It is estimated that 300,000 patients a year in England acquire a healthcare-associated infection as a result of care within the National Health Service (NHS) (National Institute for Health and Clinical Excellence [NICE] 2012).

The Nursing and Midwifery Council (NMC 2010) specified Essential Skills Clusters for 'Infection prevention and control' for student nurses, all of which are incorporated in this chapter.

This chapter includes the following topics:

- Principles for preventing healthcare-associated infection: an introduction
- Hand hygiene
- Use of personal protective equipment, including gloves, aprons and gowns
- Healthcare waste disposal and linen management
- Sharps disposal
- Healthcare environmental hygiene and multiuse equipment
- Aseptic technique
- Specimen collection: key principles
- MRSA screening and suppression procedures
- Isolation procedures (source and protective)

Recommended biology reading:

These questions will help you to focus on the biology underpinning the skills required to prevent cross-infection. Use your recommended textbook to find out the following:

- What are microorganisms? Where are they found? Are all microorganisms harmful?
- Identify some of the beneficial roles of microorganisms.
- How do microorganisms enter the body?
- How are microorganisms classified?
- What are the structure and properties of bacteria, viruses, prions, fungi, yeasts and protozoa?
- How do bacteria grow and multiply?
- What factors influence the proliferation of microorganisms?
- What is meant by the terms 'commensal', 'pathogen' and 'normal flora'?
- Distinguish between endogenous and exogenous sources of infection.
- What mechanisms does the body use to defend itself from infection? Think about non-specific defences, for example, secretions, reflexes and barriers as well as specific mechanisms. Review the structure of the skin.
- How does the body fight infections?
- What are the clinical signs of infection? What role does histamine play?
- Which cells are involved in the specific immune response? Where are they found?
- What is the difference between humoral and cell-mediated immunity?
- What are antibodies? How do they help protect us from infection?
- How do we achieve an immunological memory?
- What factors can affect an individual's immune system?

Rheumatoid arthritis

An inflammatory disease often affecting a number of joints (initially smaller joints), causing pain, swelling, stiffness and deformity. It is often accompanied by systemic ill health.

Type 2 diabetes

Type 2 diabetes develops when the body makes insufficient insulin, or when the insulin that is produced does not work effectively (known as insulin resistance). See www. diabetes. org.uk.

Infection

The successful invasion, establishment and growth of microorganisms within the tissues of the host.

Meticillin-resistant *Staphylococcus aureus* (MRSA)

A strain of *Staphylococcus aureus* that is resistant to meticillin* and other penicillin and cephalosporin antibiotics (Health Protection Agency 2012a, p. 77). *Also referred to as 'methicillin'

PRACTICE SCENARIOS

As discussed above, preventing and controlling infection is part of the nurse's role in all practice settings. The following scenarios are referred to throughout the text when discussing the practical skills covered in this chapter.

Adult

Mrs Winifred Lewis, aged 87 years, was widowed many years ago and lives in wardened accommodation. She has a history of **rheumatoid arthritis** and **type 2 diabetes**, and she recently fell and fractured her hip, which was operated on in the hospital. However, an **infection** caused by **meticillin-resistant *Staphylococcus aureus* (MRSA)** developed in the wound. She was discharged home, under the care of the district nursing team and intermediate care, but her wound deteriorated and the surrounding skin showed signs of infection. Mrs Lewis appeared unwell and dehydrated, and she had a raised body temperature, so her general practitioner (GP) requested readmission. She is now being isolated in the sideroom of a surgical ward, and an intravenous infusion and intravenous antibiotics have been commenced.

Bacteraemia

An infection in the blood caused by bacteria.

Health Action Plan

A personal action plan developed for each individual with a learning disability, which details the actions needed to maintain and improve the person's health and any help needed to accomplish these; see *Action for Health – Health Action Plans and Health Facilitation* (Department of Health 2002).

Colonise

The establishment of pathogenic microorganisms at a specific body site with little or no host response. This can lead to a large number of microorganisms, forming a reservoir for infection and cross-infection.

She has a commode in the room and can transfer with help. Blood cultures, taken on admission, showed an MRSA bacteraemia.

Learning disability

James Smith is a 59-year-old man with a learning disability who lives alone in a farm cottage and works on the adjacent farm. After an accident, James has an open wound on his lower left leg that shows signs of infection. There is a large amount of exudate, which has an offensive odour. The district nurse has been visiting the farm to carry out dressings, and a wound swab has been taken. James is keen to carry on with his usual work on the farm. The district nurse is liaising with the community nurse for learning disabilities to help to teach James how to care for his leg in between dressings. This information is now included in James's Health Action Plan. As the district nurse runs a clinic at the local GP's surgery, James is being encouraged to attend this clinic for dressings instead of receiving visits at his home.

Mental health

Stacey is 28 years old and has been addicted to opiates for 6 years. She is living with her parents, who are very supportive. Recently, Stacey began a community-based detoxification programme with support from her local drug and alcohol team. During detoxification, Stacey experienced severe withdrawal symptoms, including very high blood pressure and vomiting. As a result, she was admitted as an emergency to the acute mental health admission unit. She arrived feeling very unwell, and soon after arrival she vomited over her bed. She was prescribed intramuscular metoclopramide (an antiemetic) to stop her vomiting. Stacey is known to have hepatitis B.

PRINCIPLES FOR PREVENTING HCAI: AN INTRODUCTION

Many microorganisms exist but not all cause infection in individuals. Microorganisms that cause disease are called **pathogens**. When pathogens are acquired from another person, or from the environment, they are described as **exogenous**. The transmission of pathogens, between people and across environments, is termed **cross-infection**. When microorganisms colonise one site on the host and enter another site on the same person causing further infection, this is called self-infection or **endogenous** infection.

In the fourth national prevalence survey (Health Protection Agency [HPA] 2012a), the prevalence of HCAI in England was 6.4%, compared with 8.2% in 2006. The six most common types of HCAI, accounting for more than 80% of all HCAIs, were respiratory tract infections (pneumonia and other respiratory infections, 22.8%); urinary tract infections (UTIs, 17.2%); surgical site infections (SSIs, 15.7%); clinical sepsis (10.5%); gastrointestinal infections (8.8%); and bloodstream infections (BSIs, 7.3%). In the paediatric population, the most common HCAIs were clinical sepsis (40.2%), respiratory tract infections (15.9%) and BSIs (15.1%). Enterobacteriaceae were the most frequently reported organisms associated with HCAIs.

On completion of this section, you will be able to:
1 discuss key policies and guidance influencing infection control practices;
2 outline the composition and role of infection prevention and control teams;
3 explain the chain of infection, including the routes by which microorganisms are spread.

Learning outcome 1: Discuss key policies and guidance influencing infection control practices

Concern about HCAIs in the United Kingdom (UK) has led to many government publications and other guidance documents, providing recommendations for infection prevention and control. Here are some examples:

- *The Health and Social Care Act 2008: Code of Practice for Health and Adult Social Care on the Prevention and Control of Infections and Related Guidance* (Department of Health [DH] 2009). The Code of Practice and related guidance aim to help health and adult social care providers to plan and implement how they prevent and control infections and specifies the criteria for compliance with Care Quality Commission (CQC) standards.

- National Evidence-Based Guidelines for Preventing Healthcare-Associated Infections in NHS England (Pratt et al. 2007). In these DH-commissioned evidence-based infection control guidelines (referred to as EPIC2), the authors recommended that standard infection control precautions should be applied by all healthcare practitioners to the care of all patients. This is a requirement of the *Health and Social Care Act 2008: Code of Practice* (DH 2009), which states that registered providers must audit compliance to key policies and procedures for infection prevention. The third edition of the national evidence-based guidelines (EPIC3) is currently at final consultation stage so do access this latest version.

- *Prevention and Control of Healthcare-Associated Infections in Primary and Community Care* (NICE 2012). These guidelines (updated from the 2003 version) apply the standard precautions of hand decontamination, use of personal protective equipment and sharps disposal to community-based care and include guidance for preventing infections associated with long-term urinary catheters and vascular access devices.

- *Wipe It Out – One Chance to Get It Right: Essential Practice for Infection Prevention and Control: Guidance for Nursing Staff* (Royal College of Nursing [RCN] 2012a). This guidance document, aimed at nursing staff, highlights essential elements of good infection prevention and control practice.

New guidance to address specific infection concerns continues to be released. For example, in 2012, the DH published technical guidance aimed at those healthcare organisations providing patient care in augmented care units, such as paediatric and adult critical care, neonatal and burns units, providing advice for healthcare providers on management of *Pseudomonas aeruginosa* in water systems.

The other UK countries' administrations also provide guidance and policy on infection control: for Scotland, see Health Protection Scotland (HPS) at

Antimicrobial stewardship

Prudent prescribing of antibiotics and antimicrobial stewardship is a requirement of the 2008 Health and Social Care Act. The DH (2011a) guidance on antimicrobial stewardship outlines evidence-based criteria for antibiotic prescribing and the decision options for secondary care.

www.hps.scot.nhs.uk); for Wales, see Health in Wales (www.wales.nhs.uk) and the Welsh Healthcare Associated Infection Programme; and for Northern Ireland see the Department of Health, Social Services and Public Safety (www.dhsspsni.gov.uk).

Standard infection prevention and control precautions relevant to all areas of practice are

- healthcare environmental hygiene;
- hand hygiene;
- the use of personal protective equipment;
- isolation of patients;
- the use and disposal of healthcare waste and sharps;
- **antimicrobial stewardship**.

In this chapter, you focus on the skills that are associated with standard precautions that are based on the principle that all blood, body fluids, secretions, excretions except sweat, non-intact skin and mucous membranes may contain transmissible infectious agents. Standard precautions include infection prevention practices that apply to all patients, regardless of suspected or confirmed infection status, in any setting in which healthcare is delivered.

Learning outcome 2: Outline the composition and role of infection prevention and control teams

As you read above, there are many national infection prevention and control policies. These policies are implemented, and compliance is monitored at the local level by an **infection prevention and control team (IPCT).**

ACTIVITY

When next in the practice setting, find out who the members of the local IPCT are and where they are located. Also, find out where your local infection prevention and control policy is kept and familiarise yourself with its content.

The IPCT generally comprises an infection prevention and control nurse (IPCN) and an infection prevention and control doctor. Their roles include planning, implementing and monitoring the infection prevention and control programme. They are available to offer advice on all matters relating to infection control. They also provide education to healthcare personnel and develop local policy. An infection control committee from a variety of hospital departments provides advice and support for the IPCT.

Many community healthcare providers also employ IPCNs who work closely with their local healthcare providers and the consultant for communicable disease control. The consultant is responsible for monitoring and controlling the spread of infection in the community, as well as other environmental hazards (Wilson 2006). Trusts work proactively in multiagency collaborations with other local health and social care providers to reduce risk from infection (NICE 2012). Many healthcare settings also use infection control link nurses (or champions) to improve awareness of infection control in clinical areas. They receive basic training and help provide education, training, audit and surveillance in clinical areas. There should also be close liaison between the occupational health department and the IPCT to ensure the health and safety of patients and staff alike (Wilson 2006).

Learning outcome 3: Explain the chain of infection, including the routes by which microorganisms are spread

The chain of infection can help you to understand how to prevent spread of infection (Figure 3.1). Prevention of cross-infection is about breaking the chain of infection. Each link in the chain is discussed below.

Infectious agent

An infectious agent is a microorganism with the ability to cause disease and includes bacteria (most common in hospitals), viruses (more common in the community) and fungi (e.g. *Candida*, which causes thrush). To identify the specific infectious agent, specimens are collected and sent to the laboratory for microscopy, culture and

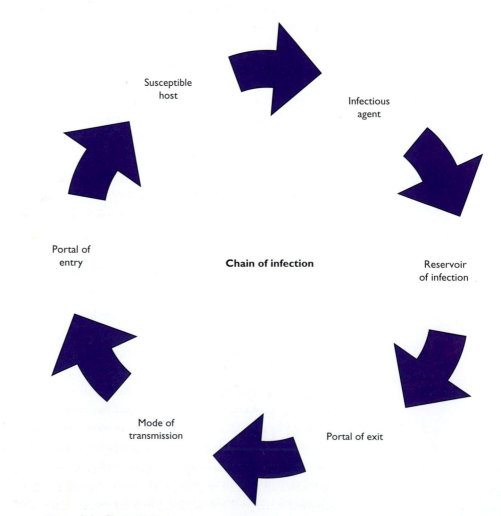

Figure 3.1: Chain of infection.

sensitivity (M, C & S). For example, if a UTI is suspected, a specimen of urine will be sent to the laboratory. A later section in this chapter focuses on the collection of a specimen. More advanced testing available in some laboratories includes molecular tests such as **polymerase chain reaction** (PCR). PCR is a biochemical technology to identify the DNA of an organism. Generally, the turnaround time is quicker for a result from a specimen sent in this way.

Two microorganisms that have caused particular concern in healthcare settings and are regularly covered in the media are MRSA and *Clostridium difficile*.

MRSA

Mrs Lewis is an example of a person who has an infection caused by MRSA, a strain of *Staphylococcus aureus (S. aureus)* that has become resistant to the antibiotic meticillin – hence the name 'meticillin-resistant *Staphylococcus aureus*'. Strains of MRSA are usually resistant to all penicillins and all cephalosporins. They may also be resistant to other first-line antibiotics. *S. aureus* commonly colonises normal skin, particularly warmer parts such as the axillae, groins, perineum and nose. Healthy people do not usually develop an infection, although they can become colonised (Wilson 2006). Serious staphylococcal infection usually occurs in people who are vulnerable because of underlying illness or medical interventions. Mrs Lewis, as a frail older person with diabetes and rheumatoid arthritis, fits into this vulnerable category.

MRSA can cause a range of superficial infections of the skin as well as hospital-acquired wound infections, as with Mrs Lewis. In the fourth national prevalence survey, less than 0.1% of the survey population had an HCAI caused by MRSA (HPA 2012a). However, in a survey of surgical site infections, *S. aureus* was the second most frequent causative microorganism, comprising 23% of the total *S. aureus* infections and 6% overall (HPA 2011). *S. aureus* can also cause boils and abscesses and serious systemic infections, such as septicaemica and pneumonia (Wilson 2006). Unfortunately, the few drugs currently available that have reliable activity against MRSA are very expensive and difficult to administer. They necessitate blood levels being monitored since they are highly toxic.

MRSA is most likely to be spread on the hands of staff as transient organisms. If staff have certain skin conditions, such as eczema or dermatitis, or have cuts on their skin, they are at increased risk of harbouring the organism and can spread it to other staff and patients. The organism can also be carried on skin scales from an infected patient or member of staff and may contaminate uniforms or clothing, especially if the clothing is damp.

Clostridium difficile

In 2009, the HPA and DH published *Clostridium difficile Infection: How to Deal with the Problem* following on from the DH's (2007) *Saving Lives: High Impact Intervention No. 7 – Care Bundle to Reduce the Risk from Clostridium difficile*. *C. difficile* produces two main toxins (A and B) that cause diarrhoea and colitis (DH and HPA 2009), and infection has led to clusters of patient deaths, which you may remember being reported in the media. *C. difficile* produces spores which are transmissible and survive for long periods in the environment (DH and HPA 2009). The normal gut flora have an important role in controlling *C. difficile*, but they are disturbed by antibiotics (DH and HPA 2009). In the fourth national prevalence survey, 0.4% of the survey population had an HCAI caused by *C. difficile* (HPA 2012a). Patients most at risk are older people and those who have recently taken antibiotics (DH and HPA 2009), so Mrs Lewis fits into this category and could be at risk.

Reservoir of infection

A reservoir of infection is a place within which microorganisms grow and reproduce and can include people (e.g. healthcare workers, patients), the environment, equipment and water. Mrs Lewis's and James's wounds provide reservoirs for infection.

Portal of exit

A portal of exit provides a way for microorganisms to leave the reservoir and includes excretions (e.g. faeces from the bowel) or droplets (via the mouth or nose by sneezing or coughing). If Stacey cut herself, the cut would provide a means for the hepatitis B microorganism to leave her body via her blood.

Mode of transmission

Microorganisms can spread through many routes.

ACTIVITY

Read Table 3.1, which presents the routes by which pathogenic microorganisms can be transmitted or spread between people. Then reread the practice scenarios. Can you work out which transmission route would feature mostly strongly for these patients?

It is likely that direct or indirect contact via hands of carers is the principal cause of spread. For Mrs Lewis, infection can be spread via the airborne route, but direct and indirect contact transmission is likely. Stacey has hepatitis B and this virus is transmitted via blood and serum-derived fluids such as vaginal secretions, so direct and indirect contact with these fluids is a major source of transmission. Without care, hands could spread infection from James's leg wound, especially since there is a large amount of exudate.

Although all routes of transmission are important, this short activity points out that the most common route of spread is via hands. Healthcare workers are a major route through which patients become infected and hence the importance of high levels of compliance with hand hygiene protocols (World Health Organization [WHO] 2009). Attention to hand hygiene has the potential to break the chain of infection and is discussed in detail later in this chapter

Portal of entry

The portal of entry is the opening allowing microorganisms to enter the body.

Table 3.1: Routes of transmission

Route	Explanation	Examples
Direct or indirect contact	Transfer from body surface to body surface directly between an infected or colonised person and a susceptible host, or indirectly via an intermediate object	Direct: Patient to patient (e.g. through touch) or staff to patient when carrying out patient care activities such as moving and handling Indirect: Patient touched by a nurse's unwashed hands or gloves that have not been changed after contact with a patient who is infected/colonised
Inanimate objects and equipment (fomites)	Susceptible host infected by an object that is contaminated with microorganisms	Beds, curtains, toys, bedpans, tables, keyboards can all be contaminated and spread infection, sometimes via hands of staff acting as transmitters
Droplet	Microorganisms transmitted through the air within droplets, mainly saliva	Coughing, sneezing, talking and singing can transmit, as well as during procedures (e.g. bronchoscopy or suctioning)
Airborne	Microorganisms carried in droplet nuclei (small particle residue) or by dust particles consisting of dead skin scales, clothing fibres, etc.	Carried by air currents in the environment and breathed in by a susceptible host, or settle on horizontal surfaces Some bacteria form spores and survive for months in such conditions
Ingestion	Ingested into the body with food or water, causing gastrointestinal infections and excreted in faeces Known as the faecal–oral route	Food may be contaminated when hands that have been in contact with faeces transfer the organisms to food
Vector	Transmission via insects or rodents	Cockroaches, rats, mice and ants cause contamination of food; mosquitoes spread malaria and yellow fever; ticks spread Lyme disease and typhus

Source: Adapted from Parker, L.J. 1999. Current recommendations for isolation practices in nursing. *British Journal of Nursing* 8: 881–7.

Identify Mrs Lewis's portals of entry.

Mrs Lewis's wound (already infected) is one portal of entry, but her intravenous site is another portal of entry. Although we have many defences to prevent microorganisms entering the body, patients/clients often have increased routes for entry because of invasive procedures (e.g. urinary catheters, vascular access devices, chest drains) and wounds. The HPA (2012a) identified that 64% of patients with a BSI had a vascular access device (peripheral or central) in the 48 hours before the onset of infection and 43% of patients with UTIs had had a urinary catheter present within 7 days before the infection onset.

Susceptible host

Most patients/clients are vulnerable to infection because of their immunity, age, underlying disease and medical interventions.

ACTIVITY Discuss with a colleague the people in the scenarios and the factors that make them susceptible to infection.

Individuals vary widely in their ability to resist infection. People are especially vulnerable to infection if they have underlying disease. Mrs Lewis's long-term conditions of rheumatoid arthritis and diabetes and Stacey's hepatitis B render them more susceptible. Mrs Lewis's impaired defence mechanisms could have led to her infection being more severe than in healthy people. Serious diseases, such as cancer, and associated treatments (e.g. powerful drugs including steroids and chemotherapy), affect the immune system too. Local factors, such as a poor blood supply to a wound, increase the likelihood of infection developing, and people who have diabetes, like Mrs Lewis, can have impaired circulation. Age (especially very young or very old people) and previous exposure to infection and vaccinations, all affect levels of risk (Wilson 2006). Mrs Lewis, as an older adult, is more vulnerable to infection.

The presence of a wound, as in the cases of Mrs Lewis and James, increases susceptibility to infection as the skin, which is an important bodily defence, is breached. Other reasons for susceptibility to infection include poor nutrition, which could apply to any of the people in the scenarios. You should look out for underlying susceptibilities when you are in clinical practice.

Children: practice points – infection prevention and control

Infection control precautions and control procedures are standard to all fields of nursing. For further information specifically to the care of children, see

Macqueen, S., Bruce, E.A. and Gibson, F. 2012. Infection prevention and control. In: *The Great Ormond Street Hospital Manual of Children's Nursing Practices*. Chichester: Wiley-Blackwell, 240–66.

Practice points: Pregnancy and birth – infection risks

Infection in pregnancy carries a risk to the mother, but even more to her foetus or newborn infant, who are especially vulnerable to infection, probably because of the immaturity of the immune system and other defence mechanisms. Viruses pose the greatest risk (e.g. abnormality, abortion, premature delivery), but bacterial infections, especially in the neonatal period, can be life-threatening and require prompt diagnosis and treatment. Some infections are bloodborne and cross the placental barrier; others can ascend via the vagina causing risk to the foetus or premature delivery. Any pregnant woman with gastrointestinal infection, rash, severe throat infection or offensive vaginal discharge requires isolation and immediate obstetric assessment.

For further reading, see

http://www.rcog.org.uk/womens-health/clinical-guidance/prevention-early-onset-neonatal-group-b-streptococcal-disease-green-

http://www.screening.nhs.uk/groupbstreptococcus

Summary

- HCAI is a major concern to governments. Infection prevention and control policies are regularly produced for implementation at local level by IPCTs.
- It is important to keep up to date with policy developments and to be familiar with local policy.
- An understanding of the chain of infection can assist in understanding the rationale behind infection prevention and control measures.

HAND HYGIENE

Adequate hand hygiene is the single most important practice in reducing the spread of infection during care delivery (HPS 2013). Pratt et al. (2007) identified standard principles for hand hygiene, and these principles are referred to throughout this chapter, with application to practice and this chapter's scenarios.

The term 'hand decontamination', used throughout these principles, is defined as 'the use of handrub or handwashing to reduce the number of bacteria on the hands' (NICE 2012, p. 13). Handwashing is the key skill used for hand hygiene. Hand decontamination can also be achieved, in some circumstances, by using an alcohol-based handrub containing isopropyl alcohol (70%).

LEARNING OUTCOMES

By the end of this section you, will be able to:

1 explain the purpose and importance of hand decontamination for the care and safety of both patients and nurses;
2 assess when hand decontamination is needed;
3 carry out hand hygiene effectively;
4 reflect on the factors that influence effective handwashing practice.

Learning outcome 1: Explain the purpose and importance of hand decontamination for the care and safety of both patients and nurses

Hungarian obstetrician Ignaz Semmelweis (1815–1865) succeeded in reducing the death rate of his patients from around 1 in 8 to 1 in 79 by persuading his colleagues and medical students to wash their hands in a solution of chlorinated lime before every patient contact (WHO 2009). Since then, it has become widely recognised that the hands of those employed in healthcare settings are an important route for the transmission of infection (Pratt et al. 2007). People requiring healthcare are often more vulnerable to infection for a variety of reasons, meaning that infection control measures, such as hand hygiene, are central to their care.

Microorganisms are important in an ecological balance on earth; some live in humans and other animals and are needed to maintain health. However, as some microorganisms cause disease, how individuals interact with the environment is important. James's work environment may not have been conducive to keeping his wound free from infection, especially if it was not adequately covered. As you will read in Chapter 7, 'Principles of Wound Care', traumatic wounds are nearly always contaminated, so infection poses a high risk in these situations.

Like everyone in the general population, James requires a basic knowledge of hygiene and infection control, including handwashing to reduce his susceptibility to infection. Now that he has an infected wound, the community nurse for learning disabilities should check that he has the cognitive ability and physical dexterity to care for his wound in between dressing changes and to carry out handwashing. The nurse could demonstrate effective handwashing to James and ensure he can carry this handwashing out. She could provide photos of the different stages in handwashing as an aide-memoire. Handwashing can help to reduce the risk of infection being transferred to other sites in his body or prevent reinfection. James's Health Action Plan should include this information and the other care associated with his leg, documenting the role of the different professionals involved in his care.

For some people with learning disabilities, a structured behavioural programme may be necessary to teach effective handwashing. Behavioural approaches are skilled interventions which use reinforcement, prompting and redirecting to help a person to learn new behaviour. The nurse would assess the individual's comprehension level and adapt the programme for the individual. Sometimes, a backward chaining technique is used, which involves teaching the final stage of the skill first, and then working consecutively backwards. Encouragement and reinforcement by nurses are very important.

Bacteria on hands

In a series of classic studies, Price (1938) discovered two populations of bacteria present on hands: resident organisms and transient organisms. Resident microorganisms, sometimes called normal flora, lie deep in the stratum corneum of the skin and are difficult to remove; therefore, they are less likely to be implicated in cross-infection. Transient microorganisms are acquired from the environment and are carried temporarily on the hands. These organisms may be transferred between nurse and patients or residents, resulting in cross-infection as the nurse moves from one person to another, or handles different sites on the same person. The aim of hand hygiene is to remove transient bacteria to below the level likely to cause infection.

Consider how you might pick up transient microorganisms on your hands during everyday nursing practice.

Some examples are

1. after the care of a person who has been incontinent;
2. when emptying urine bags and bedpans;
3. when handling the bed-linen of a person who has an infection or has been incontinent;
4. when bed-bathing and handling wash bowls;
5. when touching fomites, such as computer keyboards, patients' notes, lockers or beds;
6. during bed-making;
7. when taking a person's pulse or temperature.

Laboratory-based studies using finger impressions indicated that significant contamination can follow activities 1–4 and less so 5–7 (Ayliffe et al. 2001). However, you can pick up microorganisms in any of these ways that involve direct or indirect contact with patients/clients. Wilson et al. (2006) found that more than a third of keyboards tested in their study were contaminated with MRSA, regardless of the position of the keyboard. Hand hygiene rarely accompanied keyboard contact. Transferring bacteria from your hands to a patient can lead to them acquiring colonisation or infection. Effective hand hygiene can reduce the incidence of HCAIs in all settings.

Learning outcome 2: Assess when hand decontamination is needed

The standard principle you should adhere to is that you should decontaminate your hands immediately 'before each and every episode of direct patient contact/care and after any activity or contact that potentially results in hands becoming contaminated' (Pratt et al. 2007, S3). Pathogens are likely to be acquired on the hands in greatest numbers when handling moist, heavily contaminated substances, such as body fluids. Hand decontamination must be carried out at this time. The WHO (2009) proposes that healthcare workers remember the 'five moments of hand hygiene' (Sax et al. 2007) (Figure 3.2) and apply these moments in their practice. Storr and Kilpatrick (2012) explain how the five moments have been applied in community settings.

Consider the WHO's five moments of hand hygiene (Figure 3.2) in relation to the practice scenarios. Identify when nurses would decontaminate their hands.

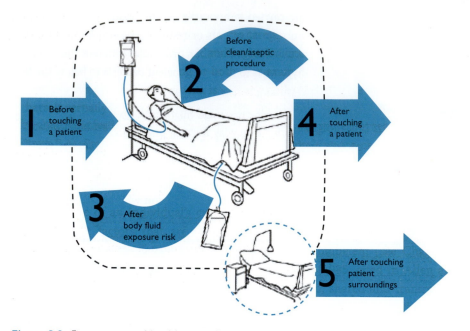

Figure 3.2: Five moments of hand hygiene. (Reprinted from Sax, H., Allegranzi, B., Uçkay, I., Larson, E., Boyce, J. and Pittet, D. 2007. My five moments for hand hygiene: A user-centred design approach to understand, train, monitor and report hand hygiene. *Journal of Hospital Infection* 67(1):9–21. With permission from Elsevier.)

Examples you could have thought of include the following:

Mrs Lewis: before and after assisting with her personal hygiene and assisting her on and off the commode, after dealing with her commode and after making her bed, before and after conducting her wound dressing.

James: before and after conducting his wound dressing.

Stacey: after dealing with her vomit and changing her bed, before giving her intramuscular injection.

Although the nurses caring for Stacey know that she has hepatitis B, in many other situations this information is not known. Therefore, following the principles of hand decontamination and the other principles, such as correct use of personal protective equipment and disposal of sharps, for each and every patient, will protect you and other patients from the unwitting transmission of dangerous pathogens such as hepatitis B. Public Health England (2013) also recommends that all appropriate healthcare staff should be up to date with immunisations for hepatitis B, tuberculosis (TB), measles, mumps and rubella, influenza and chickenpox.

Learning outcome 3: Carry out hand hygiene effectively

Most people learn about washing their hands at an early stage in their lives as part of personal health and hygiene. However, because of the susceptibility of people in healthcare settings, professionals must take particular care to decontaminate hands carefully and thoroughly. The DH (2010a) provides detailed guidance about all aspects of healthcare staff's uniform and workwear, relating to infection control and public appearance, and includes guidance relevant to hand hygiene.

Hand-cleaning preparations

Pratt et al. (2007) reviewed hand-cleaning preparations. They concluded that, generally, washing hands effectively with soap and water removes transient microorganisms and renders hands socially clean, which is sufficient for most care activities. They found that soap containing an antiseptic reduces transient and resident microorganisms and that some antiseptics have a residual effect, which is useful when carrying out surgery or other invasive procedures. Alcohol-based handrub, too, reduces both transient and resident flora, but it should not be used when hands are visibly soiled or contaminated with blood or body fluids, and it is not effective against *C. difficile*. Note, too, that norovirus is not fully susceptible to alcohol handrub (Norovirus Working Party 2012). Alcohol handrubs are advantageous in situations where handwashing facilities are absent or poor, such as in some community settings. They also reduce the need to leave patients during procedures, such as wound dressings, to carry out handwashing.

Effective handwashing technique involves three processes: preparation, washing and rinsing, and drying. The recommendations by Pratt et al. for these processes are summarised in Box 3.1. These processes are now discussed in more detail.

Box 3.1 Steps for an effective handwashing technique

At the start of each shift, remove all wrist and hand jewellery and cover all cuts/abrasions with waterproof dressings.

Preparation
- Wet hands under running water before applying liquid soap or an antimicrobial preparation.

Washing
- The handwash solution must come into contact with all the surfaces of the hands.
- The hands must be rubbed together vigorously for a minimum of 10–15 seconds.
- Particular attention must be paid to the tips of the fingers, the thumbs and the areas between the fingers.

Drying
- Hands should be rinsed thoroughly before patting dry with good-quality paper towels.

Source: Pratt, R.J., Pellowe, C., Wilson, J.A., et al. 2007. National evidence-based guidelines for preventing healthcare-associated infections in NHS, England. *Journal of Hospital Infection* 65S: S1–64.

Preparation for handwashing

ACTIVITY

What do you think you would need to do to prepare for handwashing? Consider both facilities and yourself.

Ensure you have the necessary equipment at the sink area – liquid soap and paper hand-towels. You must have your forearms exposed and should not wear false nails (they can harbour microorganisms), wristwatches, or jewellery such as rings (excluding plain wedding rings, according to local policy) and bracelets (DH 2010a). You must keep nails short, free of nail varnish and clean. Preparation also includes covering cuts and abrasions with a waterproof dressing to prevent the risk of acquiring infections such as hepatitis B and C and human immunodeficiency virus (HIV) and may also prevent infection from bacteria and fungi. Preparation before handwashing requires that you wet your hands under tepid running water before applying liquid soap or an antimicrobial cleaning agent.

Washing and rinsing

ACTIVITY

Find out whether you can access pink-dye handwashing solution. This solution may be available in the skills laboratory or via the IPCN. Wash your hands with this solution in your usual way and then take note of those areas that you have not covered with the dye. Alternatively, you may have access to germ powder and a light-box. Follow the instructions to assess your handwashing technique.

Figure 3.3 shows a diagram of the areas most commonly missed (Ayliffe et al. 2001). How does this diagram compare with your handwashing results?

Pratt et al. (2007) stressed that all surfaces of the hands must be included during handwashing. Figure 3.4 shows an example of a technique that can help you to cover all surfaces of your hands during hand decontamination. You should finish by washing your wrists.

ACTIVITY

Rewash your hands using the principles in Box 3.1 and the technique in Figure 3.4 as a guide. If available, use pink dye or germ powder for this activity, so you can note any improvement: did you manage to cover all areas of your hands this time? Ensure you time your handwashing with a watch and adhere to the recommended minimum of 10–15 seconds.

The amount of time you wash your hands is important, as the mechanical action helps to remove bacteria. As you can see, the guidelines by Pratt et al. suggest you spend a minimum of 10–15 seconds; when timing this action in the last activity, did it feel longer than usual? Hands should be rinsed thoroughly before patting dry with good-quality paper towels (Pratt et al. 2007). When disposing of paper towels, using foot-operated pedal bins reduces the risk of recontaminating hands after washing.

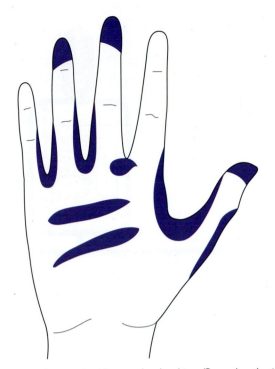

Figure 3.3: Areas commonly missed with poor handwashing. (Reproduced with permission from Ayliffe, G.A. J., Babb, J.R. and Taylor, L.J. 2001. *Hospital-Acquired Infection: Principles and Prevention*, 3rd edn. London: Arnold.)

Use of alcohol-based handrubs

Alcohol-based handrubs are quick to use and effective, although, as mentioned, they can be used only when hands are visibly clean, and they are not effective against *C. difficile* spores or fully effective against norovirus. It is also preferable that hands are washed with soap and water after glove removal (Pratt et al. 2007).

ACTIVITY

Are the principles for performing handwashing and drying that you have read about any different when using an alcohol-based handrub? If so, how?

The principles are similar. The preparatory measures for handwashing discussed also apply to decontamination of hands with alcohol-based handrubs. Pratt et al. (2007) advise that the handrub solution must come into contact with all surfaces of the hands, with the hands rubbed together vigorously, giving particular attention to the tips of the fingers, the thumbs and the areas between the fingers, until the solution has evaporated and the hands are dry. After several consecutive uses of alcohol-based handrub, the hands should be washed with soap and water.

Learning outcome 4: Reflect on the factors that influence effective handwashing practice

There are various barriers to good hand hygiene, which affect compliance. In a large hospital-wide survey, Pittet et al. (1999) identified predictors of non-compliance

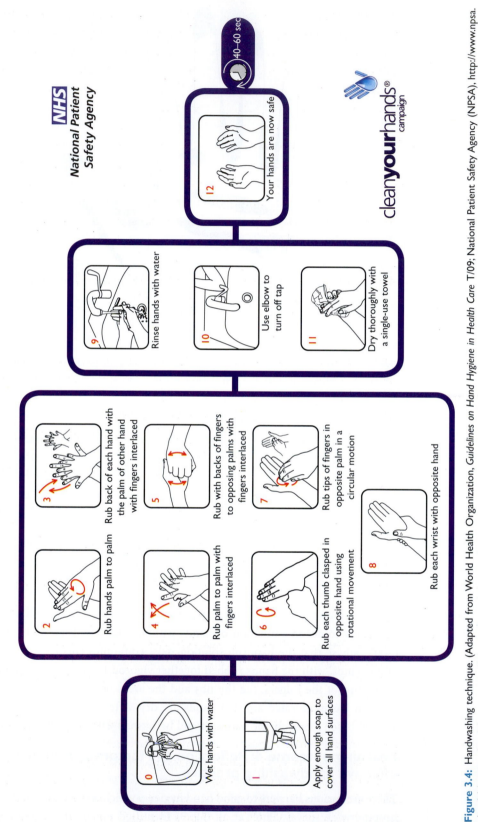

Figure 3.4: Handwashing technique. (Adapted from World Health Organization, *Guidelines on Hand Hygiene in Health Care* T/09; National Patient Safety Agency (NPSA), http://www.npsa.nhs.uk/cleanyourhands/resource-area/nhs-resources/education/training-five-moments/technique-handouts/ Accessed on September 21, 2013.)

0 Wet hands with water

1 Apply enough soap to cover all hand surfaces

2 Rub hands palm to palm

3 Rub back of each hand with the palm of other hand with fingers interlaced

4 Rub palm to palm with fingers interlaced

5 Rub with backs of fingers to opposing palms with fingers interlaced

6 Rub each thumb clasped in opposite hand using rotational movement

7 Rub tips of fingers in opposite palm in a circular motion

8 Rub each wrist with opposite hand

9 Rinse hands with water

10 Use elbow to turn off tap

11 Dry thoroughly with a single-use towel

12 Your hands are now safe

40–60 sec

NHS
National Patient
Safety Agency

cleanyourhands® campaign

with hand hygiene during routine patient care and found average compliance was 48%, being highest among nurses. Non-compliance was higher in intensive therapy units rather than medical wards, during procedures with a high risk for bacterial contamination, and when intensity of patient care was high. The results indicated that organisational factors must be considered and that hand hygiene could improve if focused on certain wards, groups of staff and patient interventions.

Staff champions or role models in hand hygiene improvement are critical to improving compliance. Each member of the staff can exert a very powerful influence on colleagues. Adequate preparation for involving patients in hand hygiene improvement is important. The need for commitment from all levels of the organisation is necessary to support this aspect of improving compliance. The DH (2009) requires that healthcare providers have adequate provision of handwashing facilities and antimicrobial handrubs.

ACTIVITY

What factors can you think of that might influence effective handwashing? In particular, think about when you would need to wash your hands either in the community or in a hospital setting. Referring to the scenarios will help you.

By referring to the scenarios you will probably have identified how frequently nurses need to wash their hands. Frequent handwashing can cause damage to skin, especially if antiseptic solutions are used, or if hands are not dried properly. Cracked skin may harbour more bacteria and increase the risk of cross-infection. Therefore, you should apply an emollient handcream regularly to protect skin from the drying effects of regular hand decontamination; if a particular soap or antimicrobial handwash or alcohol-based product causes skin irritation, then seek occupational health advice (Pratt et al. 2007).

Other reasons that could deter nurses from washing their hands include the following:

- Inadequate and inconveniently placed handwashing facilities; lack of time may deter handwashing when facilities are some distance away. Water may be too hot and no mixer taps present (Dancer 2002). Taps and dispensers should be elbow-operated, and good facilities should exist for dispensing and disposing of paper towels.
- Lack of education concerning the importance of handwashing.
- Lack of emphasis on handwashing by peers and managers.
- The use of gloves has been found to affect compliance with handwashing (Flores and Pevalin 2007; Fuller et al. 2011).

In recent years, there have been campaigns to improve hand hygiene. For Heath Protection Scotland's campaign, see www.washyourhandsofthem.com. The National Patient Safety Agency's (NPSA 2008) 'Cleanyourhands' campaign aimed to 'minimise the risk to patient safety of low compliance with hand hygiene by NHS staff through a national strategy of improvement' (see www.npsa.nhs.uk/cleanyourhands). Results from an evaluation of the Cleanyourhands campaign indicated sustained increases in hospital procurement of alcohol rub and soap, which appeared to be associated with reduced rates of some HCAIs (Stone et al. 2012). It was concluded that national interventions for infection control undertaken in the context of a high-profile political drive can reduce selected HCAIs. The WHO has launched a global hand hygiene campaign 'Save lives, Clean your hands' (see http://www.who.int/gpsc/5may/en/index.html). The WHO (2009) published an extensive evidence-based review of hand hygiene for healthcare workers and recommended a multimodal hand hygiene improvement strategy, comprising system change (access to adequate facilities), education based on the WHO's five moments, evaluation and feedback, workplace reminders and creating an environment of safety.

Summary

- Effective hand hygiene is an essential tool in preventing and controlling infection.
- There are various decontamination agents and techniques, and nurses need to be aware of which are appropriate in different situations. For example, alcohol-based handrubs are an acceptable alternative to handwashing when hands are not visibly soiled.
- Handwashing must be performed thoroughly, paying attention to preparation, washing and rinsing, and drying, and for an adequate length of time.
- Hands must be patted dry carefully with paper towels.
- There are several barriers to effective handwashing, but these barriers must be overcome to prevent cross-infection.
- An infection prevention and control champion in each clinical area can assist in improving compliance.
- Commitment from all levels of the organisation is needed to support aspects of improving compliance with hand hygiene.

USE OF PERSONAL PROTECTIVE EQUIPMENT, INCLUDING GLOVES, APRONS AND GOWNS

Pratt et al. (2007) advise that selection of protective equipment (aprons, gowns, gloves, eye protection and face masks) should be based on an assessment of the following:

> the risk of transmission of microorganisms to the patient or to the carer and the risk of contamination of healthcare practitioners' clothing and skin by patients' blood, body fluid, secretions or excretions.

This section focuses on glove and apron use as they are commonly used for protection. Masks and visors must be worn when there is a risk of blood, body fluids, secretions and excretions splashing into the face and eyes. Respiratory protective equipment (a particulate filtrate mask) must be fitted when caring for patients with some airborne respiratory infections.

Learning outcome 1: Identify the procedures for which gloves, sterile or non-sterile, are recommended and key factors in their use

Pratt et al. (2007, S20) point out that gloves are worn for two main reasons:
• to protect hands from contamination with organic matter and microorganisms;
• to reduce the risks of transmission of microorganisms to both patients and staff.

They go on to advise that gloves should not be worn unnecessarily as prolonged and indiscriminate use can lead to adverse reactions and skin sensitivity. Therefore, risk assessment should be carried out considering who is at risk and whether sterile or non-sterile gloves are needed, the potential for exposure to blood, body fluids, secretions and excretions, and the likelihood of contact with non-intact skin or mucous membranes.

In the next activities, you consider situations where sterile gloves are used, situations where non-sterile gloves are satisfactory, and situations where no gloves are needed.

Situations where sterile gloves are used

ACTIVITY

Referring to each scenario at the beginning of the chapter, write down clinical procedures and situations for which you think sterile gloves should be worn.

For Mrs Lewis and James, an aseptic technique (see later section) using sterile gloves is necessary when redressing their wounds to reduce the risk of cross-infection. For Stacey, sterile gloves are not necessary from the information given in the scenarios.

From the above-mentioned activity, you can conclude that sterile gloves are used most frequently for invasive procedures and for direct contact with non-intact skin. Another example of a procedure where sterile gloves are necessary is urinary catheterisation (for more information, see Chapter 9).

When applying sterile gloves, you must avoid contaminating the outer surface of the glove. Using the inner surface of the folded cuff, push your hand into the glove. If you line up your thumb with the thumb of the glove you will find the glove goes on more easily. The second glove is easier to put on as you can use your other, gloved, hand to help, but it must not touch ungloved areas. Figure 3.5 shows the technique required.

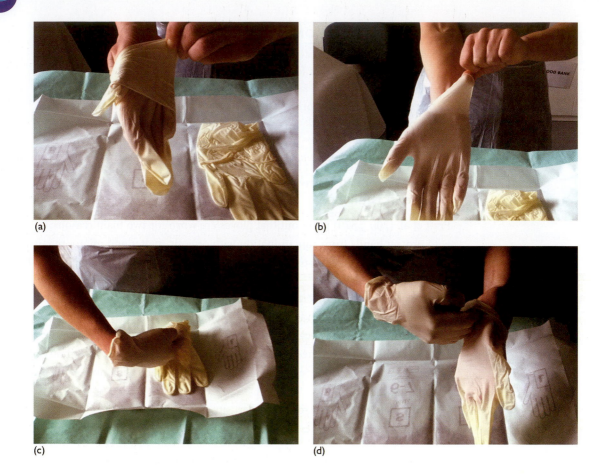

Figure 3.5: Technique for applying sterile gloves. (a) Grasp the inner surface of the folded cuff and push your hand into the glove, lining up your thumb with the thumb of the glove. (b) Pull the first glove on fully but only touch the inside of the glove to do this so the outside remains sterile. (c) Using your gloved hand, pick up the second glove under the cuff. (d) Pull the second glove on using your other, gloved, hand to help, but it must not touch ungloved areas.

Situations where non-sterile gloves are satisfactory

ACTIVITY   Look again at the practice scenarios and list those clinical procedures and situations when nurses and other staff should use non-sterile gloves.

As Mrs Lewis has MRSA, non-sterile gloves should be used by all staff entering her room (Coia et al. 2006). Gloves must always be worn when there is potential contact with faeces, urine or any other body fluid (Pratt et al. 2007), so non-sterile gloves must be worn when dealing with her commode. In addition, the domestic cleaner should be instructed to wear gloves (and apron) when cleaning the room and to dispose of them before leaving. Mrs Lewis will have blood taken regularly, for which gloves should be worn and for any other procedure where hands might be in contact with blood (WHO 2010).

For James, when the district nurse removes James's soiled dressing, any outer layers, such as a cotton bandage keeping the dressing in place, might be removed using non-sterile gloves, with sterile gloves preserved for the aseptic dressing procedure itself.

Considering Stacey, contact with vomit (a body fluid) necessitates the use of non-sterile gloves. Whether gloves would be worn for other procedures with Stacey depends on individual risk assessment and local policy. Non-sterile gloves are advised for drawing up and administering injections if there is a risk of bleeding occurring (NPSA 2007; WHO 2010), but for routine intradermal, intramuscular or subcutaneous injections, gloves are not necessary as long as skin of both patient and nurse are intact (WHO 2010). Wearing gloves also protects from potential harm to nurses during preparation of specific drugs, such as antibiotics and cytotoxic materials. *Note:* You should adhere to local policy regarding wearing of gloves in practice.

Key factors in using gloves

All gloves can perforate and should therefore be checked for defects. Keeping fingernails short helps to avoid perforations. The standard principles by Pratt et al. (2007) include the following points:

- Gloves are single-use items and must be put on immediately before an episode of care and discarded after each care activity for which they were worn to prevent the transmission of microorganisms to other sites in that individual or to other patients. However, Flores and Pevalin (2007) observed nurses wearing the same pair of gloves for more than one task, for example, making a bed and then manipulating an intravenous line.
- Hands should be decontaminated after removing gloves, preferably with soap and water. The WHO (2010) highlighted that bacterial flora colonising patients has been recovered from the hands of up to 30% of healthcare workers who wear gloves during patient contact, presumably via small defects in gloves or by contamination of the hands during glove removal.
- All gloves should be disposed of correctly (see later section).

Situations where gloves are not necessary

ACTIVITY

With reference to the scenarios, make a list of the procedures and situations for which gloves are usually unnecessary. Think particularly of all the individuals who may come into contact with the patient/client and try to decide whether they need to wear gloves.

The risk to Mrs Lewis's visitors is minimal as most do not have contact with body fluids; therefore, they do not need to wear gloves. Nevertheless, they should be instructed to wash their hands before leaving the room. If Mrs Lewis visits another department (e.g. x-ray), whether their staff require gloves depends on their level of contact with her. As porters transferring Mrs Lewis are unlikely to be in contact with her or infectious material directly, gloves are not needed.

Concerning James, gloves are needed only when changing wound dressings. For any other aspects of his care, they are not required. Similarly, for most of Stacey's care – for example, checking her blood pressure, administering oral medication and giving psychological support – gloves are not required.

Flores and Pevalin (2007) identified considerable overuse of gloves, observing them being worn for collecting equipment, answering the telephone, talking to patients, writing notes and measuring vital signs. Fuller et al. (2011) found that gloves were often worn when not indicated and vice versa.

ACTIVITY

When next in the clinical area, take note of the different types of gloves available to practitioners.

All gloves must meet the European Standard (Pratt et al. 2007). Types of disposable gloves include natural rubber latex (NRL), vinyl and nitrile. Pratt et al. (2007) make the following points about these gloves:

- NRL is the material of choice due to the degree of protection offered and level of dexterity.
- Some staff and patients have sensitivities to latex, so non-latex alternatives must be available, and allergies must be documented.
- Nitrile gloves offer good protection, but they can also cause sensitivities.
- Polythene gloves should not be used due to their permeability and tendency to damage.
- Powdered gloves should not be used.

The RCN (2012b) provides detailed guidance about glove use and prevention of contact dermatitis.

Learning outcome 2: Discuss when plastic aprons and gowns should be worn, stating the rationale

ACTIVITY

Make a list of occasions when you have seen plastic aprons worn by nurses in practice settings and when you have seen gowns worn.

You may be able to relate your experiences to the advice by Pratt et al. (2007, S21–2) about apron and gown use.

- Disposable plastic aprons must be worn when close contact with the patient, materials or equipment is expected, or when there is a risk that clothing may become contaminated with pathogenic microorganisms or blood, body fluids, secretions and excretions (with the exception of perspiration).

- Full-body gowns are worn if there is a risk of extensive splashing of blood, body fluids, secretions and excretions (with the exception of perspiration) on to the skin of the healthcare practitioner (e.g. during childbirth). Gowns are also favoured by staff handling small babies as plastic aprons provide a slippery surface.
- As with gloves, aprons and gowns must be worn as single-use items for one care activity and then disposed of.

In community settings, such as small staffed residences, there is an emphasis on social aspects of care and **normalisation**, so the use of plastic aprons is likely to be greatly reduced. However, when dealing with body fluids, they are still advisable.

In some care settings, different-coloured aprons are used for different care activities. Check your local policy about this apron use.

Summary

- Selection of appropriate personal protective equipment should be based on risk assessment.
- Gloves and aprons are single-use items and should be disposed of appropriately, followed by hand decontamination.

HEALTHCARE WASTE DISPOSAL AND LINEN MANAGEMENT

There is a statutory duty of care that applies to all those involved in the waste management chain, including nurses. European legislation has led to changes in how waste is classified and disposed of, and new methods have been established for identifying and classifying healthcare waste (DH 2011b). A revised colour-coded waste segregation and packaging system is being implemented with use of the 'List of Wastes' codes (formerly the European Waste Catalogue) (see http://www.environment-agency.gov.uk/business/topics/waste/32140.aspx). The List of Wastes provides common terminology for describing waste throughout Europe. The DH (2011b, version 2) provides detailed guidance on management of healthcare waste. For Scotland, see guidance from Health Facilities Scotland (HFS 2010).

Normalisation

The concept of normalisation, first developed by Wolfensberger, is about 'treating people with learning disabilities in ways that show that they have equal values and worth to you' (Thomas and Woods 2003, p. 75). Normalisation aims that people with learning disabilities experience normal patterns of everyday life, such as living in normal, ordinary places and undertaking normal day-to-day activities (see http://www.aboutlearningdisabilities.co.uk/normalisation-learning-disabilities.html).

LEARNING OUTCOMES

By the end of this section, you will be able to:
1 define different types of waste arising from healthcare;
2 identify how colour-coded receptacles are used for segregating different waste streams, and how waste is dealt with safely in healthcare;
3 discuss how soiled linen should be dealt with safely.

Learning outcome 1: Define different types of waste arising from healthcare

Healthcare waste is 'waste that is produced by healthcare activities, and of a type specifically related to such activities' (DH 2011b, p. 27). Different terms are used for different types of healthcare waste, according to legislation and regulations; some types are classified as **hazardous** and others as **non-hazardous**. How waste is classified affects how it is disposed of, transported and dealt with.

Clinical waste is defined by the Controlled Waste Regulations 2012 as being waste from a healthcare activity that

a. is infectious as it contains viable microorganisms or their toxins which are known or reliably believed to cause disease in humans or other living organisms, or

b. contains or is contaminated with a medicine that contains a biologically active pharmaceutical agent, or

c. is a sharp, or a body fluid or other biological material (including human and animal tissue) containing or contaminated with a dangerous substance (as defined by the Council Directive 67/548/EEC).

Most clinical waste is classified as hazardous, but some types of medicinal waste (medicines that are not **cytotoxic** or **cytostatic**) are classified as non-hazardous, although they often possess hazardous properties and, therefore, require appropriate treatment and disposal (DH 2011b). Mixing of infectious and non-infectious waste is prohibited in England and Wales, and segregation of infectious and non-infectious waste is considered best practice in Scotland and Northern Ireland. Waste is classified as infectious waste if (1) it arises from a patient known or suspected to have an infection (whether or not the causal agent is known) and where the waste may contain the pathogen; or (2) where an infection is not known or suspected, but it is considered that there is a potential risk of infection (DH 2011b). Nurses therefore need to assess whether waste generated is likely to be infectious.

Offensive/hygiene waste is non-infectious and classified as non-hazardous, but it may cause offence due to the presence of recognisable healthcare waste items, body fluids or odour.

> **Cytotoxic or cytostatic**
>
> Classification of medicinal waste used in the List of Wastes Regulations for medicinal products with one or more of the hazardous properties of toxic, carcinogenic, toxic for reproduction or mutagenic (DH 2011b, p. 27).

ACTIVITY — What types of wastes are the soiled wound dressings from Mrs Lewis and James?

You should have identified that Mrs Lewis's and James's soiled wound dressings are clinical waste as they are infectious. Both Mrs Lewis and James are known to have infections, and their soiled wound dressings are likely to contain the pathogens.

Infectious waste is classified as hazardous. Although in these scenarios we know that Mrs Lewis and James have infections, in other instances, nurses will need to assess the likelihood of an infection being present, as non-infectious soiled dressings can go into the non-hazardous, offensive/hygiene waste stream. Chapter 7 discusses recognition of a wound infection.

Learning outcome 2: Identify how colour-coded receptacles are used for segregating different waste streams and how waste is dealt with safely in healthcare

Segregation of waste is mandatory in England and Wales so that different types of waste can be managed appropriately through incineration, treatment, recycling or landfill. To facilitate segregation, the DH (2011b) recommends the use of colour-coded receptacles, advising that a national system should be in place to achieve standardisation.

ACTIVITY

What colour receptacles have you seen used in practice for waste disposal and what type of waste were they used for?

The colours you are likely to have seen will depend on the type of healthcare settings you have worked in and the type of waste produced. The DH (2011b) recommends a colour-coded system for the different waste types, which require different management (Table 3.2). *Note*: Colour coding for sharps bins is discussed in the next section.

ACTIVITY

If waste is not dealt with safely, spillage can occur, causing harm to anyone in contact with it. How can you prevent spillage from occurring?

Table 3.2: Colour-coding system for waste, recommended by the DH

Colour receptacle	Waste type and management
Yellow	Infectious waste that has an additional characteristic that means that it must be incinerated in a suitably licensed or permitted facility. Examples: anatomical waste, chemically contaminated samples and diagnostic kits, medicinally contaminated infectious waste; and Category A (as specified in the Carriage Regulations) pathogens (often when in culture form) as these are capable of causing permanent disability, life-threatening or fatal disease.
Orange	Infectious waste, for example, incontinence pads, stoma bags and soiled wound dressings where the patient has an infection and the causative agent is likely to be in the waste. For example, the stoma bag of a patient with a gastrointestinal infection. A used wound drain would always go into this waste steam. This waste stream must not contain non-infectious waste or infectious waste with additional characteristics (chemicals, medicines, anatomical waste), which mean it must be incinerated.
Purple	Waste consisting of, or contaminated with cytotoxic and/or cytostatic products.
Yellow with black stripe	Offensive/hygiene waste, such as stoma bags, incontinence pads, catheter bags and soiled wound dressings, when they are not considered infectious. In the community, a patient who is self-managing can put small amounts of these items into their domestic waste stream.
Red	Anatomical waste, which includes recognisable body parts and placenta.
Black (or clear)	Domestic waste which is similar to waste generated at home. Domestic waste should not contain any infectious materials, sharps or medicinal products.

Examples: non-recyclable packaging, such as crisp packets, polystyrene cups, flowers. |
| Blue | Medicinal waste. |

Source: Department of Health (DH). 2011b. *Safe Management of Health Care Waste*, Version 2, Gateway Reference 15645, London: DH.

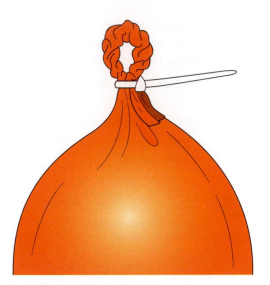

Figure 3.6: Swan-neck technique for sealing waste bags.

Appropriate receptacles must be used. For liquid waste, the receptacle should be designed to take liquids, such as a rigid leakproof plastic drum, or a receptacle with absorbing gels/materials. Sharps must only be placed in sharps receptacles. All other waste may be packaged in flexible bags. The bags or rigid containers must be no more than three-quarters full when they are sealed. The swan-neck method is recommended for sealing bags (HPS 2013) (Figure 3.6). The bags/containers must be labelled or tagged with their origin so that they can be traced back to source. Waste bags must be provided as near to use as possible. However, the DH (2011b) recommends that clinical waste receptacles are not kept in patient areas that are accessible to visitors. In the community, healthcare workers must ensure that healthcare waste awaiting collection is stored appropriately, away from children and animals.

Learning outcome 3: Discuss how soiled linen should be dealt with safely

Soiled linen requires careful handling, bagging and disposal as it can become contaminated with microorganisms from patients' body fluids or the infections that they have.

Points to remember include: when changing bed-linen, have a receptacle close by so the soiled linen can be put straight into the bag. Do not shake the linen, do not overfill laundry bags and never place soiled linen on the floor or other surface (e.g. bed table) (HPS 2013).

The laundry process decontaminates linen through the mechanical process of washing, the detergent used and the temperature of the water. The process must include sufficient time for all parts of the load to be washed at an adequate temperature. Any microorganisms that remain after washing can be destroyed by tumble drying and ironing (Wilson 2006).

Can you name three different types of linen bag and the category of linen that should be placed in each? Why are the different categories needed? Which colour would be used for Mrs Lewis's used sheets and which colour for Stacey's vomit-covered bed-linen?

The categories are needed to protect laundry staff from cross-infection. In addition, the categories protect other staff and patients by ensuring that linen is adequately decontaminated during laundering. There are three main types of linen bag. The first type of bag is white linen or clear plastic that is used for used, soiled and foul linen and will therefore be appropriate for Stacey's bed-linen. These items should be washed at 65°C for 10 minutes or at 71°C for 3 minutes for thermal disinfection. Duvets should withstand washing at 71°C and comply with DH standards of retardancy (Wilson 2006). For infected linen, a water-soluble bag with a red outer bag is required. This bag type is used for linen from patients with infectious diseases or at other times as advised by the IPCT and would be used for Mrs Lewis's bed-linen. The laundry staff do not open and sort the linen in the inner bag, and the linen is washed and thermally disinfected as for used linen. A third type of bag with an orange stripe is used for fabric likely to be damaged by thermal disinfection, for example, wool. These items are washed at 40°C, and hypochlorite is added to the penultimate wash.

Summary

- Nurses and other healthcare workers have a duty of care to ensure that they dispose of waste appropriately to prevent hazards to themselves, colleagues, patients and the public.
- It is important to differentiate between different categories of waste and to ensure that they are disposed of in the correct, colour-coded receptacle.
- Used linen must be disposed of correctly according to whether it is infectious or soiled only.

SHARPS DISPOSAL

Safe disposal of sharps, such as needles, blood glucose lancets, phlebotomy equipment, intravenous cannulae and catheter stylets, is important to maintain a safe environment and prevent cross-infection. The Council of the European Union (2010) implemented the framework agreement on prevention from sharps injuries in the hospital and healthcare sector.

In May 2013, a new European Directive (2010/32/EU) came into force in the UK, requiring employers to assess the risks of sharps injuries and where possible eliminate the use of sharps – for example, through the use of needleless systems. Where sharps cannot be eliminated, steps should be taken to reduce the risk of injuries through the use of safety-engineered sharps devices. Clinical staff and their representatives should be involved in the selection and evaluation of such devices. The directive will apply to all staff working in hospitals and wherever healthcare is delivered: NHS, private and other public sector provision, such as prisons.

Students and agency nurses are also included. The RCN (2011) produced detailed guidance on implementing the new European Directive and preventing sharps injuries in healthcare.

> **LEARNING OUTCOMES**
>
> By the end of this section, you will be able to:
> 1 appreciate the need and reasons for the safe disposal of sharps;
> 2 explain the principles for the safe use and disposal of sharps;
> 3 identify the actions required after sharps injury.

Learning outcome 1: Appreciate the need and reasons for the safe disposal of sharps

ACTIVITY

Identify two possible reasons for the importance of disposing of sharps safely.

The main reason for disposing of sharps safely is the physical prevention of cross-infection through sharps injuries, including needlesticks. Pratt et al. (2007) report that the average risk of transmission of bloodborne pathogens after a single percutaneous exposure, without post-exposure prophylaxis or prior vaccination (if available), has been estimated as

- hepatitis B virus 33.3% (1 in 3);
- hepatitis C virus 3.3% (1 in 30);
- HIV 0.31% (1 in 319).

Between 1997 and 2007, 14 healthcare workers in England contracted hepatitis C, and there have been five documented cases of HIV transmission, through sharps injuries (HPA 2008).

Staff caring for Stacey know that she has hepatitis B, but this information about patients is not always available. People may not know that they are carrying a bloodborne disease. Therefore, sharps disposal should be carried out in the same way for all patients. In the first instance, it is the injured healthcare professional who is at risk of contamination from a patient source. However, the professional may then pass the infection back to other patients if the correct procedures are not followed. All healthcare workers should be vaccinated against hepatitis B. Without immunity to hepatitis B, staff who are caring for Stacey would be at risk of acquiring this virus if they sustained a needlestick injury from her used injection needle.

A second important reason for ensuring the safe disposal of sharps is the professional responsibility of nurses to protect patients and colleagues from risk (NMC 2008). The distress that almost invariably occurs after sharps injuries is concerned with individuals' understandable fear of the blood-to-blood transmission of bacteria and viruses.

ACTIVITY

Discuss with a colleague how you would feel if you sustained a needlestick injury where the patient source was suspected of having a bloodborne infection.

You might have identified fear, anxiety and panic among your emotions. It is clearly much better to prevent needlestick or other sharps injuries.

Learning outcome 2: Explain the principles for the safe use and disposal of sharps

ACTIVITY

Make a list of the key safety factors you think you should take into account when using and disposing of sharps.

There are many factors to take into account. The RCN (2012a) includes these standard principles:

- Sharps must not be passed directly from hand to hand, and handling should be kept to a minimum.
- Needles must not be bent, recapped, dissembled or broken after use.
- Used sharps must be discarded into the designated sharps receptacle (conforming to UN3291 and BS7320 standards) immediately after use.
- Containers should be placed out of reach of children but at a height that enables safe disposal by staff.

Other important points

The responsibility for the disposal of sharps lies with the individual who has been using them. Sharps receptacles must not be overfilled; do not fill past the fill line marked on the container and never more than three-quarters full (HPS 2013). Preferably, take a sharps bin to the patient. Always place sharps carefully into the receptacle and never drop or throw them from a distance. Never put fingers into the sharps container, nor kick or shake the container to make more room. Do not attempt to clean the sharps container, particularly around the lip.

The DH (2011b) explains that, due to waste disposal legislation, sharps bins should have different-coloured lids according to their medicinal contamination, as type of medicine affects how the sharps will be managed:

- purple lid for sharps that are contaminated with cytotoxic or cytostatic medicines;
- yellow lid for sharps that are contaminated with non-cytotoxic and non-cytostatic medicines;
- orange lid for sharps not contaminated with medicines (e.g. sharps used for venepuncture).

The above applies to England and Wales. In Scotland and Northern Ireland, sharps fully discharged of medicines (non-cytotoxic and non-cytostatic), but still contaminated, can be put into orange-lidded sharps receptacles, in some circumstances.

Self-medicating community patients (e.g. people with diabetes) should be provided with a sharps receptacle and taught to seal and label it and return it to the surgery or pharmacy for disposal when it has reached the fill line. However, policies in community healthcare settings and care homes may vary, and you should ensure that you are familiar with the relevant policies for the areas that you study and work in.

ACTIVITY

What should you do when a sharps receptacle is full (i.e. reached the fill line)?

You should seal a sharps receptacle according to the manufacturer's instructions, often found on the outside of the receptacle. If you observe that a sharps box is full, be proactive about sealing it. Do not leave someone else to deal with an overfilled sharps box as this is very hazardous. Sealed receptacles should be left at identified collection points in the manner prescribed by the local policy and labelled with date and source. It is usual for facilities staff to remove the boxes and take them to a central point for transporting. The correct sealing and disposal of sharps bins are essential to protect the many people who could be injured otherwise, including porters, transport staff and waste disposal staff.

Learning outcome 3: Identify the actions required after a sharps injury

ACTIVITY

With a colleague, discuss what you think should be done after a sharps injury.

All healthcare employers are required to develop processes for dealing with sharps injuries. These processes include identifying the employee's responsibility to report the injury and their subsequent entitlement to be provided with counselling and testing services. However, before this stage is reached, emergency action is needed. Now check your ideas with Table 3.3.

The policies outlined are also used if blood or body fluid is splashed into the eyes or mouth, or onto broken skin.

ACTIVITY

When you are next in the practice setting, seek out and read the local clinical policy on the action to be taken after a sharps injury.

Table 3.3: Action after a sharps injury

Emergency action	• Encourage bleeding at the site by squeezing. • Wash the wound well with soap and running water. • For blood splashes to eyes, mouth or into broken skin, rinse thoroughly with plenty of running water. • Call for assistance. • Cover wound with waterproof dressing.
Reporting	• Inform your manager immediately. • Complete accident/incident form. • Identify patient source if possible. • Report to the occupational health department immediately, or if closed attend the emergency department for further advice.
Follow-up	• Make use of counselling if required. • Attend for testing if indicated. • Follow medical advice.

Note: You should consult and follow your local policy throughout. It is the responsibility of the member of staff involved and their manager to see that all procedures are carried out.

Summary
- Sharps pose a potential hazard to nurses, other staff and the public.
- All nurses must follow national and local policy and handle and dispose of sharps safely to prevent the risk of sharps injuries to themselves and colleagues.
- All healthcare organisations have agreed procedures to follow in the event of a sharps injury and these procedures should be adhered to carefully.

HEALTHCARE ENVIRONMENTAL HYGIENE AND MULTIUSE EQUIPMENT

The DH (2009) requires that care providers 'provide and maintain a clean and appropriate environment in managed premises that facilitates the prevention and control of infections' (p. 9). Microorganisms including MRSA have been found in the hospital environment and can be harboured by dust (Pratt et al. 2007). Cleaning removes contaminants, including dust and soil, large numbers of microorganisms and the organic matter that may harbour them such as biofilms, faeces, blood and other bodily fluids (RCN 2012a). Although cleaning cannot eradicate microorganisms from the environment, hospital environments must be 'visibly clean, free from dust and soilage and acceptable to patients, their visitors and staff' (Pratt et al. 2007, S3).

LEARNING OUTCOMES

On completion of this section, you will be able to:
1 discuss issues relating to healthcare environments and their cleanliness;
2 explain how and when communal equipment should be cleaned.

Learning outcome 1: Discuss issues relating to healthcare environments and their cleanliness

ACTIVITY

What is the environment, in relation to healthcare? List all the items you can think of.

You probably thought of the floor; furniture, such as beds and bedside lockers; and toilets. Did you identify curtains/screens, light switches, doors and door handles too? These items can easily be contaminated. The Norovirus Working Party (2012) identified 'frequently touched surfaces' as being bed tables, bed rails, the arms of bedside chairs, taps, call bells, door handles and push plates; these surfaces would all need enhanced cleaning in a norovirus outbreak. The DH (2009) clarified that the environment means the totality of a service user's surroundings when in care premises, including the fabric of the building, fittings and services, such as air and water supplies. The DH (2009) also highlighted that in community care, the suitability of the environment for the level of care needed should be considered. The RCN (2012a) provides guidelines for standard infection control precautions relating to the environment, and they advise that a well-designed environment can support effective cleaning, highlighting that high standards of cleanliness will help to reduce the risk of cross-infection and are also reassuring to patients and the public. The HPS (2013) recommends that the care environment must be free from clutter to facilitate effective cleaning and be well maintained and in a good state of repair.

ACTIVITY

Whose responsibility is it to ensure healthcare environments are clean?

You probably identified the key role that facilities staff have in ensuring that healthcare environments are kept clean, but nursing staff also have a crucial role. The DH (2009) identified that the nurse or other person in charge of any patient or resident area has direct responsibility for ensuring that cleanliness standards are maintained throughout that shift. Furthermore, the RCN (2012a) advised that all nurses, midwives and healthcare assistants have a responsibility to be aware of their local cleaning specification to ensure that any issues are highlighted immediately should they occur. The HPS (2013) advised that for routine cleaning, a fresh solution of general purpose neutral detergent in warm water should be used, which should be changed when dirty, at 15-minute intervals or when changing tasks. Pratt et al. (2007) advised that hypochlorite should be used where microorganisms are surviving for long periods in the environment and may be contributing to spread of infection. In a norovirus outbreak, enhanced environmental cleaning should be instigated, to include increased frequency of cleaning patient care areas, shared equipment and frequently touched surfaces, and increased frequency of cleaning and disinfection of toilet facilities, by using 0.1% sodium hypochlorite [1000 parts per million available chlorine (ppm av Cl)] (Norovirus Working Party 2012).

After Mrs Lewis's discharge from the sideroom, it will be the nursing staff's responsibility to request that the room and any non-disposable equipment are thoroughly cleaned and dry before other patients are in contact with them. Disposable equipment used for her care must be disposed of as infective waste. Clinical staff should be observant and proactive to ensure environments are kept clean, particularly when unexpected events occur, such as body fluids being spilt.

ACTIVITY

How should you deal with body fluid spillages, for example, blood, vomit or urine?

Blood and body fluid spillages pose cross-infection risks, so they must be dealt with immediately and appropriately; the HPS (2013) provides guidelines but also check your local policy. For any body fluid spillages, perform hand hygiene before and after, wear personal protective equipment, use recommended cleaning solutions (according to the body fluid involved) and correctly dispose of the used items. The HPS (2013) recommends the following actions, according to the body fluid involved.

- **Urine/faeces/vomit/sputum.** Initially, soak up the spillage with paper towels. *For urine*, do not use a chlorine-releasing agent; a gelling agent can be used. Decontaminate the area with a combined detergent/chlorine-producing solution of 1000 ppm av Cl. Leave the solution for 3 minutes or as per manufacturer's recommendations.
- **Blood/other body fluids.** Such fluids include cerebrospinal, peritoneal, pleural, pericardial, synovial, amniotic, semen, vaginal secretions, breast milk and other body fluids with visible blood. Apply chlorine-releasing granules to the spill or use disposable towels with a solution of 10,000 ppm av Cl. Leave the solution for 3 minutes or as per the manufacturer's recommendations and then dispose of the waste.

After application of the above-mentioned solutions, wash the area with paper towels, warm water and detergent and then dry the area.

Learning outcome 2: Explain how and when communal equipment should be cleaned

The HPS (2013) summarises the different types of equipment as follows:

Single use. Single-use equipment is used once and then discarded and not reused even on the same patient. The packaging of these items is marked with a standardised symbol (Figure 3.7).

Single patient use equipment. Single patient use equipment can be reused but only on the same patient, for example, an oxygen mask.

Reusable invasive equipment. Reusable invasive equipment is used once and then decontaminated, for example, surgical equipment.

Reusable non-invasive equipment (communal equipment). Communal equipment is reused on more than one patient after decontamination between each use.

The RCN (2012a) advised that single-use equipment should be used where available and appropriate. However, many items are communal, for example, infusion

Figure 3.7: Symbol for single use only.

Disinfection

A process to reduce the number of viable microorganisms, but it may not inactivate some microbial agents (e.g. spores).

Sterilisation

A process that renders an item free from microorganisms, including spores.

pumps, drip stands and commodes, and these items must be decontaminated between each use, after any blood or body fluid spillage, at regular predefined intervals as part of an equipment cleaning protocol, before disinfection, and before inspection, servicing or repair (HPS 2013). Wilcox et al. (2003) found that more than half of commodes were contaminated by *C. difficile*, highlighting the importance of effective decontamination. Elhasson and Dixon (2012) found that 36% of non-disposable tourniquets were contaminated with *S. aureus*, of which 12% were MRSA positive. Furthermore, 77% of staff did not clean the non-disposable tourniquets, and 66% of tourniquets were visibly soiled, some with blood. The authors argued that all staff should use disposable tourniquets.

Decontamination aims to ensure that reusable items are safe to use by other patients; equipment should be decontaminated according to manufacturers' instructions and includes cleaning, **disinfection** and **sterilisation**.

Although patients coming into contact with communally used equipment generally have intact skin and therefore infection may not be introduced by contaminated equipment, equipment may nevertheless transmit microorganisms between patients and could result in infection (Pratt et al. 2007).

ACTIVITY

Consider each of the patients in the scenarios. What communal equipment will be used in their care? How and when might you clean this equipment?

When James's wound was dressed at home, there would have been no communal equipment used in his care. At the doctor's surgery, the dressing trolley used will be in communal use. Dressing trolleys are unlikely to become contaminated during the dressing procedure, but they should be cleaned before and after use (see 'Aseptic technique'). Stacey's blood pressure monitoring equipment will be communal, although in some settings patients are allocated their own blood pressure cuff to use until their discharge. Other equipment used is single use (injection equipment) or washable (bed-linen). Her bed and bedside locker should be cleaned after her discharge and kept socially clean while in her use. As Mrs Lewis has MRSA and is isolated, any equipment that is not disposable (e.g. commode, blood pressure monitoring equipment) should be designated for her use only. After discharge, the equipment must be cleaned effectively before use by other patients.

When decontaminating equipment, check any special manufacturers' instructions and local policy. Decontamination methods are influenced by whether the patient is known to have an infection/colonisation, or whether there is body fluid contamination. Personal protective equipment must be used during decontamination, and all items used for cleaning must be disposed of safely. The HPS (2013) recommends the following methods.

- **Equipment contaminated with blood:** Use disposable cloths and fresh detergent solution, rinse, dry and follow with a disinfectant solution of 10,000 ppm av Cl, and then rinse and thoroughly dry. A combined detergent/chlorine-releasing solution can be used.

- **Equipment not contaminated by blood but contaminated by urine, vomit or faeces, or equipment that has been used by a patient with a known infection/colonisation:** Use disposable cloths and fresh detergent solution, rinse, dry and follow with a disinfectant solution of 1000 ppm av Cl, and then rinse and thoroughly dry. A combined detergent/chlorine-releasing solution can be used.
- **Equipment not contaminated by blood or other body fluid and not used by a patient with a known infection/colonisation:** Use disposable cloths and a detergent solution or detergent impregnated wipes, rinse and thoroughly dry.

The HPS (2013) advise that after decontamination, communal equipment must be rinsed and dried and then stored clean and dry.

Summary
- All healthcare workers have a duty to ensure that healthcare environments are clean.
- Body fluid spillages must be dealt with immediately using recommended procedures.
- Communal equipment must be effectively decontaminated.

ASEPTIC TECHNIQUE

NICE (2012) explains that an aseptic technique ensures that only uncontaminated equipment and fluids make contact with susceptible body sites, and the technique should be used during clinical procedures that bypass the body's natural defences, thus minimising the spread of organisms from one person to another. Aseptic technique uses a non-touch technique in which equipment is handled in such a way that the important sterile parts are not touched. Sterile gloves are used for aseptic technique in some situations, and effective hand hygiene is a fundamental aspect of aseptic technique. Ways of carrying out aseptic technique vary nationally, but a standardised approach is recommended (Aziz 2009). Aseptic Non Touch Technique (ANTT™) (Rowley et al. 2010) is an example of an aseptic technique for vascular access device maintenance, and it provides a possible framework for standardised guidance on aseptic technique (NICE 2012).

LEARNING OUTCOMES

By the end of this section, you will be able to:
1 assess when aseptic technique is required;
2 explain how to conduct an aseptic technique, with special reference to wound dressings.

Learning outcome 1: Assess when aseptic technique is required

ACTIVITY

For the items on the following list, identify whether it is true or false that an aseptic technique is required:
1. Giving food to patients
2. Removal of sutures or clips

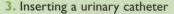

3. Inserting a urinary catheter
4. Taking a patient's temperature
5. Assisting with oral hygiene
6. Wound dressings

You should have identified that the answers for 2, 3 and 6 are true, as these are procedures that could introduce infection. For the three remaining procedures, 1, 4 and 5, hand hygiene is required but not aseptic technique. For oral hygiene, non-sterile gloves may be used (for more information, see Chapter 8).

Generally, aseptic technique should be used after surgery when skin integrity has been interrupted; after trauma to skin tissue, such as experienced by James; and during invasive procedures, such as catheterisation. Mrs Lewis would require aseptic technique during her wound care, and her intravenous cannula would have been inserted using an aseptic technique. Any other invasive techniques that may be performed as part of her investigations and treatment would require an aseptic technique. A clean, rather than aseptic, technique is sufficient in some wound care situations, such as with some chronic wounds (for further discussion, see Chapter 7).

Learning outcome 2 explains the use of aseptic technique, as applied to wound dressings, as wound dressing is a common reason for using aseptic technique.

Learning outcome 2: Explain how to conduct an aseptic technique, with special reference to wound dressings

Because hands are not sterile, forceps were traditionally used for wound dressing, but sterile disposable gloves are used for most wound dressings now. Good gloving technique is required to prevent contamination of gloves (see earlier section).

Preparing for aseptic technique

ACTIVITY

Discuss with a colleague how you would prepare James to have his wound dressed.

You would need to explain the procedure to James and gain his consent and cooperation. The accident that caused James's wound, followed by ongoing wound dressings, could cause him anxiety, so nurses should be understanding and patient with him. The community nurse for learning disabilities could help prepare James for his dressings and will be familiar with how to communicate with him effectively. Pictures and photos may be useful to aid understanding. Dressings should be changed when exudate is visible on the surface, as the dressing will no longer act as an impermeable barrier preventing bacteria from the outside reaching the open wound. If a wound is infected, then the moist exudate on the surface of the dressing will contaminate any surfaces it comes into contact with.

ACTIVITY

How might you prepare the environment before carrying out a wound dressing, either in the community as for James, or in a hospital setting, as for Mrs Lewis?

In the community, good lighting and James's comfort and privacy are key factors to consider. James has been having his dressing changed at his home near the farm, and community nurses are used to adapting within the home environment. When James attends the local surgery for his dressings, there should be a clean treatment room and good handwashing equipment. In the hospital, privacy should be maintained. Mrs Lewis is in a sideroom, but for other patients privacy will be provided by screening, or a designated treatment room may be available.

The dressing trolley or other surface should be clean and dry. Alcohol-based wipes are commonly used for decontamination but follow local policy.

ACTIVITY

Next, consider what equipment is required. Drawing on experience in practice, make a list of the equipment that you think is needed for carrying out a wound dressing.

You will have identified that you will need a dressing pack. These packs vary in content, but they typically include medium-sized sterile gloves, gauze swabs, a disposal bag, a paper towel and a container in which cleansing fluid can be poured, if required. Commercially manufactured packs often state the content on the wrapper. If there is no waste bag included, you will need to take a waste bag. If your hands are small or large, you will need separately wrapped sterile gloves in your size. You should check the dressing pack for integrity; if the pack is damaged or torn, you should discard it, as the contents can no longer be guaranteed sterile. You should also check that the pack has been sterilised and that the expiry date has not elapsed.

The choice of wound dressing depends on many factors (see Chapter 7). The wound care for each patient, including type of dressing, frequency of dressing change and cleansing agent, should all be in the care plan. If tape is needed, it should be hypoallergenic, in good condition and clean. Sterile scissors should be taken if the dressing will need cutting to size. Some wounds will need cleansing; Chapter 7 discusses when and how to cleanse wounds. As both James and Mrs Lewis have heavily exudating wounds due to their infections, cleansing will be necessary. A sterile solution such as normal saline can be used to clean and irrigate the wound, if indicated.

Carrying out aseptic technique

Before starting aseptic technique, try to ensure you will not be disturbed by telephones and so on. Box 3.2 outlines a set of guidelines that you could use to change a wound dressing by using aseptic technique. These guidelines are intended for use when alone. If available, a second nurse could, after decontaminating hands, open the pack, be available to observe and support the patient throughout the procedure and open additional items on to the sterile field when required. Before starting aseptic technique, explain that you will minimise talk during the procedure to avoid contamination. This is because, during speech, you could spread microorganisms from your oral mucosa.

You can adapt the guidelines in Box 3.2 as long as you maintain the underlying principles, and you should follow local policy for aseptic technique. In patients' own homes, where a trolley is not available, nurses can use any suitable surface.

Box 3.2 Equipment and guidelines for aseptic technique, applied to a wound dressing

Equipment

A dressing trolley or surface that can be used for the equipment

A sterile dressing pack with sterile gloves

Sterile cleansing solution (if cleansing required) and alcohol swab to clean its outer packaging

Wound dressing appropriate for wound, based on assessment, as per patient's care plan (see Chapter 7), and any additional equipment needed to apply this dressing

Hypoallergenic tape (if tape is needed)

Sterile scissors (if needed for the dressing)

Clean disposable apron

Alcohol-based handrub

Waste sack if not provided in the dressing pack

Procedure

Note: Throughout the procedure, continually observe patient's condition and take into account their comfort and privacy.

- Check patient's notes regarding wound management plan. Confirm you have the correct patient and check the patient's identity band.
- Explain the procedure, gain consent and cooperation.
- Wash hands and put on plastic apron.
- Prepare the environment. Clean the trolley surfaces.
- Collect equipment and place on bottom of trolley.
- Position the patient and adjust clothing to expose required area.
- Loosen the dressing covering the wound (wear non-sterile gloves if necessary).
- Decontaminate hands.
- Open the outer packaging of the pack and slip the inner package onto the trolley top.
- Open the dressing pack using corners only. The sterile field should lie flat on the trolley. Avoid touching sterile inner surfaces and content.

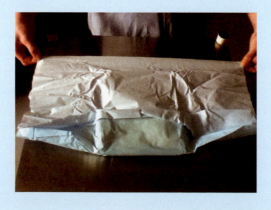

(Continued)

Box 3.2 (Continued)

- Open any additional sterile items onto the sterile field.

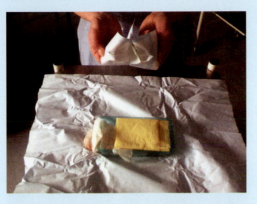

- Use the sterile disposal bag (if provided in the pack) over one hand to arrange the equipment.

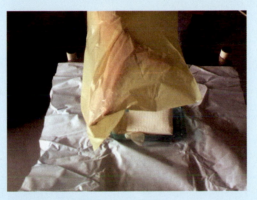

- Remove the used dressing with your hand inside the bag, invert the bag and attach it to the side of the trolley, between you and the patient.

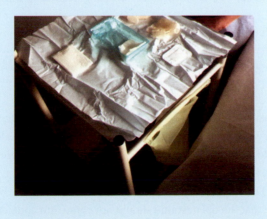

(Continued)

Box 3.2 (Continued)

- If using a sachet of cleansing solution, clean the perforation area with an alcohol swab and let it dry. Tear open and pour the solution into the dressing pack's container, avoiding splashing.

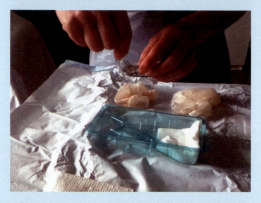

- Decontaminate hands and put on sterile gloves.

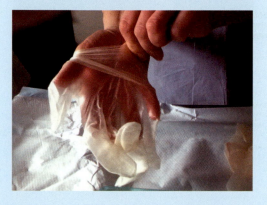

- Place sterile towel near wound.
- Irrigate/cleanse the wound, if required and apply new dressing according to manufacturer's instructions.
- Make patient comfortable.
- Dispose of all equipment safely. Remove and dispose of gloves and apron.
- Clean the trolley and wash hands.
- Document the care, reporting any significant findings or effects on the patient.

Unsworth (2011) advised that the nurse should place the sterile field at a height that prevents it from becoming contaminated by skin scales and fibres and that the sterile field should ideally be placed on a clean table. Where such placement is not possible, plastic (e.g. a plastic apron) should be placed on the surface.

The important principles of aseptic technique, when applied to wound dressings, are that the open wound should not come into contact with any item that is not sterile and that any items that have been in contact with the wound should be discarded safely or decontaminated (Wilson 2006). This same principle applies to any other procedure using aseptic technique. For example, during catheterisation (see Chapter 9) the sterile catheter, which will be inserted into the sterile urinary tract, must not be contaminated by anything that is non-sterile. Stacey's injection must also be carried out using aseptic technique. The needle will be piercing the skin (the protective barrier) and entering the sterile muscle. Therefore, the needle, syringe and drug must be sterile and should be prepared and administered using a non-touch technique (see Chapter 5), but non-sterile gloves can be worn as these will not touch sterile parts of the equipment.

ACTIVITY

If you have access to a skills laboratory and equipment, collect the equipment listed and follow the instructions in Box 3.2 to practise carrying out a wound dressing on a colleague. Take particular care to ensure that you do not contaminate the sterile gloves or your sterile field.

Summary

- There are many situations where aseptic technique is necessary to prevent cross-infection during invasive procedures.
- Effective aseptic technique requires good hand hygiene, sterile equipment and the use of a non-touch technique so that sterile items are not contaminated.
- Understanding the underlying principles of aseptic technique enables guidelines to be adapted safely to each individual situation.

SPECIMEN COLLECTION: KEY PRINCIPLES

Laboratory tests can assist with diagnosing an infection, and successful laboratory diagnosis depends on effective collection of a specimen. Successful laboratory diagnosis requires appropriate and timely collection of specimens, the correct technique and equipment, and rapid and safe transport (RCN 2012a). The sooner a specimen arrives at a laboratory, the greater the chance of organisms surviving and being identified. In general, the larger the quantity of material sent for laboratory examination, the greater the chance of isolating causative organisms. Specimens can be contaminated by poor technique, giving rise to confusing or misleading results. Ideally, samples should be collected before the beginning of treatments with, for example, antibiotics or antiseptics, or the laboratory should be informed of which antibiotics or antiseptics are being used. Both antiseptics and antibiotics affect the outcome of laboratory results.

A written local policy should be in place for the collection and transportation of laboratory specimens. You should be aware of this policy and its contents and be trained and competent to collect and handle specimens safely.

LEARNING OUTCOMES

By the end of this section, you will be able to:
1 explain the general principles relating to the collection of any specimen;
2 discuss the general principles underpinning the collection of wound swabs and pus.

Note: For urine and stool specimen collection, refer to Chapter 9. For sputum specimen collection, refer to Chapter 11.

Learning outcome 1: Explain the general principles relating to the collection of any specimen

As with any procedure you should explain the procedure to the person, gain consent and maintain privacy during the procedure.

Have you been involved in collecting any specimens? How can you ensure that you maintain safety and accuracy?

The general principles of collecting any specimen to ensure safety and accuracy include the following:

- Carry out hand hygiene before and after the procedure.
- Wear non-sterile gloves and apron if handling body fluids is likely.
- Ensure that tissue and fluid is collected from the suspected site of the infection and that the specimens are collected as aseptically as possible (see asepsis and aseptic technique) to avoid contamination with other bacteria that may influence the result.
- Preserve any microorganisms collected in the relevant medium/container and prevent it from becoming contaminated by other organisms; the microbiology laboratory may be the provider of the correct specimen container.
- Place the specimen in an appropriate and correctly labelled sterile container and seal it properly.
- Complete the specimen form using patient labels (where available):
- Check that all relevant information is included and correct.
- Take care not to contaminate the outside of the container and the request forms as this places laboratory staff at risk.
- **Do not** label the container until after the specimen is collected, to prevent contamination of the label, and mistakes.

Without full information, it is impossible to examine a specimen adequately or to report it accurately. Also, if specimens are not correctly labelled or match the request form, the laboratory cannot process the specimen and a further specimen will have to be obtained, thus delaying treatment.

Make a list of the information that you think would be essential to document and accompany the specimen. Why is full and correct information important?

You may have identified the following:

- Patient's name and location (e.g. address, ward).
- Hospital number and NHS number.
- Patient's date of birth.
- Consultant's/GP's name.
- Date and time specimen collected.
- Clinical details of relevance to the specimen, for example, signs of infection and date of onset of the illness.

- Any antibiotic therapy being taken by the patient, including information about current or recent antibiotic prescriptions.
- Type of specimen and site.
- Name and telephone/bleep number of the doctor/nurse requesting the investigation – it may be necessary to telephone the result before the report is despatched.

The specimen must be correctly labelled to ensure that it can be identified and matched with its corresponding request form, so results of the tests are related to the correct patient. Specimens are potentially hazardous to staff who could be exposed to people's body fluids. The person collecting the specimen must ensure that the specimen container is sealed securely and is leakproof, that all body fluid traces have been removed from the container's outside, that the specimen container is not overfilled, that biohazard labels are attached to the container and form if appropriate and that the container is sealed in a plastic bag (Wilson 2006). *Note*: The specimen container should never be placed into the transportation bag with the request form, to prevent contamination.

If specimens cannot be sent to a laboratory immediately, they should be stored in a dedicated specimen refrigerator at 4°C. Blood cultures, however, go in an incubator at 37°C. Cotton-wool swab sticks are used to take specimens from mucous membranes. The specimen stick is then inserted into a tube of soft agar, which preserves any microorganisms for up to 24 hours. Bottles for transporting viruses are usually acquired from the laboratory and need prompt transport to the laboratory as soon as possible after the specimen is taken.

Learning outcome 2: Discuss the general principles underpinning the collection of wound swabs and pus

Wilson (2006) states that wound infections should be recognised by clinical signs of infection rather than just isolation of bacteria from a swab. As you read in the scenarios, James had a wound swab taken from his clinically infected wound.

ACTIVITY — What would prompt you to take a swab from a wound?

You would take a wound swab when the wound shows clinical signs of infection. Chapter 7 explains in detail how to recognise a wound infection, but some signs include local heat, erythema (redness), pain, pus/purulent discharge, malodour and delayed healing. The HPA (2012b) advises that collecting samples of pus or exudate, if present, is preferable to swabbing wounds. Pus can be withdrawn using a syringe and sent to the laboratory in a universal container (Ayliffe et al. 2001). If only minute amounts of pus are present, it can be collected on a swab that is put into transport medium; swabbing dry, crusted areas is unlikely to reveal the causative organism (HPA 2012b).

When swabbing a wound, remember to follow all the principles discussed in learning outcome 1, including explaining to the patient and gaining consent. Remember that the wound may be sore, so be gentle and reassuring while taking the swab. Wound swabs or pus should be obtained at the beginning of the dressing procedure, after the dressing has been removed, and dressing material traces should be first cleansed away by irrigating using saline at body temperature. A representative part of the lesion should be swabbed (HPA 2012b). The swab should be taken from the infected site only, taking care not to touch any surrounding skin, and then placed in transport medium. Swab the wound using a zig-zag action from the centre outward, while turning the swab over in a circular manner, and ensure it is soaked with wound exudate if present (Patton 2010). Compete the accompanying information, as discussed in learning outcome 1, ensuring that you note the site of the wound so that the appropriate media can be set up for culture.

Summary
- Specimens can be important diagnostic aids and should be collected carefully, using recommended techniques.
- It is essential to prevent cross-infection and any contamination while collecting a specimen.
- Specimens should be labelled accurately, and with full accompanying information supplied.
- Clinical signs of a wound infection should be looked for. Collection of pus is preferable to wound swabs.

MRSA SCREENING AND SUPPRESSION PROCEDURES

MRSA screening is the microbiological testing of a sample taken from the potential carriage sites of a patient on or before admission to hospital. It is the process by which patients who are colonised with MRSA are identified. MRSA suppression procedures (also termed decolonisation) must then be applied, as per local protocol.

LEARNING OUTCOMES

By the end of this section, you will be able to:
1 discuss when and how MRSA screening is conducted;
2 explain how MRSA suppression (decolonisation) procedures are carried out.

Learning outcome 1: Discuss when and how MRSA screening is conducted

The guidelines of Coia et al. (2006) for the control and prevention of MRSA recommend an active approach to MRSA screening linked to isolation and cohorting facilities (see next section).

ACTIVITY

In practice, how have you seen decisions made about MRSA screening? Are you aware of a local Trust protocol on MRSA screening?

The groups of patients to be screened should be determined according to local risk assessments and practicality, but they might include the following:

- All patients previously known to be positive for MRSA.
- All elective surgical patients at preadmission clinics.
- Oncology/chemotherapy patients (as they have a high risk of MRSA bacteraemia due to immunosuppression and vascular access for treatment).
- Patients admitted from high-risk settings, including those with frequent contact with healthcare settings or who are care-home residents: 22% of care-home residents are colonised with MRSA (Barr et al. 2007).
- All emergency admissions: some NHS Trusts consider it simpler and more reliable if screening is conducted on all patients admitted through the Accident and Emergency unit or on to medical reception units. Therefore in practice, Mrs Lewis should have been screened for MRSA when she was first admitted to hospital after fracturing her hip. The screening should be carried out as soon as it is practically possible but should not delay treatment or admission.

The DH (2010b) operational guidance for screening for MRSA colonisation confirmed the requirement that Trusts should screen all people with relevant elective admissions either before or on admission. The exceptions to this rule are children, unless they are already in a high-risk group, and people having certain minor surgical procedures. The DH (2010b) also requires that all relevant emergency admissions are screened. Further guidance is available from the DH and the HPA, and the DH expects that there will be local protocols in place.

People who are emergency mental health admissions need not be screened unless they have other risk factors for MRSA (e.g. chronic wound, intravenous drug user, admitted after a surgical procedure or an admission to an acute Trust). Thus, if Stacey is an intravenous drug user, the Trust protocol may advise MRSA screening.

ACTIVITY

Have you observed or been involved in MRSA screening in the practice setting? If so, what sites were swabbed and how was this performed?

Which sites to swab will be part of locally agreed protocols. However, the essential site to swab is the nose as it is the most common site for MRSA, and most patients positive at other sites also have positive nose swabs. Secondary sites are the axilla and groin, and skin lesions should be swabbed too. Coia et al. (2006) also advised swabbing catheter sites and tracheostomies, where present, and collecting a catheter urine specimen, a sputum specimen if the patient has a productive cough, and possibly a throat swab.

You should act according to local policy when collecting specimens, but the following procedures have been recommended for swabs. A transport (culture) medium is required, and swabs taken from drier areas, such as the nose and skin, should first be moistened by dipping them into sterile saline or the culture medium. Ensure you follow the general principles of specimen collection described in the previous section, including the labelling of the swabs and completion of accompanying information.

Obtaining a nose swab

- The patient should sit facing a strong light source with the head tilted back.
- The moistened swab is rubbed several times firmly around the anterior nares of each nostril (Ayliffe et al. 2001).

Obtaining a throat swab

- A tongue depressor and a good light source are needed. This procedure is unpleasant and may cause the patient to gag.
- The swab, taken quickly but gently, should be rubbed over the pharyngeal wall, the tonsillar fossa or both. Saliva contamination should be avoided (Ayliffe et al. 2001).

Learning outcome 2: Explain how MRSA suppression (decolonisation) procedures are carried out

If MRSA is isolated from the screening, suppression procedures are commenced. Although long-term effects of the suppression procedures may be limited (Simor et al. 2007), as soon as the procedure is implemented the presence and shedding of MRSA are reduced significantly, and the risk of the patient infecting themselves or transmitting MRSA to another patient is much reduced.

For patients being admitted for routine surgery, local protocols should guide when to commence suppression, but this timeframe may be 5 days preadmission as the effect may not be sustained if started too early (Simor et al. 2007). The HPA (2009) advises the suppression regime should consist of the following:

- The use of an antibacterial shampoo and body wash daily, for 5 days. The patient should moisten their skin first and then apply the solution, giving particular attention to known carriage sites such as the axilla, groin and perineum. After washing, the person must use clean towels, sheets and clothing. The patient should wash items used separately from the family's laundry, using as high a temperature as the fabric allows.
- The application of an antibacterial nasal cream three times a day for 5 days. The patient should apply a pea-sized amount to the inner surface of each nostril and should be able to taste the ointment at the back of the throat.

ACTIVITY

What would patients need to be able to carry out MRSA suppression procedures effectively at home?

Patients will need clear explanations about what they need to do and why it is important. They will need a prescription for the antibacterial shampoo and body wash and the nasal cream and clear instructions about how to apply these materials. They will need laundry facilities and a good supply of clean bed-linen, towels and clothes. For some patients, these items may not be readily available; for example, consider what facilities a patient in a hostel might have.

Patients admitted as emergencies and then found to be colonised with MRSA are likely to need assistance to carry out suppression procedures, depending on their mobility.

Summary

- MRSA screening has been implemented to detect patients who are colonised with MRSA.
- If patients are found to be colonised with MRSA, suppression procedures should be applied, either before admission for patients having routine surgery or after emergency admission.

ISOLATION PROCEDURES (SOURCE AND PROTECTIVE)

Isolation procedures are used to prevent the spread of infection from an infected or colonised person to others in healthcare settings. This type of isolation procedure is termed 'source isolation'. 'Protective isolation' is used to protect people who are highly susceptible to infections from others in healthcare settings. In both types of isolation, standard precautions, including hand hygiene, personal protective equipment and waste disposal, are central. The DH (2007) recommends that single rooms are always preferable for isolating infected patients but that cohort nursing for a group of patients with the same organism (e.g. MRSA) is an alternative if single-room capacity is exceeded. For cohort nursing, they advise these key points:

- Patient movements for non-clinical reasons should be minimal.
- There should be designated staff for these patients.
- If there is no designated ward, use a bay within a ward – but bays should have doors that can be closed, thus physically separating them from other patients.
- In critical care, cohorting may need to occur in a specific area of the unit.

The Norovirus Working Party (2012) also advised that where single occupancy rooms are not available for people with norovirus, cohort nursing can be used.

LEARNING OUTCOMES

By the end of this section, you will be able to:
1 explain when source isolation is necessary and key principles of care;
2 discuss when protective isolation is necessary and what it entails;
3 reflect on the importance of communication and be aware of whom to inform when isolation is required.

Learning outcome 1: Explain when source isolation is necessary and key principles of care

ACTIVITY

Mrs Lewis is being nursed in isolation as she has MRSA. Why is this necessary? What infection control measures would underpin her care?

When patients, like Mrs Lewis, are identified as MRSA positive, either because they have an MRSA infection or because they were identified through screening as being an asymptomatic carrier, they should be isolated to reduce the risk of transmission to other patients. You probably identified that infection control measures underpinning Mrs Lewis's care include hand hygiene, personal protective equipment and correct waste disposal – and all these measures are important. Coia et al. (2006) advised that a standard approach to isolation should be taken using sound infection control principles rather than specific precautions for patients with MRSA.

The DH (2007) identified these key points for any patient being isolated; all are relevant to Mrs Lewis:

- Regardless of glove use, there should be high standards of hand decontamination, with hand hygiene before and after each direct patient contact.
- All staff and visitors assisting with patient care or in contact with their immediate environment should wear aprons.
- Disposable gloves should be worn when in contact with bodily fluids or contaminated items. In addition, Coia et al. (2006) advise gloves should be worn by any staff entering the isolation room of a patient with MRSA.
- Fans should not be used.
- Notes and charts should be kept outside the room/bay/area, preferably stored in washable covers or folders.
- Where possible, equipment should be single use. Multiuse equipment must be decontaminated as per manufacturer's instructions/local guidance.
- Linen should be treated as infectious.
- All waste should be disposed of as hazardous waste.
- Cleaning procedures should be rigorously applied with enhanced and terminal cleaning procedures.
- Transfer and movement of patients should be minimised and only take place for clinical reasons. The receiving area must be informed. Hand hygiene and personal protective equipment should be used when transferring. Equipment used for transferring (e.g. a trolley) should be decontaminated.

Any other special precautions used depend on the type of infection and its specific route of transmission. Check back to Table 3.1 if you need to recap on these routes of transmission. Patients with airborne infections (e.g. chickenpox, pulmonary tuberculosis) should, as a minimum, be nursed in a well-ventilated single room with the door closed, but ideally a negative-pressure ventilated isolation room would be used (Wilson 2006). In most cases, when a single room is necessary for isolation, the door should be kept shut; but the IPCT can advise concerning individual cases; for example, when a patient is confused and their safety could be jeopardised by closing the door. Patients, such as Stacey, with bloodborne infections (unless bleeding) can often be managed in the open ward using standard infection control precautions. These precautions include the safe management of sharps and the routine use of protective clothing where contact with body fluids or blood is likely.

ACTIVITY

To prevent spread of infection to other people, what precautions should be taken if someone develops diarrhoea and vomiting? Consider both small community-based units and hospital situations.

For a community setting, you might have identified the following:

- Good personal hygiene is required, particularly handwashing before eating and after using the toilet.
- Normal crockery and cutlery are usually sufficient. Bacteria are easily removed by washing in hot water and detergent. However, cleaning of crockery and cutlery is best done at high temperatures in a dishwasher.
- If dishes are washed by hand, then clean hot water should be used with detergent. The items should be rinsed and left to drain, rather than being dried with a cloth, as such cloths are easily contaminated. Dishcloths should be disposable.
- If possible, the person should be allocated a toilet for their sole use.
- If there is a suspected outbreak of gastrointestinal illness – defined as when two or more clients or staff are affected by unexplained diarrhoea or vomiting – then further action may be needed, particularly if there are other vulnerable people within the residence. In small staffed units, the other residents' GPs and the IPCT need to be informed. Stool specimens should be obtained from those affected even if they no longer have symptoms.

If gastroenteritis occurs in an institutional setting, such as a hospital, care home or prison, affected patients must be transferred to single rooms where at all possible. Standard isolation procedures should then be put in place (as previously discussed), and the infection prevention and control department should be informed.

Detailed guidance about managing specific infections is available. For norovirus, see the Norovirus Working Party (2012). For *C. difficile*, see the Department of Health and Health Protection Agency's guidance (DH and HPA 2009), which includes that healthcare professionals should remember the pneumonic SIGHT when encountering a patient with potentially infectious diarrhoea:

- **S**uspect that the person may be infective where there is no other likely cause for diarrhoea.
- **I**solate the patient and consult with the IPCT while determining the cause of the diarrhoea.
- **G**loves and aprons must be used for all contacts with the patient and their environment.
- **H**andwashing with soap and water should be carried out before and after each contact with the patient and the patient's environment.
- **T**est the stool for toxin, by sending a specimen immediately.

Learning outcome 2: Discuss when protective isolation is necessary and what it entails

Isolation is also used for patients who are extremely vulnerable to infectious diseases because their immune system is compromised. Protective isolation is used to protect patients from infection risks from themselves and others rather than to protect others from any risk that they pose.

ACTIVITY

What conditions might lead to patients being severely immunocompromised? What precautions would be necessary?

Neutropenia

Neutropenia is an abnormally low neutrophil count. Neutrophils are white blood cells and they ingest bacteria, so neutropenia affects the body's ability to fight off infections.

Examples include patients with prolonged **neutropenia** as a result of chemotherapy for leukaemia, lymphoma and bone marrow transplant (Gould and Brooker 2008). Patients in protective isolation should not be cared for by staff with infections or who are looking after people with infections on the same shift (Wilson 2006). Protective isolation requires single rooms, thorough handwashing, and use of aprons and gloves.

Management of these patients includes consideration of the food they eat. Most food contains microorganisms, and these microorganisms are not usually harmful in small numbers. Wilson (2006) advises that food for immunocompromised patients must be served without delay and must not be reheated. Eggs must be cooked thoroughly, and fresh fruit should be washed and peeled. These patients should avoid soft cheeses, undercooked meat and fish, patés and freshly made salad. Wilson (2006) advises that fresh tap water and pasteurised milk are acceptable. Bottled water is not recommended due to variable storage and manufacturing conditions.

Invasive procedures are a major threat to immunosuppressed patients, and strict protocols must be followed when these are used (Gould and Brooker 2008). Finally, visitors should have no obvious signs of infection and must decontaminate their hands before visiting the patient.

Learning outcome 3: Reflect on the importance of communication and be aware of whom to inform when isolation is required

ACTIVITY

List the key people who should be informed when a decision is made to isolate a patient. Try to link your answer to Mrs Lewis's case.

You may have identified the following: Mrs Lewis herself, her family and friends, domestic staff, the IPCT and possibly other departments (e.g. radiography, bed management teams). Further details about explanations to these key people are now discussed.

Explanations to patients and families

Infections cause emotional as well as physical distress. Webber et al. (2012) found that patients in isolation due to being colonised with MRSA had minimal knowledge about either their MRSA or why they were being isolated and, with no outward symptoms of MRSA, they found the concept difficult to grasp. They expressed that healthcare staff did not explain to their families so the task fell to them, which they found burdensome. However, in Barratt et al.'s (2011) study, some patients had received good explanations and these helped to reduce anxiety. The DH (2007) advised that staff should provide affected patients and visitors with explanations of their infection, isolation procedures and treatment. Patient information leaflets are available for certain infections, such as chickenpox and MRSA, and these leaflets can back up verbal explanations and should be available in different languages.

Some clinical areas ask that visitors enter isolation rooms only after obtaining permission and instruction from the nurse in charge. Some isolation rooms have posters informing all visiting staff what procedures they must follow. Although children and susceptible visitors should be advised of the risks of visiting, for most infections the risks are minimal, as the visitors do not have contact with body fluids (Wilson 2006). They should be advised to wash their hands before leaving the room.

Explanations to domestic staff

The facilities supervisor and their staff working in the department should be informed of any patients who are being isolated. A dedicated mop, bucket and disposable cleaning cloths should be provided for the room. The domestic will need to wear apron and gloves when cleaning, and these items must be disposed of before leaving the room. Most microorganisms are not able to survive on clean, dry surfaces for long (Wilson 2006), so the environment need not be a major factor in the transmission of infections. The normal standard of cleaning should be maintained, and domestic staff should be reassured that the risks to their own health are minimal if protective clothing is worn and careful handwashing takes place. This reassurance is very important as otherwise the standard of cleaning may suffer (Wilson 2006).

Infection prevention and control team

The clinical area will often have a list of communicable infections that indicates whether isolation is necessary and highlights which material from the patient is potentially infectious. If in doubt, the IPCT can offer advice. The IPCT must be contacted if a patient has MRSA or has been infected, colonised or transferred from a ward with MRSA cases in the recent past (usually defined as 6 months). Those patients isolated because of other infectious diseases should be notified to the IPCT too. Certain infectious diseases are notifiable to local authorities, usually by the doctor making the diagnosis (Wilson 2006).

Visits to departments

Staff in other departments and areas that the patient may need to visit should be informed so that any special arrangements can be made. If possible, investigations should be carried out immediately so that patients do not wait in communal areas in contact with other patients (Coia et al. 2006). This information would be relevant to Mrs Lewis if she requires a hip x-ray. Porters need not wear protective clothing, but they should be advised to wash their hands on completion of the journey (Wilson 2006). Any transporting staff with skin abrasions should wear gloves, and the trolley or chair should be cleaned with detergent and hot water, or in accordance with local policy. Linen use should comply with local guidelines.

Managing the psychological effects of isolation

ACTIVITY

- How might Mrs Lewis feel, being isolated in a sideroom?
- What might nurses do to reduce the effects of isolation?

Studies of patients' experiences of being in isolation for MRSA revealed many negative feelings, for example, anger, fear of contaminating others, fear of telling others, apathy and depression (Webber et al. 2012). Feelings of stigmatisation associated with MRSA and isolation have been expressed (Barratt et al. 2011; Webber et al. 2012). One patient said, 'You don't feel like a human being' (Webber et al. 2012, p. 45). In the study by Barratt et al. (2011), some patients' families were reluctant to visit because of fear of catching MRSA, causing patients to feel hurt and abandoned. Patients viewed isolation as lonely and boring, especially long-term patients and patients with few visitors (Webber et al. 2012) and being in a single room prevented socialisation with other patients (Barratt et al. 2011). However, some did appreciate the benefits of a single room (Barratt et al. 2011; Webber et al. 2012).

Nurses should be sensitive to the psychological implications of being labelled infectious and of being isolated. Patients who are isolated may receive less attention and contact from nurses as they are not in immediate view, and because nurses must put on gloves and apron before entering, quick casual contact is reduced. In the study by Barratt et al. (2011), patients gave various examples of how they felt that their contact with healthcare professionals and access to care were reduced due to being in isolation with MRSA. It is important for nurses to try to reduce patients' fears and problems of isolation and to ensure that they approach people in an understanding manner (see Chapter 2).

Summary

- Although standard precautions are sufficient to prevent cross-infection in many circumstances, in some situations additional measures are necessary in the form of source isolation.
- Source isolation requires correct use of hand hygiene, gloves, aprons and waste disposal and usually a single room for the person who is identified as a source of infection – with, if possible, equipment for their sole use.
- For patients who are severely immunocompromised, protective isolation may be required.
- When isolation is necessary, good communication with patients, relatives and staff is essential.
- Nurses should be aware of the psychological impact of isolation and provide support and information.

CHAPTER SUMMARY

This chapter has highlighted the problem of healthcare-associated infection and covered important practices for preventing cross-infection. Infection prevention and control polices and principles underpinning cross-infection were introduced. Standard principles and precautions for preventing cross-infection were outlined, and each chapter section has focused on the practical skills involved and how they can be applied in different situations. Having worked your way through this chapter, you should now be aware of the fundamental principles that underpin the prevention of cross-infection. The principles are relevant to all other practical nursing skills, and this chapter is therefore referred to within many other chapters in this book.

The Code of Professional Conduct (NMC 2008) demands that nurses protect and support the health of individual patients and clients and the health of the wider community, while being personally accountable for their practice. Therefore, there is a professional as well as moral imperative to assist the prevention of cross-infection, which is of fundamental importance to the health, safety and well-being of patients, nurses and other healthcare practitioners alike.

REFERENCES

Ayliffe, G.A.J., Babb, J.R. and Taylor, L.J. 2001. *Hospital-Acquired Infection: Principles and Prevention,* 3rd edn. London: Arnold.

Aziz, A.M. 2009. Variations in aseptic technique and implications for infection control. *British Journal of Nursing* 18(1): 26–30.

Barr, B., Wilcox, M., Brady, A., Parnell, P., Darby, B. and Tompkins, D. 2007. Prevalence of methicillin-resistant *Staphylococcus aureus* colonization among older residents of care homes in the United Kingdom. *Infection Control and Hospital Epidemiology: The Official Journal of the Society of Hospital Epidemiologists of America* 28: 853–9.

Barratt, R., Shaban, R. and Moyle, W. 2011. Behind barriers: Patients' perceptions of source isolation for methicillin-resistant *Staphylococcus aureus* (MRSA). *Australian Journal of Advanced Nursing* 28(2): 53–9.

Coia, J.E., Duckworth, G.J., Edwards, D.I., et al. 2006. Guidelines for the control and prevention of meticillin-resistant *Staphylococcus aureus* (MRSA) in healthcare facilities. *Journal of Hospital Infection* 63: S1–44.

Council of the European Union 2010 Council Directive 2010/32/EU. Implementing the framework agreement on prevention from sharps injuries in the hospital and healthcare sector concluded by HOSPEEM and EPSU. *Official Journal of European Union.* Available from: http://eur-lex.europa.eu/LexUriServ/LexUriServ.do?uri=OJ:L:2010:134:0066:0072: EN:PDF (Accessed on 14 January 2013).

Dancer, S.J. 2002. Handwashing hazard? *Journal of Hospital Infection* 52: 76.

Department of Health (DH). 2002. *Action for Health – Health Action Plans and Health Facilitation.* London: DH.

Department of Health (DH). 2007. *Isolating Patients with Healthcare-Associated Infection: Summary of Best Practice.* London: DH.

Department of Health (DH). 2009. *The Health and Social Care Act 2008: Code of Practice for Health and Adult Social Care on the Prevention and Control of Infections and Related Guidance.* Gateway Reference 13072. London: DH.

Department of Health (DH). 2010a. *Uniforms and Workwear: Guidance on Uniform and Workwear Policies for NHS Employers.* Gateway Reference 13712. London: DH.

Department of Health (DH). 2010b. *MRSA Screening – Operational Guidance 3.* Gateway Reference 13482. London: DH. Available from: http://webarchive.nationalarchives. gov.uk/20130107105354/http://www.dh.gov.uk/en/Publicationsandstatistics/ Lettersandcirculars/Dearcolleagueletters/DH_114961 (Accessed on 21 September 2013).

Department of Health (DH). 2011a. *Antimicrobial Stewardship: Start Smart – Then Focus.* Gateway Reference 16853. London: DH.

Department of Health (DH). 2011b. *Safe Management of Health Care Waste.* Version 2. Gateway Reference 15645. London: DH.

Department of Health (DH). 2012. *Water Sources and Potential Pseudomonas Aeruginosa Contamination of Taps and Water Systems — Advice for Augmented Care Units.* Gateway Reference 17334. London: DH.

Department of Health and Health Protection Agency (DH and HPA). 2009. *Clostridium difficile Infection: How to Deal with the Problem.* Gateway Reference 9833. London: DH.

Elhassan, H.A. and Dixon, T. 2012. MRSA contaminated venepuncture tourniquets in clinical practice. *Postgraduate Medical Journal* 88(1038): 194–7.

Flores, A. and Pevalin, D.J. 2007. Glove use and compliance with hand hygiene. *Nursing Times* 103(38): 46–8.

Fuller, C., Savage, J., Besser, S., Hayward, A., Cooper, B. and Stone, S. 2011. "The dirty hand in the latex glove": A study of hand hygiene compliance when gloves are worn. *Infection Control & Hospital Epidemiology* 32(12): 1194–9.

Gould, D. and Brooker, C. 2008. *Infection Prevention and Control: Applied Microbiology for Healthcare*, 2nd edn. London: Macmillan.

Health Facilities Scotland (HFS). 2010. *Scottish Health Technical Note 3 NHS Scotland Waste Management Guidance Part A. Best Practice Overview.* Available from: http://www.hfs. scot.nhs.uk/publications-1/environment/shtns/ (Accessed on 14 January 2013).

Health Protection Agency (HPA). 2008. *Eye of the Needle: United Kingdom Surveillance of Significant Occupational Exposures to Bloodborne Viruses in Healthcare Workers.* London: HPA.

Health Protection Agency (HPA). 2009. *Meticillin Resistant Staphylococcus aureus (MRSA) Screening and Suppression.* Quick reference guide for primary care – for consultation and local adaptation. HPA. Available from: http://www.hpa.org.uk/webc/HPAwebFile/ HPAweb_C/1194947336805 (Accessed on 15 January 2013).

Health Protection Agency (HPA). 2011. *Surveillance of Surgical Site Infections in NHS Hospitals in England, 2010/2011.* London: HPA.

Health Protection Agency (HPA). 2012a. *English National Point Prevalence Survey on Healthcare-Associated Infections and Antimicrobial Use, 2011.* Available from: http:// www.hpa.org.uk/Publications/InfectiousDiseases/AntimicrobialAndHealthcareAsso ciatedInfections/1205HCAIEnglishPPSforhcaiandamu2011prelim/ (Accessed on 12 January 2013).

Health Protection Agency (HPA). 2012b. *UK Standards for Microbiology Investigations: Investigation of Skin, Superficial and Non-Surgical Wound Swabs.* B 11 Issue 5.1. Available from: http://www.hpa.org.uk/webc/HPAwebFile/HPAweb_C/1317132856530 (Accessed on 14 January 2013).

Health Protection Scotland (HPS). 2013. *National Infection Prevention and Control Manual.* Available from: http://www.documents.hps.scot.nhs.uk/hai/infection-control/ic-manual/ ipcm-p-v2.1.pdf (Accessed 30 October 2013).

National Institute for Health and Clinical Excellence (NICE). 2012. *Prevention and Control of Healthcare-Associated Infections in Primary and Community Care.* Clinical Guidelines 139. London: NICE.

National Patient Safety Agency (NPSA). 2007. *Promoting Safer Use of Injectable Medicines: NPSA Template Standard Operating Procedure for Use of Injectable Medicines.* London: NPSA. Available from: http://www.nrls.npsa.nhs.uk/resources/?entryid45=59812 (Accessed on 14 January 2013).

National Patient Safety Agency (NPSA). 2008. *Clean Hands Save Lives: Patient Safety Alert.* London: NPSA.

Norovirus Working Party. 2012. *Guidelines for the Management of Norovirus Outbreaks in Acute and Community Health and Social Care Settings.* Available from: http://www.hpa.org.uk/webw/HPAweb&HPAwebStandard/HPAweb_C/1317131647275 (Accessed on 11 January 2013).

Nursing and Midwifery Council (NMC). 2008. *The Code: Standards of Conduct, Performance and Ethics for Nurses and Midwives.* London: NMC.

Nursing and Midwifery Council (NMC). 2010. *Standards for Pre-Registration Nursing Education.* London: NMC.

Parker, L.J. 1999. Current recommendations for isolation practices in nursing. *British Journal of Nursing* 8: 881–7.

Patton, H. 2010. Identifying wound infection: Taking a swab. *Wound Essentials* 5: 64–6.

Pittet, D., Mourouga, P., Perneger, T.V. et al. 1999. Compliance with handwashing in a teaching hospital. *Annals of Internal Medicine* 130(2): 126–30.

Pratt, R.J., Pellowe, C., Wilson, J.A., et al. 2007. National evidence-based guidelines for preventing healthcare-associated infections in NHS, England. *Journal of Hospital Infection* 65S: S1–64.

Price, P.B. 1938. The classification of transient and resident microbes. *Journal of Infectious Disease* 63: 301–8.

Public Health England. 2013. *Immunization against Infectious Disease: The Green Book.* Available from: https://www.gov.uk/government/organisations/public-health-england/series/immunisation-against-infectious-disease-the-green-book (Accessed on 21 September 2013).

Rowley, S., Clare, S., Macqueen, S. and Molyneux, R. 2010. ANTT v2: An updated practice framework for aseptic technique. *British Journal of Nursing* (Intravenous Supplement) 19(5): S5–11.

Royal College of Nursing (RCN). 2011. *Sharps Safety: RCN Guidance to Support Implementation of the EU Directive 2010/32/EU on the Prevention of Sharps Injuries in the Health Care Sector.* London: RCN.

Royal College of Nursing (RCN). 2012a. *Wipe It Out – One Chance to Get It Right: Essential Practice for Infection Prevention and Control: Guidance for Nursing Staff.* London: RCN.

Royal College of Nursing (RCN). 2012b. *Tools of the Trade: Glove Use and Prevention of Contact Dermatitis.* London: RCN.

Sax, H., Allegranzi, B., Uçkay, I., Larson, E., Boyce, J. and Pittet, D. 2007. My five moments for hand hygiene': A user-centred design approach to understand, train, monitor and report hand hygiene. *Journal of Hospital Infection* 67(1): 9–21.

Simor, A.E., Philip, I., McGreer, A. et al. 2007. Randomized controlled trial of chlorhexidine gluconate for washing, intranasal mupirocin, and rifampin and doxycycline versus no treatment for the eradication of methicillin-resistant *Staphylococcus aureus* colonization. *Clinical Infectious Diseases* 44: 178–85.

Stone, S.H., Fuller, C. and Savage, J. 2012. Evaluation of the national Cleanyourhands campaign to reduce *Staphylococcus aureus* bacteraemia and *Clostridium difficile* infection in hospitals in England and Wales by improved hand hygiene: Four year, prospective, ecological, interrupted time series study. *British Medical Journal* 344 e3005. doi: 10.1136/bmj.e3005

Storr, J. and Kilpatrick, C. 2012. Hand hygiene improvement in the community: A systems approach. *Wound Care* (March): S24–29.

Thomas, D. and Woods, H. 2003. *Working with People with Learning Disabilities: Theory and Practice.* London: Jessica Kingsley.

Unsworth, J. 2011. District nurses and aseptic technique: Where did it all go wrong? *British Journal of Community Nursing* 16(1): 29–34.

Webber, K.L., Macpherson, S., Meagher, A., Hutchinson, S. and Lewis, B. 2012. The impact of strict isolation on MRSA positive patients: an action-based study undertaken in a rehabilitation center. *Rehabilitation Nursing* 37(1): 43–50.

Wilcox, M.H., Fawley, W.N., Wigglesworth, N., et al. 2003. Comparison of the effect of detergent versus hypochlorite on environmental contamination and incidence of *Clostridium difficile* infection. *Journal of Hospital Infection* 54: 109–14.

Wilson, A., Hayman, S., Folan, P., et al. 2006. Computer keyboards and the spread of MRSA. *Journal of Hospital Infection* 62(3): 390–2.

Wilson, J. 2006. *Infection Control in Clinical Practice,* 3rd edn. London: Baillière Tindall.

World Health Organization (WHO). 2009. *WHO Guidelines on Hand Hygiene in Health Care.* Geneva: WHO.

World Health Organization (WHO). 2010. *WHO Best Practices for Injections and Related Procedures Toolkit.* Geneva: WHO.

4 Measuring and Monitoring Vital Signs

Sue Maddex

Measuring and monitoring the five vital signs of temperature, pulse, respiration, blood pressure and oxygen saturation are essential parts of many nurses' roles each day. All student nurses should learn to measure and record vital signs accurately (Nursing and Midwifery Council [NMC] 2010), as acting upon patients' vital sign measurements in a timely and appropriate manner can contribute to patients' well-being. Vital signs measurement is part of the overall nursing assessment of patients; it establishes a baseline for future comparison and helps to identify abnormalities. Patient Safety First (2008) stresses the importance of physiological observations being recorded and interpreted accurately for all adult patients admitted to acute hospitals so that deterioration is recognised early. This chapter aims to prepare you to undertake these measurements skilfully, based on best evidence, and to begin to interpret findings.

Vital signs monitoring forms part of early-warning track and trigger systems that alert staff to patients' potential deterioration (see Chapter 11). Pain assessment is also important to assess when recording vital signs (see Chapter 12).

This chapter includes the following topics:

- Key principles in vital signs measurement
- Measuring and recording temperature
- Measuring and recording the pulse
- Measuring and recording respirations
- Measuring and recording blood pressure
- Measuring oxygen saturation by pulse oximetry
- Neurological assessment

Recommended biology reading:

The following questions will help you to focus on biology underpinning this chapter's skills. Use your recommended textbook to find answers to the following questions:

• What is homeostasis and why is it important?

Temperature control

• Which body systems are involved in thermoregulation?
• How is heat generated within the body?

• How is heat lost from the body?
• What effect does temperature have on cellular function?
• What happens if the body starts to get too hot or too cold?
• Why do we appear flushed when too warm?

Cardiovascular system
• What are the components of the cardiovascular system?
• Which vessels usually carry oxygenated blood?
• Why does blood travel in one direction?
• Name the four chambers of the heart, the great vessels and valves. Draw a diagram of the heart and label these structures. Indicate the direction in which oxygenated and deoxygenated blood flows through the heart.
• What are the layers of the heart wall and what types of tissue are they composed of?
• How does the heart contract in such a coordinated way? Explore the route taken by impulses through the myocardium.
• Myocardial tissue needs its own blood supply. Where are the coronary vessels located? What would result from their blockage?
• Compare the structures of arteries, capillaries and veins. Which vessels permit gaseous exchange and why? Which vessels contain valves?
• When tissues are damaged, an inflammatory process is initiated to repair the damage. What are the clinical signs of inflammation? What role does histamine play in inflammation? Why is inflammation of brain tissue potentially life-threatening?
• What role does blood play in maintaining cellular homeostasis?
• What are the components of blood and what specific roles do they play?
• Where are blood cells produced?
• What is haemostasis? Why is it important?
• What is blood pressure and how is it maintained?

Respiratory system
• What are the components of the respiratory system (e.g. airways, respiratory muscles, control mechanisms) and what are their functions?
• How do these functions contribute to maintaining homeostasis?
  • What is the main function of the respiratory system?
  • How is ventilation controlled?
  • How is oxygen transported in the body?
• Where does gaseous exchange occur? Which gases are being exchanged?
• Why does this exchange occur? What may affect this exchange?
• How does inspiration occur? What is the stimulus for us to breathe?
• What are the proportions of gases in atmospheric, alveolar and expired air?
• What factors are required for adequate tissue oxygenation to occur? Consider the role blood plays in this oxygenation.

Nervous system
• What are the different areas of the brain?
• What are the components of the nervous system?
• What is the role of the autonomic nervous system?
• What do the parasympathetic and sympathetic nervous systems do?

PRACTICE SCENARIOS

Observation and recording of a person's vital signs are carried out for many reasons. The following scenarios are used to assist you to relate your learning of these skills to people you might encounter in practice settings.

Adult

Mrs Anne Parkinson is a 56-year-old woman who has been taken to the Accident and Emergency unit by ambulance after a head injury received by falling from her bicycle. She cannot remember the accident but was apparently unresponsive for 2–3 minutes afterwards. She is alert but appears disorientated. Her husband is present.

Learning disability

Ken O'Reilly is a 49-year-old man with **Down's syndrome** and a moderate learning disability. He has some verbal communication difficulties. He lives in a small group home with a live-in staff team. Ken is known to the community learning disability nurse (CLDN) as he is prone to chronic chest infections. He has oxygen therapy and a nebuliser at home, which the staff team have been trained to support him with. The nurse, while carrying out routine **health facilitator's** training with the staff team, is informed that Ken is unwell and is asked for advice. The nurse records Ken's vital signs and advises the staff to arrange for the general practitioner (GP) to visit to carry out further health assessment.

Mental health

Natalie Turney is 21 years old. She has been admitted as a voluntary patient to an acute mental health ward with severe depression. After going home for a day, she returns to the ward, appearing unsteady on her feet and she has a strong smell of alcohol. Her speech is very slurred and she is quite uncommunicative. When the staff ask her if she has taken any tablets, she mentions some little yellow pills and paracetamol. However, she won't give details about the quantity or when she took them.

EQUIPMENT REQUIRED FOR THIS CHAPTER

Before working through this chapter, find out what vital signs recording equipment is available within the skills laboratory or your practice area. Look for:
- thermometers: may be tympanic, electronic probes, chemical disposable;
- sphygmomanometers: electronic and/or manual equipment;
- pulse oximeter for recording oxygen saturations;
- electronic monitoring devices which record temperature, pulse, blood pressure, oxygen saturation – check your local Trust to identify which devices are regularly used and check that you are aware of how these should be operated.

You also need a watch with a second hand or stopwatch device, a pen torch and observation charts for temperature, pulse, respiration, pulse oximetry, blood pressure and neurological assessment. You may wish to work through the sections with a colleague so that you can practise this chapter's skills.

Down's syndrome

Down's syndrome is a congenital condition caused by an extra chromosome, often leading to a characteristic physical appearance and a low intelligence quotient (IQ). Other physical effects (e.g. heart disease) are often associated with it. There is an increased risk of dementia at a younger age.

Health facilitator

The role of the health facilitator focuses on an individual's health outcomes and can be undertaken by a range of people, including support workers, family carers, friends and advocates as well as health professionals; see *Health Action Planning and Health Facilitation for People with Learning Disabilities: Good Practice Guidance* (DH 2009).

KEY PRINCIPLES IN VITAL SIGNS MEASUREMENT

When measuring, monitoring and recording vital signs, there are some key principles that you should always apply. These principles are explored in this first section, before the later sections that focus on specific vital signs.

LEARNING OUTCOMES

By the end of this section, you will be able to:
1 explain key principles that apply to the measurement of vital signs;
2 reflect on how the nurse's approach will affect vital signs measurement;
3 consider how technological developments are influencing vital signs measurement.

Learning outcome 1: Explain key principles that apply to the measurement of vital signs

As explained in the introduction to this chapter, vital signs measurement is a key aspect of a patient's assessment. The results contribute to decisions about further investigations and treatment, including medication prescriptions. Therefore, accurate measurement is crucial.

ACTIVITY   What might affect the accuracy of vital signs measurement?

You might have considered the following:

The equipment used. It is crucial that equipment in use works correctly. The National Institute for Health and Clinical Excellence (NICE 2011a) highlights that electronic devices used for vital signs measurement should be properly validated, maintained and regularly recalibrated according to manufacturer's instructions. This point also applies to manual equipment. When new devices are introduced into clinical settings, staff must be trained to use them correctly, in accordance with manufacturers' instructions.

The competence of the person recording vital signs. Although these skills are frequently used, they may not always be performed in a competent manner (Rose 2010). Competence includes how to practically carry out the skill, including documentation, the approach of the nurse (discussed further in learning outcome 2) and the underpinning knowledge and understanding of how to interpret the results and plan appropriate actions. Documenting the skills and reporting the measurements are crucial to ensure that abnormalities or potential problems are identified and addressed promptly. In any practice setting, ensure that you become familiar with the documentation in use, including early-warning score/track and trigger systems (see Chapter 11). After recording the observations, discuss them with a qualified nurse, so that appropriate actions can be taken if observations fall outside the normal parameters.

It is essential that you learn and then rehearse vital signs measurement frequently to develop competence and confidence. Practising vital signs skills within simulated environments can help you to contextualise these skills (Everett and Wright 2011) and support the acquisition of your clinical skills (Meechan et al. 2011). Take every opportunity to practise vital signs measurement in different situations, for example, emergencies, and with people across the life span. Ensure that you practise with both manual and electronic equipment; Lewis (2011) warns of overreliance of technology in vital signs monitoring, causing deskilling.

Vital signs measurement across the life span. The Royal College of Nursing (2007) highlighted that practitioners who assess, measure and monitor vital signs in infants, children and young people should be competent in observing their physiological status and be aware of vital signs parameters for different age ranges. This book focuses on adults but in each section, you will be advised about the normal parameters across the age range and guided to further resources. How vital signs may alter during pregnancy and key factors in interpreting vital signs in pregnancy are also highlighted, as a nurse may care for pregnant women when they have other health issues.

Learning outcome 2: Reflect on how the nurse's approach will affect vital signs measurement.

ACTIVITY

Reflect on how the nurse's approach to a person might affect both the accuracy of vital signs measurement and the person's care experience.

When carrying out nursing observations, effective non-verbal and verbal communication skills are essential (covered in Chapter 2). You may be aware that heart rate, respiratory rate and blood pressure are affected by emotions, for example, fear, anxiety or anger. Therefore, for accurate measurements, patients need to feel comfortable with you and well-informed. Ensure that you introduce yourself, are friendly and kind, gain consent (e.g. 'Is it ok if I check your blood pressure?') and explain what you are doing. Taking this approach will promote accurate measurements and dignity in care. You must also foster patients' confidence in your ability to perform these skills accurately, hence the need to develop your competence. Displaying uncertainty in your skills may produce fear and anxiety in people, thus altering their vital signs measurements.

Learning outcome 3: Consider how technological developments are influencing vital signs measurement

The future of vital signs monitoring lies in further development and production of electronic devices that will record, interpret and analyse vital signs. The goal is to enhance the care of patients.

ACTIVITY

Are you aware of any technological developments relating to vital signs measurement?
Consider: What might be associated advantages and safety issues?

In the increasing world of technology, smartphone and tablet applications will undoubtedly assist healthcare professionals in their care delivery. Wireless technology for healthcare enables practitioners to offer immediate advice regarding vital signs readings to patients or other healthcare professionals. For example, patients being monitored for hypertension (high blood pressure) can send their blood pressure readings to GP surgeries for monitoring and interpretation. Paramedic crews can liaise with emergency departments regarding patients' vital signs when caring for critically ill patients. An inpatient can have vital signs results sent to the doctor's smartphone or tablet device to ensure that critically ill patients are assessed and treated in a timely manner. Safety issues include the validity of devices and applications; only those tools that are validated and accepted within your practice area should be used. Security of patient data and confidentiality must be maintained when using technology. You are advised to seek your mentor's guidance regarding the local use of technological devices in practice.

Summary

- Accuracy of vital signs measurement is crucial; equipment used must be well maintained and used correctly and competently.
- The nurse's approach to patients when recording vital signs should promote their comfort, confidence and dignity.
- Technological advances are affecting how vital signs are recorded, monitored and communicated; any devices should be validated and used safely.

MEASURING AND RECORDING TEMPERATURE

Nurses frequently measure temperature to assess whether body temperature is within the normal range. A person's body temperature is measured by a thermometer in degrees Celsius (°C). Body temperature results from a balance between heat production within the body and heat loss from the body (Marieb and Hoehn 2013). In a healthy individual, the normal core body temperature – the temperature of the organs within the cranial, thoracic and abdominal cavities – is maintained within a range of 35–37.5°C (Montague et al. 2005). This process is called **thermoregulation** and is controlled by the hypothalamus, which acts as a thermostat (Tortora and Derrikson 2011). There may be times when this process is ineffective for various reasons. Body temperature which is higher than 37.5°C is termed **pyrexia,** and a body temperature lower than 35°C is termed **hypothermia** (Montague et al. 2005).

LEARNING OUTCOMES

By the end of this section, you will be able to:

1 explain the rationale for monitoring temperature;

2 identify the sites and equipment used for measuring temperature;

3 accurately measure a person's temperature.

Learning outcome 1: Explain the rationale for monitoring temperature

ACTIVITY

What factors might influence a person's body temperature?

You may have identified the following factors:

- **Age.** Older people often have a lower body temperature as metabolic rate falls after the age of 50 years (Childs 2011). Newborn infants' ability to regulate temperature is not fully developed. Young children grow rapidly, producing heat as a by-product of metabolism, so they have a slightly higher temperature.

- **Environment.** Heat loss is influenced by environmental temperature and humidity. The body's ability to thermoregulate cannot accommodate extremes of heat and cold for long periods. Hence, hypothermia may result from prolonged exposure to cold, and heat exhaustion can arise in a very hot environment. If thermoregulation is impaired, people become susceptible to overheating or cooling. Older people are less able to respond metabolically to falling body temperature and may have decreased perception of cold (Tortora and Derrikson 2011), increasing risk for hypothermia. People with impaired cognitive function, confusion or perceptual disturbance may be unable to recognise and respond appropriately to environmental temperature changes; for example, they may go out inadequately dressed in cold weather.

- **Level of physical activity.** Muscular activity produces heat energy that contributes to maintaining body temperature; changes to muscle activity are an important part of thermoregulation (Marieb and Hoehn 2013). Muscle movement brings about heat production in the body (Norris and Siegfried 2011). In the adult, the body's natural response to cold brings about shivering leading to a large amount of heat being produced. This shivering is a physiological response to cold and is the body's attempt to raise its temperature. In the young child, however, the underdeveloped hypothalamus inhibits this action. Strenuous exercise may lead to a higher core body temperature for several hours afterwards due to heat production by muscles (Childs 2011). People with diminished mobility, due to conditions such as cerebral palsy or arthritis, may be susceptible to cold and unable to respond behaviourally by, for example, adding extra clothing, without assistance.

- **Metabolic rate.** The body's metabolic processes are a source of heat production. People with an excessive metabolic rate, for example, people with an overactive thyroid gland, may have a higher than normal body temperature. Underactivity of the thyroid gland results in a condition termed **myxoedema** and a low metabolic rate. Low metabolic rates may cause low body temperatures (see http://www.hormone.org/Thyroid/).

- **Time of day.** A roughly 24-hour cycle in a physiological process in living human beings, such as body temperature, is referred to as a circadian rhythm. Body temperature normally falls during sleep and so tends to be lowest at night and rises during the day, peaking in the early evening.

- **Drugs.** Alcohol diminishes perception of cold, impairs shivering and causes vasodilation, thus predisposing an individual to a lowered body temperature. Sedative and narcotic drugs may reduce perception of cold and thus the likelihood of appropriate behavioural responses (Marieb and Hoehn 2013).
- **Infection.** One of the body's responses to infection is to raise body temperature; the thermostat of the hypothalamus is reset, causing increased heat production and inhibition of heat loss (Marieb and Hoehn 2013).
- **Menstrual cycle.** Many women have higher body temperature around ovulation (Childs 2011).
- **Eating.** Digesting and metabolising food can produce enough heat to raise body temperature slightly (Childs 2011).

Nurses must take all these factors into account when interpreting temperature measurements.

ACTIVITY

For each of this chapter's scenarios, explain reasons why you might record the person's temperature.

You would measure Anne's temperature during her initial patient assessment and as a baseline for future recordings. Also, she may have become hypothermic if she was lying on the ground outside in very cold weather. Ken's temperature would be recorded as part of his general assessment, particularly if he feels hot or cold to touch. He may have an infection, causing him to feel unwell. Natalie's temperature would have been recorded during her admission assessment; this temperature acts as a baseline against which future measurements can be compared. Her body temperature may be lower due to alcohol consumption.

Body temperature is routinely recorded when a person is admitted to hospital, pre- and postoperatively, after invasive procedures and during various treatments. For people with learning disabilities, recording body temperature can help identify whether behavioural changes are due to a physical health problem. Also, recording temperature regularly for people with learning disabilities, perhaps during routine health checkups, promotes familiarity with the equipment and procedure so that temperature measurement should not cause undue distress during ill health. Frequency of measurements may range from just one recording on admission to hourly in a person with a high temperature.

Learning outcome 2: Identify the sites and equipment used for measuring temperature

Ideally, the same site and method should be used for a person's temperature measurement each time to promote greater consistency. However, different sites and methods are appropriate in different circumstances.

ACTIVITY

From your experience in practice, as well as personal experience of having your temperature taken, list the equipment and sites that can be used to record body temperature. What might be their advantages and disadvantages?

Sites

You are likely to have seen the following sites used:

- Mouth
- Axilla (armpit)
- Tympanic membrane (in the ear)

The rectum can also be used to measure temperature, but this site is rarely used, except in a few special circumstances. Taking temperatures rectally is invasive and can cause patients embarrassment. Temporal artery temperature measurement is sometimes used. The device is held over the forehead and senses infrared omissions to note the temperature (Davie and Amoore 2010). Oral measurements are unsuitable for people who are confused, unconscious or breathless. A breathless person tends to mouth breathe so oral temperature measurement would then be both distressing and inaccurate. Axillary temperature measurement requires good contact between the two skin surfaces, so this site will probably be inaccurate with very thin people. The person must be able to keep the arm still by the side of the chest. The axillary temperature is not an accurate indicator of core body temperature if the person is vasoconstricted or chilled, as Anne may be if she has been outside for a prolonged period. The tympanic membrane is a convenient site for temperature recording and can be used with most people if the equipment is available.

ACTIVITY

When you are next in the practice setting, observe which routes are used for temperature measurement for different people and identify the rationale for their choice.

Equipment

You may have seen chemical disposable, electronic and infrared light reflectance thermometers. In the past, mercury thermometers were used, but they are no longer used due to concerns about the potential risks of mercury spillage from broken glass thermometers. The World Health Organization (WHO 2011) has made recommendations for mercury-free healthcare due to the potential hazards; for further information, see http://www.mercuryfreehealthcare.org.

Chemical disposable thermometers

Chemical disposable thermometers are thin plastic strips with small dots of thermosensitive chemicals that change colour with increasing temperature and may be used in the mouth or axilla (Figure 4.1). They are disposed of after use, so there is no cross-infection risk. Accuracy depends on correct technique in relation to timing and positioning. Also, they must be stored at under 30°C. When using these thermometers, ensure the mouth is closed for 60 seconds and leave them *in situ* no longer than 2 minutes. In the axilla, the thermometer should be placed against the torso and completely covered by body surfaces for 3 minutes (3M 2007). If the thermometer is left in the mouth for longer than 2 minutes or in the axilla longer

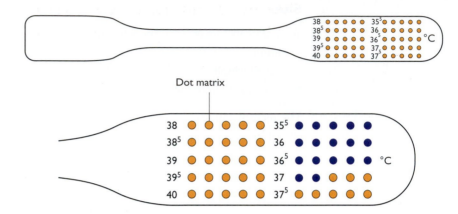

Dot matrix

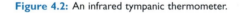

Figure 4.1: A chemical dot matrix thermometer showing 37.1°C.

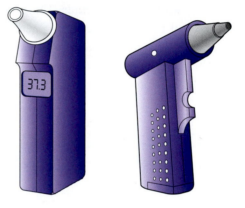

Figure 4.2: An infrared tympanic thermometer.

than 5 minutes, it must be rerecorded with a new thermometer (3M 2007) as it could be inaccurate otherwise.

Electronic thermometers

Electronic thermometers consist of a probe that is placed in the mouth, the axilla or the rectum, usually connected to a power supply and display unit. The purchase cost is significant, as are the ongoing costs of probe covers needed for each use. Most of these thermometers produce an auditory signal after a preset time or when maximum temperature is reached, so the user does not determine the timing.

Infrared thermometers

Infrared thermometers detect heat radiated as infrared energy from the tympanic membrane (Figure 4.2). Temperature is recorded within a few seconds, causing little inconvenience or discomfort. The thermometers are designed to detect heat from the tympanic membrane, but they also detect heat from the ear canal (which may be 2°C lower) if not correctly placed to provide a snug fit (Medicines and Healthcare Regulatory

Agency [MHRA] 2009); therefore, correct placement of the probe is essential. Bridges and Thomas (2009) warned against taking a patient's temperature immediately after a patient has been lying on the ear that you use to record a temperature in as this can affect the reading. If a patient is lying on their ear, use the upward facing ear if possible, but if this is not possible, due to surgery or trauma for example, wait 3 minutes before recording the temperature in the ear that the patient has been lying on.

ACTIVITY	Which method and site are most appropriate for each of the people in this chapter's scenarios, and why?

Compare your answers with the points below:

- **Adult** – For Anne, a tympanic thermometer would probably be used. The oral route is not appropriate as she is disorientated, and she may be in pain, anxious and receiving oxygen via a mask. A tympanic thermometer would record her temperature without affecting her other treatments and observations.
- **Learning disability** – Ken's temperature could be measured in the axilla using either a disposable or an electronic thermometer. A tympanic thermometer could be used if the equipment is available. Ken may have preferences about the type of equipment used and method, and these preferences should be respected if at all possible. The nurse should explain carefully first, especially if the equipment used is unfamiliar to him.
- **Mental health** – Natalie's temperature could be recorded tympanically if a tympanic thermometer is available. The oral route is not suitable as she is not fully conscious. The axilla route could be used, using a disposable thermometer or electronic thermometer. The nurse would need to help her keep her arm by her side for the required length of time.

Learning outcome 3: Accurately measure a person's temperature

Oral measurements

ACTIVITY	Find a willing volunteer with whom to practise this activity. You will need a chemical disposable thermometer. Carefully work through the instructions in Box 4.1.

Factors that might affect the oral temperature measurement include:

- eating or drinking hot or cold substances shortly before the procedure;
- smoking;
- talking;
- breathing through the mouth;
- incorrect positioning of the thermometer;
- thermometer in the mouth for too short a time.

An oral temperature should not be recorded within 15 minutes of the patient eating, drinking or smoking.

Box 4.1 Oral temperature measurement using chemical disposable thermometer

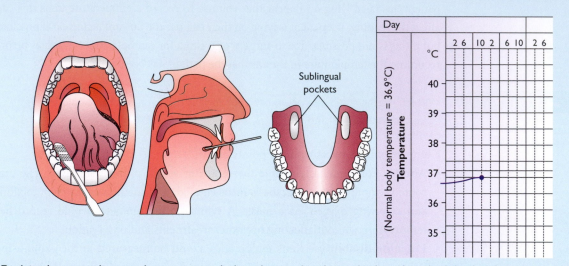

Explain the procedure to the person, including the need to keep the lips closed while the thermometer is in position.

• Position the plastic strip in the person's mouth under the tongue to the side; see the diagram for correct positioning. The face with the dots on (dot matrix) can be placed either way up and must be left in for 1 minute.

• Remove the thermometer. Wait 10 seconds and read the last blue dot, ignoring any dots in between that have not changed colour (3M 2007). Dispose of the thermometer.

• Record the measurement on an observation chart, as per example, of a temperature of 36.8°C. Report abnormal temperatures.

Axilla measurements

ACTIVITY

Now try using a chemical disposable thermometer to measure axillary temperature using the instructions in Box 4.2. Compare this reading with the previous oral measurement.

Electronic devices

Box 4.3 lays out instructions for using electronic thermometers. You may be able to practise using these devices if the equipment is available. Note that the tympanic temperature should not be taken with a hearing aid in place, in an ear that is infected or after ear surgery (Molton et al. 2001). If the patient has experienced any trauma in and around the ear, then seek medical advice as to whether the tympanic thermometer is suitable. Consideration of ottorhoea (discharge from the ear) also needs to be made. Several manufacturers of tympanic thermometers advise not using a tympanic thermometer in an ear that has been operated on for a week postoperatively, so check the manufacturer's instructions regarding this issue.

ACTIVITY

Using a thermometer will give you an accurate measurement of temperature, but what other observations could help you to assess body temperature?

Box 4.2 Measurement of a temperature in the axilla, using a chemical, disposable thermometer

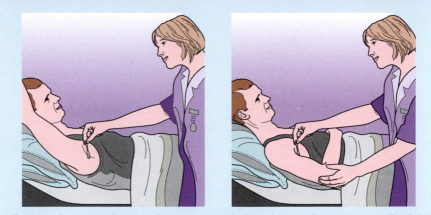

- Explain the procedure to the person, including the need to remain still while the thermometer is in position.
- Raise the person's arm. Place the thermometer in the centre of the person's axilla (see the diagram), positioning it with the dot matrix against the torso.
- Check to ensure there is good contact with the skin when the arm is lowered.
- Rest the person's arm across the chest and maintain the thermometer in position for a minimum of 3 minutes.
- Remove the thermometer, read and record the result described as in Box 4.1.
- Dispose of the chemical thermometer.
- Report abnormal temperatures.

Box 4.3 Temperature measurement using electronic devices

Using an electronic thermometer to record oral or axilla temperature

- The positioning of electronic probes in the mouth or the axilla is the same as for chemical disposable thermometers (see Boxes 4.1 and 4.2).
- A new probe cover should be used for each person.
- Devices have either an auditory (e.g. bleeping sound) or visual (e.g. flashing) indicator when maximum temperature is reached; the probe should remain in place until this indicator is noted.

Using an infrared tympanic membrane thermometer

- The speculum is covered with a disposable cover.
- The ear is pulled gently but firmly to straighten the ear canal, pulling the ear up and back.
- The speculum is inserted gently into the ear canal, ensuring a snug fit.
- The start button is pressed.
- The reading is obtained within 1–2 seconds, indicated by a bleeping sound.

You can feel whether the person has cold extremities or is hot to touch, whether the person is shivering or sweating and ask them how they feel. It is particularly important to use these observations if people are unable to communicate verbally about whether they feel cold or hot. Your observations may prompt you to record their temperature.

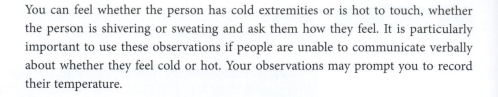

Children: practice points – temperature measurement

All children who attend a healthcare setting should have their temperature taken as part of their assessment. Children can present with mottled skin, feel hot or cold to touch or may have a rash, so it is appropriate to take a temperature within the assessment using a measurement device suitable for the child's age.

Gormley-Fleming (2010, p.111) recommends the following choices:

Infants under 4 weeks: Axilla route using an electronic thermometer

4 weeks to 5 years: Axilla route using an electronic or chemical dot thermometer, or tympanic, using an infrared tympanic thermometer

5 years and over: oral or axilla (with electronic or chemical dot thermometer) or tympanic, using an infrared tympanic thermometer

see

Gormley-Fleming, E. 2010. Assessment and vital signs: A comprehensive overview. In: Glasper, A., Aylott, M. and Battrick, C. (eds.) *Developing Practical Skills for Nursing Children and Young People*. London: Hodder Arnold, 109–147.

Macqueen, S., Bruce, E.A. and Gibson, F. 2012. Assessment. In: *The Great Ormond Street Hospital Manual of Children's Nursing Practices*. Chichester: Wiley-Blackwell, 1–35.

Royal College of Nursing. 2011. Standards for assessing, measuring and monitoring vital signs in infants, children and young people. Available from: http://www.rcn.org.uk/__data/assets/pdf_file/0004/114484/003196.pdf

Pregnancy and birth: practice points – body temperature

- The hormone progesterone as well as a raised metabolic rate during pregnancy increases the amount of heat generated by the body by 30–35%. Even though the body compensates for this incresae by losing heat, maternal temperature can be increased by 0.5°C.
- A high maternal temperature raises the foetal temperature and heart rate, which can lead to serious complications for the foetus, such as preterm labour and hypoxia (Centre for Maternal and Child Enquiries 2011).
- A newborn baby's inability to thermoregulate effectively as well as a large surface area and little subcutaneous fat to insulate them makes them vulnerable to cold air and draughts. In addition, care must be taken with overheating, which is one of the risk factors for cot death. See http://fsid.org.uk.

Summary

- Choice of route and equipment for measuring temperature should consider individual factors such as physical and mental conditions as well as the devices available.
- For each route and device used, the measurement should be conducted and recorded carefully and accurately.
- Abnormal measurements should be reported and appropriate action taken.
- As temperature can vary between body sites, the measurement site should be recorded and the same site used for subsequent recordings whenever possible.

MEASURING AND RECORDING THE PULSE

When the left ventricle of the heart pumps blood into the already full aorta and out into the arterial system, this causes a wave of expansion throughout the arteries. Where arteries are near the surface of the body, this expansion – the pulse – can be felt when lightly pressing (palpating) the artery against bone. The pulse thus represents each ventricular contraction of the heart, and in the healthy heart one heart beat corresponds to one pulse beat.

Disease can affect the cardiac cycle, leading to a difference between the heart rate and the pulse rate. The pulse rate is the number of heart beats in a 60-second period. Pulse measurement provides very useful information about health status. As with temperature, pulse rate will be recorded on admission to hospital as a baseline, and subsequent measurements may be performed for monitoring purposes.

LEARNING OUTCOMES

By the end of this section, you will be able to:

1 explain the rationale for monitoring pulse rate and the normal values of the pulse;
2 locate pulses in different areas of the body and identify which area might be palpated in specific situations;
3 accurately measure a person's pulse rate.

Learning outcome 1: Explain the rationale for monitoring pulse rate and the normal values of the pulse

ACTIVITY

Look again at the definition of a pulse, and then identify what a person's pulse might actually tell you about their body.

The pulse is measured to identify the rate and strength of the ventricular contraction and to gain information regarding a person's health. For example, in the case of trauma and severe bleeding, the pulse rate might be weak and fast. When measuring a pulse, the following should be observed:

- **The frequency of the pulse.** The frequency of the pulse indicates the rate of contraction of the left ventricle. It is affected by numerous factors, including age, exercise, stress, injury and disease. The normal adult heart rate ranges from 60 to 100 beats per minute (bpm), but at rest is usually between 60 and 80 bpm (Waugh and Grant 2010). The heart rate is influenced by the autonomic nervous system during sleep, producing sinus bradycardia (a slow heart rate); the heart rate can diminish during sleep by about 10–20 bpm (Waugh and Grant 2010). An abnormally slow pulse is termed **bradycardia**, and in an adult, would usually be a pulse rate below 60 bpm. An underactive thyroid gland, hypothermia and some drugs slow the pulse. An abnormally fast pulse is termed **tachycardia** – usually a pulse rate above 100 bpm in an adult. There are many reasons for a fast pulse – for example, a fever, an overactive thyroid gland and certain drugs. The thickness and tension of a person's arteriole walls influence the pulse. Atherosclerosis develops in many people over the age of 40 years and can lead to structural changes in the arteries, thus altering the pulse rate.
- **The volume.** Volume indicates the strength of the ventricular contraction. A weak contraction produces a pulse that feels weak, or it may not be strong enough to produce a pulse at the periphery – such as the wrist – at all. A lack of blood volume also leads to a weak pulse. For example, loss of blood due to trauma could lead to **hypovolaemia** (low blood volume) and thus eventually affect the volume of the pulse.
- **The rhythm.** Rhythm helps to establish whether the heart is beating regularly. An irregular pulse indicates a possible abnormality in the heart's conduction system. NICE (2006) recommends that manual pulse palpation should be performed to identify an irregular pulse, which can indicate **atrial fibrillation**. Electronic devices may not be able to record irregular pulse rates, so learn how to record a pulse manually.

Atrial fibrillation

Fibrillation of the atria leading to irregular and often fast ventricular contraction and thus a highly irregular pulse rate.

Learning outcome 2: Locate pulses in different areas of the body and identify which might be palpated in specific situations

It is important to know the sites where a pulse can be found.

ACTIVITY

Here is a list of pulses that can be palpated (Figure 4.3). How many can you find on yourself?

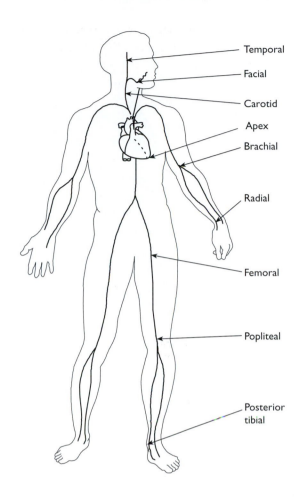

Figure 4.3: Location of pulses within the body.

- Temporal artery – on the side of the forehead
- Facial artery – on the side of the face
- Carotid artery – at the neck
- Brachial artery – in the antecubital fossa of the arm
- Radial artery – at the wrist
- Femoral artery – in the groin
- Popliteal artery – behind the knee
- Posterior tibial artery – at the inner side of each ankle.

The choice of site for pulse measurement depends on the individual and the situation. For adults in a non-emergency situation, the radial pulse is usually recorded because this site is non-invasive and easily accessible. Anne, Ken and Natalie could all have their radial pulses taken. It may be difficult to palpate some pulse sites in people with contractures. Pulses in the lower legs are usually only palpated when assessing the presence of circulation to the limbs, which might be after trauma or surgery.

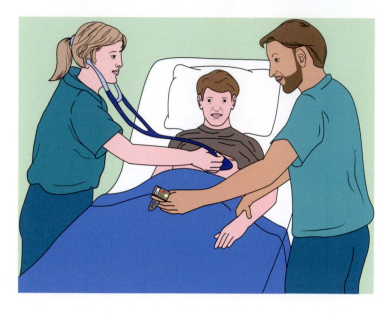

Figure 4.4: Measurement of the apex beat and radial pulse together.

Some pulses are easier to palpate and more accessible than others. In an emergency situation when a person has collapsed, it is often difficult to locate peripheral pulses (including the radial pulse), so the carotid or femoral pulse may be checked. You may see these pulses being checked during prolonged resuscitation attempts and monitoring of patients who have deteriorated in a clinical area. However, the Resuscitation Council (UK) (2010) guidelines specify that only staff who are trained and experienced in clinical assessment should check the carotid pulse when assessing signs of life in a collapsed person. Checking a patient's pulse as part of basic life-support guidelines is not advised as this check is time-consuming and slows down the response time for resuscitation attempts.

Note that the apex beat (site shown in Figure 4.3) can be listened to with a stethoscope, and it is located to the left side of the sternum over the heart. The apex beat may be measured when the patient has a cardiac condition and is usually measured along with the radial beat. Two nurses are required to perform this skill. With the patient either sitting or lying still, they use the same watch over 1 minute. Nurse 1 counts the radial pulse and nurse 2 counts the apex beat of the heart, listening with a stethoscope (Figure 4.4). The measurement is usually recorded as apex (A) and radial (R), for example, A72, R72. The numbers should be the same but in some instances, the pulse will differ, for example, A80, R72. This situation is known as a pulse deficit. People who have atrial fibrillation sometimes show these observation variations.

Learning outcome 3: Accurately measure a person's pulse rate

With all individuals, the person's psychological state needs to be considered, and cooperation sought, before measuring the pulse. This cooperation involves explaining why the pulse needs to be measured.

ACTIVITY

You need a willing volunteer, a watch with a second hand or a digital watch and an observation chart from your skills laboratory. Now, follow the steps in Box 4.4 to measure and record the radial pulse.

When measuring the pulse rate, nurses often count the pulse for 30 seconds and multiply by two. With a regular pulse, this count gives a reasonably accurate measurement, but an irregular pulse should always be counted for a full minute – and the word 'irregular' should be written by the recorded rate.

ACTIVITY

Now ask your volunteer to jog on the spot for 1 minute and then record the pulse rate again. You will probably find that their pulse rate has risen, due to the extra oxygen demands caused by exercise. Can you remember any other reasons why the pulse may be faster in a healthy person?

Anxiety or stress raise the pulse rate. Thus, Anne's pulse rate could be raised due to the anxiety about her situation. As discussed earlier, you need to put people at

Box 4.4 Measuring a radial pulse

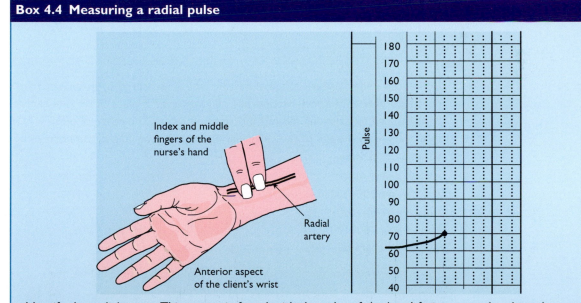

- Identify the radial artery. This artery is found with the palm of the hand facing upward and gently pressing at the wrist region at the thumb side (see the diagram).
- Press the artery gently against the bone with your fingers (not your thumb, which itself has a pulse) and feel the pulse bounding.
- Using your watch, count the beats of the pulse for 1 minute. The number of beats corresponds to the pulse rate. For example, 70 beats indicates the person's pulse rate is 70.
- Using the example, which shows a pulse rate of 70 beats per minute (bpm), record the pulse on the observation chart.

ease when recording vital signs, thereby relieving anxiety and gaining an accurate measurement.

Electronic measurement of the pulse rate

The following devices can electronically record the pulse rate:

- **Oscillometer.** An oscillometer can be used for blood pressure measurement (discussed later in this chapter) and the pulse rate is usually displayed too.
- **Pulse oximeter.** A pulse oximeter (discussed later in this chapter) measures oxygen saturation, and the pulse rate is usually displayed too.
- **Cardiac monitor.** A cardiac monitor displays the heart rate as well as the rhythm of the person's heart. Chapter 11 discusses cardiac monitoring.

Although these devices provide a pulse rate, they will not all indicate either the volume of the pulse or its regularity. With the pulse oximeter and cardiac monitor, movement may cause an artefact, leading to an inaccurate figure being displayed. Ensure that the pulse rate accurately represents your patient's physical appearance and your own assessment. If during measuring vital signs an electronic device shows a low reading or that the pulse is unrecordable, always attempt to record a pulse manually. If you doubt the accuracy of any observation, rerecord it manually and inform a qualified member of the healthcare team.

Children: practice points – pulse measurement

In children under 2 years of age, the heart rate is measured by listening to the apical beat with a stethoscope. For children over 2 years, heart rate can be measured by palpating the radial or carotid artery. The range of pulse rates vary with the age of the child. Having an understanding of the normal parameters is vital.

- <1 year 110–160
- 1–2 years 100–150
- 2–5 years 95–140
- 5–12 years 80–120
- Over 12 years 60–100

For further guidance on pulse measurement for infants and children, see

Gormley-Fleming, E. 2010. Assessment and vital signs: A comprehensive review. In: Glasper, A., Aylott, M. and Battrick, C. (eds.) *Developing Practical Skills for Nursing Children and Young People.* London: Hodder Arnold, 109–47.

Macqueen, S., Bruce, E.A. and Gibson, F. 2012. Assessment. In: *The Great Ormond Street Hospital Manual of Children's Nursing Practices.* Chichester: Wiley-Blackwell, 1–35.

Royal College of Nursing. 2011. Standards for assessing, measuring and monitoring vital signs in infants, children and young people. Available from: http://www.rcn.org.uk/__data/assets/pdf_file/0004/114484/003196.pdf.

Pregnancy and birth: practice points – pulse measurement

You should ascertain what the woman's normal pulse rate is and use this rate as a guide. The technique for assessing and recording the pulse is the same as for any other adult. Until 32 weeks of pregnancy, maternal heart rate increases by 10–20 bpm (healthy non-pregnant female value = 65–85 bpm) as cardiac output has to cope with the increased blood volume that occurs. This can adversely affect women with associated pre-existing cardiac disease due to the additional stress on the cardiovascular system (CMACE 2011).

Summary

- Measuring a person's pulse is minimally invasive and uses little equipment but is a useful vital sign giving insight into health status.
- Nurses must be able to palpate a range of pulses and be aware of which pulse is appropriate to measure in different situations.
- It is important to be aware of the normal pulse range and to assess the volume and regularity of the pulse as well as the rate.

MEASURING AND RECORDING RESPIRATIONS

The major function of the respiratory system is to supply the body with oxygen and remove carbon dioxide. When the respiratory rate is measured, it is the act of ventilation that is observed. One respiration consists of one inspiration (breathing in) and one expiration (breathing out). Respiratory rate measurement is an important aspect of patient assessment. Deterioration of respiratory effort leads to low levels of oxygen in the blood and raised levels of carbon dioxide. Chapter 11 provides further detail about respiratory assessment.

LEARNING OUTCOMES

By the end of this section, you will be able to:

1 explain when and why observation of respiration is performed and state the range of normal respiratory rates for adults;
2 discuss other aspects of breathing to observe when measuring respiratory rates;
3 accurately measure and record the respiratory rate.

Learning outcome 1: Explain when and why observation of respiration is performed and state the range of normal respiratory rates for adults

ACTIVITY

Why would a person's respiration be observed? The practice scenarios will give you some clues. List the possible reasons.

You may have thought of the following situations:

- To provide a baseline for future comparison, for example, when a person is admitted to hospital or has a preoperative assessment
- To monitor a person in hospital or in the community following injury or during an illness, for example, loss of consciousness, chest injury, difficulty with breathing, chest pain (so Anne, Ken and Natalie should all have their respiration rates measured)
- To monitor a patient's condition – for example, after surgery, or during treatment, such as a morphine infusion
- To monitor a patient's response to treatments or medication that affects the respiratory system

When assessing respiratory rate, you should know the expected normal rate; if a baseline reading is available, you can make a comparison with this rate. The respiratory rate varies according to age, size and gender and can fluctuate in well people, for example, if metabolic demands change. The normal adult respiratory rate is about 12–18 breaths per minute (Blows 2012). Exercise, stress and fear all increase the respiratory rate; this increase is a normal bodily response. If you count people's respiratory rates when they have just arrived at the hospital, anxiety may lead to a raised respiratory rate, which would not be an accurate baseline. In deep (referred to as stage 4) sleep, respiratory rate drops to its lowest normal level. Knowledge of normal biological functioning will help you to recognise abnormalities and causes for concern.

An increased respiratory rate is termed **tachypnoea**. The respiratory rate is often the first vital sign to alter when a patient is deteriorating, so it is imperative that this vital sign is monitored and recorded. Ken's respiratory rate may increase due to his chest infection. A decreased respiratory rate is termed **bradypnoea**. Natalie's respiratory rate may decrease owing to the drugs she has taken. A serious side effect of opioid drugs, such as morphine, is a depressed respiratory rate.

In healthy people, the relationship between pulse and respiration is fairly constant, being a ratio of one respiration to every four or five heart beats. Very rapid respirations, such as over 40 per minute in an adult (in the absence of exercise), or very slow respirations, such as 8 per minute, are cause for alarm and should be reported promptly.

Learning outcome 2: Discuss other aspects of breathing to observe when measuring respiratory rates

ACTIVITY

When you are counting the respiratory rates of the people in the scenarios, what else about their respiration should you observe?

You should observe the difficulty, sound, depth and pattern of breathing, as discussed next.

Difficulty in breathing

Respirations are normally effortless, and you should therefore observe whether breathing is difficult (termed **dyspnoea**). Dyspnoeic patients may use accessory muscles of respiration, such as their neck and abdominal muscles. When Ken has a chest infection, he is likely to experience dyspnoea. People with dyspnoea often mouth breathe because there is less resistance to airflow through the mouth than the nose. Mouth breathing can lead to drying of the oral mucus membrane and so oral hygiene (discussed in Chapter 8) is essential.

People with dyspnoea need to sit up, either in an armchair or in bed well supported by pillows, to optimise ventilation. **Orthopnoea** is the term used when people cannot breathe unless they are upright. Dyspnoea is frightening and psychological support is essential.

Sound of breathing

You should also observe the sound of breathing, which is normally quiet. You may hear a variety of abnormal breath sounds. A **wheeze**, often heard in people with **asthma**, is a high-pitched sound occurring when air is forced through narrowed respiratory passages. A wheeze may also occur with chest infections. A **stridor** is a harsh, high-pitched sound that is heard during respiration when the larynx is obstructed.

> ### Asthma
>
> A respiratory disorder characterised by recurrent episodes of difficulty in breathing, wheezing on expiration, coughing and viscous mucoid bronchial secretions.

Depth of breathing

The person's depth of breathing should be observed, which relates to the volume of air moving in and out of the respiratory tract with each breath – the **tidal volume**. An adult's tidal volume should be about 500 mL (Blows 2012). The term **hyperventilation** refers to prolonged, rapid and deep ventilations that can occur during an anxiety attack, causing dizziness and fainting as the resulting low carbon dioxide level causes cerebral vasoconstriction.

Hypoventilation is the term used for slow and shallow breathing, which could lead to inadequate gaseous exchange. You should also observe whether the chest expands equally on both sides, particularly if there is a history of chest injury.

Pattern of breathing

The pattern of breathing should be observed. Terms are given to certain abnormalities.

Apnoea. Apnoea is a period without breathing. It could occur during hypoventilation, with another breath only occurring when arterial carbon dioxide levels rise and breathing is stimulated.

Cheyne–Stokes respirations. Cheyne–Stokes respirations are when there is a gradual increase in the depth of respirations leading to an episode of hyperventilation, followed by a gradual decrease in the depth of respirations, and then a period of apnoea lasting about 15–20 seconds.

Kussmaul's respiration. Kussmaul's respiration is very deep and laboured breathing, sometimes associated with people in a diabetic coma. The deep breathing is due to metabolic acidosis.

The person's respiratory rate should be equal between each breath, with a short pause at the end of inspiration and expiration. Irregularities of breathing rate may indicate respiratory disease.

Learning outcome 3: Accurately measure and record the respiratory rate

For the following activities, you need a willing volunteer. If a colleague is not available, another friend or family member may oblige!

> **ACTIVITY**
>
> Measure your volunteer's respiratory rate, using the instructions in Box 4.5.

Respiratory rates, particularly on admission, may be recorded simply as a number (the number of respirations per minute). If the person's respiratory rate is recorded regularly over a period of time, an observation chart is used. Frequency of recordings varies but may be every 15 minutes (for a patient with acute breathing difficulties), hourly, four-hourly or twice daily.

> **ACTIVITY**
>
> Ask your volunteer to spend a couple of minutes exercising (e.g. jogging on the spot) and then count the respiratory rate again. Using the example in Figure 4.5 as a guide, record on an observation chart the two respiratory rates that you have taken.

Box 4.5 Measuring respiratory rate

Note the placement of the second hand of your watch or zero your timing device

• Count each rise and fall of the chest for 1 minute.

In practice you should do this count when people are unaware that they are being observed, as otherwise they may alter their breathing pattern. For an unresponsive person, this precaution is not relevant.

Tip: In an alert individual, the respiratory rate may be counted directly after the pulse, while still outwardly counting the pulse.

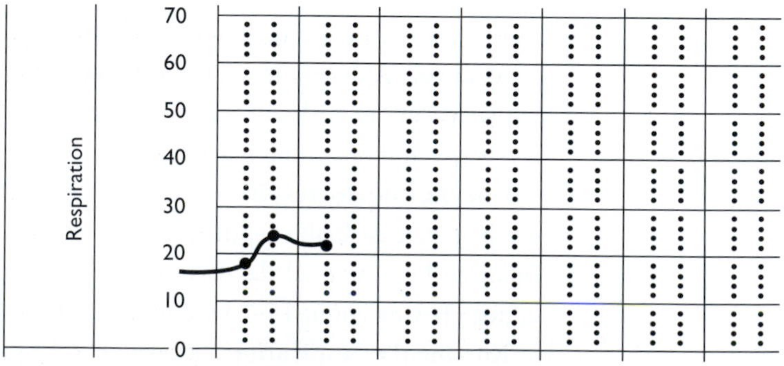

Figure 4.5: Observation chart, showing how respirations could be recorded.

Children: practice points – respiration

It is important to observe the child's breathing when they are not aware that you are doing so which will allow for a more accurate assessment. Thorough assessment of the child's respiratory function is vital as children deteriorate very quickly if left unmanaged. The range of respiratory rates varies with the age of the child so having an understanding of the normal parameters is vital:

- <1 year 30–40
- 1–2 years 25–35
- 2–5 years 25–30
- 5–12 years 20–25
- Over 12 years 15–20

For further guidance on respiratory assessment of infants and children, see

Gormley-Fleming, E. 2010. Assessment and vital signs: A comprehensive review. In: Glasper, A., Aylott, M. and Battrick, C. (eds.) *Developing Practical Skills for Nursing Children and Young People*. London: Hodder Arnold, 109–47.

Macqueen, S., Bruce, E.A. and Gibson, F. 2012. Assessment. In: *The Great Ormond Street Hospital Manual of Children's Nursing Practices*. Chichester: Wiley-Blackwell, 1–35.

Royal College of Nursing. 2011. Standards for assessing, measuring and monitoring vital signs in infants, children and young people. Available from: http://www.rcn.org.uk/__data/assets/pdf_file/0004/114484/003196.pdf.

Pregnancy and birth: practice points – respiration

During pregnancy, women are encouraged to adopt the left lateral position when lying down, to prevent caval decompression. If the woman lies on her back, then her blood flow may be affected and in turn affect her general well-being, which will impact on her vital signs. During pregnancy, some women experience fluid retention that can seriously affect, amongst other things, respiratory function. Fluid retention may affect gaseous exchange, and changes to oxygen saturation and respiratory rate may be seen. Seek midwifery advice regarding positioning of a pregnant woman once she is in your care.

In later pregnancy, breathing becomes largely diaphragmatic due to the enlarging uterus. However, the respiration rate remains unchanged. Therefore, breathlessness (RR > 20) is one of several significant symptoms in pregnancy or the postnatal period indicating deteriorating health or signs of puerperal sepsis that will require accurate regular monitoring (Dawson and Robson 2012). The use of Early Warning Scores for obstetrics (MEOWS) is strongly recommended (see Chapter 11).

Summary

- Respirations are measured as part of an acutely ill person's assessment, as a baseline for future comparison, and to monitor and evaluate a person's condition and response to treatment.
- It is important to be aware of normal respiratory rates and of possible abnormalities that can occur.

MEASURING AND RECORDING BLOOD PRESSURE

Blood pressure is the pressure that the blood exerts on the walls of the blood vessels (Waugh and Grant 2010). Blood pressure is different in different blood vessels, but in everyday clinical practice the term *blood pressure* is used to mean systemic arterial blood pressure (Webster and Thompson 2011). Blood pressure is regulated by complex neural and hormonal systems (Tortora and Derrikson 2011). Blood pressure is a key vital sign to assist in monitoring general health, so an accurate recording is imperative (Nicholas 2012).

LEARNING OUTCOMES

By the end of this section, you will be able to:

1. explain what makes up blood pressure and when blood pressure should be measured;
2. discuss the equipment used for blood pressure measurements and the meaning of the reading obtained;
3. identify the normal values for blood pressure and factors affecting blood pressure recordings;
4. accurately measure a person's blood pressure using manual and electronic equipment.

Learning outcome 1: Explain what makes up blood pressure and when blood pressure should be measured

Understanding blood pressure and its effects on the body is complex. Tuggle (2009) explains that blood pressure results from cardiac output (CO), multiplied by systemic vascular resistance (SVR), which is opposition to blood flow from friction between blood and blood vessel walls. CO is the production of heart rate and stroke volume (SV), which is the amount of blood ejected with each beat. SV is determined by preload (volume of blood in the ventricle waiting to be ejected), afterload (resistance of moving the preload) and contractility (strength of heart muscle). If a person's blood pressure is high or low, then some of these factors are out of balance.

Currently, blood pressure is measured in millimetres of mercury (mmHg) using a sphygmomanometer or electronic device (O'Brien et al. 2003).

A blood pressure reading has two values, systolic and diastolic. Systolic blood pressure is primarily determined by CO and diastolic by SVR.

- The **systolic** pressure occurs during ventricular contraction and is the maximum pressure of the blood against the wall of the artery. This pressure is recorded as the top figure when documenting the blood pressure.
- The **diastolic** pressure is the minimum pressure of the blood against the wall of the artery, which occurs following closure of the aortic valve. This measurement assesses the pressure when the ventricles are at rest and is recorded as the bottom figure. ·

Thus, a blood pressure recorded as 120/70 means that the systolic pressure is 120 mmHg and the diastolic pressure is 70 mmHg. The measurements of systolic and diastolic pressure should be judged as one reading. The difference between systolic and diastolic readings is termed the **pulse pressure** (Webster and Thompson 2011).

ACTIVITY

How often should routine blood pressure be measured?
Ask older members of your family when they last had their blood pressure measured.

Health Action Plan

A personal action plan developed for each individual with a learning disability, which details the actions needed to maintain and improve the person's health and any help needed to accomplish these actions; see *Action for Health – Health Action Plans and Health Facilitation* (DH 2002).

According to Williams et al. (2004), blood pressure recording should be carried out routinely at least every 5 years until the age of 80, but people with high blood pressure should have more frequent measurements – at least annually. For people with learning disabilities, regular health checks should be carried out as part of their health promotion, and these checks should include blood pressure measurement.

Blood pressure checks are now increasingly performed twice, once on each arm, to detect any differences (Skerrett 2012). Ambulatory recording of blood pressure, where patients take a device home to record their blood pressure over a period of time, can be beneficial and has also become more popular; see later discussion (Learning outcome 3). Ken's **Health Action Plan** should include his blood pressure measurement, and an ambulatory blood pressure device may well be used for him.

Learning outcome 2: Discuss the equipment used for blood pressure measurements and the meaning of the reading obtained

ACTIVITY

What equipment have you seen used to measure blood pressure? If you are not familiar with the sphygmomanometer ('sphygmo'), try to access one in the skills laboratory or the practice setting. If possible, look at electronic equipment too, as many devices are now used in the clinical setting.

There are two main ways of measuring blood pressure:

- **Indirect method.** Pressure can be measured indirectly, using electronic/digital equipment – for example, an oscillometer. An oscillometer is a machine that is attached to the patient's arm by means of a cuff. The cuff is inflated by the machine, which then reads the pressure within the artery. The result is displayed as two readings – the systolic and the diastolic pressure. In clinical practice, blood pressure recording is most frequently performed using an electronic device; however, it is important that you learn to use both manual and electronic devices.
- **Non-invasive auscultation method.** The pressure is taken manually by using a sphygmomanometer and stethoscope

Blood pressure was traditionally recorded manually but is increasingly recorded electronically. Mercury sphygmomanometer use is discouraged, due to the risks of mercury spillage (MHRA 2012) and drive to reduce mercury use in healthcare (WHO 2011). Mercury sphygmomanometers have been largely replaced with aneroid sphygmomanometers (Figure 4.6), but there is debate about their accuracy; these devices must be calibrated and serviced as per manufacturer's guidelines. Oscillometric devices are increasingly used for measurement, although their accuracy continues to be critically debated. Nurses need to learn how to record a blood pressure manually, as electronic devices are not always available, particularly in community and non-acute settings.

On oscillometers and monitoring devices you will notice the term *MAP*, which refers to mean arterial pressure, or the average blood pressure during the cardiac cycle. MAP can indicate when a patient is deteriorating (for more information, see Chapter 11).

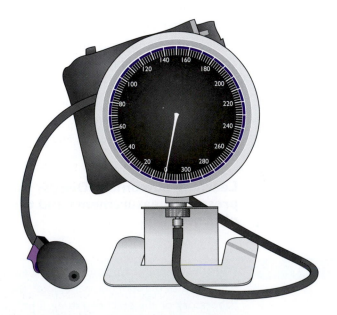

Figure 4.6: An aneroid sphygmomanometer.

Learning outcome 3: Identify the normal values for blood pressure and factors affecting blood pressure recordings

When measuring blood pressure, as with any other vital signs, you should be aware of expected normal ranges. O'Brien et al. (2003) highlight the variability in blood pressure from person to person. Normal adult blood pressure is generally considered to range from 100/60 to 140/90. However, the NICE guidelines CG 127 (2011a) for hypertension, written in conjunction with the British Hypertension Society (BHS), offer more detailed classification of blood pressure levels to indicate acceptable/unacceptable parameters. The term used for high blood pressure is **hypertension,** and the term used for low blood pressure is **hypotension**. The physiological changes that occur during hypotension and hypertension are outlined by Marieb (2012).

ACTIVITY	What factors do you know of that might affect blood pressure measurements? Would any of these apply to the people in this chapter's scenarios?

Age, disease, injury and medicines all influence blood pressure and could be factors relevant to all three scenarios. There are many other factors too.

- **Blood volume.** Regulatory mechanisms can cope with minor fluctuations in circulating blood volume, but losses of 10% or more – due to trauma, haemorrhage or severe dehydration – result in a fall in blood pressure (Tortora and Derrikson 2011).
- **Age.** Blood pressure increases from birth and throughout life (Marieb 2012). Anne and Ken may have a higher blood pressure than Natalie, who is a younger adult.
- **Disease.** Elasticity of the arteries is affected directly by diseases such as atherosclerosis (Webster and Thompson 2011). Many other diseases can raise blood pressure, including heart disease, kidney disease, endocrine disorders and neurological conditions (Marieb 2012). In these instances, high blood pressure is termed secondary hypertension.
- **Posture and gravity.** A decrease in blood pressure may occur from lying to sitting or standing position, but O'Brien et al. (2003) asserted that this positioning is unlikely to lead to significant error in recording, provided the arm is supported at the patient's heart level. Some people's blood pressure falls more significantly on standing (termed **orthostatic hypotension**). This effect is more common in older people (Marieb 2012) and is a complication of immobility (see Chapter 6).
- **Drug use.** Some prescribed drugs affect blood pressure; examples are diuretics and tranquillisers (Tortora and Derrikson 2011). If Natalie has taken an overdose of a tranquilliser, depending on the quantity, this drug intake could lower her blood pressure. It may be beneficial when a patient is taking medication to note the time of drug ingestion in association with the blood pressure being monitored.

- **Emotional factors.** Stress, fear and anxiety all increase blood pressure. Staff who fail to explain the procedure or rush the procedure and patients who are anxious about the outcome are factors that can affect the reading (O'Brien et al. 2003). In people with dementia, remember to explain the procedure, show the person the equipment and allow the person time to comprehend what you are doing.
- **Weight.** An obese person's heart has to work harder, so the blood pressure may be higher (Marieb 2012).
- **Diet.** High salt and low calcium dietary intakes may lead to a rise in blood pressure (Marieb 2012).
- **Exercise.** People who take regular exercise may have a lower blood pressure (O'Brien et al. 2003).
- **Arm support and position.** Diastolic blood pressure may increase by 10% if the arm is left unsupported (O'Brien et al. 2003). An overestimation of blood pressure can result if the arm is placed below the heart level.
- **Arm used.** During a patient's initial assessment, bilateral blood pressure measurements should be recorded to identify any differences in the readings (BHS 2012a,b; Clark et al. 2012). It is normal to have a small difference in blood pressure readings between arms, but a big difference is a cause for concern. Differences could indicate abnormalities or disease of the aorta, such as **coarctation** or an **aneurysm**. Surgical and cardiac procedures, for example, cardiac catheterisation, may also result in differences. Clark et al. (2012) found that people with big differences in systolic pressure between arms were more likely to die from heart attack, stroke or other causes.
- **White coat hypertension.** White coat hypertension is a term used when a person's blood pressure is consistently higher when recorded in a medical situation, such as a hospital, clinic or GP's surgery, than at home (O'Brien et al. 2003). It is a common phenomenon, affecting up to 25% of those who appear to have hypertension (O'Brien 2001). NICE (2011a) highlighted that patients' treatment regimes could be based upon false readings and therefore recommended that patients with long-term hypertension should have their blood pressure measured at home, using ambulatory devices, over a period of time before treatment regimes are commenced.
- **Observer bias.** When recording routine observations, healthcare professionals may be at risk of expecting the measurement to be normal. For example, when recording blood pressure for a patient who they know well or when recording several blood pressure measurements in a shift.

Aortic coarctation

A congenital narrowing of the aorta.

Aneurysm

A weakness in the arterial wall leading to a bulge, with the risk of rupture.

Learning outcome 4: Accurately measure a person's blood pressure using manual and electronic equipment

Attaining accurate results for blood pressure recordings, both manual and electronic, is very important. Many treatment regimes and clinical decisions are made based upon blood pressure monitoring.

Although many clinical settings predominantly use electronic devices, it is imperative to learn the technique of manual blood pressure and ensure you are

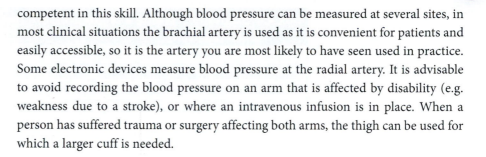

competent in this skill. Although blood pressure can be measured at several sites, in most clinical situations the brachial artery is used as it is convenient for patients and easily accessible, so it is the artery you are most likely to have seen used in practice. Some electronic devices measure blood pressure at the radial artery. It is advisable to avoid recording the blood pressure on an arm that is affected by disability (e.g. weakness due to a stroke), or where an intravenous infusion is in place. When a person has suffered trauma or surgery affecting both arms, the thigh can be used for which a larger cuff is needed.

Recording Korotkoff sounds in manual blood pressure measurement

The Korotkoff sounds are heard through the stethoscope when you manually record a blood pressure (Table 4.1). These sounds are not audible using electronic/ digital devices. The sounds are named after Nikolai Korotkoff, who first identified the audible sounds of blood pressure in 1905 (Korotkoff 1905, cited by O'Brien et al. 1999). There may be a period between phases 2 and 3 where no sounds are audible, but they become audible again at a lower pressure. This phenomenon is known as an **auscultatory gap** (O'Brien et al. 2003) and is the reason that correct procedure involves palpation to find systolic blood pressure before using the sphygmomanometer. This technique is explained later.

There is debate about whether the diastolic pressure should be recorded at phase 4 or phase 5. Generally, guidelines recommend phase 5 as the point of diastolic pressure (BHS 2012a; O'Brien et al. 2003).

Steps in recording blood pressure

Blood pressure recording is frequently carried out by nurses and is a common experience for most people, but remember that for some people it will be their first time. Always give adequate explanation and warning about the tightness of the cuff, which some people find quite uncomfortable. Box 4.6 provides the steps in measuring blood pressure using both manual and electronic equipment. Selection of correct cuff size is essential for an accurate reading. There are a variety of sizes of cuffs available: small adult, standard and large adult as well as a thigh cuff. Ensure that you note the size of the patient's arm and use an appropriate cuff (Table 4.2).

Table 4.1: Korotkoff sounds

Phase	Sound	When they are normally heard (mmHg)
1	Clear tapping	Usually above 120
2	Blowing or whistling	Around 110
3	Soft thud	Around 100
4	Low-pitched, muffled sound	Around 90
5	Disappearance of all sounds	Around 80

Source: Korotkoff 1905, cited by O'Brien, E., Petrie, J., Littler, W. et al. 1999. *Blood Pressure Measurement Recommendations of the British Hypertension Society*. London: BMJ Publications.

Box 4.6 Steps in recording a blood pressure manually and electronically

Blood pressure measurement with manual blood pressure monitors	Blood pressure measurement with electronic blood pressure monitors
The patient should be seated for at least 5 minutes, relaxed and not moving or speaking.	
• The arm must be supported at the level of the heart. Ensure no tight clothing constricts the arm.	
• Place the cuff on neatly with the centre of the bladder over the brachial artery. The bladder should encircle at least 80% of the arm (but not more than 100%).	
• Estimate the systolic beforehand: a) Palpate the brachial artery. b) Inflate cuff until pulsation disappears. c) Deflate cuff. d) Estimate systolic pressure. • Then, inflate to 30 mmHg above the estimated systolic level needed to occlude the pulse. • Place the stethoscope diaphragm over the brachial artery and deflate at a rate of 2–3 mm/second until you hear regular tapping sounds. • Measure systolic (first sound) and diastolic (disappearance) to nearest 2 mmHg.	• Some monitors allow manual blood pressure setting selection where you choose the appropriate setting. Other monitors will automatically inflate and reinflate to the next setting if required. • Repeat three times and record measurement as displayed. Initially, test blood pressure in both arms and use arm with highest reading for subsequent measurement.

Source: Reproduced with kind permission from British Hypertension Society. 2012a. *Blood pressure measurement with manual blood pressure monitors*. Available from: http://www.bhsoc.org/files/9013/4390/7747/BP_Measurement_Poster_-_Manual.pdf; British Hypertension Society. 2012b. *Blood pressure measurement with electronic blood pressure monitors*. Available from: http://www.bhsoc.org/files/8413/4390/7770/BP_Measurement_Poster_-_Electronic.pdf

Table 4.2: Selection of cuff size

	Indication	Width (cm)[a,b]	Length (cm)[a,b]	BHS Guidelines Bladder width and length (cm)[a]	Arm circumference (cm)[a]
Cuff size	Small adult/child	10–12	18–24	12 × 18	<23
	Standard adult	12–13	23–35	12 × 26	<33
	Large adult	12–16	35–40	22 × 40	<50
	Adult thigh cuff[c]	20	42		<53

[a] The range for columns 2 and 3 are derived from recommendations from the British Hypertension Society (BHS), European Hypertension Society (ESH) and the American Heart Association. Columns 4 and 5 are derived from only the BHS guidelines.
[b] Bladders of varying sizes are available, so a range is provided for each indication (applies to columns 2 and 3).
[c] Large bladders for arm circumferences >42 cm may be required.

Source: Reproduced from British Hypertension Society. 2012a. *Blood pressure measurement with manual blood pressure monitors*. Available from: http://www.bhsoc.org/files/9013/4390/7747/BP_Measurement_Poster_-_Manual.pdf; British Hypertension Society. 2012b. *Blood pressure measurement with electronic blood pressure monitors*. Available from: http://www.bhsoc.org/files/8413/4390/7770/BP_Measurement_Poster_-_Electronic.pdf. With permission.

ACTIVITY

If you can access manual blood pressure recording equipment – a sphygmomanometer and a stethoscope – practise measuring and recording a blood pressure with a colleague, using the guidance in Box 4.6. Ensure you choose a correct size cuff (see Table 4.2).

Table 4.3: Common problems with manual blood pressure measurement and suggested solutions

Problem	Solution
Incorrect blood pressure reading	Ensure that the measurement is made to the nearest 2 mmHg.
Incorrect size and position of cuff for the patient	Use the appropriate size of cuff for the individual: the cuff bladder should cover 80% of the arm's circumference.
	A too large or too small cuff will give a false reading.
Confusion about diastolic blood pressure reading	Diastolic measurement taken at cessation of sounds.
Poorly maintained equipment causing errors in measurement	Ensure that the manometer starts at zero and that the machine is calibrated according to the manufacturer's instructions.
	The tubing and all connections should be carefully checked before use.

Source: O'Brien, E., Petrie, J., Littler, W. et al. 1999. *Blood Pressure Measurement Recommendations of the British Hypertension Society.* London: BMJ Publications.

Errors in blood pressure measurement

Errors in blood pressure measurement, including equipment failure and operator error, can significantly affect a person's investigations and treatment. Nurses should be aware of the potential pitfalls in recording and overcome the risk of errors. Table 4.3 lists possible problems you may encounter and how to resolve them.

Ambulatory blood pressure monitoring (ABPM)

Ambulatory blood pressure devices are now used frequently. NICE (2011a) guidelines recommend ambulatory devices are used to identify, measure and monitor patients' blood pressure in the home setting before treatment regimens are commenced. Ambulatory blood pressure devices consist of an electronic device that is worn on the person's arm for 24 hours while they continue their normal daily routine. Such monitoring allows the healthcare team to review the person's blood pressure over a longer period than their hospital visit, providing a more accurate view of their blood pressure measurement. Ambulatory devices are used for people with an unusual variability of readings, possible white coat hypertension, to decide treatment regimes, review drug therapy effectiveness, review hypertension treatment in pregnancy and evaluate symptomatic hypotension.

Recording blood pressure in patients with postural hypotension or requiring sitting and standing blood pressure recordings

Some people experience a drop in blood pressure when they suddenly stand up. For example, older people often experience postural drops in blood pressure that may lead to falls or injury, and some women experience postural drops while pregnant. Identifying postural drop in blood pressure and managing these drops appropriately is essential, thus recordings of lying and standing blood pressures are needed. To record lying and standing blood pressures, first lie the patient down for 5 minutes, ensuring they are as relaxed as possible and not eating, drinking or talking. Measure the blood pressure using an appropriate device. Stand the patient up for a minute taking care of your own and your patient's safety. Measure the blood pressure again. Seat your patient or lie them down again before documenting your findings. Remember that the patient may feel dizzy, faint or sick at this time, so have someone on hand to assist you. If you are concerned about your own or your patient's safety, abandon the procedure and safeguard your patient. Repeat the procedure with colleagues on hand to assist you.

Self-monitoring of blood pressure

In the United Kingdom, approximately 10% of the population now monitor their own blood pressure at home, work or elsewhere using electronic devices (www.bhsoc.org). McManus et al. (2012) report how this growing trend allows patients to be more aware of their own blood pressure, and the blood pressures recorded

Pregnancy and birth: practice points – blood pressure

Blood pressure is measured regularly throughout pregnancy as an indication of maternal health. Pregnancy itself is not normally associated with significant changes in arterial blood pressure because any potential rise due to increased blood volume as pregnancy progresses is counterbalanced by the hormone progesterone, which reduces resisitance in blood vessel walls. This effect results in a lowering of systolic pressure of 5–10 mmHg and diastolic pressure of 10–15 mmHg up to 24 weeks of pregnancy However, serious conditions can occur. Blood pressure is monitored at every antenatal appointment and very frequently during labour. Some women develop high blood pressure alone during pregnancy with no other symptoms. NICE (2011b) offers 'Hypertension in pregnancy' guidelines to ensure that these conditions are recognised, monitored and treated. An even more serious complication, *pre-eclampsia* can occur, where the mother's blood pressure may be raised along with protein detected in the urine, after 20 weeks gestation and over. If symptoms are not recognised, this condition can lead to reduced oxygen through the placenta to the foetus (hypoxia) and, in its severest form, lead to *eclampsia* and *eclamptic seizures*, potentially life-threatening for mother and foetus.

during self-monitoring can often be lower than those taken by medical personnel. However, there are some inaccuracies in measuring devices and / or techniques used by people who monitor their own blood pressure. The British Hypertension Society (www.bhsoc.org) offers guidance on which ambulatory devices should be used for these purposes. It is important to be aware that some patients will be well informed about their own blood pressure, and obtaining the patient's views and understanding of this procedure will be beneficial. Normal parameters of the person's blood pressure will be obtained, and potential home monitoring problems with blood pressure recording can be reduced or avoided.

Children: practice points – blood pressure

When measuring blood pressure for an infant or child, the correct size cuff must be used to obtain an accurate reading. For children, blood pressure readings vary with age; see ranges below.

Systolic blood pressure (mmHg)
- <1 year 70–90
- 1–2 years 80–95
- 2–5 years 80–100
- 5–12 years 90–110
- >12 years 100–120

For further guidance on blood pressure in infants and children, see

Gormley-Fleming, E. 2010. Assessment and vital signs: A comprehensive review. In: Glasper, A., Aylott, M. and Battrick, C. (eds.) *Developing Practical Skills for Nursing Children and Young People*. London: Hodder Arnold, 109–47.

Macqueen, S., Bruce, E.A. and Gibson, F. 2012. Assessment. In: *The Great Ormond Street Hospital Manual of Children's Nursing Practices*. Chichester: Wiley-Blackwell, 1–35.

Royal College of Nursing. 2011. Standards for assessing, measuring and monitoring vital signs in infants, children and young people. Available from: http://www.rcn.org.uk/__data/assets/pdf_file/0004/114484/003196.pdf.

Summary
- Blood pressure is an important indicator of health.
- Readings can be affected by psychological, physical and environmental factors, but technique and equipment are also important aspects.
- Electronic devices are increasingly used for recording pulse, blood pressure and oxygen saturation. However, an understanding of how to use manual equipment accurately remains important for nurses.
- There is increasing use of ambulatory devices and self-monitoring of blood pressure, which can lead to greater accuracy as blood pressure is measured over time, rather than as a one-off, and patients may be more relaxed.

MEASURING OXYGEN SATURATION BY PULSE OXIMETRY

Pulse oximetry enables continuous non-invasive monitoring of the oxygen saturation of haemoglobin (SpO_2) in arterial blood, updated with each pulse wave, via a microprocessor with a probe attached to the patient. Haemoglobin (Hb) is a molecule present in erythrocytes (red blood cells) that transports gases – especially oxygen – around the body. About 98% of the oxygen in the blood is transported and attached to these Hb molecules, then called oxyhaemoglobin (HbO_2), and about 2% of the oxygen is carried and dissolved in the plasma. Pulse oximetry measures how saturated with oxygen are the Hb molecules.

LEARNING OUTCOMES

By the end of this section, you will be able to:
1 explain how pulse oximetry works and how it is used;
2 identify when pulse oximetry is used and discuss its advantages and limitations.

You may be able to access a pulse oximeter in the skills laboratory or your practice setting.

Learning outcome 1: Explain how pulse oximetry works and how it is used

ACTIVITY

Have you seen pulse oximetry used in practice? If so, can you remember what the equipment looked like, and do you know how it works? What is a normal reading?

Pulse oximeters range from small hand-held devices, displaying the percentage of oxygen saturation and the pulse rate, to more substantial devices that also show the pulsatile waveform (Figure 4.7). The box has a wire leading to the sensor or probe – a clip or sleeve that is placed on a finger, toe or earlobe. Probes can be disposable or reusable and are available in different sizes. Ambulatory devices allow the patient to be monitored while still maintaining some independence and mobility. The diagram in Figure 4.8 shows how the sensor works.

Pulse oximeters monitor only light absorption from tissue with a pulsatile flow, thereby preventing false readings from fat, bone, connective tissue and venous blood. It is essential that the patient has sufficient arterial blood flow to the extremities to produce a reliable reading.

ACTIVITY

If you have access to a pulse oximeter, measure your oxygen saturation using the instructions in Box 4.7.

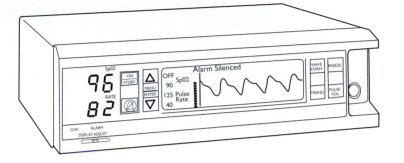

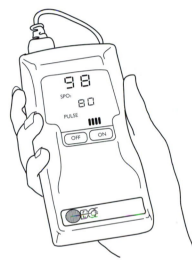

Figure 4.7: Examples of pulse oximeters.

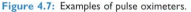

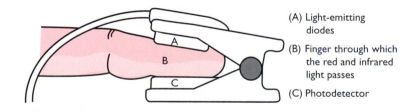

(A) Light-emitting
diodes

(B) Finger through which
the red and infrared
light passes

(C) Photodetector

Figure 4.8: Diagram showing how a pulse oximeter works.

Hypercapnic respiratory failure

Inadequate gas exchange by the respiratory system where there is a buildup of carbon dioxide.

The normal value of oxygen saturation is 95–100%, so hopefully your reading was within that range. This figure refers to the percentage of Hb molecules fully saturated with oxygen. O'Driscoll et al. (2008) suggest that the recommended target saturation range for acutely ill patients not at risk of **hypercapnic respiratory failure** is 94–98%. However, some people, especially if aged 70 years, may have oxygen saturation measurements below 94% and do not require oxygen therapy when clinically stable. Repositioning the person to a more upright position, if not

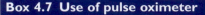

Box 4.7 Use of pulse oximeter

Turn the pulse oximeter on and allow the device to go through its checking and calibration procedure.

- Select the appropriate probe; ensure correct fitting and positioning on the digit. Avoid placing probe on false nails, or nail-polished fingernails.
- Allow several seconds for the oximeter to detect your pulse and calculate your reading.
- Look at the waveform displayed.
- Read percentage (%) displayed and record this number on the observation chart.
- In practice you should record whether the patient is receiving oxygen (and if so, the percentage) or breathing air.

Source: Adapted from Hill, E. and Stoneham, M., *Practical Applications of Pulse Oximetry,* 2000, http://www.nda.ox.ac.uk.

contraindicated, may provide significant improvement. Pulse oximeters have alarm systems that sound if the measurement falls below a normal level.

Most manufacturers claim that their devices are accurate to ±2% at oxygen saturations of 70–99%. The ability of pulse oximeters to detect **hypoxaemia** (insufficient oxygenation of blood) was confirmed by a systematic review (Pedersen et al. 2009). However, as hypoxaemia rises, pulse oximetry becomes less accurate. An SpO_2 of less than 80% can lead to inaccurate readings, so at 80–85% a more detailed assessment is necessary. If there is any doubt about the accuracy of pulse oximetry, blood gas analysis (analysis of a sample of arterial blood) should be performed (see Chapter 11, Box 11.3). If a patient is peripherally shut down or has a weak pulse, pulse oximetry readings will not be precise. Cardiac arrhythmias such as atrial fibrillation can interfere with capture of the pulsatile signal and thus reduce accuracy.

Fingertips, toes, earlobes and the bridge of the nose can be used to measure oxygen saturation. Movement of the fingers or toes can cause artefact leading to inaccurate readings, so, if possible, the sensor should be attached to a part of the body that the patient is most likely to keep still. Higgins (2005) warns how pulse oximetry does not provide information on Hb concentration, oxygen delivery to the tissues or ventilatory function, so patients may have normal oxygen saturations yet still be **hypoxic**. In the clinical setting, you are advised to ensure that you observe, monitor and report any changes in your patient's appearance along with measuring their oxygen saturation.

> **Hypoxia**
> A condition in which inadequate oxygen is available to the tissues to allow normal function.

Learning outcome 2: Identify when pulse oximetry is used and discuss its advantages and limitations

O'Driscoll et al. (2008) recommended that oxygen saturation should be checked by pulse oximetry for all breathless and acutely ill patients and that pulse oximetry should be available wherever emergency oxygen is used. Assessing hypoxaemia through observation is notoriously inaccurate and unreliable, but hypoxaemia can rapidly lead to tissue damage. The brain is very sensitive to oxygen depletion, and visual and cognitive changes can occur when oxygen saturation falls to 80–85%. Other signs of hypoxaemia include restlessness, agitation, hypotension and tachycardia. However, all these signs can be missed or wrongly interpreted.

Cyanosis is the visible sign of hypoxaemia, but it is only detected at a saturation of about 75% in normally perfused patients. Pulse oximetry should therefore be a more accurate and objective measure of hypoxaemia, alerting health professionals at an early stage. It is an inexpensive and non-invasive method that allows for monitoring during the transfer of a patient.

> **Cyanosis**
>
> A bluish, greyish or purple discoloration of the skin due to presence of abnormal amounts of reduced haemoglobin in the blood.

ACTIVITY

Think about your practice placement experiences. In what situations have you seen pulse oximetry being used?

- **Acute illness.** Pulse oximetry is part of the assessment of anyone who is acutely ill, particularly during initial assessment and management.
- **Investigations and surgery.** Pulse oximetry is used during and after procedures and investigations involving general anaesthesia, or sedation.
- **Respiratory and circulatory problems.** Patients with respiratory disease, particularly if receiving oxygen therapy, will have SpO_2 monitoring. The amount of oxygen administered may be adjusted according to the SpO_2. O'Driscoll et al. (2008) recommend that oxygen should be prescribed to achieve 94–98% oxygen saturations for most acutely ill patients, or 88–92% for those patients at risk of hypercapnic respiratory failure – and the target saturation should be written on the drug chart. Any patients who are at risk of hypoxaemia – such as those with pneumonia, congestive heart failure, **chronic obstructive pulmonary disease** (COPD) exacerbation or acute lung injury – may have continuous SpO_2 monitoring via a pulse oximeter. Patients whose cardiorespiratory status is unstable, and who are undergoing transfer, often have pulse oximetry *in situ*.
- **Chronic Illness.** Pulse oximetry can be used in the community with people who are at risk of hypoxaemia, for example, with chronically ill patients such as those with **cystic fibrosis**.

> **Chronic obstructive pulmonary disease**
>
> A chronic disease that includes conditions such as emphysema, chronic bronchitis and chronic asthma. It causes debilitating breathlessness, which affects day-to-day living.

> **Cystic fibrosis**
>
> A genetic disease causing oversecretion of a viscous mucous, thus predisposing to respiratory infections.

Limitations of pulse oximetry

Although pulse oximetry has allowed for non-invasive measurements of arterial oxygen saturation, monitoring of pulse oximetry should be viewed with caution. Pulse oximetry complements measurement of other vital signs, but it does not replace them; oxygen saturations are only a single physiological variable and should not be overrelied upon. Pulse oximeters cannot differentiate between different forms of saturated Hb and therefore cannot identify hypoxaemia. When carbon monoxide is inhaled, carboxyhaemoglobin (COHb) is formed and is absorbed and registered as oxyhaemoglobin, leading to overestimation of oxygen saturation. Thus, for people who have been involved in accidents where there was smoke, or who are affected by carbon monoxide poisoning, pulse oximetry is not recommended. COHb readings are also high in tobacco smokers.

Holmes and Peffers (2009) highlight various conditions that can influence pulse oximetry, such as anaemia, including sickle cell anaemia and peripheral vascular disease in older people, and also some antiretroviral medication (HIV drugs). They also identify that nail polish, dirt or artificial nails on the finger tip, movement leading to artefacts and dark or pigmented skin can alter readings. Barnett et al. (2012) describe the choice of sites in pulse oximetry readings and note that ear and finger sites may offer different readings. Therefore, it is important that you identify which site is used routinely in your clinical area, in an attempt to eliminate errors of reading. If you consider the factors mentioned above, you can try to increase accuracy in measurement of pulse oximetry, and you must report any abnormal findings immediately to a qualified nurse or doctor.

Note that it is the quality of oxygen delivery to the tissues that is of most importance – which depends on cardiac output, tissue perfusion and Hb concentration – not just oxygen saturation of arterial blood. Oxyhaemoglobin saturation could be 99%, but this saturation is of no value if the heart cannot deliver it to the tissues.

ACTIVITY

What signs and symptoms might indicate a lack of oxygen to the tissues (hypoxia)?

Signs that you could observe for include the warmth of peripheral areas of the body, colour of skin and tongue, urine output and mental state.

Children: practice points – measuring oxygen saturation

For infants and children, smaller probes are used. Different sizes are available, and for infants, the device used is usually wrapped around the foot. The normal values are the same across the life span. For further guidance on measuring oxygen saturations for infants and children, see

Gormley-Fleming, E. 2010. Assessment and vital signs: A comprehensive review. In: Glasper, A., Aylott, M. and Battrick, C. (eds.) *Developing Practical Skills for Nursing Children and Young People*. London: Hodder Arnold, 109–47.

Macqueen, S., Bruce, E.A. and Gibson, F. 2012. Assessment. In: *The Great Ormond Street Hospital Manual of Children's Nursing Practices*. Chichester: Wiley-Blackwell, 1–35.

Royal College of Nursing. 2011. Standards for assessing, measuring and monitoring vital signs in infants, children and young people. Available at http://www.rcn.org.uk/__data/assets/pdf_file/0004/114484/003196.pdf.

Summary

- Pulse oximetry is widely used and has many applications.
- Pulse oximetry is non-invasive and easy to apply and provides a continuous measurement.
- It is important to understand the limitations of pulse oximetry and to be aware of its role as complementary to the overall clinical picture.

NEUROLOGICAL ASSESSMENT

Neurological assessment is performed to assess a person's neurological status and is appropriate whenever there is impaired consciousness, a history of loss of consciousness or a risk that the level of consciousness might deteriorate. Neurological assessment consists of either a quick review of a patient's neurological state using the **AVPU Scale**, or an evaluation of the level of consciousness using the Glasgow Coma Scale (GCS), pupil size and reaction, motor and sensory function and vital signs. The GCS is now included in many clinical areas as part of the physiological track and trigger assessment or early warning score process in the care of acutely ill people, as recommended by NICE (2007a). See Chapter 11 for more information.

AVPU Scale

A = Alert
V = (responds to) Voice
P = (responds to) Pain
U = Unresponsive

LEARNING OUTCOMES

By the end of this section, you will be able to:

1 appreciate why a neurological assessment would be needed and what instruments are used;
2 accurately perform and record an assessment of an adult's neurological status.

Learning outcome 1: Appreciate why a neurological assessment would be needed and what instruments are used

ACTIVITY

For which of the people in the scenarios would a neurological assessment be appropriate, and why?

Neurological assessment would be particularly important for Anne and Natalie because they have histories of impaired consciousness. Anne has a head injury and was unconscious briefly. Natalie is not fully alert, and she has ingested an unknown quantity and variety of drugs that may affect her neurological function.

A head injury (as in Anne's case) is a particularly important reason for performing neurological assessment. In 2007, NICE published guidelines for assessing and managing people who have head injuries. Neurological observations should be conducted only by professionals competent in assessment of head injury (NICE 2007b). The GCS, which forms part of this assessment, directly affects subsequent investigations and management for such patients.

Box 4.8 Signs of raised intracranial pressure

- Headache – which is worse in morning and increases in severity with coughing, straining and bending
- Vomiting – which may be projectile; usually worse in morning; often associated with nausea
- Papilloedema – swelling of the optic disc, leading to blurred vision and potential vision loss
- Decrease in level of consciousness
- Seizures
- Changes in pupil size and reaction of the pupils to light; could be enlargement, asymmetry, oval shape or decreased reaction

If any of the above-mentioned changes occur, it is extremely important that you report these immediately to a qualified nurse or doctor.

Source: Mestecky, A. 2011. Assessment and management of raised intracranial pressure. In: Woodward, S. and Mestecky, A. (eds.) *Neuroscience Nursing Evidence Based Practice*. Oxford: Wiley Blackwell, 87–106.

Extradural haematoma

Extradural haematoma is an accumulation of blood between the dura and the skull. The meningeal artery passes through the extradural space and can become torn after a head injury, resulting in an arterial bleed into the extradural space. The brain then becomes compressed and displaced. This condition is life-threatening and requires urgent treatment.

Subdural haematoma

Blood accumulates in the subdural space and gradually builds up to produce a haematoma. This haematoma can lead to compression of the brain, which in turn can result in loss of brain function.

Accurate neurological assessment is particularly important where there is a concern about the development of raised intracranial pressure (Box 4.8). Being a rigid vault, the skull (cranium) cannot accommodate any swelling without the function of the brain being impaired. In disease or injury, the brain tissue, blood or cerebral spinal fluid (CSF) can increase in volume or size, causing a rise in intracranial pressure and thereby affecting cerebral blood flow (Suadoni 2009). In some situations, particularly with a head injury where an **extradural** or **subdural haematoma** can develop, detection of deteriorating consciousness level is paramount because life-saving treatment could be needed. Neurological observations should be carried out under supervision of a registered nurse, and any concerns should be reported immediately.

Instruments used to assess neurological status

The GCS was developed by Jennett and Teasdale (1974) and is widely used and recognised, often being incorporated into trauma assessment charts (Skinner et al. 2002). The GCS is recommended by NICE (2007b).

ACTIVITY

Access a neurological observation scale from your local practice setting. Look at the sections and how they are laid out. They should include the GCS, pupil reactions and limb movements and a section for charting vital signs.

The GCS is used to assist nurses in providing a consistent and standard measurement of people's neurological status (NICE 2007b). Scoring using the GCS is done in three sections: eye opening, motor response and verbal response (Figure 4.8). Each section is given a score, and these scores are totalled to give a score ranging from 15 (best) to 3 (worst). As a person's neurological condition improves, their GCS score should improve.

The severity of a head injury can be indicated by the score attained (Jennett 2005; Jennett and Teasdale 1974). A score of 8 or less indicates a severe head injury, and the person will be in a coma. The rhyme 'If the Glasgow score is 8, then it's time to intubate' may help you to remember that a GCS score of 8 or below is a serious clinical situation where the patient is unconscious. Maintenance of the patient's airway by intubation of the trachea or nasopharyngeal airway using an advanced airway is a specialised clinical skill, performed by advanced practitioners who have undergone training for this procedure. You may, however, be required to observe or assist with this skill in an emergency (for more information, see Chapter 11).

A GCS score of more than 8 indicates that the person is conscious. People with a minor head injury might have a score between 13 and 15. Use of the GCS for people with head injuries is well documented, but it can be used for anyone who requires a neurological assessment, regardless of the underlying cause – so it may be relevant for Natalie and Ken, as well as for Anne.

Learning outcome 2: Accurately perform and record an assessment of an adult's neurological status

When assessing any person in your care the first priorities are to check responsiveness, ensure the patient has an open airway, check breathing and maintain adequate circulation after the basic life-support algorithms (Resuscitation Council [UK] 2010). Systematic assessment of acutely ill patients is discussed further in Chapter 11. It should be quickly established whether the person lost consciousness at any stage and appears to be deteriorating, particularly after an accident (NICE 2007b). Thus, the person and any bystanders should be asked about the incident. Witnesses to a cardiac or respiratory event can be a valuable source of information regarding a person's condition (Resuscitation Council [UK] 2010), so it will be essential to gain a detailed history from Anne's husband about exactly what he observed. The onset and duration of signs and symptoms, previous medical history and any recent illnesses are all useful to note. After taking a history, the person's neurological status can be assessed using the GCS. This assessment provides a quantitative score for assessing eye opening, verbal response and motor response.

ACTIVITY

Find a willing adult volunteer to help you to work through the GCS. Look at the scale in Figure 4.9 and consider how you might assess whether your volunteer's GCS score was 15 – the best response.

A person with a GCS score of 15 will have airway, breathing and circulation that is present and normal and will speak to you and answer questions appropriately. In brief, a talking, breathing, alert, coherent and orientated person will have a score of 15. Hopefully your volunteer attained this score!

Jennett (2005) and NICE (2007b) recommend that the scores for each of the three sections – eye opening (E), motor response (M) and verbal response (V) – should be documented separately to explain exactly what score has been awarded in each category.

	Score
Eye opening	
Spontaneous	4
To speech	3
To pain	2
None	1
Motor response	
Obeys commands	6
Localises to pain	5
Withdraws to pain	4
Abnormal flexion to pain	3
Extensor response to pain	2
No movement	1
Verbal response	
Oriented	5
Confused	4
Inappropriate words	3
Incomprehensible speech	2
None	1

Figure 4.9: Glasgow Coma Scale. (Adapted from Jennett, B. 2005. Development of Glasgow coma and outcome scales. *Nepal Journal of Neuroscience* 2(1): 24–8.)

Each section of the scale is now be explained in more detail via linking to how you might assess Anne, who has sustained a head injury.

Eye opening (E)

Assessment of Anne's eye opening response indicates the arousal mechanisms found within her brainstem. When observing her eye opening response, gently touch her arm when you ask a question. Touch is an important way of communicating non-verbally and is particularly important for people with hearing and visual deficits. Anne's husband could inform you if these deficits apply to Anne. Some people with a head injury might have difficulty opening their eyes due to eyelid swelling, particularly if there is an accompanying facial injury.

- **Spontaneous** (score 4). Anne will score 4 if she opens her eyes or already has her eyes open when you approach her.
- **To speech** (score 3). It is important to differentiate between a person sleeping and being unresponsive. This distinction can be done by asking a simple question, such as 'Can you open your eyes?'

- **To pain** (score 2). If Anne does not open her eyes to speech, you should assess whether she responds to pain. How pain should be inflicted remains controversial. You may only use appropriate touch and must take care not to cause damage such as bruising. Cook and Woodward (2011) suggest that squeezing the trapezius muscle is the most suitable method, achieved through grasping approximately 3 cm of muscle between the thumb and forefinger, where the neck meets the shoulder, and gently twisting for 30 seconds. Alternatively, you can apply supraorbital pressure by pressing the skin just below the eyebrow, or apply the sternal rub by using the knuckles of a clenched fist to apply pressure to Anne's sternum. Underlying injuries must be considered when applying these techniques to avoid causing more pain or injury to people. For example, do not press over the sternum if you know the person has fractured ribs, and do not apply supra-orbital pressure if there is an injury in this area. Only the minimum stimulus to elicit a response should be used. You should discuss the accepted practice within your area with your supervising practitioner.
- **None** (score 1). This score is recorded where applying pain causes no eye opening response.

ACTIVITY

If your volunteer agrees, you could try out the different techniques for applying painful stimuli, or even try them on yourself!

Motor response (M)

When assessing motor response, you should consider pre-existing disabilities and also any new injuries, which in Anne's case could have been sustained in her fall. Motor response assessment is performed in relation to upper limbs, because lower limb responses can reflect spinal function. *Note*: Assessment of limb movement (discussed later) is carried out on both upper and lower limbs.

- **Obeys commands** (score 6). When you are carrying out Anne's other observations, you can assess whether she coordinates her actions in response to your requests. For example, you might ask Anne to roll up her sleeve for blood pressure measurement. Alternatives would be to ask her to close/open her eyes or stick out her tongue. If Anne were unable to obey commands, you would next apply painful stimuli (as discussed previously) and note her motor response to pain.
- **Localises** (score 5). Anne would move her hand towards the pain. For example, if you apply supraorbital pressure, she would try to push your hand away.
- **Withdraws** (score 4). If Anne's limb flexes normally to pain, this response scores a 4.
- **Abnormal flexion** (score 3). Anne's flexion to pain would be slow and abnormal.
- **Extensor response** (score 2). Anne would straighten her arm as a response to painful stimuli.
- **No movement** (score 1). Here, no motor response to any painful stimulus is made.

Verbal responses (V)

The verbal response should be assessed in relation to a person's usual communication, so you need to be aware of how they would communicate normally. Anne's neurological status is being assessed by staff who do not know her and how she communicates, so her husband's input would be particularly helpful.

- **Orientated** (score 5). If Anne is fully orientated, she should be able to answer your questions appropriately. She will tell you her name, where she is and the date.
- **Confused** (score 4). In this case, Anne can discuss something with you but may not give accurate information. For example, when asked 'Where are you?' she may respond: 'I'm in the town'.
- **Inappropriate words** (score 3). Here, Anne will use words that do not make sense. She may appear agitated and at times aggressive when you ask questions.
- **Incomprehensible speech** (score 2). Anne will not use any understandable words but will make verbal noises such as mumbling, moaning or groaning.
- **None** (score 1). Anne will not respond verbally at all. If a person is intubated, they will be unable to talk and should be recorded as 'I'.

ACTIVITY

When assessing a person's GCS score, what factors could affect the accuracy of the assessment and how could you overcome these?

- **Hearing loss.** If the person has impaired hearing, it may be difficult to communicate verbally, which could affect the accuracy of the result in all three categories. Sign language could be used or a communication board, provided that this is appropriate to the person's level of consciousness and that their vision is not impaired. The person may lip-read and therefore be able to communicate effectively with you. Written responses are also valuable in this situation.
- **Language barrier.** If a person cannot understand or speak English, it could lead to difficulties with obtaining an accurate response, for example, assessing orientation or whether commands are obeyed. A communication board may help, or assistance from a professional interpreter.
- **Speech difficulties or physical impairment.** A person with learning disabilities, for example, may communicate by a signing system, in which case information from family or carers would be important.
- **Alcohol use.** If a person has ingested alcohol and has a suspected head injury, it is difficult to assess accurately. However, nurses should always err on the side of caution. A person's neurological assessment should never be assumed to be due to alcohol until other causes, for example, a head injury, have been ruled out.

A nurse carrying out neurological assessment of any of the people in the scenarios would need to be aware of all of the above-mentioned factors. For example, any of them could have impaired hearing. Involvement by family or significant others who know the person's usual level of response is invaluable.

Pupil reaction

Assessment of pupil reaction usually forms part of neurological observation, as alteration in pupil sizes and reaction could indicate a rise in intracranial pressure. Look at the pupil sizes shown in Figure 4.10. You will see that they are shown in varying sizes from 1 to 8 mm. The person should be examined in dim light because bright light affects pupil reactions to the torchlight.

ACTIVITY

Ask your willing volunteer to walk into a brightly lit room, and observe what happens to their pupils. Now observe the pupils in a dimly lit room. When did the pupil size appear the greatest?

When recording pupil reactions, the size and reaction of each eye are checked and recorded individually, for example, L5 for left eye and R5 for right eye. A light beam (usually from a pen torch) is directed into the eye to assess the reaction to the light and the size of the pupil against the chart.

- **Pupil sizes and equality.** Before shining the light in the eyes consider the following: Are the pupils equal? Do they look between 2 and 5 mm? Do they look round?

- **Reaction.** What happens when a light is shone into the eyes? Are the reactions brisk? (If yes, record **B**.) Are they sluggish? (If yes, record **SL**.) Is there no reaction? (If so, record **None**.)

Always note whether a person is wearing contact lenses or has a false eye because these conditions will affect the results. In Figure 4.10, both the left and right pupils have been recorded as 4B, meaning that the pupils are approximately 4 mm in size and react to light briskly.

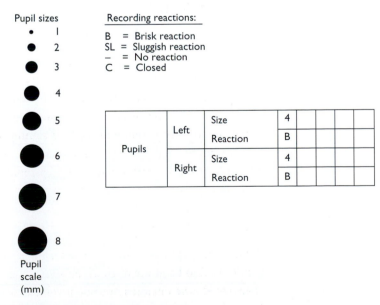

Figure 4.10: Pupil sizes and recording reactions.

Now assess the size and reaction of your volunteer's pupils.

Glaucoma

An increase in the intraocular pressure of the eye causing reduced vision in the affected eye.

People with visual impairment or people who have had ocular surgery or disease may have altered pupil reactions, so you should establish what is normal for this person. For example, a person who has **glaucoma** may use eyedrops that constrict the pupil.

Limb movements

A neurological chart contains a section for recording limb movements. There are different versions used in practice, and Box 4.9 gives one example. Verbal commands are used to examine these movements. For example, the nurse may ask the person to push and pull against them with each limb. The responses are recorded for arms and legs separately. If there is a difference between the limbs, they are recorded separately.

In Box 4.9, the assessment indicates normal power in both legs, a mild weakness in the left arm and normal power in the right arm. **Normal power** is recorded when the person responds appropriately to commands and shows normal function and strength of the limb. **Mild weakness** implies that the limb can be moved but with reduced power. The arm weakness recorded on the chart shown may be due to a stroke or other pre-existing condition, such as cerebral palsy. **Severe weakness** implies movement is possible but with no real strength. **Flexion** is recorded when the knee or elbow is bent, and **extension** is recorded when the arm or leg straightens, when a painful stimulus is applied. **No response** is recorded when no stimulus (as used in best motor response) obtains any motor response from the person.

Box 4.9 Recording limb movements

Arms	Normal power	R		
	Mild weakness	L		
	Severe weakness			
	Flexion			
	Extension			
	No response			
Legs	Normal power	R/L		
	Mild weakness			
	Severe weakness			
	Flexion			
	Extension			
	No response			

(Limb Movements)

Practise all the skills included in this chapter by recording a full set of neurological observations with your willing volunteer. This full set should include vital signs as well as level of consciousness, pupil reactions and limb movements.

Consistency and frequency of neurological recordings

Neurological assessment is complex and requires practice in the clinical setting (NICE 2007b). You should first observe a qualified nurse recording a neurological assessment and then take part under supervision, according to local policy. The first set of neurological observations forms the baseline for future assessment. To improve reliability before a new nurse takes over the care of the person, the previous nurse should demonstrate a neurological assessment.

NICE (2007b) recommended that neurological assessment is conducted on a half-hourly basis until a GCS score equal to 15 has been achieved. The minimum frequency of observations for patients with a GCS score equal to 15 should be half-hourly for 2 hours, then hourly for 4 hours and 2-hourly thereafter.

Children: practice points – neurological assessment

Neurological assessment of children is a complex procedure that must be conducted by a skilled, experienced person. Eye movement, motor responses and vocal responses are measured using a scale of 15/15 with a modified GCS chart (Kirkham et al. 2008). If you have opportunity, compare the different charts used for different age groups in practice. NICE (2007b) guidelines for head injury include infants and children as well as adults.

For further guidance on neurological assessment of infants and children, see

Gormley-Fleming, E. 2010. Assessment and vital signs: A comprehensive review. In: Glasper, A., Aylott, M. and Battrick, C. (eds.) *Developing Practical Skills for Nursing Children and Young People*. London: Hodder Arnold, 109–47.

Macqueen, S., Bruce, E.A. and Gibson, F. 2012. Assessment. In: *The Great Ormond Street Hospital Manual of Children's Nursing Practices*. Chichester: Wiley-Blackwell, 1–35.

Pregnancy and birth: practice points – neurological assessment

In pregnancy, neurological assessment remains the same as in the adult; however, consideration must be given to the parameters of vital signs, as discussed earlier in this chapter. Remember to seek advice about the positioning of the pregnant woman who has become unwell. The unborn child and the life of the mother will be of urgent concern if a neurological condition develops as a rise in vital signs can be harmful to both.

Summary

- Neurological observations are frequently performed by nurses and are very important when monitoring the condition of a person with actual or potential neurological impairment.
- The GCS has been developed to promote consistency in assessment. Nevertheless, slight variations of terminology in the categories of eye opening, motor responses and vocal responses can be found, and there may be variation in how the scale is used in practice. To promote reliability between readings, one nurse should carry out the observations and demonstrate how they were carried out to any other nurse who is taking over the care.
- The GCS score can be highly influential in terms of treatment, further investigation and predicting a patient's eventual outcome. Therefore, students carrying out these observations should be working under supervision and report immediately any concerns.
- Most head injuries are mild, but a few patients suffer serious injuries to their brain, resulting in severe disability or death. Nurses who observe, measure and record neurological observations must be aware that people who have experienced neurological trauma can deteriorate very quickly. Noticing any changes in neurological function and notifying senior nursing and medical colleagues of these changes are imperative so that life-saving procedures can be carried out.

CHAPTER SUMMARY

This chapter aimed to help you develop your skills in assessing vital signs within the practice setting. These observations should not be considered in isolation but as part of a person's holistic assessment, which will include a range of other observations and information from various sources. It is imperative that you observe, question, discuss and practise vital signs first in a simulated environment and then in a clinical area. It is necessary to become familiar with clinical equipment used for vital signs monitoring to ensure that this equipment is used correctly. Overreliance of electronic equipment should be avoided because there is a potential to become deskilled in monitoring vital signs. Observation, rehearsal and supervised practice will initially develop your confidence in performing this set of skills.

Vital signs must be assessed and recorded accurately, using the appropriate equipment in the recommended manner, as per Trust protocols and manufacturers' instructions. They must also be reported and guidance sought in their interpretation. Some vital signs can change quickly along with the person's level of consciousness, so they must be carried out at the required frequency. Chapter 11 offers further guidance regarding the assessment of patients whose condition is deteriorating. It can take considerable practice with a range of people in a variety of settings to become really confident and competent in these skills. See it, record it and report it should be your motto in vital signs monitoring.

REFERENCES

3M™. 2007. *3M Tempa DOT™ Single-use Clinical Thermometers: How to Read 3M Tempa DOT Thermometers.* US: 3M Medical Division. www.3M.com/healthcare

Barnett, E., Duck, A. and Barraclough, R. 2012. Effect of recording site on pulse oximetry readings. *Nursing Times* 108(1–2): 22–3.

Blows, W.T. 2012. *The Biological Basis of Nursing: Clinical Observations,* 2nd edn. London: Routledge.

Bridges, E. and Thomas, K. 2009. Noninvasive measurement of body temperature in critically ill patients. *Critical Care Nurse* 29: 94–7.

British Hypertension Society. 2012a. Blood pressure measurement with manual blood pressure monitors. Available from: http://www.bhsoc.org/files/9013/4390/7747/BP_Measurement_Poster_-_Manual.pdf

British Hypertension Society. 2012b. Blood pressure measurement with electronic blood pressure monitors. Available from: http://www.bhsoc.org/files/8413/4390/7770/BP_Measurement_Poster_-_Electronic.pdf

Centre for Maternal and Child Enquiries (CMACE). 2011. Saving mothers' lives: Reviewing maternal deaths to make motherhood safer: 2006–08. The Eighth Report on Confidential Enquiries into Maternal Deaths in the United Kingdom. *BJOG* 118 (Suppl.1):1–203.

Childs, C. 2011. Maintaining body temperature. In: Brooker, C. and Nicol, M. (eds.) *Alexander's Nursing Practice: Hospital and Home,* 4th edn. Edinburgh: Churchill Livingstone, 617–32.

Clark, C.E., Taylor, R.S., Shore, A.C., et al. 2012. Association of a difference in systolic blood pressure between arms with vascular disease and mortality: A systematic review and meta-analysis. *The Lancet* 379(9819): 905–14.

Cook, N. and Woodward, S. 2011. Assessment, interpretation and management of altered consciousness. In: Woodward, S. and Mestecky, A. (eds.) *Neuroscience: Evidence-Based Practice.* Chichester: Blackwell Science, 107–22.

Davie, A. and Amoore, J. 2010. Best practice in the measurement of body temperature. *Nursing Standard* 24(42): 42–9.

Dawson, G. and Robson, F.D.E. 2012. Puerperal sepsis: a case study. *British Journal of Midwifery* 20(7): 472–6.

Department of Health (DH). 2002. *Action for Health – Health Action Plans and Health Facilitation.* London: DH.

Department of Health (DH). 2009. *Health Action Planning and Health Facilitation for People with Learning Disabilities: Good Practice Guidance.* London: DH.

Everett, F. and Wright, W. 2011. Measuring vital signs: An integrated teaching approach. *Nursing Times* 107(27): 16–17.

Higgins, D. 2005. Pulse oximetry. *Nursing Times* 101(6): 34.

Hill, E. and Stoneham, M. 2000. Practical applications of pulse oximetry. Available from: http://www.nda.ox.ac.uk (Accessed on 7 February 2013).

Holmes, S. and Peffers, S. 2009. PCRS-UK opinion sheet No 28 pulse oximetry in primary care. Available from: http://www.pcrs-uk.org (Accessed on 1 February 2013).

Jennett, B. 2005. Development of Glasgow coma and outcome scales. *Nepal Journal of Neuroscience* 2(1): 24–8.

Jennett, B. and Teasdale, G. 1974. Assessment of the coma and impaired consciousness. *The Lancet* 2: 81–4.

Kirkham, F., Newton, C., and Whitehouse, W. 2008. Paediatric coma scales. *Developmental Medicine & Child Neurology* 50(4): 267–74.

Lewis, S. 2011. The nursing week: Deteriorating patient special. *Nursing Times* 107(3): 2–4.

Marieb, E. 2012. *Essentials of Human Anatomy and Physiology,* 10th edn. San Francisco, CA: Benjamin Cummings.

Marieb, E.N. and Hoehn, K. 2013. *Human Anatomy and Physiology,* 9th edn. London: Pearson Education.

McManus, J., Glasziou, P., Haye, A., et al. 2012. Self-monitoring: Question and answers from a national conference. *British Medical Journal* 337(10): 2732.

Medicines and Healthcare Products Regulatory Agency (MHRA). 2009. Kid's stuff – paediatric special. *One-liners* (73). Available from: http://www. mhra. gov.uk (Accessed on 1 February 2013).

Medicines and Healthcare Products Regulatory Agency (MHRA). 2012. *Device Bulletin: Blood Pressure Measurement Devices.* Available from: http://www. mhra. gov.uk (Accessed on 1 February 2013).

Meechan, R., Jones, H. and Valler-Jones, T. 2011. Students' perspectives on their skills acquisition and confidence. *British Journal of Nursing* 20(7): 445–50.

Mestecky, A. 2011. Assessment and management of raised intracranial pressure. In: Woodward, S. and Mestecky, A. (eds.) *Neuroscience Nursing Evidence Based Practice.* Oxford: Wiley Blackwell, 87–106.

Molton, A., Blacktop, J. and Hall, C. 2001. Temperature taking in children. *Journal of Child Health Care* 5(1): 5–10.

Montague, S.E., Watson, R. and Herbert, R. 2005. *Physiology for Nursing Practice,* 3rd edn. Edinburgh: Elsevier.

National Institute for Health and Clinical Excellence (NICE). 2006. *Atrial Fibrillation. The Management of Atrial Fibrillation.* Clinical Guidelines 36. London: NICE.

National Institute for Health and Clinical Excellence (NICE). 2007a. *Quick Reference Guide. Acutely Ill Patients in Hospital: Recognition of and Response to Acute Illness in Adults in Hospital.* Clinical Guidelines 50. London: NICE.

National Institute for Health and Clinical Excellence (NICE). 2007b. *Head Injury: Triage, Assessment, Investigation and Early Management of Head Injury in Infants, Children and Adults.* Clinical Guidelines 56. London: NICE.

National Institute for Health and Clinical Excellence (NICE). 2011a. *Hypertension: Clinical Management of Primary Hypotension in Adults.* Clinical Guidelines 127. London: NICE.

National Institute for Health and Clinical Excellence (NICE). 2011b. *Hypertension in Pregnancy: The Management of Hypertensive Disorders during Pregnancy.* Clinical Guidelines 107. London: NICE.

Nicholas, A. 2012. Oscillometric sphygmomanometers: A critical appraisal of current technology. *Blood Pressure Monitoring Journal* 17(2): 80–8.

Norris, M. and Siegfried, D. 2011. *Anatomy and Physiology for Dummies,* 2nd edn. Indianapolis, IN: Wiley.

Nursing and Midwifery Council (NMC). 2010. *Standards for Pre-Registration Nursing Education.* London: NMC.

O'Brien, E. 2001. Blood pressure measurement is changing. *Heart* 85(1): 3–5.

O'Brien, E., Asmar, R., Beilin, L., et al. 2003. European Society of Hypertension recommendations for conventional, ambulatory and home blood pressure measurement. *Journal of Hypertension* 21: 821–48.

O'Brien, E., Petrie, J., Littler, W., et al. 1999. *Blood Pressure Measurement Recommendations of the British Hypertension Society.* London: BMJ Publications.

O'Driscoll, B.R., Howard, L.S. and Davison, A.G. 2008. Guideline for emergency oxygen use in adult patients. *Thorax* 63 (Suppl VI): vi1–vi68.

Patient Safety First. 2008. The 'How to Guide' for reducing harm from deterioration. Available from: http://www.patientsafetyfirst.nhs.uk/ashx/Asset.ashx?path=/How-to-guides-2008-09-19/Deterioration%201.1_17Sept08.pdf) (Accessed on 21 September 2013).

Pedersen, T., Hovhannisyan, K. and Møller, A.M. 2009. Pulse oximetry for perioperative monitoring. *Cochrane Database of Systematic Reviews Issue* (4): Art. No.: CD002013. DOI: 10.1002/14651858.CD002013.pub2.

Resuscitation Council (UK). 2010. *Resuscitation Guidelines.* Available from: http://www.resus.org.uk (Accessed on 1 February 2013).

Rose, L. 2010. Vital signs. *American Journal of Nursing* 110(5): 11.

Royal College of Nursing. 2007. Standards for assessing, measuring and monitoring vital signs in infants, children and young people. Available from: http://www.rcn.org (Accessed on 7 February 2013).

Skerrett, P.J. 2012. *Different Blood Pressure in Right and Left Arms Could Signal Trouble.* Available from: http://www.health.harvard.edu/blog/different-blood-pressure-in-right-and-left-arms-could-signal-trouble-201202014174 (Accessed on 21 September 2013).

Skinner, D., Driscoll, P. and Earlam, P. 2002. *ABC of Major Trauma,* 3rd edn. London: BMJ.

Suadoni, M.T. 2009. Raised intracranial pressure: Nursing observations and interventions. *Nursing Standard* 23(43): 35–40.

Tortora, G. and Derrikson, B. 2011. *Principles of Anatomy and Physiology,* 11th edn. New York: John Wiley.

Tuggle, D. 2009. Hypotension and shock: The truth about blood pressure. *Nursing Critical Care* 4(6): 29–35.

Waugh, A. and Grant, A. 2010. *Ross and Wilson's Anatomy and Physiology in Health and Illness,* 11th edn. London: Churchill Livingstone.

Webster, R. and Thompson, D. 2011. Nursing patients with cardiovascular disorders. In: Brooker, C. and Nicol, M. (eds.) *Alexander's Nursing Practice Hospital and Home,* 4th edn. Edinburgh: Churchill Livingstone, 9–50.

Williams, B., Poulter, N.R., Brown, M.J., et al. 2004. British Hypertension Society guidelines for hypertension management: Summary. *British Medical Journal* 328: 7440–634.

World Health Organization (WHO). 2011. Mercury-free healthcare: An initiative to substitute mercury-based medical devices around the world. Available from: http://www.mercuryfreehealthcare.org (Accessed on 1 February 2013).

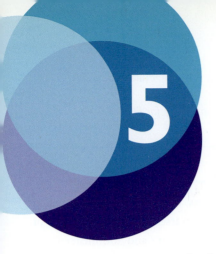

5

Administering Medicines

Kirsty Andrews and Martina O'Brien

In almost every healthcare setting, nurses administer medicines or supervise their administration. To administer and supervise medicines safely, nurses require a breadth of knowledge, including pharmacology and legal and policy issues. They also need to know how to administer medicines via a variety of routes and how to perform medicine dose calculations. Nurses must have the skills to work in partnership with patients and colleagues (such as the pharmacist). To administer medicines safely requires considerable experience and practice. Therefore, students should take every opportunity to develop their knowledge and skills during the preregistration nursing programme. The Nursing and Midwifery Council's (NMC 2010a) Essential Skills Clusters for medicines management are represented in this chapter's content.

This chapter includes the following topics:

- Legal and professional issues in medicine administration
- Safety, storage and general principles of medicine administration
- Administering oral medication
- Applying topical medication
- Administering medication by injection routes
- Administering inhaled and nebulised medication
- Intravenous fluid and blood administration
- Calculating medicine and intravenous fluid administration doses
- Preventing and managing anaphylaxis

Recommended pharmacology reading:

It is important that you have an understanding of the pharmacology of medicines; this understanding includes how medicines work in the body (pharmacodynamics) and how medicines are absorbed into the body, distributed to body tissues, metabolised and excreted from the body (pharmacokinetics). There are pharmacology books available that are applied to nursing and healthcare practice, and you may find these helpful. Examples are as follows:

- Greenstein, B. 2009. *Trounce's Clinical Pharmacology for Nurses*, 18th edn. Edinburgh: Churchill Livingstone.

- Karch, A.M. 2008. *Focus on Nursing Pharmacology*, 4th edn. Philadelphia, PA: Lippincott Williams and Wilkins.
- McGavock, H. 2011. *How Drugs Work: Basic Pharmacology for Health Care Professionals*, 3rd edn. Radcliffe: Oxford.

PRACTICE SCENARIOS

The following practice scenarios illustrate situations where medicines are being administered via several different routes and where nurses require knowledge of these drugs' actions and side effects, as well as how to store and administer them safely. These scenarios are referred to throughout the chapter.

Adult

Mercy Makumbe is 72 years old. She has recently had a below-knee amputation of her leg, has a long history of cardiovascular disease and has now been transferred to her local community hospital, where she is currently receiving subcutaneous (SC) **heparin**, as well as oral morphine solution for pain. For years, she has taken **diuretics** and other medication for her cardiac problems, and she is concerned about having to take regular strong pain-relieving medicines too. She has had a known penicillin allergy for some time. She has also been prescribed **fucidin** cream for a small infected area behind one ear. A recent urinalysis showed blood in her urine.

Learning disability

Carol Lee is a 57-year-old woman who has mild learning disability and has been diagnosed as having symptoms of early-onset **dementia**. She lives with one other person with a learning disability, and they are now supported by a sleep-in support worker. Over the past year, she has experienced two seizure-like episodes and has been prescribed **anticonvulsant medication**. She wishes to maintain her independence and self-medicate. The community learning disability nurse is working with her and her support worker to enable her to manage this. They are using a **Dosett box system** and pictures as prompts. They are also helping her to record any side effects.

Mental health

Malcolm Barber is 49 years old and has a long history of schizophrenia. His main carer is his wife. His condition was stabilised on oral medication, until he experienced side effects of weight gain and akathesia (an inability to sit still). Because of these side effects, he stopped taking the medication, began to neglect himself and developed symptoms of psychosis. This deterioration led to his admission to an acute mental health unit as a voluntary patient. On admission, he was given a test dose of a depot, which is a slow-release injection of an antipsychotic drug. This treatment led to an improvement in his mental state, with minimal side effects. The plan is for him to continue with these injections administered twice-monthly by his community mental health nurse. Malcolm also has mild asthma and has a salbutamol inhaler that he uses occasionally.

Heparin

An anticoagulant that works by prolonging the anticoagulation time. It is not absorbed orally and is given either subcutaneously or intravenously.

Diuretics

Medicines that cause increased excretion of urine by the kidneys. There are many types of diuretic medicine.

Fucidin

A topical antibiotic cream used for treatment of a wide variety of infected skin conditions.

Dementia

The term *dementia* is used to describe the symptoms that occur when the brain is affected by specific diseases and conditions. Dementia is progressive; symptoms include loss of memory, confusion and problems with speech and understanding. See http://alzheimers.org.uk for more information.

Anticonvulsant medication

Medicines used to treat or control seizures particularly in individuals who have epilepsy.

Dosett box system

An aid to support medication compliance. A pre-prepared box of medication with identified doses for each day. Nomad is another similar system.

LEGAL AND PROFESSIONAL ISSUES IN MEDICINE ADMINISTRATION

Nurses must adhere to many legal and professional issues relating to safe medicine administration.

LEARNING OUTCOMES

By the end of this section, you will be able to:
1 identify key aspects of legislation, policies and professional issues governing medicine administration;
2 discuss important professional issues for nurses who are administering medicines;
3 discuss the importance of working in partnership with patients;
4 understand what Patient Group Directions are and how they are used in practice.

Learning outcome 1: Identify key aspects of legislation, policies and professional issues governing medicine administration

ACTIVITY

Who do you think might provide rules about medicine administration? Discuss this issue with one of your colleagues. Consider abuse of drugs and related regulations. What have you seen about drug safety in the media?

All major issues related to managing the prescribing and safety of medicines are regulated by government legislation. Therefore, all issues connected with medicines management involve legal as well as professional issues (Ogston-Tuck 2011). The National Reporting and Learning System (NRLS), formerly the National Patient Safety Agency (NPSA), monitors and advises on many issues related to medicines administration.

Traditionally, medicines were prescribed only by doctors or dentists. Legislation now permits non-medical staff, including nurses and pharmacists, to prescribe from the *British National Formulary* (BNF) if they have received special training (Department of Health [DH] 2005a). This type of prescribing is called **non-medical prescribing** (Nuttall and Rutt-Howard 2011).

ACTIVITY

Find a nurse who is able to prescribe and ask him or her about what prescribing involves.

You are probably aware that there is government legislation covering abuse of drugs, sale of medicines over the counter, labelling of medicines and pharmacies in supermarkets. Two important acts of Parliament, the Misuse of Drugs Act 1971 and the Medicines Act 1968, provide public protection in these and related matters

189

and infringement of these acts is a criminal offence. There are other related acts and reports too. The main acts are introduced below.

- *The Misuse of Drugs Act 1971* lists and classifies controlled drugs (CDs). It also details special controls for the manufacture, supply and possession of CDs.
- The *Misuse of Drugs Regulations 2001* identifies five schedules for CDs and specifies requirements for their import, export, manufacture, supply, possession, prescribing and record keeping.
- The *Medicines Act 1968* controls the manufacture, importation, exportation, labelling, sale and distribution of all medicines and established a licensing system.
- The *Mental Capacity Act 2005* defines and advises on a patient's capacity to understand treatment, including medicine administration. It also covers the role of professionals in protecting such patients. Chapter 2 explains more about this act and assessment of mental capacity.
- The revised *Duthie Report* (RPSGB 2005) provides further guidance on storage and administration of medicines.
- The *Health Act 2006* requires the appointment of an accountable officer for each healthcare organisation who is responsible for the safe use and management of CDs.

Categories of medicines defined in the Medicines Act 1968

- **Prescription-only medicines (POMs).** POMs can be obtained only on prescription from any registered independent prescriber. In hospitals, almost all medicines are POMs. Each patient has a medicines administration chart where the medicines to be administered are detailed. If you have any medicines prescribed by your general practitioner (GP), in many cases you will see POM printed on the packet.
- **Pharmacy-only medicines (P).** Pharmacy-only medicines can be sold only in the presence of a pharmacist, but they do not require a prescription. The pharmacist may ask the customer questions relating to their symptoms to ascertain that the medicine they are requesting is appropriate. These medicines are identified by the letter 'P' on the packaging
- **General sale list (GSL).** GSL medicines are a restricted list of medicines that can be freely sold through almost any outlet, for example, garages and supermarkets. Although there are no general restrictions on their sale, as with any medicine, there is potential to misuse them. The Medicines and Health care products Regulatory Agency (MHRA) provides guidance for some medicines. For example paracetamol may only be sold in packets of 16 tablets/capsules as a GSL (MHRA 2009). However, in hospital settings, there is control over these medicines too.

ACTIVITY

Can you think of an example for each of the above-mentioned three categories of medicines?

Suggested examples are antibiotics (POM), cough mixtures (P) and aspirin (GSL). There are many other examples, of course. Note that the category into which a medicine is placed can change; for example, ibuprofen was a pharmacy-only medicine but is now a GSL medicine.

Controlled drugs

ACTIVITY

CDs were mentioned briefly above. Why would a drug need to be controlled in some special way? What might make a drug particularly dangerous if people could access it easily?

A controlled drug is addictive, because of the dependency that could result. Medicines such as pethidine, morphine or any other medicines of the opiate family (derived from opium) can cause addiction, with all its consequences, very quickly if taken for non-therapeutic reasons. These medicines are therefore dangerous, and their sale is controlled because of their addictiveness. They are controlled by the legislation detailed above. Since the Shipman Inquiry (DH 2005b), their control has been tightened still further, including electronic prescribing in primary healthcare settings with the move to implementing this system in acute healthcare settings in the future. Anyone collecting CDs also now has to provide official identity before collection. Mercy, like many other patients, may be anxious about taking morphine because of this view of potentially addictive drugs.

The Misuse of Drugs Act 1971 and the Misuse of Drugs Regulations 2001 identify five categories of CDs, with category 1 being those drugs requiring the most control because of their serious addictive qualities and category 5 drugs requiring the least control. It also underlines that CDs must be kept in a separate locked cupboard with no other medicines in them and supplied with a key that is different from any other key in that setting. It does not stipulate the need for a locked cupboard within a locked cupboard, although this practice is common in acute healthcare settings for additional safe storage. In addition, a light is situated on the outside of the cupboard to alert staff when the cupboard is open or has not been locked. In people's homes, too, drugs must be kept very securely, with decisions based on an assessment of local risk (NMC 2010b). The level of safety has to be negotiated with the person concerned, because it is within their property. Carol's nurse will have to consider this negotiation and either carry out a risk assessment or work with the support staff to complete a risk assessment.

CDs can be ordered only by a registered nurse. They must be administered by a registered nurse with a second checker, who fits the local medicines management policy criteria for a checker. Criteria may vary in community settings and where people are self-medicating. You should check these details in every setting you work in and try to access the appropriate medicines management policy (Royal Pharmaceutical Society of Great Britain [RPSGB] 2005). Checking administration of CDs requires an understanding of the gravity of the issue, as detailed above. Thus, student nurses may be able to check these medicines, but in some areas a student nurse check may not be permitted. You will need to check your hospital or Trust medicines management policy in conjunction with your university medicines management policy to ascertain whether you are allowed to act as a second checker.

Checking during administration involves the whole procedure from preparing the medicine, each checker individually calculating the dose, administration of the medicine and disposal of any remaining medicine and equipment (NMC 2010b). Therefore, if you were the second checker when Mercy receives her morphine, you would have to accompany the registered nurse throughout the procedure. As a student nurse, you need to feel confident to check and give such medicines. You may decide that you need more observational practice and knowledge before being prepared to take on this role.

CD registers must include details of stock and medicines administered and must be signed by both persons providing such detail. They should be kept for at least 2 years. Once electronic ordering records are in widespread use, the requirement will be to preserve secure copies of the records for up to 11 years (DH 2008).

ACTIVITY

As you are now aware, there are laws that govern medicine administration. What other organisations may be involved in medicine regulation?

You should have included professional bodies and employers.

Professional bodies

Professional bodies involved in medicine regulation in the United Kingdom (UK) include the British Medical Association (BMA), the Royal Pharmaceutical Society (RPS) (formerly the RPSGB) and the NMC.

Pharmacists provide expert knowledge about medicines and often have an information adviser who can provide instant and accurate advice. The NMC issues guidance via statements of principles on many issues, including administration of medicines, to all its registered nurses in all fields. It is vital that nurses read these statements of principles and abide by them, to protect patients/clients and themselves professionally. The booklet *Standards for Medicines Management* (NMC 2010b) clarifies that administration is about thought and judgement as well as a task and that registered nurses must take personal accountability for their actions. The NMC also expects newly qualified graduate nurses to work within legal and ethical guidelines, thus ensuring safe and effective management of medicines (NMC 2010a). Approximately 100 people die or are seriously harmed each year due to medication incidents (NPSA 2009).

ACTIVITY

Access and familiarise yourself with the NMC's (2010b) *Standards for Medicines Management* and the NMC's (2008) 'The code: Standards of conduct, performance and ethics for nurses and midwives' (both downloadable from www.nmc-uk.org).

Employers

Employers, both private healthcare employers (e.g. care homes) and National Health Service (NHS) Trusts, produce medicine policies. Independent care providers will each have their own medicine administration policies, which Carol's community nurse must comply with. Similarly, Malcolm's Mental Health Trust will have a policy about patients' mental capacity to understand and adhere to prescribed treatments.

Staff must work to the regulations set out in their particular employer's policy. These policies contain useful information in a usually readable format. They refer to the student role and other issues too. They are particularly useful where administration is not straightforward, as in all three scenarios in this chapter.

Learning outcome 2: Discuss important professional issues for nurses who are administering medicines

Professional issues of particular relevance are personal accountability, knowledge and honesty.

Personal accountability

When administering medicines, a registered nurse takes personal accountability for his or her actions, as with all interventions carried out by registered nurses (NMC 2008). Therefore, if you as a student give out medication under supervision, the registered nurse is accountable for what you do, as well as their own actions. There are no legal frameworks governing who can actually administer medicines, although local policies will stipulate how medicines should be administered. The Royal Pharmaceutical Society of Great Britain (RPSGB 2005) states that the person administering medication (e.g. Carol's sleep-in support worker) can be someone suitably trained.

ACTIVITY

Who do you think would take accountability for Carol's medication arrangements?

Accountability may vary according to local policy and arrangements. Carol's support worker is likely to have operational responsibility for supervising her self-medication, understanding medication use and side effects and reporting to the community nurse or senior support worker. The NMC (2010b) recommends that, ideally, compliance aids (e.g. Dosett or Nomad boxes) should be dispensed, labelled and sealed by a pharmacist, who then takes accountability for this aspect. The community learning disability nurse is likely to be accountable for educating Carol and the support worker about her medication, using the picture prompts. She also has overall responsibility as the registered nurse for ensuring processes are carried out properly, according to Carol's level of capacity (Mental Capacity Act 2005), in view of her dementia.

Although as a student you are not professionally accountable, you should consider these issues in preparation for becoming a registered nurse (NMC 2010b).

Knowledge of medicines

Nurses need a working understanding of medicines administered, therapeutic dosages and side effects (Dougherty and Lister 2011a), coupled with due thought and professional judgement (Watkinson and Seewoodhary 2008). As a student, you need basic knowledge of the medicines you are involved in administering, and you should continue to develop this basic knowledge throughout your preregistration programme and after registration. New medicines are constantly being developed, and knowledge about existing medicines is expanding.

ACTIVITY

Review the scenarios. Are there any particular issues about side effects of medicines? Why should nurses know about side effects of the medicines they administer? Where can you find out about these side effects?

The side effects from Malcolm's oral medication were so unpleasant that he stopped taking these medicines, leading to a recurrence of his mental health symptoms. A urinalysis showed blood in Mercy's urine (haematuria). Nurses caring for her should be aware that this could be a side effect of her prescribed heparin, which is an anticoagulant. Morphine has various unpleasant side effects, including constipation, so these might cause Mercy's reluctance to take them. People like Carol with learning disabilities may be hypersensitive to medication or may experience side effects different from those commonly expected. Staff such as Carol's support worker should be extra vigilant for any unusual effects when medication is prescribed.

There is a compendium called the BNF which provides up-to-date information about all aspects of medicines, including side effects. This book should be available in all clinical settings, but it can also be accessed at www.bnf.org. This compendium would help you understand why Malcolm's medication has been changed and would also assist in Mercy's case; she is taking various medicines together, so you need to know about their interactions.

Honesty about possible errors

If you suspect a medicine administration error, always report it immediately to the nurse in charge. Similarly, if you do not agree with a dosage or any other aspect of a prescription, always have the courage to speak up. Errors cannot be retracted, and the patient is the one who ultimately suffers. An atmosphere of openness and honesty is now being positively encouraged in this respect at all times (NMC 2010b).

Learning outcome 3: Discuss the importance of working in partnership with patients

The NMC (2010a) Essential Skills Clusters for medicines management include the requirement for nurses 'to work in partnership with people receiving medical treatments and their carers'. **The Medicines Partnership** is a DH-supported initiative which aims to enable patients to get the most out of medicines, by involving them as partners in decisions about treatment and supporting them in medicine taking. The Medicines Partnership defines concordance as 'a new approach to the process of successful prescribing and medicines taking, based on partnership between patients and health care professionals'. Its key message is the importance of two-way communication between patients and healthcare professionals to enable patients to better understand their medicines.

The term *adherence* is also a relevant concept to medicines management. Banning (2008) identifies that adherence can be considered as the aim of medicine prescribing, whereas concordance is the process used. Guidelines are offered by the National Institute for Health and Clinical Excellence (NICE 2009) to support the involvement of patients in decisions about their medicines and adherence.

ACTIVITY

Reread the scenarios. What signs are there that healthcare professionals are working in partnership with Mercy, Malcolm and Carol, in relation to their medicines?

There is no obvious indication of partnership working with Mercy from the scenario provided; in particular, it does not appear that pain management methods were discussed with her and an agreement reached as she apparently remains concerned about taking opiates. As with any medication prescribing, Mercy should be encouraged to discuss her values and beliefs about her medicines. Banning (2008) reviewed the literature about patients' beliefs, perceptions and views in relation to medication adherence, highlighting the need for shared decision-making between older people and prescribers. With Carol, partnership working seems much more evident as the community learning disability nurse is working with her and her support worker. In Malcolm's scenario, a lack of partnership working could have underpinned his decision to stop taking his oral anti-psychotic medication, when he experienced side effects, rather than an alternative treatment plan being developed with him. Hopefully, this time, the acute mental health unit staff have worked in partnership with Malcolm in relation to his depot injections, so that medication adherence is more likely.

Learning outcome 4: Understand what Patient Group Directions are and how they are used in practice

Although as a student you cannot administer Patient Group Directions (PGDs), not even under the direct supervision of a registered nurse, you should understand what PGDs entail. In certain circumstances, healthcare professionals can administer prescription-only drugs without a prescription, using a PGD; see National Prescribing Centre (NPC 2009). This is a legal framework allowing certain healthcare professionals (e.g. nurses and therapists) to supply and administer medicines to groups of patients who fit certain criteria, laid down in a previously agreed PGD. Their use is limited to certain patient conditions where it will benefit the patient in terms of speed and continuity of care (because the patient does not need to wait to see a doctor) without compromising patient safety. They are very useful for supplying or administering medicines such as vaccines, analgesics, antibiotics and emergency contraception. A prescription is not required, but there are strict considerations that must be adhered to when you are supplying or administering medicines to your patients under a PGD. For example, certain travel vaccines can be administered to groups of people who fit certain criteria – people who are medically fit, blood pressure within normal limits or no known allergies. The medicine does not need to be prescribed by a doctor or a non-medical prescriber, but it can be given by someone trained in the use of PGDs and related pharmacology, for a particular patient group. PGDs are often used in areas where there is not always a doctor, such as clinics or some emergency settings.

PGDs are not suitable for those patients whose care needs are more complex. In these situations, individuals would need to see the prescriber for a thorough assessment and a prescription based on the outcome of this assessment.

ACTIVITY	Consider what would be needed for safety in PGDs.

You may have thought of the following:
- A clear framework that identifies who can be given the medicine, and in what circumstances.
- Extra training for professionals in pharmacology, understanding the patient group.
- Ongoing effective monitoring of processes and personal competency.

You might wonder about the difference between PGDs and non-medical prescribing. The non-medical prescriber assesses an individual's suitability and issues a medicine prescription for them. PGDs are in a legal framework where a specific medicine can be given to a group of patients who fit certain criteria, without the need for a prescription.

Pregnancy and birth: practice points – medicine administration

The Medicines Act 1968 stipulates that medicines are supplied and administered under direction of a medical practitioner. Midwives are exempt from this requirement for specified medicines under the *Prescription Only Medicines Order 1997; Amended in 2010*. This allows midwives to supply and administer on their own initiative, all GSL and P medicines in their professional practice either as Midwives Exemptions (ME) or as PGDs. The ultimate aim to ensure timely, safe and effective care of women and their babies and to respond aprropriately in an emergency.

Summary

- Medicine administration by a student must be under the direct supervision of a registered nurse.
- Medicine administration must comply with both legal and professional requirements. Therefore, nurses must be familiar with the relevant legislation and NMC guidance and work within their employers' policies.
- Nurses must take responsibility for developing their knowledge about the medicines they are administering, recognising their personal accountability in relation to medicine administration.
- Nurses and other professionals must work in partnership with patients for effective medicine management.
- Appropriately trained nurses can initiate medicine administration using PGDs and non-medical prescribing.

SAFETY, STORAGE AND GENERAL PRINCIPLES OF MEDICINE ADMINISTRATION

LEARNING OUTCOMES

By the end of this section, you will be able to:

1 discuss issues concerning the safety and storage of medicines;

2 understand the general principles of medicine administration, including recording of administration.

Learning outcome 1: Discuss issues concerning the safety and storage of medicines

The revised Duthie Report (RPSGB 2005) reaffirms safety procedures for storing and handling medicines.

ACTIVITY

When you are next in practice, ask a practitioner what these safety procedures are and check them with the points below.

Safe storage

Safe storage varies depending on the setting. In a hospital, there will be a locked cupboard or immobilised medicine trolley; these items must conform to the British Standard for Medicines Storage (BS2881). In a person's home, it could be the kitchen table, if a patient is immobile and lives alone. Even lotions and cleaning agents must be stored like medicines, in a locked or safe place, especially where there are children around. The RPSGB (2005) states that, in care settings, there should be separate locked cupboards for CDs and internal and external medicines.

In some settings, for example, community hospitals, where Mercy is a patient, patients may have their own locked receptacles, where they can access their medication themselves (NMC 2010b). These receptacles must not be readily portable (RPSGB 2005). Continuous assessment of patients' competency to self-medicate must be performed and appropriate documentation completed.

A cool place

Medicines are often quite unstable chemically and may even be manufactured with a stabiliser included in the chemical compound. They generally become more unstable if they are warm; hence, a cool, dark place, away from direct sunlight, is most suitable for storage and this is why medicines are usually stored in dark bottles. Some medicines must be stored in a refrigerator, for example, insulin. In residential settings of any kind, separate locked drug fridges should be used which have a visible temperature gauge on the outside; the temperature is regulated to 8°C (Greenstein 2009).

Stock rotation

As with food storage, medicines should be kept in chronological order, with new items put to the back, and the older items used first. Where the expiry date is given as a month and year, the medicine can be used until the last day of that month.

Labelling of medicines

Most UK medicines have an approved (non-proprietary) name and a brand (proprietary) name. The approved name is the chemical name, and it is used by all prescribers. The brand name may be different, depending on the company who produced it. For example, cold remedies may contain the same constituents but be marketed under different names. These differences in naming can cause confusion, so all prescriptions should display the approved name (O'Brien et al. 2011), and this name is strictly controlled under the Medicines Act 1968.

European law now requires use of the recommended International Non-proprietary Name (rINN) for medicines (available in BNF 2012). Most British approved names (BANs) are the same as the rINNs, but a few BANs have had to be altered and are listed in the BNF. For example, frusemide, a commonly prescribed diuretic, is now known as furosemide.

Medicine containers are labelled with a number specific to a batch of medicines produced at the same time. Thus, medicines should never be transferred from one container to another. Labels could also be misread and different medicines be mixed in the same container.

Holding drugs keys

Keys should always be held by a registered nurse, preferably the nurse in charge (NMC 2010b). As a student, you should never hold the drug keys.

In areas where there is no registered nurse, as in some settings for people with learning disabilities (like Carol), you may be advised not to be involved in medicine administration. This decision is because staff will be unable to comply with professional regulations – although, as discussed earlier, there will be a different policy in place. Talk to your lecturers about this situation.

Learning outcome 2: Understand the general principles of medicine administration, including recording of administration

Medicine administration must be under direct supervision of a registered nurse until you qualify; even then, your employer may require you to undergo assessments to ensure you are competent in all aspects of medicines management before allowing you to administer independently. Good patient/client assessment is vital before administering medicines of any kind.

You may be familiar with the rights that should be considered when administering medicines. There are several variations on how many rights to consider. This section discusses six rights (commonly referred to as the 6 Rs) that must be taken into account when administering medicines. The 6 Rs ensure that the *right* patient receives the *right* medicine and *right* dose via the *right* route at the *right* time ensuring that the *right* documentation procedure is used to record medicines administered or not (O'Brien et al. 2011). Standard 8 of the NMC's Standards for medicines management also clearly details the standard for practice of medicines administration (NMC 2010b).

Right patient

How do you know that this person is the correct person for the medicine? For hospital inpatients in acute hospitals, identity bands are recommended (NPSA 2005); the bands' design and the information on them should be standardised, to improve patient safety (NPSA 2007c). However, the person may not have a name band, for example, in outpatient settings, when a patient is newly admitted, or long-term residents in settings for older people or people with a learning disability (like Carol). You will need to ask the person, or a friend or relative, to tell you their name and date of birth, where possible as well. If you merely ask the person to acknowledge what you think their name is, they may agree regardless, because of their developmental level of functioning or if they are too unwell to think clearly. Up-to-date photos may be used for identity in some settings, attached to the medicines administration chart (NMC 2010b).

You must also gain informed consent from your patient before administering their medicines. You will come across some situations where it may be difficult to obtain informed consent. For example, does Carol understand what the medicine is for and agree to it being given? Only in rare circumstances does consent not need to be given – for example, if the medicine is considered essential (e.g. life-saving) and the person is unconscious, very unwell or unable to understand for developmental reasons.

The Mental Capacity Act 2005 states that, when working with potentially incapacitated people for whatever reason, the healthcare professional must assess their individual capacity at that moment when making decisions on their behalf regarding their care, which includes medicine administration. In some instances, it is necessary to organise a meeting to discuss what medication is in the person's best interests. If Carol's dementia increased and she eventually lacked capacity to make decisions about her medication, the community learning disability nurse would coordinate such a meeting, ensuring the relevant people are invited (e.g. Carol's GP, a family member or advocate).

People who are detained under Section 3 of the Mental Health Act 1983 may be administered medicines to treat their mental health condition without consent, even if they have declined this treatment, for up to 3 months. However, it is only the medication required for their mental health condition, as specified on their section papers, that can be given without consent. A clear explanation about the medicine and rationale for its prescription is essential – see earlier discussion about working in partnership with patients. The explanation should take into account level of understanding and developmental stage, as in Carol's case using picture prompts.

Right medicine

It is vital that you have a good understanding of all medicines that you are administering to your patients. You must ensure that it is suitable for your patient's condition and that it is not contraindicated because of any other medicines they are taking or treatments they are undergoing. The name of the medicine must be written clearly, avoiding abbreviations. Care should be taken to match the name of the prescribed medicine against that on the medicine packaging. Any allergies should be noted and clearly visible on the medicines administration chart and in their patient records. It is recommended that patients wear only one wristband to avoid confusion (NPSA 2007c). Rather than a patient wearing a separate wrist band to indicate an allergy, some Trusts may use a red wrist band detailing the patient's identification details to alert the nurse that the patient has a known risk. The nurse should check the patient's records to establish the type of risk (NPSA 2007c). For example, Mercy is allergic to penicillin. An allergic reaction to a medicine could produce a serious local or systemic reaction – anaphylaxis. Anaphylaxis is a potentially life-threatening condition.

Right dose

Nurses must decide or advise how much of a medicine to give to a patient if the prescription gives a varied dose (e.g. 5–10 mg), thus exercising professional judgement. The nurse should consider whether the dose seems correct for the person and if it falls within the normal dose range for that particular medicine. Some medicines are used for different conditions and will fall outside the normal dose range. The preparation of the medicine may also determine its dose (O'Brien et al. 2011). You must also consider whether the dose involves a complex calculation because then two nurses will be needed. If a calculation has to be done, both nurses need to work it out separately and then compare their answers; otherwise, it is really only one calculation (NMC 2010b).

Right route

It is important to administer the medicine by the correct route. Doing so will ensure that the medicine is used appropriately within the body. Consideration also needs to be given to the preparation of the medicine; for example, clearly a tablet cannot be prescribed for intravenous administration.

Right time

Medicines must be administered at the correct time. Malcolm and his wife need to understand the importance of him receiving his depot injection on exactly the correct day. Some medicines should be taken with food if they need an acid medium in which to be metabolised, whereas others (e.g. the antibiotic flucloxacillin) should be taken on an empty stomach because an acid medium would break the medicine down before it can be absorbed in its useful form. Mercy is taking diuretics, which are usually prescribed in the morning to prevent a diuresis late in the day or at night. She needs to understand that it is preferable to take morphine at regular intervals, instead of waiting until the pain is already severe.

Right documentation

It is vital that all medicines administered are recorded on the patient's medicine administration chart as soon as each is taken.

ACTIVITY

What could the consequences be of failing to record if a patient has taken their medicine?

You may have realised that the nurse who is next to administer the patient's medicines will be faced with the dilemma of whether to administer the medicine or not. If he or she decides to administer it, based on the assumption that it has not been given, the patient could end up receiving an additional dose.

You should note that dispensing a medicine is not the same as administering it. It is therefore not appropriate to sign that you have given a medicine if you have simply just dispensed it into a medicine pot. The registered nurse must follow the correct procedure for his or her organisation in terms of how this information is recorded. The NMC (2010b) states that any medicine refused by the patient or intentionally withheld must also be clearly recorded. A single signature is permitted for administration of any GSL, POM or P medicines (although local policies may require two signatories). Student nurses must always have any medicines they administer under direct supervision of a registered nurse, countersigned by that individual. For CDs, a second signatory is recommended, although when drawing up local policies, appreciation to administering CDs by lone workers in settings such as people's own homes must be taken into consideration. The second signatory is usually another registered healthcare professional, such as a doctor or pharmacist. Student nurses may also act as second signatories, depending on local and university policies (NMC 2010b). Any alteration to a prescription must be signed and dated by the doctor.

Verbal orders

In an emergency, verbal messages may be taken over the phone by a registered nurse. However, a verbal order is not acceptable on its own. Information technology such as fax, e-mail or text message from the prescriber must be attached to the patient's medicines administration chart prior to the medicine being administered.

The verbal order should be signed by the prescriber normally within 24 hours (NMC 2010b). Student nurses should not become involved in verbal messages; always check local medicines policy on these issues.

Abbreviations

You may find that abbreviations are used on medicines administration charts for routes and frequency of administration. The BNF (2012) states that, although generally directions on prescriptions should be written in English without abbreviations, it is recognised that some Latin abbreviations are used. Increasingly frequently, you will see electronic prescribing and administration used in hospital settings. However, facilities must still exist to do prescribing and administration manually if technological breakdown occurs.

ACTIVITY

The BNF recognises all the following abbreviations. Do you know what they mean? Answers are at the end of the chapter.
b.d., o.d., o.m., o.n., q.d.s., t.d.s., stat, e/c, i/m, m/r, mL, p.r.n.

Children: practice points – medicine administration

Nurses administering prescribed medicine to children must ensure that the dose is correct for the individual child's weight. Calculation of children's medicine doses is more complex than for adults because the doses are calculated according to either the child's weight (mg/kg) or body surface area (mg/m²), although body weight is more common in practice. When nurses administer medicines to children, they must take into account the child's developmental stage and find out how the child usually takes medicines (e.g. from a spoon) and continue familiar processes.

Administration of medicines to children is specifically addressed in

Hall, C. 2010. Medicines administration. In: Glasper, A., Aylott, M., and Battrick, C. (eds.) *Developing Practical Skills for Nursing Children and Young People*. London: Hodder Arnold, 148–66.

Macqueen, S., Bruce, E.A. and Gibson, F. 2012. Administration of medicines. In: *The Great Ormond Street Hospital Manual of Children's Nursing Practices*. Chichester: Wiley-Blackwell, 357–95.

Summary

- Nurses need to be familiar with legislation and local policies concerning medicine storage and be aware of issues that could affect safe storage.
- It is crucial that medicines are stored safely, whether in a hospital or in the community, and in appropriate conditions, thus maintaining their effectiveness.
- There are many key safety principles that apply to medicine administration by any route to any individual, and it is very important to adhere to these principles, to uphold safety of patients/clients.

ADMINISTERING ORAL MEDICATION

> **LEARNING OUTCOMES**
>
> By the end of this section, you will be able to:
> 1 identify the different types of oral medication available;
> 2 discuss how to administer oral medication safely.

Learning outcome 1: Identify the different types of oral medication available

ACTIVITY
What types of oral medication have you seen? Devise a list with a colleague.

- **Tablets.** Tablets come in a variety of shapes, sizes, colours and types. They often contain additives to prevent disintegration in the gastrointestinal tract. An enteric coating is used if the drug is a gastric irritant. Some tablets are formulated to control the rate of release; these preparations are referred to as 'sustained-release', 'controlled-release' and 'modified-release' (Dougherty and Lister 2011).
- **Capsules.** Capsules are oval-shaped, with a coat of hard gelatin. They are useful for bitter drugs and for unpleasant liquids, such as chlormethiazole. *Remember*: Never open capsules because they are made to be swallowed whole (Greenstein 2009).
- **Elixirs and syrups.** Elixirs and syrups are flavoured and sweetened liquids particularly useful for children, and many of these liquids are sugar free.
- **Emulsions.** Emulsions are a mixture of two liquids, one dispersed through the other (Greenstein 2009), for example, oil and water. They need to be shaken well to mix the contents.
- **Linctus.** Linctus is a sweet syrupy preparation, for example, cough linctus (Greenstein 2009).

Below are two other forms of medicines that, although taken into the mouth, are not swallowed:

- **Sublingual medication.** These medicines are produced as sprays or as tablets and are absorbed through the mucosa under the tongue. Because the sublingual area is very vascular, absorption and effect of the drug occur rapidly.
- **Buccal medication.** These medicines are usually produced as tablets and are put on to the gum under the lip. Again, the effect of the drug is rapid.

When these routes are used, careful instructions should be given so that the person understands that sublingual and buccal tablets should not be swallowed straight away.

Learning outcome 2: Discuss how to administer oral medication safely

Before administering any medicine, you should know:
- what the medicine is;
- how it works;

- the normal dosage;
- any known side effects;
- any extra precautions you should tell the person.

We are now going to look at how you would administer oral medication to a patient. Hand hygiene and gaining patient consent must always be the first consideration. You should identify the appropriate bottle or packet of medicine that corresponds with the prescription. Check all the prescription details with the medicine label, the expiry date and any special instructions. Think about the person's positioning before administering because sitting up well (if not contraindicated) makes swallowing easier and safer.

Liquids

For people with swallowing difficulties, most oral medicines prescribed will be in liquid form. Many suspensions are sold with a double-ended spoon, which can measure 2.5- and 5-mL volumes, but 5-mL special oral medicine syringes can be obtained from chemists.

First, shake the bottle for even distribution. Then, hold the bottle with the label uppermost, so that the medicine cannot flow over the label and deface it. Now, carefully pour the medicine into a measuring pot; place at eye level on a flat surface to measure the amount dispensed, for accuracy.

If the dose is 1 mL or less, use a 1-mL syringe and aspirate it directly from the bottle or via a quill. It may be useful to use a syringe for withdrawing larger quantities too because they are more accurate than medicine pots. This approach would be appropriate for measuring Mercy's morphine. The BNF (2012) recommends that, for any oral medication prescribed in doses other than multiples of 5 mL, an oral syringe should be used. Oral syringes have a different appearance from usual syringes, and they should be used for all oral liquid medication, to reduce risk of mistakes (NPSA 2007a). They are often coloured and well labelled and have a different connection, preventing them from being attached to intravenous cannulae.

Tablets

If the tablets are in a bottle, tip the correct amount into the lid and then tip into a medicine pot or spoon. Many tablets are supplied in blister packs, so that they can be individually sealed and then pushed out through a foil backing into a medicine pot without being touched (O'Brien et al. 2011).

ACTIVITY

Consider the following scenario. A patient has difficulty swallowing her tablets. A colleague suggests to you that the tablets could be crushed and given to the patient in food. How might you respond and why?

Crushing tablets is **not recommended** for the following reasons:

- Crushing tablets could alter the medicine's therapeutic action, making it ineffective or causing adverse effects. For example, slow-release tablets which are crushed will no longer be released in the way intended. Crushing enteric-coated tablets (e.g. prednisolone) would remove the protective coating and could cause tissue damage. Particles of crushed tablets might be inhaled.
- Crushing tablets has legal consequences because it changes the product's licence (marketing authorisation) – if an adverse action resulted, then the person crushing the tablet will be responsible. Crushing must only occur if underwritten by a pharmacist who has determined that the medicine will not be compromised by crushing and that crushing is in the patient's best interest (NMC 2010b).

Putting medicines in food is also not recommended for the following reasons:

- It can be difficult to know how much of the tablets have been taken, when given in food.
- The food might affect the medicine's actions.
- Patients may not realise they are taking medication if it is given in food or drink.

So what should you do? Having explained to your colleague that you cannot crush tablets to be put in food for the above reasons, you should discuss the situation with the pharmacist. Most medicines are now available in liquid form or there may be another alternative such as the topical route.

Administering the medicine

Next, consider how to administer the medicine. Can the person self-administer or do you need to administer it on a spoon? Is the medicine best put into the mouth from a syringe? For obvious reasons (prevention of cross-infection), never touch medication with your hand. Always provide adequate fluids, about 50 mL for an adult, to ensure medication has been swallowed, and offer a choice of fluid. Ensure that the person has swallowed all the medication before documenting. A patient may pocket tablets, spit them out when you have gone or be unable to totally clear them from the mouth. Following administration, nurses/carers need to evaluate whether the medication has been effective and whether side-effects have occurred, as in Mercy's case, and document this.

Medicines not used should be disposed of immediately, for whatever reason, in accordance with standard operating procedures for the organisation (RPSGB 2005). In both community and hospital settings, unwanted medicines should be returned to the pharmacy. Medicines should never be disposed of in a waste bin where someone else could have access to them. Following administration, nurses/carers need to evaluate whether the medication has been effective and whether side-effects have occurred, as in Mercy's case, and document this.

ACTIVITY

Look in your local medicines policy and find out the guidance for disposal of medicines.

Summary

- Both preparation and administration of oral medicines should be performed systematically, ensuring that policy is adhered to, promoting safety and prevention of cross-infection.
- Careful assessment should ensure that the oral medicine administration is performed in an acceptable and appropriate manner for each individual, taking into account factors such as swallowing ability.

APPLYING TOPICAL MEDICATION

The topical route consists of medicine administration via the epidermis (outer layer of the skin) and external mucous membranes, therefore including administration into eyes and ears. These preparations may also affect the patient systemically, so they must be treated as all other medicines (Watkinson and Seewoodhary 2008).

LEARNING OUTCOMES

By the end of this section, you will be able to:
1. understand the indications and preparations used for the topical route;
2. show awareness of how topical medication is administered.

Learning outcome 1: Understand the indications and preparations used for the topical route

ACTIVITY

Mercy is prescribed fucidin cream for the small infected area behind her ear. Why might a topical antibiotic cream have been prescribed for her?

The topical route permits local rather than systemic absorption of the medicine and reduces its side effects on the body generally. In Mercy's case, it would have been considered appropriate because the lesion is small and superficial.

Medications are increasingly available in topical form. Common examples are patches applied to the skin being used for pain relief (fentanyl) or angina (glyceryl trinitrate). Many topical medications are designed to give a 24-hour slow release of the drug and therefore continuous action. Topical preparations also include drops into eyes and ears, where absorption occurs through the mucous membranes. There must be enough absorption from the site of application to be effective.

Topical preparations

- **Pastes.** Pastes contain a large amount of powder and a little water in their composition; thus, they are fairly stiff and may be difficult to spread. Lids must be carefully secured to prevent drying when exposed to the air, which would make them even drier in texture.

- **Creams.** Creams are easier to spread and less prone to solidification because they are emulsions – either oil dispersed in water (e.g. aqueous cream) or water dispersed in oil.
- **Ointments.** Ointments may be water- or oil-based, are semisolid and are usually available in a tube. They are occlusive and therefore better for dry lesions. Creams and ointments should be applied exactly as prescribed; for example, steroid creams are always applied very sparingly. Sometimes, directions are given as a weight in grams; as a rough guide, 2 g is a 10-cm length from a standard nozzle (Greenstein 2009).
- **Patches.** Medication in patch form is sealed in a small patch, with a peel-off sheet, which exposes the adherent part to be placed on the skin. You must follow the instructions for where it should be placed, but most patches are applied to the abdomen or chest, in a relatively hairless region if possible. The site is alternated each time the patch is changed, usually every 24 hours. The skin needs to be sufficiently permeable to allow absorption, so areas with good vascularity, such as the trunk, are preferable (Greenstein 2009).
- **Drops.** Drops are presented in solution in either single-use containers called minims, or in a larger bottle with a pipette-type end or dropper. Care must be taken to ensure that they are used for one person only; that the expiry time once opened is observed, usually 28 days; and that they are refrigerated if indicated. Drops facilitate relatively rapid absorption compared with ointment, which provides a more sustained drug action and less systemic toxicity.
- **Sprays.** Sprays are produced in containers under pressure and enable a fine spray to be directed on to the area requiring it, for example, nasally.

Learning outcome 2: Show awareness of how topical medication is administered

Applying medication to eyes, ears and nose

Eyedrops and eye ointments should be applied with the face horizontal, the person preferably lying flat. Looking up reduces the blink reflex, as well as making it easier to apply the drops or ointment into the correct place.

Slowly squeeze the bulb when applying drops and drop vertically, from as near to the patient as possible, without actually touching the eye. Always put the drop inside the lower lid (Figure 5.1) (Watkinson and Seewoodhary 2008). Ensure the eye is kept shut for 60 seconds after application, and always instil drops before an ointment if both are being used, as the ointment leaves a film over the eye, preventing the drops being absorbed. Eye ointment should be applied to the inside of the lower lid (Figure 5.2), and the eye held closed afterward for a short time, where possible, enabling the ointment to settle. Vision may be blurred afterwards for a while. Excess medication should be wiped away with a clean tissue.

If eye medication is being applied to both eyes, use separate products for each eye, ensuring bottles and tubes are labelled R and L (Watkinson and Seewoodhary 2008). Apply to the least affected eye first, to reduce the risk of spreading the infection. If more than one medication is being used, leave at least 3–5 minutes between applications (Watkinson and Seewoodhary 2008).

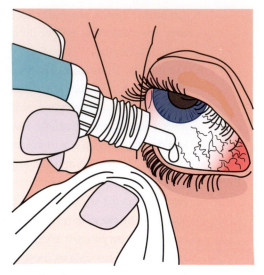

Figure 5.1: Administration of eyedrops.

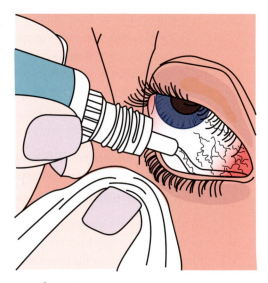

Figure 5.2: Administration of eye ointment.

For application into ears, lying with the ear to be treated uppermost is most effective. For nasal sprays, the person should be upright. Nasal medication should be administered 20 minutes before food so that the nasal passages are clear, which makes eating easier. Ensure the patient has blown their nose or cleared their mouth or throat before administration and follow closely any special instructions accompanying the spray.

Applying topical medication to the skin

For application of ointment or cream to the skin, gloves should be worn if someone other than the patient is applying the medication. Wearing gloves partly prevents cross-infection from you to the patient and vice versa and also prevents you absorbing any of the medication applied into your own skin.

Encourage people to apply topical medication themselves to promote independence and reduce the risk of cross-infection, although self-medication will not always be possible. For example, in Mercy's case it might be difficult with the sore area being behind her ear. Often, some manual dexterity is necessary to apply topical medication, so people should be assessed for their ability to manage this treatment themselves. All stages of the skill will need to be taught, with handwashing explained carefully so that the medicine is not inadvertently transferred to other parts of the body. Creams and ointments should be gently massaged in the direction of the hair flow. Steroid creams thin the skin, so apply them sparingly.

After application, the patient should remain still for several minutes, and the type of covering to be applied, if any, must be considered. People may require advice about clothing and instructions about possible staining or soiling. Remember to always evaluate the effectiveness of the treatment and report and document progress or deterioration to the doctor or nurse in charge.

Children: practice points – topical medicines

Children can be susceptible to several skin conditions, which will require topical medication. Atopic eczema is particularly common and is a chronic, dry and itchy condition, necessitating emollient application.

For detailed information about administering topical medicines to children, see

Keeton, D. 2010. Skin Health Care A) Normal skin conditions and managing common skin conditions. In: Glasper, A., Aylott, M., and Battrick, C. (eds.) *Developing Practical Skills for Nursing Children and Young People*. London: Hodder Arnold, 312–23.

Macqueen, S., Bruce, E.A. and Gibson, F. 2012. Administration of medicines. In: *The Great Ormond Street Hospital Manual of Children's Nursing Practices*. Chichester: Wiley-Blackwell, 357–95.

Summary

- Topical medicines are prepared in many different formats and have several advantages, such as direct action on the affected area and slow absorption through the skin.
- Specific instructions should be followed carefully.
- Measures to prevent cross-infection when administering topical medication are particularly important.

ADMINISTERING MEDICATION BY INJECTION ROUTES

Nurses in most settings give injections, but intramuscular (IM) injections are being used less often nowadays, so you should make the most of any opportunity to gain this experience.

Learning outcome 1: Explain the rationale for using the injection route

ACTIVITY

What injection routes have you seen used? Why do you think these routes were chosen?

You may have seen injections into muscle (**intramuscular**), into the fat layer under the skin (**subcutaneous**), into veins through a cannula (**intravenous**) or under the skin (**intradermal**). Injections can also be given into joints, into the epidural space or directly into the heart. As a student nurse, you can give only intramuscular (IM) and subcutaneous (SC) injections, and these injections must be given under direct supervision. Injections must always be given by the person who has drawn them up (NMC 2010b) – this includes you as a student nurse.

To use the intravenous route, you will require further training and supervised practice as a registered nurse. The intradermal route is used mainly for local anaesthetic before invasive procedures. Registered nurses in some specialities undergo preparation to give intradermal injections. The other injection routes mentioned are mainly used by medical staff.

Rationale for injections

Here are some situations in which an injection will be used rather than other routes for medicine administration:

* When speed of effect is required – medicines are more rapidly absorbed into the circulation when they avoid the gastrointestinal tract completely (O'Brien et al. 2011)
* When patients are 'nil by mouth'
* When the drug is destroyed by digestive enzymes in the gut – for example, insulin
* When long-term release of a drug is required – for example, depot injections for mental health clients, as in Malcolm's case (Wynaden et al. 2006)

Key features of the IM route

* The effects are more rapid than the SC route because of the good blood supply to skeletal muscles.
* Absorption can last for 2–5 weeks if desired, using oil-based, slow-release preparations, as in Malcolm's scenario.

Key features of the SC route

- A large variety of sites are available because any SC tissue can be used (Greenstein 2009).
- The speed of action is slower than with the IM route because of the poorer blood supply. The medication administered therefore has a longer duration, which can be useful.
- The person's ability to absorb needs to be considered. If peripheral circulation is poor, the drug may stay in the SC region and not be absorbed.

Learning outcome 2: Outline the principles of, and issues relating to, administering medicine by injection

Remember, all safety procedures for the oral route apply to injections too.

ACTIVITY

Consider the following issues in relation to IM and SC injections. What have you seen in practice regarding: skin cleaning, injection sites, syringe and needle selection? Compare what you have observed with the points made below.

Skin cleaning

Views vary considerably about skin cleaning (O'Brien et al. 2011), with some studies suggesting that social cleanliness is sufficient (Royal College of Paediatrics and Child Health [RCPCH] 2002). Skin cleaning before injections for patients who are immunocompromised and thus susceptible to infection continues to be recommended.

The Vaccination Administration Taskforce (VAT 2001) advised that skin cleansing is unnecessary in socially clean patients and that, if cleansing is required, soap and water is adequate. They warn that if spirit swabs are used, the site must be left to dry because vaccines can be inactivated by alcohol. The Royal College of Paediatrics and Child Health (RCPCH 2002) estimated the rate of abscess formation to be 1 per 1–2 million injections. They commented that skin preparation has been largely abandoned with no sudden increase in abscess occurrence and that formal skin preparation is not necessary before injection administration. You should check your local policy on this issue. Always allow skin to dry for 30 seconds if swabs are used (DH 2007). Alcohol swabs are always contraindicated when SC insulin and heparin are administered, because alcohol interferes with the medicines' action and hardens the skin (King 2003).

Injection sites

The site used is influenced by such factors as age, medication to be injected and general client condition. Figure 5.3 shows skin, SC and muscle layers and needle insertion.

Intramuscular sites

IM sites are shown in Figure 5.4. In adults, up to 4–5 mL can be given into most sites but only 1–2 mL in *deltoid* muscle.

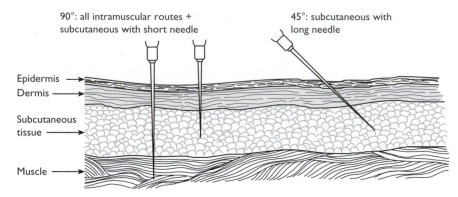

Figure 5.3: Subcutaneous (SC) and intramuscular injections: diagram showing skin, SC and muscle layers and needle insertion.

The *gluteus maximus* muscle has the slowest uptake of medication, whereas the *deltoid* has the fastest (Greenstein 2009). The *deltoid* is excellent for small volumes because the site area is small and minimal undressing is required; VAT (2001) recommended this site for vaccines in children >1 year and adults. The anterolateral aspect of the thigh, the *vastus lateralis*, is easy to access, has few major blood vessels in the area and is suitable for all age groups. The *ventrogluteal* site is a fairly new area to be used for injections; it is free of penetrating blood vessels and nerves and contains a large muscle mass, making it a good site to use for adults (Donaldson and Green 2005).

If the *gluteus maximus* muscle in the buttock is used, it is important to quarter the buttock first and then administer in the upper outer quarter, thus avoiding the **sciatic nerve** totally. Any other quarter could cause nerve injury. When injecting intramuscularly, spreading the skin 2–3 cm sideways (Figure 5.5) to provide a Z-track reduces the chance of leakage and pain (Cocoman and Murray 2006). This method will be advantageous when giving Malcolm his injection, because depot injections can cause discomfort.

Subcutaneous sites

SC sites are numerous, but the main sites are shown in Figure 5.6. When administering by this route, ensure a skin fold is gently pinched to free the adipose tissue from the underlying muscle (King 2003).

Syringe and needle selection

Syringes are selected according to the volume to be given. Volumes of ≤1 mL must be given in a 1-mL syringe, because of the smaller units of graduation, usually 0.1 mL. Some drugs require a special syringe. For example, insulin needs a syringe that is marked in units, which is how insulin is prescribed. Insulin syringes incorporate a needle as well. Some injections (e.g. low-molecular-weight heparin) are pre-prepared, and these syringes also have a needle attached.

Otherwise, needles are selected according to the route and sometimes according to the body adipose of the person. For example, for an IM injection, if there is a large amount of adipose, a longer needle will be required to ensure the drug enters the muscle. Nurses sometimes underestimate the required needle length by trying to be

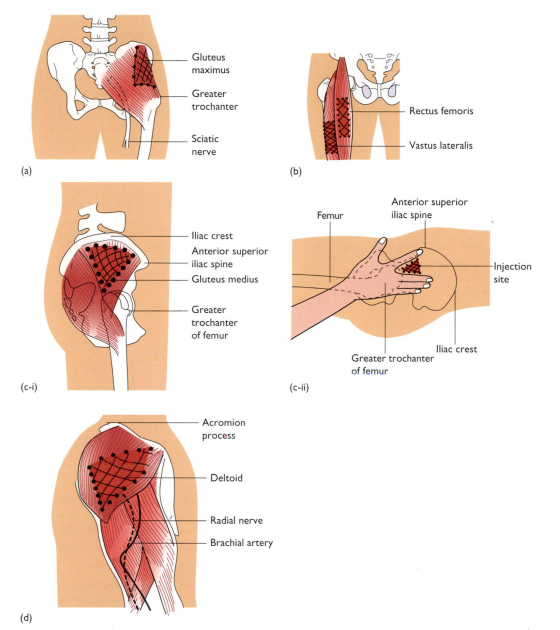

Figure 5.4: Intramuscular injection sites: (a) *gluteus maximus* site (upper outer quadrant of buttock); (b) *quadriceps* sites – *vastus lateralis* (outer middle third of thigh), *rectus femoris* (anterior middle third of thigh); (c-i) *ventrogluteal* site (hip); (c-ii) locating the *ventrogluteal* site; (d) *deltoid* site (upper arm).

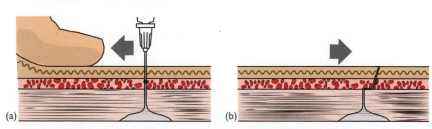

Figure 5.5: The Z-track technique: (a) skin spread to the left on administration of intramuscular medication; (b) skin released afterwards, showing formation of Z-track as a result.

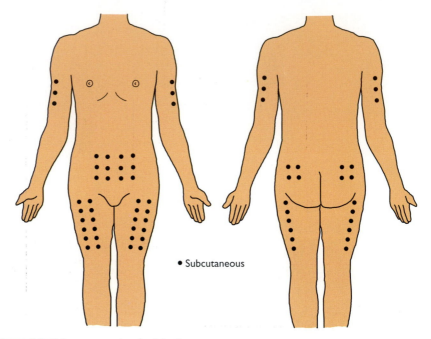

• Subcutaneous

Figure 5.6: Subcutaneous sites for injection.

kind to patients, but using too short a needle means that the drug does not enter the muscle (Zaybak et al. 2007).

Needles are colour-coded according to their gauge (G); the higher the gauge, the narrower the lumen of the needle. VAT (2001) identifies standard UK sizes as follows:

- **Green:** 21 G and 38-mm ($1\frac{1}{2}$-in.) length
- **Blue:** 23 G and 25-mm (1-in.) length
- **Orange:** 25 G and 10-mm ($\frac{3}{8}$ in.), 16-mm ($\frac{5}{8}$ in.) or 25-mm (1 in.) length

In general, green needles (21 G) are used for adult IM injections, so the nurse should use a green needle for Malcolm's depot injection. Orange needles are used for SC injections, although the most commonly given SC injections have a short thin needle already attached to the syringe (for insulin or low-molecular-weight heparin). When drawing up liquids from glass ampoules, use a needle that has a built-in filter where possible, to prevent possible particles of glass being withdrawn (NPSA 2007b).

Learning outcome 3: Discuss health and safety issues, especially for nurses, when giving injections

ACTIVITY

What hazards might nurses encounter when administering injections?

Drug contamination

There can be a danger of contact dermatitis, particularly if there is frequent exposure to a certain drug. For example, a nurse preparing a penicillin solution for injection could contaminate his or her hands with the drug. Repeated contact can cause skin sensitisation, so gloves should be worn.

Needlestick injury

Remember that you should never resheath used needles (O'Brien et al. 2011). These needles are contaminated and should be left uncovered on the injection tray and disposed of immediately into a designated sharps container. Never overfill the sharps box. Despite these precautions, needlestick injuries can still occur (particularly when sharps boxes are overloaded), so what should you do if this happens?

- Remove the needle from your skin quickly.
- Encourage the wound to bleed by applying indirect pressure.
- Then, place the injured area under cold running water.
- Cover with a dressing or plaster if required.
- Complete an incident form.

The Occupational Health Department policy will advise you about further action. You should also follow your university policy regarding managing and reporting sharps injuries.

Note: The needle can be changed to a new, sheathed needle after drawing up, using a non-touch technique. Follow local policy on this issue.

Learning outcome 4: Identify key principles of practice for administering intramuscular and subcutaneous injections

The steps to take when giving an IM or SC injection are set out below.

1. Ensure that the injection is due to be given and is written up correctly and that the patient has given consent.
2. Perform hand hygiene and put on disposable gloves (NPSA 2007b).
3. Assemble equipment: cleaned reusable injection tray (DH 2007), or equivalent, appropriate syringe and needle, alcohol swab (if local policy), medication and diluent if required.
4. Check details of the medication, and then draw it up either directly from the vial or, if powder, by mixing according to the manufacturer's instructions.
   - Always use the exact volume and diluent recommended to provide the most therapeutic concentration. Holding the syringe at eye level ensures you get the exact volume.
   - Remember to check the vial for cracks, precipitation or cloudiness.
   - Clean the rubber septum on vials with an alcohol wipe and allow to dry for 30 seconds. Inject an equal volume of air to that of the volume being withdrawn, to make withdrawal easier (NPSA 2007b).
5. Recheck the person's details and medication, consent and name band. Your approach to the person is very important in developing rapport and reducing anxiety about the injection.
6. Position the person comfortably, supporting the limbs if necessary. Depot injections like Malcolm's can be very uncomfortable.
7. Identify the site. Take into account the volume to be administered and convenience to the person when choosing the site. You should also rotate sites if repeated injections are being given.

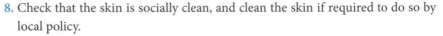

8. Check that the skin is socially clean, and clean the skin if required to do so by local policy.

9. For IM injections, spread the skin in a Z-track manner to prevent seepage (see Figure 5.5). For SC injections, bunch the skin to release the SC tissue from the muscle. Hold the needle at approximately 90° for all IM and most SC injections (as for insulin or low-molecular-weight heparin) (Dougherty and Lister 2011). Having first warned the patient, gently insert two thirds of the needle into the skin.

10. With IM injections, pull back on the plunger. If blood appears in the syringe, support the skin, withdraw the needle and discard the medication. Blood indicates that the needle must have entered a capillary, and the route would then be intravenous rather than IM. Repeat the above-mentioned process. If no blood appears, administer the injection slowly (especially when giving a depot as with Malcolm). Use the recommended rate if one is given, or at 1 mL/10 seconds.

11. Observe the person carefully throughout the procedure, providing reassurance as necessary.

12. Quickly withdraw the needle, supporting the skin with the swab and apply gentle pressure over the site. Do not rub the skin as you will cause local irritation and may alter the drug absorption rate.

13. Ensure the person is comfortable. Check that there is no untoward form of reaction, either systemic or local. All nurses should be aware of signs of anaphylaxis, a severe allergic reaction. Some drugs are known to be more likely to cause a severe allergic reaction, for example, pabrinex (Greenstein 2009).

14. Dispose of equipment according to local policy.

15. Document on the medicines administration chart and in the person's notes or wherever is required.

16. Return to the patient about 15 minutes later to check the effectiveness of the drug. The site itself should be checked 2–4 hours after administration.

ACTIVITY

What would be the IM sites of choice for

a. a fully dressed woman who is prescribed an IM tetanus injection (0.5 mL); and

b. a patient lying on his back in bed, who has abdominal pain that is worse on movement, and is prescribed an IM injection of 100 mg of pethidine (2 mL) and 10 mg of metoclopramide (2 mL)?

EMLA cream

EMLA (eutectic mixture of local anaesthetics) contains local anaesthetic and when applied to the skin enables an intravenous cannula to be inserted or blood to be taken (venepuncture) without causing pain. It is used extensively with children but can also be used for adults with needle phobia. At least 45 minutes must be allowed after application to produce adequate analgesia.

For case a, the obvious site would be the *deltoid*, because this muscle can take an injection of 1–2 mL and is less intrusive for this woman, who need only roll her sleeve up. You will remember from earlier that this muscle is the preferred site for vaccinations. In case b, the volume for injection is too great for the *deltoid*. Because this man has pain on movement, it would be better to inject into his thigh (*vastus lateralis*) or the *ventrogluteal* site so that he does not have to move.

Main problems associated with injections

Pain

Pain may be unavoidable but can be reduced by using distraction techniques. Applying a local anaesthetic cream (**EMLA**) will reduce the pain. However, VAT

(2001) advises that generally using local anaesthetic cream before vaccinations is impractical but can be used if needle phobia is preventing vaccination. Keeping the skin taut helps to reduce pain because it stretches the small nerves and reduces sensitivity (Greenway et al. 2006). With an IM injection, try to encourage the person to relax by choosing a comfortable position for them, because injecting into a tense muscle will be more painful.

Tissue damage

Damage can be caused by the drug being administered. This damage can be avoided by ensuring correct dilution according to the manufacturer's instructions and by using the appropriate technique; for example, always use the Z-track technique for depot injections like Malcolm's. Bruising may sometimes be unavoidable especially when giving SC anticoagulants. The nurses administering Mercy's injections should rotate the site to prevent local damage. You should never inject into an already bruised area.

Infection

Using an aseptic technique in the preparation and administration of an injection and ensuring that skin is socially clean should reduce the risk of infection.

Hypersensitivity

It is important to obtain a clear allergy history from patients before giving a medicine for the first time. Observe the patient/client carefully during administration and after, especially during the first few doses. Because of the first-pass effect, the action and therefore reaction to the drug will be faster than when it is given orally.

Staining of the skin

Staining of the skin may occur with pigmented drugs such as iron. Using the Z-track method should leave intact tissue above the injected material in an indirect line, thereby preventing leakage to the surface tissue (Cocoman and Murray 2006).

Summary
- Student nurses can give IM and SC injections under supervision. It is advisable to take opportunities to observe and then practise injection administration so that skill and confidence develop.
- It is important to understand the sites, equipment and hazards involved in IM and SC injections and to be aware of how complications can be avoided.

ADMINISTERING INHALED AND NEBULISED MEDICATION

The inhaled route permits medication to go directly to where it is needed in the mucous membranes of the bronchioles, providing an effective method of absorption. Examples of drugs commonly inhaled are bronchodilators, and steroids for their anti-inflammatory effect.

The nebulised route is the passage of medication to the bronchioles directly, as with inhalers, but by vapourising the particles in a stream of air or oxygen.

Nebulised particles are much smaller in diameter than inhaled particles (British Thoracic Society and Scottish Intercollegiate Guidelines Network 2009). Medication for nebulisers is normally supplied in solution in single-use plastic sealed containers called **nebules**. As with inhalers, the most common drugs given by nebuliser are bronchodilators and steroids.

> ### LEARNING OUTCOMES
>
> By the end of this section, you will be able to:
> 1 explain why inhalers are used and how they can be used effectively;
> 2 demonstrate knowledge of various types of inhaler;
> 3 identify indications for nebulised rather than inhaled therapy;
> 4 administer nebulised therapy safely and effectively.

Learning outcome 1: Explain why inhalers are used and how they can be used effectively

ACTIVITY

For what reasons, and by whom, have you seen inhalers used?

Chronic obstructive pulmonary disease

A chronic respiratory disease, including conditions such as emphysema, chronic bronchitis and chronic asthma. It causes debilitating breathlessness.

You have probably seen inhalers used by both children and adults. Asthma is probably the commonest reason for inhaler use: one in five households has someone with asthma (Asthma UK 2012). Inhalers are also used in **chronic obstructive pulmonary disease (COPD).** Inhalers may be used as maintenance therapy (called **preventers**), as well as in emergency situations where acute breathlessness occurs (called **relievers**). Malcolm's inhaler is therefore a reliever. Inhalers can be used as prophylactic (preventative) treatment, for example, before coming into contact with animal fur, grass, pollen, etc., which may be **allergens** to people with asthma, or before taking strenuous activity where extra oxygen is needed. If steroid inhalers are being used, they need to be taken first and then bronchodilators.

ACTIVITY

Instructions for using an inhaler are listed in Box 5.1. Think about how you would actually explain this to somebody.

Allergen

A foreign substance that initiates an allergic response.

To ensure concordance and maximum benefit, take into account the patient's ability to understand instructions (Leyshon 2007). Demonstration is a useful teaching strategy. Duerden and Price (2001) propose that frequent reassessments and re-education are needed as correct technique usually deteriorates over time. You can now get a haleraid device from pharmacists, which fits over the traditional inhaler so that a squeezing rather than pushing-down action can be used (Leyshon 2007).

Measuring the effectiveness of inhalers

Peak flow measurements can be helpful in monitoring effects of inhaled medication. Observations of respiration, including difficulty, rate and sound, are important

Box 5.1 Instructions for inhaler use

- The person should be sitting or preferably standing, to maximise lung expansion, with their head slightly tilted to give them a clear airway. They should clear the respiratory tract by coughing if necessary and then inhale and exhale deeply before commencing.
- Check inhaler details (medication and dose) and prescription.
- Remove the cap and shake the inhaler.
- Place the mouthpiece into mouth and at the start of a slow deep inspiration, press the canister down and continue to inhale deeply.
- Remove the inhaler from mouth and hold breath for 10 seconds, or as long as possible (Vines et al. 2000).
- Wait several seconds before repeating for a second time if prescribed (note that most people are prescribed two puffs at a time).
- Record administration on the prescription chart.
- Wash and dry mouthpiece twice weekly (Vines et al. 2000).

indicators of whether the medication has been effective. You can also ask the person how they are feeling and observe their colour, mental state and how well they are able to talk.

Learning outcome 2: Demonstrate knowledge of various types of inhaler

ACTIVITY

Think back to inhalers that you have seen and identify different types of devices currently in use.

The most commonly used is the **pressurised metered-dose inhaler** (pMDI), which contains liquid medication under pressure. This medication is released in the form of a mist when the inhaler is used. pMDIs are widely available and comparatively cheap. Other examples you might have remembered include the **diskhaler** and the **rotohaler**. With a diskhaler, the inhaled particles are contained within a disk, and with a rotohaler, the particles are enclosed in a capsule. The disk or capsule is then inserted into the inhaler to deliver a metered amount and is activated by inspiration. Patient preference regarding device is crucial, so a good assessment is very important. **Autohalers** and the **Easi-breathe** are alternative types, both of which are breath activated, removing the need for good coordination, but the range of drugs is restricted in these devices (Leyshon 2007). Another device you have probably seen is a spacer (Figure 5.7).

Spacers

Spacers, sometimes referred to as a holding device, can be large (e.g. the Volumatic), or small (e.g. the Aerochamber). They are often more effective than any other hand-held inhaler (British Thoracic Society and Scottish Intercollegiate Guidelines Network [BTS/SIGN] 2007) and preferred by many patients (Leyshon 2007).

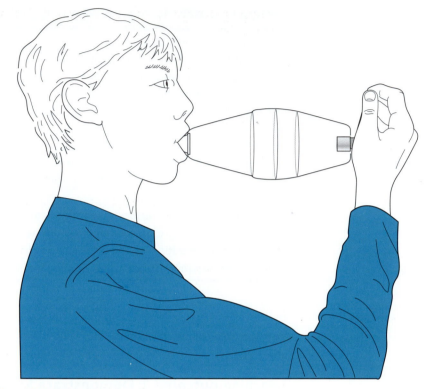

Figure 5.7: The volumatic inhaler.

The spacer holds the medication that has been released, allowing time for the drug to be inhaled through a mouthpiece by activating a one-way valve. By filling the chamber with inhaled particles of drug, the person can then breathe these particles in at their own rate, usually two breaths per inhaled dose, and the particles are less likely to be lost into the atmosphere.

Learning outcome 3: Identify indications for nebulised rather than inhaled therapy

ACTIVITY   Can you identify the advantages of nebulised therapy over inhaled therapy?

The nebulised route enables bronchodilators to be transported more effectively than inhalers to the bronchioles because the oxygen or air in which it is converted into a vapour reduces the size of the particles, preventing them from sticking to the oral mucosa, and therefore being lost to the respiratory tract (Booker 2007). The smaller particles can also travel more easily into the respiratory tract.

Nebulisers are useful for people who cannot manage to hold and coordinate a metered-dose inhaler. Nebulised medication can be delivered without a high degree of patient cooperation, for example by a mask, or holding a nebuliser mouthpiece between the lips and breathing normally. Thus, nebulisers tend to be given in emergency situations, or where high doses of drug need to be administered in a situation where a person is unable to use other forms of inhaler device.

Learning outcome 4: Administer nebulised therapy safely and effectively

ACTIVITY

Are there any special instructions you would need to give a patient receiving nebulised therapy?

The following points are all important:

- Sitting upright to ensure an optimum position for ventilation.
- Safety measures if oxygen is being used.
- The need to explain the noise of the nebuliser and the sensation within the mouth.

Figure 5.8 shows nebuliser equipment; either a mask or mouthpiece can be used with the nebuliser.

ACTIVITY

Before administering a nebuliser, what questions would you need to ask yourself?

Does the peak flow need to be measured first?

This measurement would serve as a baseline for comparison afterwards (see Chapter 11, for peak flow measurement technique).

Should the person use a mouthpiece or a mask?

Mouthpieces are used where patients are physically and cognitively able to cooperate with holding it in the mouth. They should sit with their chest in a vertical position to ensure good ventilation, and mouth breathe to gain maximum effect. A very breathless patient may find this too difficult and prefer to use a mask. However, masks can be distressing to patients. There is no difference in effectiveness when applied correctly.

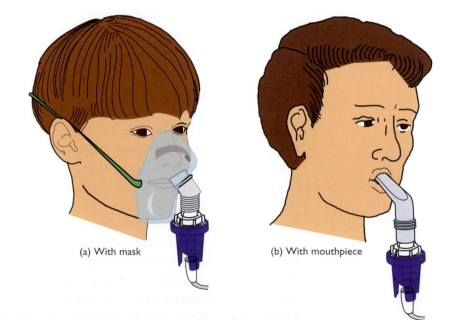

(a) With mask   (b) With mouthpiece

Figure 5.8: Nebuliser equipment.

If using a cylinder (either air or oxygen) or piped oxygen/air, what flow rate would be set on the flow meter?

The flow rate must at least 6 L per minute (BTS/SIGN 2007), otherwise the particles will not be reduced to the appropriate size for inhalation.

Should the nebuliser be administered via air or oxygen?

Some patients with chronic respiratory disease continually have a high level of carbon dioxide in their blood, and their breathing is only stimulated by lack of oxygen. Nebulisers for such patients should therefore be administered via air (Jevon 2007), either through an air cylinder, a piped air outlet or by using an air compressor if available. If a patient requires ongoing nebulisers at home, these portable air compressor machines are much more convenient. They extract air from the atmosphere and are available on prescription.

What instructions would I need to give to the person?

The person will need to understand that the mouthpiece or mask must be kept in place and that nebulisation only occurs on inhalation, so it is important to inhale well. There is no need to remove to exhale. The nebuliser unit must be kept vertical throughout administration and continued until all the liquid disappears from the unit, usually within 10 minutes (Booker 2007).

ACTIVITY After administering a nebuliser, what questions might you ask yourself?

What should be done with the equipment?

You need to check the manufacturer's instructions as to whether the equipment is single-use only or single-patient use. If it is single-use only, it is not suitable for reusing. However, if it is single-patient use, the nebuliser unit and mouthpiece or mask are washed in warm tap water at least once daily, dried well and kept covered in a clean place, and the set can last for a maximum of 3 months (Booker 2007). Tubing should not be washed because it cannot be dried properly.

How can I evaluate the nebuliser's effectiveness?

You can observe whether the person is still breathless, whether their colour has improved and whether peak flow readings have increased. You should also consider whether there are any apparent side effects. Nebulised therapy can produce unpleasant side effects.

Adverse side effects of nebulised medicines can include giddiness, tremor, palpitations, wheeziness and irritable coughing. These side effects may be related to the drugs, and then dosage may need adjustment. It is also important that the nebules are not too cold because cold nebules would cause bronchoconstriction. Mouth infections (e.g. candidiasis) may occur after prolonged use of steroid inhaled drugs, so rinsing the mouth after use is beneficial in this case. If a nebulised steroid is being administered, delivery via a mask may cause irritation to the eyes and skin. Ipratropium bromide, a quite commonly prescribed bronchodilator, can also be irritating to the eyes when given via a mask, so washing the face afterward may help.

> ## Children: practice points – inhalers and nebulisers
>
> Children under 5 years who need inhaler administration will need to use a spacer and facemask because they will not be able to make a good seal around a mouthpiece or coordinate their inhalation with the inhaler's use. Inhalers are more effective when the child is relaxed rather than distressed, which affects respiratory patterns. Children over 5 years should be able to use a mouthpiece. Consideration of age, motor skills and understanding needs to be considered with each individual child for the appropriate technique. For a detailed review of inhaler and nebuliser administration to children, see
>
> Aylott, M. 2010. Non-invasive respiratory therapy: A) Aerosol therapy. In: Glasper, A., Aylott, M. and Battrick, C. (eds.) *Developing Practical Skills for Nursing Children and Young People*. London: Hodder Arnold, 312–23.
>
> Macqueen, S., Bruce, E.A. and Gibson, F. 2012. Administration of medicines. In: *The Great Ormond Street Hospital Manual of Children's Nursing Practices*. Chichester: Wiley-Blackwell, 357–95.

Summary

- Inhaled medication is frequently prescribed, particularly for people with chronic obstructive pulmonary disease and asthma. Many different devices are available.
- Inhaled medication is taken both prophylactically and as an emergency measure.
- Inhalers act directly on the respiratory tract, so doses can be lower than when medication is taken systemically.
- Inhaler technique must be effective so that the correct dose of medication is inhaled.
- Nebulised therapy is widely used, particularly for people with acute respiratory disease.
- Appropriate decisions must be made as to whether to administer a nebuliser with a mask or a mouthpiece, and via air or oxygen.
- Nurses should be aware of side effects and how these side effects can be prevented or reduced.

INTRAVENOUS FLUID AND BLOOD ADMINISTRATION

As a student or healthcare assistant, you are not allowed to administer intravenous fluids or blood in any way. So, you cannot connect up a bag of infusion fluid, or alter the flow rate, because both actions mean you are administering the intravenous fluid. However, you may well be caring for patients receiving infusions, so you need to know how to care for them safely, general precautions (e.g. how to ensure the infusion site is kept clean) and signs to look for if the infusion is causing the patient problems.

By the end of this section, you will be able to:

1 appreciate the main indications for administration of intravenous fluids and medicines;
2 know how to care for a patient with an infusion or a transfusion;
3 recognise some of the common problems and safety issues surrounding intravenous fluid and blood administration, and understand your role.

Learning outcome 1: Appreciate the main indications for administration of intravenous fluids and medicines

Intravenous infusions can be given peripherally into a vein (Dougherty and Lamb 2008) or centrally into the right atrium.

ACTIVITY

Why do you think fluids and medicines are administered intravenously?

You might have identified that intravenous administration is used to:

- provide large volumes of fluid, blood or other nutritional supplements;
- provide fluids when other routes are not appropriate, as with patients who are nil by mouth;
- provide a route for certain drugs (e.g. chemotherapy, drugs destroyed by the gut).

Whole blood is now rarely given to patients, because there are alternative products that can be used that are less difficult and costly to collect but are just as effective. So, packed cells, plasma and platelets are given where there is a specific need (e.g. a patient with low platelets after chemotherapy), but if the patient has lost blood but is still medically stable, intravenous fluids may provide sufficient replacement while their body manufactures more blood cells.

Learning outcome 2: Know how to care for a patient with an infusion or a transfusion

Cannulae should be sited in the non-dominant arm where possible (Dougherty and Lamb 2008; Royal College of Nursing 2005) and not in the antecubital fossa unless necessary. Where the infusion is connected to a drip stand, make sure the stand is lightweight and has wheels that run smoothly, to preserve independence of mobile patients. Ensure that clothing worn is loose and that tubing is fed through sleeves to provide maximum normality. This approach would have helped maintain some of Mercy's independence after surgery.

Useful tip: When putting on clothing, put the bag and tubing through the sleeve, followed by the affected arm. Reverse this order when removing clothing.

Ensure the patient understands why they have an infusion and to be careful not to knock it. Patients will have a medicines administration chart with details of their regime and a fluid chart to monitor fluid balance.

Learning outcome 3: Recognise some of the common problems and safety issues surrounding intravenous fluid and blood administration, and understand your role

ACTIVITY

What problems and safety issues are you aware of relating to intravenous and blood transfusion?

Key problems relate to infection risk and systemic reactions.

Infection risk

One of the main risks of infusions is infection, particularly at the site of cannula insertion (DH 2006). The DH's (2007) 'Saving Lives' campaign focuses on issues of safe care, especially infection prevention in line management (Box 5.2).

Systemic reactions and care

Patients may have more central or systemic reactions to infusion management, so you need to observe for these reactions and report them to a registered nurse. Reactions include breathlessness, which could indicate either an overinfusion of fluid (i.e. a bag that has been administered too quickly, causing some cardiac failure) or an allergic reaction to an infusion fluid (e.g. blood or a drug). Postoperatively, while receiving intravenous infusions, Mercy should have been observed carefully for breathlessness because of her previous cardiac history. Also, watch and report alarms sounding on pumps and any untoward discomfort, including rashes (Dougherty and Lamb 2008), which could be a sign of an allergic reaction too.

Ensure that you document observations or care provided and report any changes. Many patients with infusions will have their intake and output monitored on a fluid balance chart, so then ensure all oral input and all forms of output, including vomit, are measured.

Safety issues regarding blood transfusions

Blood cells are very fragile, so bags need careful handling, and some such as platelets are therefore never put through a pump, which would crush them further. They are

---

Box 5.2 Infection prevention in intravenous line management

- Always wash hands and put on gloves before and after each patient contact.
- Check the cannula site locally at least daily for local inflammation (erythema), swelling around site (extravasation) and any inflammation along the line of the blood vessel (phlebitis) – and document this.
- Ensure that a dry adherent transparent dressing is intact over the insertion site.
- Ensure trained staff change administration sets at least every 72 hours – and document this.
- Cannulae should be changed at least every 72 hours by trained staff, who should be encouraging discontinuation as soon as possible, to reduce infection risks.

Source: Adapted from Department of Health (DH). 2007. *Saving Lives: Reducing Infection, Delivering Clean and Safe Care.* London: DH.

all infused through filtered giving sets, and blood products must also be used within 30 minutes of removal from the designated blood fridges they are kept in, otherwise the cells start to become damaged; see British Committee for Standards in Haematology (BCSH 2009).

The main problem with blood products is that they carry different antigens on their cell surfaces, which are described by the different blood groups (A, B, AB and O) and by the rhesus factor. If the patient is not matched or given the correct blood group (incompatibility), the patient will quickly become ill with a haemolytic reaction and could die if not treated fast (Serious Hazards of Transfusion 2008).

ACTIVITY

You may have observed the process involved in administering blood. When do you think the main errors in the process are likely to occur?

You may not have been aware that these occur when the blood is collected from the designated blood fridge and also when the bedside checks are done immediately before administering the blood (BCSH 2009). It is important that the patient's identity is checked properly before administering blood products.

The person's temperature, pulse and blood pressure must be taken before administration and 15 minutes after the start of each component transfusion (BCSH 2009). You must report any rise in temperature and pulse or drop in blood pressure immediately to a registered nurse. You must monitor the patient for shivering, breathlessness, loin pain, rashes and fever because these are all signs of reaction. If you see any of these signs, tell the nurse in charge immediately who will stop the transfusion, and call the doctor. The patient will need close observation and further treatment. Be prepared to resuscitate if anaphylaxis occurs.

As a student nurse or healthcare assistant, you cannot administer any fluid, blood or drug intravenously. However, you may well be the person caring for patients undergoing these therapies at the bedside, so you need to know how to recognise and report unusual signs and symptoms, while providing them with as much safe independence as possible.

Children: practice points – Intravenous therapy

For intravenous fluid therapy for children, see

Chalk, S., Harvey, J., Watson, N. and Kelsey, J. 2010. Venesection, cannulation and the care of children requiring intravenous infusions. In: Glasper, A., Aylott, M. and Battrick, C. (eds.) *Developing Practical Skills for Nursing Children and Young People*. London: Hodder Arnold, 590–607.

For administration of blood and blood products to children, see

Agacy-Cowell, D. 2010. Administration of blood and blood products. In: Glasper, A., Aylott, M. and Battrick, C. (eds.) *Developing Practical Skills for Nursing Children and Young People*. London: Hodder Arnold, 295–311.

Macqueen, S., Bruce, E.A. and Gibson, F. 2012. Administration of blood components and products. *The Great Ormond Street Hospital Manual of Children's Nursing Practices*. Chichester: Wiley-Blackwell, 74–86.

Summary

- Students and healthcare support workers are not permitted to administer intravenous fluids, blood or drugs but often care for patients with infusions or transfusions in progress.
- Good intravenous care requires holistic care of patients.
- There are important safety aspects related to intravenous fluid administration and blood transfusion; students must be able to recognise problems and report these promptly.

CALCULATING MEDICINE AND INTRAVENOUS FLUID ADMINISTRATION DOSES

Nurses often worry about their ability to calculate medicine doses. Therefore, if you have a problem with basic maths, talk to a friend or family member, and ask them to help you solve it and/or access maths support sessions in your university. There are also many online maths packages available to practice your numeracy skills. BBC Skillswise offers useful packages to help you to learn or refresh essential mathematical principles. These packages can be found at http://www.bbc.co.uk/skillswise/topic-group/calculation. MathCentre also offers online packages that can be accessed via http://www.mathcentre.ac.uk/.

Tip: Try to be involved in doing calculations in the clinical setting whenever possible. Many nurses find this easier than doing calculations from a book or in the classroom.

For further explanations and more practice exercises, there are many books specifically focusing on this topic. An example is *Drugs Calculations for Nurses: A Step-By-Step approach*, 3rd edn. (Lapham and Agar 2009).

LEARNING OUTCOMES

By the end of this section, you will be able to:

1 appreciate the need for effective numeracy skills in practice;
2 perform calculations using decimal numbers;
3 understand units of weight and volume and their equivalences;
4 apply a variety of formulae to calculate medicine doses;
5 use formulae to calculate intravenous administration rates and volumes for pumps and giving sets.

Learning outcome 1: Appreciate the need for effective numeracy skills in practice

ACTIVITY

Consider what the outcome of occasionally getting a calculation slightly wrong would be. Can you ever be justified in giving a person an inaccurate dose?

The answer must always be no. You have to be 100% accurate all the time. Even a small discrepancy will mean that the patient will not receive the prescribed dose, which could be very harmful. It is also a requirement that to qualify as a registered nurse you must demonstrate proficiency with your calculations (NMC 2010a,b). Of all medication incidents reported to the NPSA in 2007, 3674 (5%) occurred as a result of the wrong dose of medicine being administered (NPSA 2009).

There is great debate about the use of calculators for working out medicine doses. They can increase accuracy and are certainly useful for complex calculations. However, there may be occasions when a calculator is unavailable or not working. It is also only as good as its operator; hence, if the wrong numbers, or for some calculations, the wrong order of sequence, are put in by mistake, the answer will be incorrect. Also, if you are totally unable to work without a calculator, you cannot estimate easily what the right answer will be and therefore have no way of checking that the calculator answer is about right (Lumsden and Doodson 2003). Having a 'sense of number' is crucial when dealing with calculations (Lapham and Agar 2009, p. 1) The NMC (2010b) advises that using calculators should not act as a substitute for arithmetical knowledge and skill.

It is therefore sensible to be able to calculate medicine doses manually and by calculator, to prevent any chance of error.

Learning outcome 2: Perform calculations using decimal numbers

Decimals or decimal fractions are often used in calculating medicine doses where less than a whole number is involved. Whole numbers and fractions of a whole number are separated by a decimal point. Numbers to the left of the decimal point are whole numbers and will always be at least 1 or greater than 1. Numbers to the right of the decimal point are fractions of a whole number and are expressed in measurements of tenths, hundredths, thousandths and so on. Each number in a decimal is 10 times larger than the number to its immediate right. In other words, each number represents a different numerical value depending on where it is positioned in relation to the decimal point.

The number 1234.567 is made up of the following values:

Whole numbers				Decimal point	Decimal fractions		
Thousands	Hundreds	Tens	Units	.	Tenths	Hundredths	Thousandths
1	2	3	4	.	5	6	7

When dealing with whole numbers only, the decimal point is omitted but when dealing with decimal fractions that involve numbers less than 1, it is necessary to place a '0' to the left of the decimal point so as not to mistake a fraction of a number with a whole number. For example, .567 should be written as 0.567.

Rounding off decimal numbers

When using decimal numbers in calculations, sometimes answers will result in a lot of numbers after the decimal point; this is often impractical to manage and in most cases it is not necessary to use all of these numbers since their value may be negligible. With such calculations it is necessary to round up or round down the answer, usually to the second or third decimal place. Number digits below five are usually rounded down and digits above five are rounded up. Caution should be exercised as some drug doses are so small that to round them off may adversely affect the dose a patient receives and could result in your patient being under- or overdosed.

Calculation exercise I

Round off the following decimal numbers (answers are at the end of the chapter):

a) 3.666 to 1 decimal place

b) 423.12 to 1 decimal place

c) 1001.6772 to 2 decimal places

d) 964.9814 to 3 decimal places

e) 6.6666666 to 2 decimal places

Most calculations will divide into relatively easy numbers because nurses have to be able to give that portion of the drug without dividing into complicated amounts. For example, a dose of 3/8th of a tablet or 0.0065 mL of a liquid would be unrealistic to administer and unsafe. A sensible rule to follow is if your calculation requires you to administer a fraction of a tablet or a very small amount of a liquid, it is worthwhile rechecking your calculation; equally, if your calculation results in a large number of tablets or liquid to administer please recheck. You should also recheck the dose prescribed as this may be wrong!

To add and subtract decimals

The same mathematical principles of addition and subtraction apply when using decimal numbers as when using whole numbers. The only additional action to consider is ensuring that the decimal point is inserted into the correct place in your answer.

Calculation exercise 2

Calculate the following (answers are at the end of the chapter):

a) 154 + 36.21

b) 98.4 + 106.2

c) 456.789 − 45.67

d) 200 − 145.98

e) 5723. 9 + 47.8 − 4056.438

To multiply and divide decimals

When dealing with calculations that require you to multiply or divide decimals, it is usually easier to convert the decimals to whole numbers. This conversion will involve multiplying and dividing by units of 10. Since decimals represent fractions in tenths, this representation makes these processes very easy.

- To multiply by 10, move the decimal point one place to the right. For example, $0.05 \times 10 = 0.5$; $5.8 \times 10 = 58$.
- If you want to multiply by a different unit of ten (e.g. 1000), move the decimal point to the right by the number of 0's – in the case of 1000, three places, in the case of 100, two places. For example, $0.06 \times 1000 = 60$; $5.23 \times 1000 = 5230$; $0.67 \times 100 = 67$.

- If there are no more figures to move the point over, add 0 to fill the spaces. For example, $5.8 \times 100 = 580$.

  When multiplying using two decimal numbers, it is not necessary to multiply each decimal number by the same amount (i.e. 10, 100, 1000). Only multiply enough to reach a whole number. For example, to calculate 0.05×1.3, do the following:

  $0.05 \times 100 = 5$

  $1.3 \times 10 = 13$

  $5 \times 13 = 65$

  At this stage, your answer now needs to reflect its correct value; therefore, the decimal point needs to be placed in the correct position. To do this, you must count how many digits there were to the right of the decimal point in both the numbers used in your calculation and place the decimal point with this number of digits to its right. Since 0.05 has two digits and 1.3 has one digit, this totals three digits to the right of the decimal point. Therefore, the answer to this calculation is 0.065.

- To divide by 10, or multiples of, do the reverse. For example, $63 \div 100 = 0.063$; $25 \div 1000 = 0.025$.

  Division of a decimal by a whole number is a relatively straightforward process. The same principles of dividing whole numbers apply with the additional step of ensuring that the decimal point is correctly placed. The decimal point in the answer is positioned directly above the number being divided. For example, to calculate $8.6 \div 2$

$$\begin{array}{r} 4.3 \\ 2\overline{)8.6} \end{array}$$

Division of a decimal number by another decimal number requires the number you are dividing by to be converted into a whole number first. It will therefore be necessary to multiply the dividing number by 10, 100, 1000, and so on to reach a whole number. It is also essential to multiply the number being divided by the same amount to ensure the numerical value in the answer is correct. For example, to calculate $10.55 \div 0.5$.

Multiply the dividing number 0.5×10 to give a whole number of 5.

Multiply the number being divided 10.55×10 to give 105.5.

Then, carry out the calculation as follows:

$$\begin{array}{r} 21.1 \\ 5\overline{)105.5} \end{array}$$

Calculation exercise 3

Calculate the following. Where necessary round off your answers to two decimal places (answers are at the end of the chapter).

a) 2.5×3.06

b) 678.98×3

c) $78 \div 3.2$

d) $0.032 \div 0.6$

e) $156.1 \div 9.87$

Learning outcome 3: Understand units of weight and volume and their equivalences

Medicine doses are expressed in units of weight (e.g. grams, micrograms) or volume (e.g. litres, millilitres). It is essential to use the same units throughout a medicine calculation – you cannot work with both micrograms and milligrams, or millilitres and litres. Therefore, you need to convert the medicine doses in the calculation into the same units. It does not matter which unit you change them into. There is a simple rule for conversion which is the rule of thousands: everything that needs converting is achieved by either dividing or multiplying by a thousand. In Table 5.1, you can see the most common units of weight and volume and their abbreviations. Each unit has been multiplied by 1000 to give its equivalent unit of weight or volume.

With a few exceptions, these are the units used in medicine prescriptions. So, to convert 5 milligrams (mg) into micrograms (mcg), you need to multiply by 1000 (equals 5000 micrograms). To convert the other way, you need to divide by 1000. For example, 50 micrograms to milligrams equals 0.05 mg. In essence, to convert to a larger unit, you need to divide the figure, so there will be less numerical digits. To convert to a smaller unit you need to multiply, so there will be more numerical digits. Nanograms and micromoles are rarely used in medicine doses for adults; however, they are used for children's doses. When dealing with plurals in a dose abbreviation, the 's' is not included (write 8 mg and not 8 mgs). Also, when writing litres or millilitres, you may see the letter 'L' in both abbreviations written as a capital letter 'L' rather than in lowercase, that is, 'l'.

Note: Recommended practice is to write micrograms and nanograms in full, rather than their abbreviated terms (BNF 2012), to prevent such abbreviations being misread, which could result in a patient receiving the wrong dose of a medicine.

Calculation exercise 4

Convert the following to their equivalent units (answers are at the end of the chapter):

(a) 2000 mg = __ g   (d) 3 mg = __ microgram

(b) 2 L = __ mL   (e) 3500 mL = __ L

(c) 50 mg = __ g   (f) 125 mg = __ g

Table 5.1: Common units of weight and volume and their abbreviations

Unit	Abbreviation	Multiply by 1000	Equivalent	Abbreviation
1 kilogram	kg	× 1000	1000 grams	g
1 gram	g	× 1000	1000 milligrams	mg
1 milligram	mg	× 1000	1000 micrograms	mcg
1 microgram	mcg	× 1000	1000 nanograms	ng
1 litre	l or L	× 1000	1000 millilitres	ml or mL
1 mole	mol	× 1000	1000 millimoles	Mmol
1 millimole	mmol	× 1000	1000 micromoles	Mcmol

Learning outcome 4: Apply a variety of formulae to calculate medicine doses

Tablets and capsules

The formula to use for these calculations is as follows:

$$\frac{\text{What you want}}{\text{What you've got}} \quad \text{or} \quad \frac{\text{Dose prescribed}}{\text{Stock dose}}$$

This means that the prescribed dosage needs to be divided by the stock dose that is available.

For example, 80 mg of furosemide (a diuretic) is needed for Mercy, and the stock dose is 40 mg tablets. Thus, to follow the formula:

Dose prescribed = 80 mg

Stock dose = 40 mg

$$\frac{80}{40} = 2 \text{ tablets.}$$

Liquids

The formula to use for these calculations is as follows:

$$\frac{\text{Dose prescribed}}{\text{Stock dose}} \times \text{the volume of the stock dose}$$

A useful mnemonic to remember this formula is NHS:

N – What you **N**eed (i.e. dose prescribed)

H – What you **H**ave (i.e. stock dose)

S – The **S**olution (i.e. stock volume

$$\frac{N}{H} \times S$$

Now try exercise 5. Remember that in each calculation you must ensure that the medicines are in the same units before you apply the formula.

Calculation exercise 5

How much would you dispense for the following (answers are at the end of the chapter)?

(a) 200 mg of trimethoprim required; stock dose is 100 mg tablet

(b) 100 mg of chlorpromazine required; stock dose is 25 mg tablet

(c) 10 mg of diazepam elixir required; stock dose is 5 mg per 5 mL

(d) 1.2 g of augmentin required; stock dose is 600 mg tablet

(e) 240 mg of paracetamol elixir required; stock dose is 120 mg per 5 mL

(f) 50 mg of morphine elixir required; stock dose is 10 mg per 5 mL

(g) 40 mg of pethidine required; stock ampoule contains 50 mg per mL

(h) 6 mg of morphine is required; stock ampoule contains 10 mg per mL

(i) heparin, 2000 units required; stock ampoule contains 5000 units per mL

Doses based on body weight

Sometimes doses of medicines are calculated according to how much the patient weighs. The patient's weight must always be recorded in kilograms (kg) to enable you to apply the correct calculation formula to check that the correct dose has been prescribed and to work out how much of the medicine needs to be administered to your patient. Common medicines include heparin and gentamicin, which are prescribed in this way. The medicine dose will be prescribed in milligrams/micrograms/nanograms per kilogram of body weight.

To calculate the correct dose simply multiply the prescribed dose by the patient's body weight in kilograms. For example, a patient is prescribed 2 mg of a medicine per kilogram of their body weight; this is commonly written as 2 mg/kg. The patient weights 64 kg. To calculate how much the patient should be prescribed:

$$64 \times 2 = 128$$

The patient should be prescribed 128 mg of the medicine.

It is important to note that if the medicine is prescribed in divided doses, then it is necessary to divide the total amount by the number of doses. In the example above, if the patient was to be given this medicine twice daily, then divide 128 mg by 2. Therefore,

128 ÷ 2 = 64 mg. The patient would receive 64 mg per dose.

Calculation exercise 6

How much would you give (answers are at the end of the chapter)?
(a) Furosemide 0.5 mg/kg. The patient weighs 60 kg.
(b) Heparin 250 units/kg. The patient weighs 88 kg.
(c) Tinzaparin sodium 175 units/kg. The patient weighs 74 kg.
(d) Gentamicin 3 mg/kg. The patient weighs 65 kg.
(e) Heparin 250 units/kg every 12 hours. The patient weighs 55 kg. How many units of heparin should they be administered in a 24-hour period?

Learning outcome 5: Use formulae to calculate intravenous administration rates and volumes for pumps and giving sets

Intravenous infusions are often used for fluid replacement therapy, to administer electrolytes such as sodium and potassium, as a medium for administering medicines and to deliver blood products. This section will enable you to understand how to calculate drip rates (an amount per unit of time) to ensure your patients receive the correct volume in a prescribed period of time.

Pump rates

Look at a pump and see how fluid rates are measured. They are all in millilitres (mL) per hour. Per means divided by, so you need to divide the total volume prescribed by the number of hours it has been prescribed over and that will give you the pump rate.

Example

Prescribed: 1 litre (1000 mL) of normal saline over 8 hours:

$$\frac{\text{Total volume in mL}}{\text{Time in hours}} \quad \frac{1000}{8} = 125 \text{ mL per hour}$$

Like calculators, its accuracy in its rate of delivery will depend on the correct information inputted by the administering nurse.

Calculation exercise 7

How many millilitres per hour should be administered (answers are at the end of the chapter)?

(a) 500 mL of normal saline in 6 hours

(b) 1 litre of dextrose in 10 hours

(c) 50 mL of normal saline in 2 hours

Manual giving sets

Depending on the type of giving set used (the device used to deliver the infusion), the drop factor will vary.

A standard giving set for administering a crystalloid (such as normal saline) will hold 20 drops in 1 mL and for infusion of a colloid (such as blood or blood products) will hold 15 drops per mL. Other giving sets such as a microdrop giving set (or burette) can hold 60 drops in 1 mL. It is therefore necessary to use the correct giving set for fluids being administered and to know their drop factor to ensure the correct numbers are used in the calculation.

The formula to use when calculating how many drops per minute should be infused is

$$\frac{\text{Total volume (mL)} \times \text{drop factor}}{\text{Time (minutes)}}$$

Example:

To calculate how many drops per minute should be infused when delivering 1 litre of fluids in 6 hours, with a drop factor of 20 drops per mL:

$$\frac{1000 \times 20}{360} = 55.5 \text{ drops per minute}$$

Since it is not possible to count half a drop, the answer should be rounded off to 56 drops per minute

Calculation exercise 8

Calculate these rates in drops per minute, all with a drop factor of 20 drops per mL. Answers are at the end of the chapter.

(a) 500 mL in 4 hours

(b) 1 litre in 10 hours

(c) 1000 mL in 12 hours

Summary
- All nurses must be able to calculate medicine doses accurately, so a basic understanding of fractions and decimals is needed.
- There are formulae that can be used when a calculation is required, and it is important to develop skill in their application.
- Students do not carry out medicine calculations unsupervised. However, it is advisable to start working on this skill at an early stage, in preparation for registration, because students may be asked to be second checkers for a calculation at some stage during the preregistration programme.

PREVENTING AND MANAGING ANAPHYLAXIS

Anaphylaxis is a severe allergic reaction that is potentially fatal (Bryant 2007) and, therefore, requires rapid recognition and treatment (Resuscitation Council [UK] 2012). The allergen which is the substance causing the reaction may be a drug, so it is important that when medicines are being administered (especially straight into a vein), nurses observe the patient closely. It often occurs after the second dose rather than the first, when the body has already become sensitised to the drug. Such allergic reactions may also be caused by plaster, tape, dressings and food.

Useful reading: The Resuscitation Council (UK) (2012) details guidelines on the emergency treatment of anaphylactic reactions (available from www.resus.org.uk). NICE (2011) provides guidelines for assessment and referral following a suspected anaphylactic episode.

LEARNING OUTCOMES

By the end of this section, you will be able to:

1 identify how to prevent anaphylaxis;
2 know how to recognise and manage anaphylaxis.

Learning outcome 1: Identify how to prevent anaphylaxis

When you assess a new patient, always ask about any allergies they may have. These allergies must be written clearly in the patient's records and on the medicines administration chart and checked before any medicine is given. Mercy is an example of someone with a known allergy to penicillin, and this should be recorded and checked so that there is no possibility that penicillin is administered to her.

Knowing how to recognise anaphylaxis and when it is most likely to occur will help you respond promptly and effectively.

Learning outcome 2: Know how to recognise and manage anaphylaxis

Recognition is often difficult because the symptoms can vary so much. With drugs, the speed of onset is usually linked to the route; for example, if intravenous it will be

> **Box 5.3 Recognising and managing anaphylaxis**
>
> **Recognition of symptoms**
> - Early call for help
> - Airway problems – swelling, stridor
> - Breathing problems – shortness of breath, wheeze, cyanosis
> - Circulation – shock, blood pressure drop, pulse raised, consciousness reduced
> - Disability – neurological status – confusion, agitation, loss of consciousness
> - Exposure – flushing, urticarial (similar to nettle rash), angioedema (swelling of deeper tissues most often of eyelids or lips, sometimes mouth or throat)
>
> **Management**
> - Positioning – *airway/breathing problems:* sit-up; *low blood pressure:* lie down and raise legs where possible; *unconscious:* recovery position.
> - Remove triggering source where possible, for example, stop infusion of medication.
> - Give high-concentration oxygen.
> - Get intramuscular epinephrine ready, or get patient to administer their Epi-pen.
> - Be prepared to resuscitate.
>
> *Source*: Summarised from Resuscitation Council (UK). 2012. *Emergency Treatment of Anaphylactic Reactions: Guidelines for Healthcare Providers.* Revised edition (First published 2008) Available from: http://www.resus.org.uk/pages/reaction.pdf.

much quicker (10 minutes) than if oral (several hours) (Finney and Rushton 2007). The body's reaction to an allergen is to produce histamine in large quantities, which can induce severe bronchospasm and swelling of the bronchioles and face.

Box 5.3 summarises the Resuscitation Council's (UK) guidelines for recognising and managing anaphylaxis; you can read these in detail on the website and remember, they are regularly updated.

Children: practice points – anaphylaxis

The Resuscitation Council (UK) advise that treatment of anaphylaxis for adults and children is mainly the same but provides different drug does for children <6 months, 6 months–6 years, 6–12 years and >12 years, and fluid regimes differ from adults. Anaphylaxis is more likely to be caused by food in children than it is in adults. Some children in anaphylaxis may present with signs and symptoms very similar to severe asthma. For full details and algorithm, see http://www.resus.org.uk/pages/reaction.pdf.

Also see

Macqueen, S., Bruce, E.A. and Gibson, F. 2012. Allergy and anaphylaxis. *The Great Ormond Street Hospital Manual of Children's Nursing Practices.* Chichester: Wiley-Blackwell, 38–51.

Summary
- All patients/clients must be asked about allergies and the information recorded.
- Anaphylaxis can be rapidly fatal, so be sure you know how to recognise it.
- The body may react more severely to a second dose of a drug where the antibodies remember the allergen.
- Epinephrine (adrenaline) is the main medicine used to correct anaphylaxis, but be prepared to resuscitate too. Medical help will be needed.

CHAPTER SUMMARY

This chapter has explained the importance of having a basic understanding of the laws concerning medicine administration and of ensuring that local drugs policies are adhered to in practice. You should now be able to understand the need for a working knowledge of the medicines you are giving and be able to calculate doses accurately. The chapter has stressed the importance of safe practice with regard to medicine administration and the student role and should have helped you to understand the reasons for different routes of administration and key principles for safe and evidence-based practice. It should have prepared you to administer medicines safely in a variety of clinical settings.

Remember: The golden rule in medicine administration is to be honest to yourself. If you do not understand or agree with what is being given for any reason, you must challenge the situation you find yourself in.

ACKNOWLEDGEMENT

With thanks to Veronica Corben for her contributions to the first three editions of this book.

ANSWERS TO EXERCISES

Drug calculation exercises

Exercise 1

(a) 3.7

(b) 423.1

(c) 1001.68

(d) 964.981

(e) 6.67

Exercise 2

(a) 190.21

(b) 204.6

(c) 411.119

(d) 54.02

(e) 1715.262

Exercise 3

(a) 7.65

(b) 2036.94

(c) 24.38

(d) 0.05

(e) 15.82

Exercise 4

(a) 2 g

(b) 2000 mL

(c) 0.05 g

(d) 3000 micrograms

(e) 3.5 L

(f) 0.125 g

Exercise 5

(a) 2 tablets

(b) 4 tablets

(c) 10 mL

(d) 2 tablets

(e) 10 mL

(f) 25 mL

(g) 0.8 mL

(h) 0.6 mL

(i) 0.4 mL

Exercise 6

(a) 30 mg

(b) 22,000 units

(c) 12,950 units

(d) 195 mg

(e) 27,500 units

Exercise 7

(a) 83 mL per hour

(b) 100 mL per hour

(c) 25 mL per hour

Exercise 8

(a) 42 drops per minute

(b) 33 drops per minute

(c) 28 drops per minute

Abbreviations

b.d. = twice daily;

o.m. = every morning;

q.d.s = to be taken 4 times daily;

stat = immediately;

i/m = intramuscular;

mL = millilitre;

o.d. = daily;

o.n. = every night;

t.d.s. = to be taken 3 times daily;

e/c = enteric-coated;

m/r = modified release;

p.r.n = when required.

(Source: www.bnf.org)

REFERENCES

Asthma UK. 2012. Home page. Available from: http://www.asthma.org.uk (Accessed on 31 August 2012).

Banning, M. 2008. Older people and adherence with medication: A review of the literature. *International Journal of Nursing Studies* 45: 1550–61.

Booker, R. 2007. Correct use of nebulisers. *Nursing Standard* 22(8): 39–41.

British Committee for Standards in Haematology (BCSH). 2009. Guideline on the administration of blood components. Available from: http://www.bcshguidelines.com/documents/Admin_blood_components_bcsh_05012010.pdf (Accessed on 10 February 2013).

British National Formulary (BNF). 2012. Available from: http://www.bnf.org (Accessed on 10 February 2013).

British Thoracic Society and Scottish Intercollegiate Guidelines Network (BTS/SIGN). 2007. *British Guidelines on the Management of Asthma,* Revised edn. SIGN Publication 63. Edinburgh: BTS/SIGN.

British Thoracic Society and Scottish Intercollegiate Guidelines Network. 2009. *British Guidelines on the Management of Asthma.* SIGN Publication. Edinburgh: BTS/SIGN. Available from http://www.brit-thoracic.org.uk/Portals/0/Guidelines/AsthmaGuidelines/ sign101%20revised%20June%2009.pdf. (Accessed on 31 August 2012).

Bryant, H. 2007. Anaphylaxis: Recognition, treatment and education. *Emergency Nurse* 15(2): 24–8.

Cocoman, A. and Murray, J. 2006. IM injections: how's your technique? *World of Irish Nursing* 14(4): 50–1.

Department of Health (DH). 2005a. *Written Ministerial Statement on the Expansion of Independent Nurse Prescribing and Introduction of Pharmacists Independent Prescribing.* London: DH.

Department of Health (DH). 2005b. *Shipman Inquiry Sixth Report.* London: DH. Available from: http://webarchive.nationalarchives.gov.uk/20050129173447/http://the-shipman-inquiry.org.uk/6r_page.asp?ID=3391.

Department of Health (DH). 2006. The Health Act 2006: *Code of Practice for the Prevention and Control of Healthcare Associated Infections.* London: DH.

Department of Health (DH). 2007. *Saving Lives: Reducing Infection, Delivering Clean and Safe Care.* London: DH.

Department of Health (DH). 2008. *Safer Management of Controlled Drugs (CDs): Changes to Record Keeping Requirements.* Guidance (For England Only). London: DH.

Donaldson, C. and Green, J. 2005. Using the ventrogluteal site for intramuscular injections. *Nursing Times* 101(16): 36–8.

Dougherty, L. and Lamb, J. 2008. *Intravenous Therapy in Nursing Practice,* 2nd edn. Oxford: Blackwell.

Dougherty, L. and Lister, S. 2011a. *The Royal Marsden Hospital Manual of Clinical Nursing Procedures,* 8th edn. East Sussex: John Wiley.

Dougherty, L. and Lister, S. (eds.) 2011b. *The Royal Marsden Manual of Clinical Nursing Procedures Student Edition,* 8th edn. Chichester: Wiley-Blackwell.

Duerden, M. and Price, D. 2001. Training issues in the use of inhalers. *Disease Management Health Outcomes* 9: 75–87.

Finney, A. and Rushton, C. 2007. Recognition and managements of patients with anaphylaxis. *Nursing Standard* 27(37): 50–9.

Greenstein, B. 2009. *Trounce's Clinical Pharmacology for Nurses,* 18th edn. Edinburgh: Churchill Livingstone.

Greenway, K., Merriman, C. and Statham, D. 2006. Using the ventrogluteal site for intramuscular injections. *Learning Disability Practice* 9(8), 34–7.

Health Act 2006. London: HMSO. Available from: http://www.legislation.gov.uk/ ukpga/2006/28/contents (Accessed on 13 October 2013)

Jevon, P. 2007. Respiratory procedures. Part 3: use of a nebuliser. *Nursing Times* 103(34): 24–5.

King, L. 2003. Continuing professional development: Injection management. *Nursing Standard* 17(34): 45–52.

Lapham, R. and Agar, H. 2009. *Drugs Calculations for Nurses: A Step-by-Step Approach,* 3rd edn. London: Hodder Arnold.

Leyshon, J. 2007. Correct technique for using aerosol inhaler devices. *Nursing Standard* 21(52): 38–40.

Lumsden, H. and Doodson, M. 2003. Neonatal drug calculations: A practical approach. *Journal of Neonatal Nursing* 9(1): 14–18.

Medicines Act, 1968. London: HMSO.

Medicines and Healthcare Products Regulatory Agency (MHRA). 2009. *Best Practice on the Sale of Medicines for Pain Relief.* Available from: http://www.mhra.gov.uk/home/groups/pl-p/documents/websiteresources/con065560.pdf (Accessed on 24 July 2012).

Mental Capacity Act, 2005. London: HMSO.

Misuse of Drugs Act, 1971. London: HMSO.

Misuse of Drugs Regulations, 2001. London: HMSO.

National Institute for Health and Clinical Excellence (NICE). 2009. *Medicines Adherence: Involving Patients in Decisions about Prescribed Medicines and Supporting Adherence.* Clinical Guidelines 76. London: NICE.

National Institute for Health and Clinical Excellence (NICE). 2011. *Anaphylaxis: Assessment to Confirm an Anaphylactic Episode and the Decision to Refer after Emergency Treatment for a Suspected Anaphylactic Episode.* Clinical Guidelines 134. London: NICE.

National Patient Safety Agency (NPSA). 2005. Safer practice note wristbands for hospital inpatients improves safety. Available from: http://www.nrls.npsa.nhs.uk/resources/?EntryId45 = 59824 (Accessed on 25 August 2012).

National Patient Safety Agency (NPSA). 2007a. Patient safety alert 19: Promoting safer measurement and administration of liquid medicines via oral and other enteral routes. Available from: http://www.nrls.npsa.nhs.uk/resources/?entryid45=59808 (Accessed on 22 September 2013).

National Patient Safety Agency (NPSA). 2007b. Promoting safer use of injectable medicines: NPSA template standard operating procedure for use of injectable medicines. London: NPSA. Available from: http://www.nrls.npsa.nhs.uk/resources/?entryid45=59812 (Accessed on 22 September 2013).

National Patient Safety Agency (NPSA). 2007c. Safer practice note: Standardising wrist bands improves patient safety. Available from: http://www.nrls.npsa.nhs.uk/resources/?EntryId45 = 59824 (Accessed on 25 August 2012).

National Patient Safety Agency (NPSA). 2009. *Safety in Doses: Improving the Use of Medicines in the NHS.* Available from: http://www.nrls.npsa.nhs.uk/resources/?entryid45=61625 (Accessed on 22 September 2013).

National Prescribing Centre (NPC). 2009. *A Practical Guide and Framework of Competencies for all Professionals Using Patient Group Directions.* Liverpool: NPC.

Nursing and Midwifery Council (NMC). 2008. *Code: Standards of Conduct, Performance and Ethics for Nurses and Midwives.* Available from: http://www.nmc-uk.org/Publications/Standards/The-code/Introduction/ (Accessed on 26 August 2012).

Nursing and Midwifery Council (NMC). 2010a. *Final: Standards for Pre-Registration Nursing Education–Annexe 3: Essential Skills Clusters (2010) and Guidance for Their Use.* (Guidance G7.1.5b). Available from: http://standards.nmc-uk.org/Documents/Annexe3_%20ESCs_16092010.pdf (Accessed on 24 July 2012).

Nursing and Midwifery Council (NMC). 2010b. *Standards for Medicines Management,* Revised edn. (First published 2007). London: NMC.

Nuttall, D. and Rutt-Howard, J. 2011. *The Textbook of Non-Medical Prescribing.* Chichester: Wiley-Blackwell.

O'Brien, M., Spires, A. and Andrews, K. 2011. *Introduction to Medicines Management in Nursing*. Exeter: Learning Matters.

Ogston-Tuck, S. 2011. *Introducing Medicines Management*. Harlow: Pearson.

Resuscitation Council (UK). 2012. *Emergency Treatment of Anaphylactic Reactions: Guidelines for Healthcare Providers*. Revised edition (First Published 2008). Available from: http://www.resus.org.uk/pages/reaction.pdf (Accessed on 10 February 2013).

Royal College of Nursing. 2005. *Right Blood, Right Patient, Right Time*. London: RCN.

Royal College of Paediatrics and Child Health (RCPCH). 2002. *Position Statement on Injection Technique*. London: RCPCH.

Royal Pharmaceutical Society of Great Britain (RPSGB). 2005. *The Safe and Secure Handling of Medicines: A Team Approach* (Revised Duthie Report). London: RPSGB.

Serious Hazards Of Transfusion. 2008. *SHOT Toolkit*. Version 3. Available from: http://www.shotuk.org/wp-content/uploads/2010/03/SHOT-Toolkit-Version-3-August-2008.pdf (Accessed on 31 August 2012).

Vaccination Administration Taskforce (VAT). 2001. *UK Guidance on Best Practice in Vaccine Administration*. London: Shirehall Communications.

Vines, D.L., Shelledy, D.C. and Peters, J. 2000. Questions and answers about inhalers. *Journal of Critical Illness* 15: 563–4.

Watkinson, S. and Seewoodhary, R. 2008. Administering eye medications. *Nursing Standard* 22(18): 42–8.

Wynaden, D., Landsborough, I., McGowan, S., et al. 2006. Best-practice guidelines for the administration of intramuscular injections in the mental health setting. *International Journal of Mental Health Nursing* 15(3): 195–200.

Zaybak, A., Gunes, Y., Tamsel, S., et al. 2007. Does obesity prevent the needle from reaching the muscle in intramuscular injections? *Journal of Advanced Nursing* 58(6): 552–6.

6 Caring for People with Impaired Mobility

Glynis Pellatt

The National Institute for Health and Clinical Excellence (NICE 2008) defined physical activity as any force that is exerted by skeletal muscle resulting in energy expenditure above resting level. This includes the full range of human movement from activities of daily living such as housework to competitive sport. Mobility is a multidimensional concept, encompassing physical, cognitive, emotional and social dimensions.

Impaired mobility affects not only the ability to move about. It can also impact upon a person's ability to independently carry out activities of daily living with resulting reduction in quality of life (Kneafsey 2007). Nurses in many healthcare settings encounter people who have impaired mobility and are therefore susceptible to complications. Nurses have an important role, therefore, in actively preventing complications as well as promoting mobility safely whenever possible.

Correct moving and handling techniques are necessary when caring for people with impaired mobility, and some key principles are highlighted in this chapter. You must remain up to date with these techniques and attend organised sessions. As a registered nurse, you will also need yearly updates. The Nursing and Midwifery Council (NMC 2008) requires that nurses collaborate with patients/clients as partners in care, so when caring for people with mobility problems nurses should actively involve them in the assessment process and care planning.

This chapter includes the following topics:

- Pressure ulcer risk assessment
- Pressure ulcer prevention
- Prevention of other complications of immobility
- Key principles of moving and handling people
- Assisting with mobilisation and preventing falls

Recommended biology reading:

The questions below will help you understand the biology underpinning this chapter's skills. Use your recommended textbook to find answers.

- What systems are involved in movement and posture? Do not forget that individual cells need oxygen and nutrients.

- Which cells actually shorten and lengthen? What controls their activity?
- What are joints? What are the different types of joints?
- Are all joints moveable?
- What are tendons and ligaments?
- Why does damage to these tissues take so long to heal?
- How do we maintain flexibility?
- What are the functions of our muscles and bones?
- What happens to them if we are immobile?
- What other body systems are affected by immobility?
- How does immobility affect metabolic rate and energy balance?
- How would you feel if you were unable to move about?

Note: You should also revise the layers of the skin.

PRACTICE SCENARIOS

The following scenarios illustrate situations where nurses need to assist with and promote mobility, and implement measures to prevent complications of impaired mobility.

Adult

Diane Beck is a 50-year-old woman with **multiple sclerosis** who lives at home with her husband and two teenaged children. She has difficulty walking. She has tingling and burning pains and **spasms** in her legs, so she uses walking sticks or a wheelchair. She has a suprapubic catheter for her bladder problems.

Learning disability

Marion Pearce is a 42-year-old woman with a severe learning disability who lives in a community home. Due to accompanying physical disabilities, she uses a wheelchair for mobilising. She is underweight and incontinent of urine and faeces; her skin tends to be dry. Joint deformities make it very difficult to position her comfortably in the wheelchair. She has a poor appetite and is unable to eat independently or manage her own hygiene needs. Marion's **health facilitator** is her keyworker who liaises closely with the community nurse for learning disabilities. Marion's **Health Action Plan** includes input from many different health professionals including the general practitioner, the occupational therapist and the physiotherapist. She has also been assessed by the speech and language therapist.

Mental health

John Barnes, aged 52 years, is a client on an acute mental health admission ward. He has severe depression and also has a history of limited mobility and chronic pain after an accident 10 years ago. He needs a walking frame for support but unfortunately fell on the ward recently and sustained a fractured wrist, which is now in a plaster cast.

Multiple sclerosis

A condition where the autoimmune system attacks the myelin sheath (nerve coating) in the central nervous system. This demyelination causes transmission of impulses along the nerves to become slow and erratic.

Spasm

Stiff muscles that resist passive movement.

Health facilitator

The role focuses on an individual's health outcomes and can be undertaken by a range of people, including support workers, family carers, friends and advocates as well as health professionals [see *Health Action Planning and Health Facilitation for people with Learning Disabilities: Good Practice Guidance* (DH 2009)].

Health Action Plan

A personal action plan developed for each individual with a learning disability, which details the actions needed to maintain and improve the person's health and any help needed to accomplish these; see *Action for Health – Health Action Plans and Health Facilitation* (DH 2002).

PRESSURE ULCER RISK ASSESSMENT

A **pressure ulcer** (sometimes termed a bedsore, pressure sore or decubitus ulcer) is defined by the European Pressure Ulcer Advisory Panel (EPUAP) and National Pressure Ulcer Advisory Panel (NPUAP) as 'localised injury to the skin and/ or underlying tissue, usually over a bony prominence, as a result of pressure, or pressure in combination with shear' (EPUAP and NPUAP 2009). Although pressure ulcers most commonly occur over bony prominences (Anton 2006; Dinsdale 2007), pressure damage can occur in other areas in some circumstances. *The Essence of Care* (Department of Health [DH] 2010) identified benchmarks of best practice for pressure ulcer screening, risk assessment and prevention.

LEARNING OUTCOMES

By the end of this section, you will be able to:
1 explain how pressure ulcers are formed and the areas of the body that are most at risk;
2 discuss why some people are more likely to develop pressure ulcers;
3 use a pressure ulcer risk calculator to identify people at risk of pressure ulcers;
4 discuss the importance of accurate documentation of pressure ulcer risk assessment.

Learning outcome 1: Explain how pressure ulcers are formed and the areas of the body that are most at risk

ACTIVITY

Hold a clear plastic tumbler in your hand using your fingertips. Press with your fingers and notice how your fingertips have become very pale. Now release the pressure and look at your fingertips: they will have a red flush.

The red flush, called **reactive hyperaemia,** is one of the first signs of pressure damage when skin and other tissues are compressed between bone and another surface. Body cells die if the blood flow in the capillary bed is insufficient to supply oxygen, carbohydrates and amino acids for metabolism and to remove carbon dioxide and the products of catabolism (Anton 2006). Capillary closing pressure is the degree of external pressure required to occlude blood vessels. External pressures above the mean capillary blood pressure can cause capillary closure. The average mean capillary blood pressure in healthy people is 16–32 mmHg, but it can be much lower in ill health (Hampton and Collins 2005). If the pressure is not relieved, vessels become inflamed and microthrombi form in the capillaries (Hampton 2003).

The time taken for irreversible changes to occur, leading to tissue death, varies. Researchers have attempted to produce mathematical models of pressure–time thresholds, but more research is needed to produce a valid and reliable

Non-blanching hyperaemia

The term *non-blanching* means that when you apply light finger pressure to the red area, it remains red rather than whitening, as in blanching hyperaemia where the microcirculation remains intact. The damage present in non-blanching hyperaemia progresses to deeper layers if the pressure is not relieved.

model (Gefen 2009). If the pressure is relieved while the capillary and lymphatic circulation are intact, there is a sudden increase in blood flow to the area as the buildup of metabolites acts on the arteriole sphincters. However, if the capillaries and lymphatic circulation have been irreversibly damaged, the hyperaemia will be **non-blanching**. The reddening is then caused by blood leaking from damaged capillaries. In patients with darker skin, warmth, oedema or hardness can indicate non-blanching hyperaemia (Vanderwee et al. 2007; EPUAP and NPUAP 2009).

There is an inverse relationship between time and intensity of pressure; a pressure ulcer may develop in less time with strong intensity or in response to a longer duration at lower intensity (Jaul 2010).

ACTIVITY

What areas of the body are most at risk of developing pressure ulcers? Which of these sites are risk areas for the people in the scenarios at the start of the chapter?

The skin over bony prominences is particularly at risk of pressure ulcers (Figure 6.1). The sacrum, hips, heels, elbows, knees and malleoli are at risk for patients who are confined to bed, visiting the x-ray department or undergoing surgery. Lying on a trolley, x-ray table or operating table adds to the risk to vulnerable areas due to

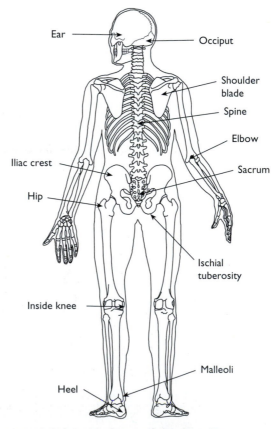

Figure 6.1: Skin areas particularly at risk of pressure ulcer formation.

> ### Box 6.1 Signs of early pressure ulcer development
>
> - Non-blanching redness of a localised area usually over a bony prominence.
> - Darkly pigmented skin may not have visible blanching. Its colour may differ from the surrounding area.
> - The area may be painful, firm, soft, warmer or cooler compared with adjacent tissues.
>
> *Source*: European Pressure Ulcer Advisory Panel and National Pressure Ulcer Advisory Panel (EPUAP and NPUAP). 2009. *Pressure Ulcer Prevention Quick Reference Guide*. Available from: http://www.npuap.org/wp-content/uploads/2012/02/Final_Quick_Prevention_for_web_2010.pdf (Accessed on 22 September 2013)

immobility, people who are being operated on will be unable to feel the pain caused by pressure and shearing forces, and anaesthetic agents lower blood pressure and alter tissue perfusion, also increasing risk of tissue damage (Thompson 2011).

When seated, the body weight causes greatest pressure over the ischial tuberosities (buttocks and thighs) (EPUAP and NPUAP 2009). Marion and Diane use wheelchairs; therefore, the skin areas over their ischial tuberosities and the inner aspects of their knees are vulnerable. Patients who are immobile in the seated position have a more rounded shape, allowing them to rock backward on to the sacrum – posterior pelvic tilt – creating friction and shear forces (Collins 2002).

The shoulder blades, iliac crests, sides of feet, ears and spine are also at risk. However, pressure ulcers can occur anywhere there is pressure exerted by equipment or clothing – such as tight clothes, shoes, splints, ill-fitting plaster casts, cervical collars, oxygen masks, pulse oximeters, intravenous lines or catheters. The device itself may produce pressure, or humidity and warmth between the device and the skin changes the microclimate of the skin (Black et al. 2010). Nurses caring for John should be aware that his plaster cast could rub, particularly if it becomes too loose or too tight, and so should advise him to report any discomfort. Skin covered by antiembolic stockings is also vulnerable (NICE 2005).

Inspection of vulnerable areas

Areas of the body at risk of pressure ulcers are usually termed 'pressure areas'; nurses should be vigilant about checking these for early signs of pressure. Vulnerable areas of risk for each patient should be inspected regularly. People can also be taught to inspect their own skin, using a mirror where necessary. See Box 6.1 for signs of early pressure ulcers. Figure 6.2 shows an example of a category 1 pressure ulcer (for details about grading of pressure ulcers and related wound management, see Chapter 7).

Learning outcome 2: Discuss why some people are more likely to develop pressure ulcers

ACTIVITY

Sit in a straight-backed chair. Now see how long you can sit there without moving.

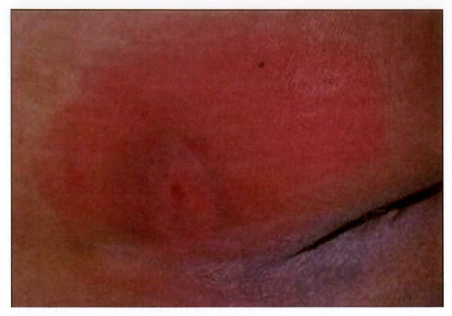

Figure 6.2: A category I pressure ulcer.

How long did you manage: 5 minutes, 10 minutes or longer? What made you move? You probably found that your pressure areas became uncomfortable and eventually you had to move position. Immobility is the most important factor in the development of pressure ulcers. Reenalda et al. (2009) suggest that people who are not disabled move about eight times an hour to relieve pressure when they are sitting. The body's defence against pressure therefore is to shift weight frequently, whether asleep or awake, in response to sensory stimulation. Therefore, anyone with reduced mobility, including people with impaired consciousness, have an increased risk of developing pressure ulcers.

Some people have reduced sensation to pressure and pain neurologically induced by medical conditions such as multiple sclerosis (like Diane), **spinal cord injury** or **stroke**. Some medication, such as sedatives, may cause chemically induced reduction in sensitivity to pressure and pain. Sedation from hypnotic and psychotropic drugs can cause people to be too drowsy to move around (Dinsdale 2007). Critical care patients on vasopressor therapy such as adrenaline are at risk of developing pressure ulcers (Cox 2011). John is depressed and could lack motivation to move, or pain may prevent him moving. Some people (e.g. people with dementia) are unable to respond to pressure stimuli and cannot spontaneously alter their position (Jaul 2010). People receiving epidural analgesia for postoperative pain management may have leg weakness or complete motor block, or there may be some sensory loss without motor block. In maternity, women who have epidural analgesia will have sensory loss during and shortly after labour and are therefore at risk of pressure ulcer development. Patients should therefore be encouraged to change position regularly (Weetman and Allison 2006; Reenalda et al. 2009).

> **Spinal cord injury**
>
> Damage to the spinal cord, causing paralysis and loss of sensation below the injury.

> **Stroke**
>
> Cerebral damage caused either by decreased blood flow or haemorrhage. Effects vary but it often causes paralysis down one side of the body (hemiplegia) and speech and swallowing difficulty.

Factors that render people at increased risk of pressure ulcers are often classified as **extrinsic** (outside the person, e.g. environmental) or **intrinsic** (to do with individuals themselves). Reduced mobility and sensation are therefore intrinsic factors.

ACTIVITY

Think about factors other than reduced sensation and mobility that may make people susceptible to pressure ulcers. Try to think of some extrinsic factors and some other intrinsic factors.

Box 6.2 lists the main factors contributing to pressure ulcer formation; these factors are discussed below.

Extrinsic factors

We have already considered the role of pressure in causing pressure ulcers. *Shear* occurs when a person begins to move or slide due to gravity. The bone and subcutaneous layer move in the opposite direction to the stationary skin. This results in twisting or angulation of capillary blood vessels causing them to be starved of oxygen and nutrients. Ageing skin is particularly vulnerable because it is less elastic (Jaul 2010). *Friction* damage is caused by skin rubbing against a support surface (Fernandez 2007). Diane has spasm which may cause uncontrolled movement of limbs, thus causing friction. Immobile and/or critically ill patients are reliant on care givers for repositioning and transfers, and friction damage may occur due to poor moving and handling techniques (Cox 2011). Shear and friction could be a problem for Marion and Diane because they may slide if not properly

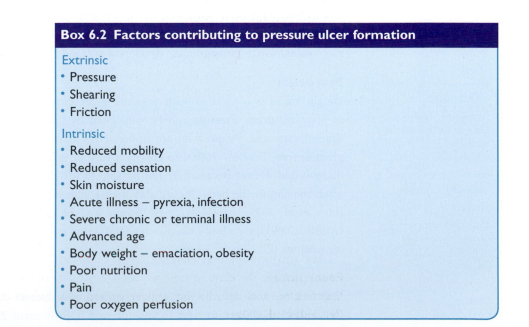

Box 6.2 Factors contributing to pressure ulcer formation

Extrinsic
- Pressure
- Shearing
- Friction

Intrinsic
- Reduced mobility
- Reduced sensation
- Skin moisture
- Acute illness – pyrexia, infection
- Severe chronic or terminal illness
- Advanced age
- Body weight – emaciation, obesity
- Poor nutrition
- Pain
- Poor oxygen perfusion

positioned in their chairs. *Moisture* makes skin more vulnerable due to greater risk from maceration, friction and shearing. Contamination by urine and faeces adds to the vulnerability, so Marion is particularly at risk; however, other body fluids such as sweat, drainage from a fistula or a wound may also increase risk (Jaul 2010). The risk of pressure ulcer development can be increased fivefold by the presence of moisture (Black et al. 2010). Chapter 9 has further discussion of how incontinence affects skin integrity.

Intrinsic factors

Intrinsic factors that cause pressure ulcers are based on vascular, degenerative, inflammatory or metabolic changes.

Acute illness

> **Metabolic rate**
>
> The overall rate at which heat is produced in the body.

Acutely ill people are vulnerable to pressure ulcer formation for various reasons. Pyrexia increases the **metabolic rate**, particularly the demand for oxygen, which endangers ischaemic areas. Severe infection can also cause nutritional disturbances, with bacteria increasing demand on local metabolism by both their own requirements and the response of the body's defence mechanism. NICE (2005) and EPUAP and NPUAP (2009) stress that patients should be assessed for conditions that might affect perfusion and oxygenation.

Severe chronic or terminal illness

Patients are at risk of pressure ulcers due to multiorgan failure, poor perfusion and immobility.

Ageing

Pressure ulcers are more common in older people for several reasons. As skin ages, there is a slower turnover of skin cells, loss of elasticity, thinning of subcutaneous layers, reduced muscle mass and decreased intradermal vascular perfusion and oxygenation (Jaul 2010). Loss of sweat and sebaceous glands may make older people more vulnerable to pressure ulcer development (Lindgren et al. 2004).

Bodyweight

> **Obese**
>
> People who weigh 20% or more above their normal body weight.

> **Body mass index**
>
> Measure of body fat based on height and weight.

Weight status is associated with pressure ulcer development and poor healing of pressure ulcers. Pressure can be calculated by considering body weight and skin contact area. People who are underweight have less cushioning over bony prominences (Benbow 2008), so this is a further risk factor for Marion who is underweight. **Obese** people may not be able to lift clear and experience friction when moving in the bed. Obesity also makes wheelchair transfers more difficult (Liou et al. 2005). Morbidly obese people and bariatric patients (Hignett and Griffiths 2009) have a **body mass index (BMI)** that exceeds 40 (for details on BMI, see Chapter 10).

Poor nutrition

Malnutrition and dehydration are recognised risk factors for pressure ulcers (NICE 2005; NHS Institute for Innovation and Improvement 2009); many people are already malnourished on admission to hospital (Thompson 2011). Marion has a poor appetite, and nutrition – including adequate hydration – is important in pressure ulcer prevention (Thompson 2011). Jaul (2010) suggests that protein contributes to preventing pressure ulcers. Fractured neck of femur is a common injury in older people, and the fracture increases nutritional requirements as well as reducing mobility.

Pain

Pain prevents patients from repositioning themselves, particularly at night. John has chronic pain and could have difficulty moving, especially with his arm in a plaster cast. Diane has burning pains in her legs, which could affect movement.

Poor oxygen perfusion

Patients who have poor oxygen perfusion due to conditions such as heart disease, respiratory disease, anaemia and diabetes have a lower peripheral capillary pressure (Cox 2011). Evidence suggests that smoking reduces the hyperaemic response to pressure (Noble et al. 2003).

Learning outcome 3: Use a pressure ulcer risk calculator to identify people at risk of pressure ulcers

NICE (2005) recommends that patients should be assessed for pressure ulcer risk using both formal and informal procedures and that assessment should take place within 6 hours of admission to a care episode. Pressure ulcer risk calculators can help identify people at risk of developing pressure ulcers. They use scoring systems based on risk factors for pressure ulcers, as discussed earlier.

ACTIVITY

Have you seen any pressure ulcer risk calculators used in the practice setting? If so, which ones have you seen?

There are many pressure ulcer risk calculators in use, including those explained below. The calculator used should be appropriate to the clinical setting, and research with a similar care group should support the calculator's accuracy.

The Waterlow scale

The Waterlow risk assessment card was developed for use with general adult populations (Waterlow 1985, 1988). It identifies three degrees of risk status: at risk, high risk and very high risk. The tool also provides guidelines on nursing care, preventive aids and equipment, wound assessment and dressings (Waterlow 2005). It is widely used in the United Kingdom (UK), sometimes in adapted forms; the revised 2005 version can be seen in Figure 6.3. The developer of this tool emphasises that education to accompany its use is essential and has set up a web page (www.judy-waterlow.co.uk) and developed a Pressure Ulcer Prevention Manual – the 'Waterlow Manual' – for this purpose.

Anaemia

Reduced haemoglobin concentration in the blood, or abnormal haemoglobin, resulting in reduced oxygen-carrying capacity.

Diabetes (mellitus)

A disease caused by deficient insulin release leading to inability of the body cells to use carbohydrates, and an elevated blood glucose.

WATERLOW PRESSURE ULCER PREVENTION/TREATMENT POLICY

RING SCORES IN TABLE, ADD TOTAL. MORE THAN 1 SCORE/CATEGORY CAN BE USED

BUILD/WEIGHT FOR HEIGHT	◆	SKIN TYPE VISUAL RISK AREAS		SEX AGE	◆	MALNUTRITION SCREENING TOOL (MST) (Nutrition Vol. 15, No. 6, 1999 – Australia)		
AVERAGE		HEALTHY	0	MALE	0	A–HAS PATIENT LOST	B –WEIGHTLOSS SCORE	
BMI = 20–24.9	0	TISSUE PAPER	1	FEMAL E	2	WEIGHT RECENTLY	0.5 – 5 kg = 1	
ABOVE AVERAGE		DRY		14 – 49	1	YES – GO TO B	5 – 10 kg = 2	
BMI = 25–29.9	1	OEDEMATOUS	1	50 – 64	2	NO – GO TO C	10 – 15 kg = 3	
OBESE		CLAMMY, PYREXIA	1	65 – 74	3	UNSURE – GO TO C	> 15 kg = 4	
BMI > 30	2	DISCOLOURED		75 – 80	4	AND		
BELOW AVERAGE		GRADE 1	2	81+	5	SCORE 2	unsure = 2	
BMI < 20	3	BROKEN/SPOT S						
BMI = Wt(kg)/Ht(m)^2		GRADE 2 – 4	3			C – PATIENT EATING POORLY OR LACK OF APPETITE 'NO' = 0; 'YES' SCORE = 1	NUTRITION SCORE If > 2 refer for nutrition assessment/intervention	

CONTINENCE	◆	MOBILITY		SPECIAL RISKS			
COMPLETE/ CATHETERISED	0	FULLY	0	TISSUE MALNUTRITION	◆	NEUROLOGICAL DEFICIT	◆
URINE INCONT.	1	RESTLESS/FIDGETY	1	TERMINAL CACHEXIA	8	DIABETES, MS, CVA	4 – 6
FAECAL INCONT.	2	APATHETIC	2	MULTIPLE ORGAN FAILURE	8	MOTOR/SENSORY	4 – 6
URINARY+ FAECAL INCONTINENCE	3	RESTRICTED	3	SINGLE ORGAN FAILURE (RESP, RENAL, CARDIAC)	5	PARAPLEGIA (MAX OF 6)	4 – 6
		BEDBOUND, for example, TRACTION	4	PERIPHERAL VASCULAR DISEASE	5	MAJOR SURGERY or TRAUMA	
SCORE		CHAIRBOUND, for example, WHEELCHAIR	5	ANAEMIA (Hb < 8)	2	ORTHOPAEDIC/SPINAL	5
10+ AT RISK				SMOKING	1	ON TABLE > 2 HR#	5
15+ HIGH RISK						ON TABLE > 6 HR#	8
20+ VERY HIGH RISK				MEDICATION – CYTOTOXICS, LONG-TERM/HIGH-DOSE STEROIDS, ANTI–INFLAMMATORY MAX OF 4			

Scores can be discounted after 48 hours provided patient is recovering normally

REMEMBER TISSUE DAMAGE MAY START PRIOR TO ADMISSION, IN CASUALTY. A SEATED PATIENT IS AT RISK ASSESSMENT (See Over) IF THE PATIENT FALLS INTO ANY OF THE RISK CATEGORIES, THEN PREVENTATIVE NURSING IS REQUIRED A COMBINATION OF GOOD NURSING TECHNIQUES AND PREVENTATIVE AIDS WILL BE NECESSARY
ALL ACTIONS MUST BE DOCUMENTED

PREVENTION
PRESSURE-REDUCING AIDS ©

Special
Mattress/beds: 10+ Overlays or specialist foam mattresses
15+ Alternating pressure overlays, mattresses and bed systems
20+ Bed systems: Fluidised bead, low air loss and alternating pressure mattresses
Note: Preventative aids cover a wide spectrum of specialist features. Efficacy should be judged, if possible, on the basis of independent evidence

Cushions : No person should sit in a wheelchair without some form of cushioning. If nothing else is available, use the person's own pillow. (consider infection risk)
10+ 100mm foam cushion
15+ Specialist Gell and/or foam cushion
20+ Specialised cushion, adjustable to individual person

Bed clothing: Avoid plastic draw sheets, inco pads and tightly tucked in sheet/sheet covers, especially when using specialist bed and mattress overlay systems
Use duvet - plus vapour permeable membrane

NURSING CARE
General HAND WASHING, frequent changes of position, lying, sitting. Use of pillows
Pain Appropriate pain control
Nutrition High protein, vitamins and minerals
Patient Handling Correct lifting technique - hoists, monkey poles Transfer devices
Patient Comfort Aids Real Sheepskin - bed cradle
Operating Table
Theatre/A&E Trolley 100 mm(4ins) cover plus adequate protection

Skin Care General hygene, NO rubbing, cover with an appropriate dressing

WOUND GUIDELINES
Assessment odour, exudate, measure/photograph position

WOUND CLASSIFICATION - EPUAP
GRADE 1 Discolouration of intact skin not affected by light finger pressure (non-blanching erythema) This may be difficult to identify in darkly pigmented skin
GRADE 2 Partial thickness skin loss or damage involving epidermis and/or dermis The pressure ulcer is superficial and presents clinically as an abrasion, blister or shallow crater
GRADE 3 Full thickness skin loss involving damage of subcutaneous tissue but not extending to the underlying fascia The pressure ulcer presents clinically as a deep crater with or without undermining of adjacent tissue
GRADE 4 Full thickness skin loss with extensive destruction and necrosis extending to underlying tissue.
Dressing Guide Use Local dressings formulary and/or www.worldwidewounds

IF TREATMENT IS REQUIRED, FIRST REMOVE PRESSURE

Figure 6.3: The Waterlow card (revised version 2005). (Reproduced from Waterlow, J. 2005. The Waterlow score card. Available from: http://www.judy-waterlow.co.uk (Accessed on 18 January 2013). With permission.)

The Braden scale

This scale was developed to predict pressure ulcer risk due to intrinsic factors (Bergstrom et al. 1987). It comprises six subscales; the first three subscales reflect primary factors (sensory perception, activity, mobility) contributing to pressure. The other three subscales (moisture, nutritional status, friction and shear) reflect factors contributing to diminished tissue tolerance. Although less common in the UK, it is widely used in other countries.

ACTIVITY

Use either the Waterlow scale in Figure 6.3 or the pressure ulcer risk assessment tool used in your practice setting to assess the people in the scenarios for pressure ulcer risk. Ask a colleague to undertake the same exercise and compare your answers. Did you both arrive at the same score for each person?

In the above-mentioned activity, you were assessing reliability of the tool, which concerns whether different people using the tool arrive at the same score. The many risk calculators are all based on factors known to predispose people to pressure ulcer formation. Many studies have reviewed these scales. To be accurate, risk calculators need to demonstrate predictive validity – that is, **sensitivity** (the ability to predict patients who will develop pressure ulcers) and **specificity** (the ability to predict patients who will not develop pressure ulcers) (Papanikolaou et al. 2007). Some calculators may overpredict pressure ulcer risk, which has cost implications when pressure-relieving equipment is provided. However, if a scale underpredicts, there is the human cost of pain and suffering from a pressure ulcer as well as cost implications if a patient's stay in hospital is prolonged.

The role of pressure ulcer risk calculators has been the subject of much debate. Pancorbo-Hidalgo et al. (2006) and Anthony et al. (2008) suggested that nurses' clinical judgement has an important place in the assessment of risk, and NICE (2005) advised that pressure ulcer risk calculators should be used only as an *aide-memoire* and should not be a substitute for clinical judgement. Papanikolaou et al. (2007) argued that, if assessment scales have such limitations, they may have little to offer and more reliable tools need to be developed. Kelly (2005) suggested that, if risk assessment tools are used only as *aides-memoire*, then perhaps they should only identify a patient's at risk status rather than the degree of risk. A key point is that all staff carrying out pressure ulcer risk assessment should be properly trained in the factors to be considered in their particular clinical setting (Papanikolaou et al. 2007).

Learning outcome 4: Discuss the importance of accurate documentation of pressure ulcer risk assessment

ACTIVITY

Consider why it is important to record information relating to pressure ulcer risk in nursing documentation.

The care plan is the principal means of communication between the nurses caring for a patient and other healthcare professionals. What is written or omitted may seriously affect the care a person receives (Taylor 2003), which has important implications for patient safety. Therefore, best practice guidelines require risk assessment and documentation in the patient's care plan. This assessment should be ongoing, and if the patient is transferred to another clinical area, the assessment should be handed over to the receiving staff (Thompson 2011). *The Essence of Care* (DH 2010) best practice indicator states that the plan of care should be continuously evaluated and revised to meet individual needs.

Pressure ulcer development may be construed as medical negligence and is an increasing cause of compensation claims; therefore, in some countries, hospital-acquired pressure ulcers have been deemed adverse patient safety events or 'never events' that can be prevented by implementing evidence-based prevention (Cox 2011). There are regular cases and complaints involving poor standards of communication, which include inadequate documentation and non-reflective practice, and pressure ulcers are used as quality indicators in healthcare systems (Bosch et al. 2011). Therefore, evidence of risk assessment and pressure ulcer prevention must be recorded in patient records. NICE (2005) highlighted that all formal risk assessments should be documented and readily available to all members of the multidisciplinary team and patients, and carers and relatives where appropriate should be involved in care decisions.

Children: practice points – pressure ulcer risk assessment scales

For a review of pressure ulcer risk assessment scales with application to children, see

Macqueen, S., Bruce, E.A. and Gibson, F. 2012. Personal hygiene and pressure ulcer prevention. In: *The Great Ormond Street Hospital Manual of Children's Nursing Practices.* Chichester: Wiley-Blackwell, 167–220.

Willock, J. 2010. Skin Health Care: B) Managing pressure ulcer risk in healthcare settings. In: Glasper, A., Aylott, M. and Battrick, C. (eds.) *Developing Practical Skills for Nursing Children and Young People.* London: Hodder Arnold, 324–7.

Summary

- There are many factors rendering people vulnerable to pressure ulcer formation.
- Pressure ulcer risk calculators may help nurses to identify those at risk but should not replace clinical judgement.
- There are a range of pressure ulcer risk calculators available. Nurses need to choose one suitable for their patient/client group after considering available evidence.
- Documentation of pressure ulcer risk assessment is essential for medicolegal reasons and to promote good communication.

PRESSURE ULCER PREVENTION

It has been suggested that most pressure ulcers that develop in NHS settings are avoidable and that they usually occur because of failure of the processes that should prevent them (Thompson 2011). However, the drive towards early

Incidence rate of pressure ulcers

The number of new patients with pressure ulcers in a population during a specified timespan – usually expressed per 1000 population per year.

Prevalence rate of pressure ulcers

The total number of patients with pressure ulcers occurring at a specific time (e.g. on a certain day) in a particular population – usually expressed per 1000 population.

hospital discharge, expansion in day care, and technologies that lengthen the survival of patients who previously would not have survived have resulted in more very ill hospital patients (Gould et al. 2000). Therefore, comparisons between the **incidence rate** and **prevalence rate** of pressure ulcers made several years apart are not valid.

LEARNING OUTCOMES

By the end of this section, you will be able to:

1 explain why pressure ulcer prevention is an important aspect of the nurse's role;
2 discuss ways of preventing pressure ulcers in people at risk.

Learning outcome 1: Explain why pressure ulcer prevention is an important aspect of the nurse's role

ACTIVITY

Why is it important that pressure ulcer prevention is implemented for people identified at risk of pressure ulcers?

You may have thought of some or all of the following points.

- Pressure ulcers can have serious physical effects. They can lead to infections including osteomyelitis (infection of bone) and sepsis (Jaul 2010), which can result in amputation, and they can be life-threatening (Fernandez 2007). The scar tissue resulting from pressure ulcers predisposes patients to further pressure ulcers owing to the reduced tissue strength.
- Pressure ulcers can markedly affect health-related quality of life (Clark 2002). They can cause pain, depression, loss of independence, social isolation and loss of earnings with severe effects on people's relationships. They are chronic wounds and can adversely affect body image and self-esteem (Hopkins et al. 2006; Kelly and Isted 2011).
- Patients with pressure ulcers remain in hospital longer than necessary and often need intensive treatment (Bosch et al. 2011).
- Pressure ulcers are a financial drain on the NHS with an estimated cost in the UK of between £1.4 billion and £2.1 billion a year (Bennett et al. 2004). There has been considerable government pressure to reduce the incidence of pressure ulcers, and guidelines have been developed to inform prevention and treatment (Stephen-Haynes 2006). A Nurse Sensitive Outcome indicator has been developed for pressure ulcers. The indicator measures the number of newly acquired pressure ulcers in any given clinical setting per month (NHS Institute for Innovation and Improvement 2009).

There are therefore many reasons why pressure ulcers must be prevented. Prevention of pressure ulcers has always been a nursing role – Florence Nightingale believed that good nursing care could prevent pressure ulcers. However, there should also be a multidisciplinary team approach, with effective communication and efficient coordination of tasks and responsibilities (Bosch et al. 2011), a view also supported by *The Essence of Care* (DH 2010). Nevertheless, as nurses assess, plan, implement and evaluate care to meet all aspects of patients/clients' needs, they are in a key position to minimise pressure ulcers.

Learning outcome 2: Discuss ways of preventing pressure ulcers in people at risk

ACTIVITY

List some methods of pressure ulcer prevention that you have observed in practice. Consider which might be suitable for patients/clients in the scenarios.

Care bundle

A care bundle is a set of evidence-based interventions which, used together, improve patient outcomes.

Pressure ulcer prevention can take several forms. It includes maintaining and improving tissue tolerance to pressure; protection against pressure, shear and friction forces; and education of staff, patients/clients and carers. The NHS Institute for Innovation and Improvement (2009) identified four key elements in the SKIN **care bundle**: Surface, keep moving, incontinence and nutrition.

Pain control

Uncontrolled pain will prevent patients from moving, so adequate pain control is essential. Diane has tingling and burning pains in her legs, and John has chronic pain from his previous injury and acute pain from his newly fractured wrist. Nurses caring for them, in conjunction with the multidisciplinary team, must implement appropriate pain management strategies and promote their comfort. You can read more about pain management strategies in Chapter 12.

Nutrition

Nutritional status should be assessed; a Malnutrition Universal Screening Tool (MUST) score 2 or above requires referral to a dietician (Thompson 2011). This referral may be necessary for Marion; the staff who are caring for her need to understand the importance of nutrition in maintaining her skin integrity. Some people's dietary intake may need to be supplemented, particularly to increase vitamin and trace elements. Chapter 10 focuses on assessing and meeting nutritional needs in detail, including explanations about using MUST.

Promotion of continence and skin care

Marion is incontinent. There is an association between moisture and pressure ulcers. The normal pH of the skin is between 4.0 and 5.5, but the breakdown of urea in urine produces ammonia which will increase skin pH. Frequent washing with soap can change skin pH from acidic to alkaline causing dryness and cracking plus it can remove natural lipids that help to create a barrier. The skin should be washed with a non-soap cleanser or low pH soap (Lloyd Jones 2012). Superabsorbent incontinence pads help to keep skin dry, and faecal incontinence must be dealt with promptly. Chapter 9 explores this topic in detail.

Patient handling techniques and repositioning

The patient handling sessions you attend will prepare you to use good moving and handling techniques, which prevent people being dragged up the bed, thus avoiding friction and shear. Patient handling education aims to teach the principles of good practice and problem-solving skills so that you have the flexibility to apply, modify and adapt the principles to different situations (Pellatt 2005). There is a vast range of patient handling equipment available, which is designed either to help a patient move independently or, with help, to move a patient who is totally dependent. New equipment is constantly being developed; therefore, nurses need to keep up to date with new equipment and recent developments in best practice. Equipment includes transfer boards, sliding sheets and hoists (Rinds 2009). Specialised equipment is required for bariatric patients as most beds, mattresses, hoists and other equipment are not safe for use by very heavy patients; however, this equipment will often require more space and the load-bearing capacity of floors might need to be considered (Hignett and Griffiths 2009). Marion's carers need instruction on correct patient handling techniques and how to use the necessary equipment.

Pressure damage can be avoided by repositioning patients regularly to ensure tissue perfusion. This repositioning will be necessary for Marion, who has a high risk of pressure ulcers. However, as there is no satisfactory time–pressure model available, the time limits for particular point pressures need to be considered on an individual basis for each patient (EPUAP and NPUAP 2009). *The Essence of Care* benchmark for best practice recommends that patients'/clients' needs for repositioning should be assessed and documented and that there should be ongoing reassessment (DH 2010). NICE (2005) advises that turning schedules should be devised on an individual basis rather than ritualistically.

Repositioning schedules must consider a range of patient factors, such as their breathing and the patient's total care management (e.g. treatment by other healthcare professionals, meal times). People often develop their own routines and strategies to prevent pressure ulcers, especially when living with long-term conditions, which should be appreciated by healthcare professionals. For example, Diane has probably been living with her condition for some years and has developed her own routine.

Regular turning of patients also helps to prevent chest infections, osteoporosis, deep vein thrombosis (DVT) and contractures (Pellatt 2007a). Therefore, repositioning should occur even when patients are on pressure-relieving devices (NICE 2005). The EPUAP and NPUAP (2009) recommend that repositioning should be undertaken using the 30-degree tilted side lying position (alternately, right side, back, left side) and that positions that increase pressure (e.g. a 90-degree side-lying position or semi-recumbent position) should be avoided. Moore et al. (2011) in a multicentre randomised control trial found that using the 30° tilt and three-hourly repositioning reduced pressure ulcers by 67%.

Pressure-relieving devices

A wide range of pressure-relieving devices has been developed to assist in protecting skin against pressure damage. *The Essence of Care* benchmark for best practice states that 'People are cared for on pressure redistributing support surfaces to reduce the risk, and manage the care, of pressure ulcers' (DH 2010, p. 8). NICE (2005) uses the term 'pressure relieving' for all types of devices and support systems. Support surfaces can redistribute weight in two ways: (1) pressure reduction by spreading pressure evenly around the body, for example, static gel or air-filled cushions; and (2) pressure relief by very low localised pressure such as alternating air pressure mattresses (Finucane 2006).

Devices are available as mattresses, bed systems, overlays and seat cushions and are designed to either reduce or redistribute pressure.

Seat cushions

Marion and Diane spend a lot of time in their wheelchairs and need appropriate wheelchair cushions that will relieve pressure. Sitting time in wheelchairs may need to be restricted to less than 2 hours for people with a high risk of pressure ulcers (NICE 2005). However, this restriction is not always achievable in all care settings, especially in the community, with limited resources (Benbow 2008). Wheelchair cushions should fit the seat and the user; be at the right height; be stable, promote symmetrical posture and positioning; and be comfortable. The cushion's ability to reduce the **interface pressure** and promote the ideal sitting posture is equally important. There are different types of cushion:

- Foams, in a variety of densities, reduce friction and shear by acting as a barrier between the skin and the chair. They are lightweight and can be cross cut, convoluted or contoured but will deteriorate if exposed to heat or ultraviolet light. Although foam can provide ventilation for the skin, it can act as an insulator and increase skin temperature, making the skin more susceptible to damage.
- Gel cushions provide even distribution of weight and conform to body shape, stabilising the pelvis and supporting the thighs, enhancing comfort and reducing shear and friction. They conduct heat away from the body. However gel can be heavy and may leak, if punctured.
- Combination-filled cushions such as foam in combination with gel can provide stability and are lighter. They can provide aeration and reduce shear.
- Air-filled cushions distribute pressure evenly, but if underfilled they will not relieve pressure, and if overfilled they can be unstable. They require regular maintenance to check they are inflated correctly.

An alternative means of positioning is to use a moulded chair to fit the person's body shape (Finucane 2006; Fernandez 2007).

Marion and Diane need to be correctly positioned in their chairs. The joints of the lower limbs should be in the mid-range of movement. The weight of the upper body should be supported evenly by both ischial tuberosities with the pelvis in a slight anterior tilt. The pelvis should rest at 90° of flexion, the knees should be flexed to 90° and the feet placed flat on the footplates. The head should be directly over the pelvis to encourage normal spinal curvature (Collins 2002). EPUAP and NPUAP (2009) suggest that positioning can be complex as it is important that the person is able to maintain their full range of activities.

Interface pressure

The pressure between a hard surface and weight-bearing bony prominences (Hampton and Collins 2005).

Mattresses

A standard foam mattress will not be a suitable surface for Marion and may not be appropriate for Diane or John either. The minimum provision for people assessed as vulnerable to pressure ulcers should be a higher specification foam mattress with pressure-relieving properties; this provision should be instigated for patients undergoing surgery too (NICE 2005; EPUAP and NPUAP 2009). There are two main categories of pressure-relieving mattress systems:

- *Systems that increase the area of the body in contact with the support surface.* These systems use materials that mould or contour to the body shape, distributing the load more widely and reducing pressure at bony prominences. These mattress systems are also known as static or low-tech equipment. Examples include foam mattresses and gel or air-filled mattresses (Finucane 2006).

- *Systems that relieve the source of pressure from the surface of the body.* These systems do so by alternately inflating cells in a cyclical manner so that the body is supported on one set of cells while the remaining cells deflate away from the body. These systems may be in the form of mattresses, overlays or beds. These systems are also known as dynamic or high-tech equipment (Finucane 2006; Benbow 2008). Examples include alternating-pressure, air-fluidised or low-air-loss devices and turning beds.

There is little good-quality data to support the selection of any one particular piece of equipment, and more research is needed (NICE 2005). However, dynamic or active support surfaces (overlay or mattress) are recommended for people who are at high risk of pressure ulcers, where frequent manual repositioning is not possible (EPUAP and NPUAP 2009). Air-fluidised and low-air-loss beds have been found to promote pressure ulcer healing better than standard beds.

When choosing a surface, other criteria need to be considered too. Patient acceptability is very important. If the equipment is uncomfortable, increases pain or disturbs sleep, then its use must be reconsidered. The small study by Hopkins et al. (2006) found that alternating-pressure air mattresses increased their patients' pain, and a review of 15 randomised controlled trials was unable to draw conclusions about their comfort (Vanderwee et al. 2008).

Another vital consideration is effects on **mobility.** The goal is to increase mobility, so using a support system that reduces mobility is inappropriate. Reduced mobility may occur for several reasons.

- Lack of a firm edge to the bed gives insufficient support for people transferring in and out of bed. Lack of stability can make transferring on and off surfaces difficult. The person needs to push down on the surface to obtain leverage; the contents will move when the body weight is lifted and support disappears.
- Increased height of the bed or chair may reduce access, particularly for wheelchair users.
- Loss of balance can occur with alternating-pressure systems, and low-air-loss and fluidisation beds. A hoist may be needed to transfer on/off these beds (Disabled Living Foundation [DLF] 2006).

Other criteria when choosing a support system include the size and weight of the equipment, the patient's weight, the patient's lifestyle, cost implications, availability of carers/healthcare professionals to reposition the patient and ease of use (NICE 2005). An *Essence of Care* (DH 2010) best practice indicator states that arrangements should be in place for the cleaning, maintenance and storage of equipment.

Some people may need joint protectors for comfort, protection and pressure relief. Examples are fleece joint protectors or booties, polyester fibre, air-filled, fluid-filled or foam joint protectors. Pads are available for walking equipment and to line prostheses to protect the skin (DLF 2006); their fastenings must not exert pressure.

NICE (2005) has produced evidence-based clinical guidelines for pressure ulcer prevention (www.nice.org.uk). However, many organisations have developed their own evidence-based local guidelines. Clinical guidelines are gaining increased support from the NHS Executive and other healthcare organisations. The NMC (2008) requires nurses to keep their knowledge and skills up to date, and this will include knowledge of evidence-based clinical guidelines.

ACTIVITY

In your clinical setting, find out about
- any local guidelines for pressure ulcer prevention;
- whether there are locally based tissue viability specialist nurses and how they can be contacted for advice;
- how pressure-relieving equipment is ordered locally.

Children: practice points – pressure ulcer prevention

NICE (2005) includes guidelines for preventing pressure ulcers in children as well as adults.

For further reading, see

Macqueen, S., Bruce, E.A. and Gibson, F. 2012. Personal hygiene and pressure ulcer prevention. In: *The Great Ormond Street Hospital Manual of Children's Nursing Practices*. Chichester: Wiley-Blackwell, 167–220.

Children with spinal injuries are particularly at risk of pressure ulcers due to impact on mobility and sensation. For further detail about preventing pressure ulcers in children with spinal injuries, see

O'Donnell, K. 2010. Care of the child with spinal injury. In: Glasper, A., Aylott, M. and Battrick, C. (eds.) *Developing Practical Skills for Nursing Children and Young People*. London: Hodder Arnold, 576–8.

Summary
- Pressure ulcers can have serious consequences. When a person has been identified as being at risk of pressure ulcers, effective measures must be taken to prevent pressure ulcer formation.
- Appropriate preventive measures for people at risk of pressure ulcers must be planned. These measures should include a suitable support surface that does not

impair mobility, correct moving and handling techniques, promoting adequate nutrition, carer/patient education, pain management and appropriate skin care.
● Patients/carers should be involved in decision-making processes about pressure ulcer prevention.

PREVENTION OF OTHER COMPLICATIONS OF IMMOBILITY

Pressure ulcers are a significant potential problem for people with impaired mobility, but there are many other possible complications.

LEARNING OUTCOMES

By the end of this section, you will be able to:
1 identify physical and psychosocial problems arising from impaired mobility;
2 explain ways in which nurses can prevent complications of immobility.

Learning outcome 1: Identify physical and psychosocial problems arising from impaired mobility

ACTIVITY

Think of people you have cared for whose mobility was reduced for some reason. They may have been confined to bed or were dependent on a wheelchair, or physical or psychological problems may have made walking difficult. What problems did their limited mobility cause them?

Compare your answers with the list of problems in Box 6.3. You may observe that immobility affects many bodily functions, as well as having psychosocial effects; this list highlights the multidimensional nature of immobility. Some of the problems are discussed below.

Circulatory and respiratory problems

There are many circulatory and respiratory problems which can occur; some are discussed below.

Box 6.3 Physical and psychosocial problems caused by reduced mobility

- Cardiovascular – deep vein thrombosis, orthostatic hypotension
- Respiratory – pneumonia, pulmonary embolism
- Gastrointestinal – loss of appetite, constipation, faecal impaction
- Urinary – renal calculi, urinary tract infection, incontinence
- Musculoskeletal – osteoporosis, muscle wasting, contractures
- Psychosocial – loss of self-esteem, depression, frustration, boredom, isolation

Source: Goldhill, D.R., Imhoff, M., McLean, B., et al. 2007. Rotational bed therapy to prevent and treat respiratory complications: A review and meta-analysis. *American Journal of Critical Care* 16(1): 50–62.

Deep vein thrombosis (DVT): Normally, movement of the legs contracts the muscles, which press on the veins and cause them to empty. Legs that are not mobile cannot maintain this pumping action, so the venous blood pools, causing a blood clot (DVT). The blood clot or part of it may break off and travel to the lungs, causing a pulmonary embolism (PE) which may be fatal (Nutescu 2007; Anderson et al. 2009). There are many risk factors for DVT, but active malignancy, pregnancy and the puerperium, surgery, acute medical illness, recent fractures and plaster immobilisation of the lower limb carry a particularly high risk (Carter 2009). NICE (2010) sets out the risk factors for venous thromboembolism (VTE) in detail and recommends that risk should be assessed in all patients admitted to hospital.

Orthostatic hypotension (when blood pressure falls on moving to an upright position) can quickly develop in patients confined to bed or chair. Marion, for example, may feel faint and dizzy when she is transferred from bed to wheelchair. The act of lying down shifts 11% of the blood volume away from the legs, with most going to the chest. Normally, about 30% of circulating blood volume is in the thoracic cavity. When moving to an upright position, the effect of gravity causes a volume drop of about one-third, reducing venous return to the heart and consequently reducing blood pressure. This reduction triggers physiological responses to return the blood pressure to normal. Certain conditions – such as spinal cord injury, diabetes mellitus, ageing and prolonged bedrest – can prevent normal compensatory mechanisms from functioning adequately (Clayden et al. 2006; Vollman 2010).

Decreased cardiac output and reduced tissue perfusion related to immobility can cause venous leg ulcers, particularly if there is associated poor calf muscle function or venous obstruction (Tyrrell 2002). Leg ulcers will limit a person's mobility as standing and walking may cause pain. Wound dressings, swollen legs, leakage and the need to wear large shoes compromise mobility too (Persoon et al. 2004).

Impaired mobility can cause *reduced ventilation of the lungs* and *reduced stimulation for coughing*, leading to a buildup of secretions in the bronchi and bronchioles, which can become infected. If the person is on bed rest, the normal lung clearing functions of the mucociliary escalator, cough reflex and drainage are compromised by the supine position. Oxygen uptake is reduced, with the danger of pneumonia (Lindgren et al. 2004; Vollman 2010). Marion could be at risk of chest infections. Patients with paralysis of their abdominal and intercostal muscles, for example, patients with spinal cord injury, will have reduced lung ventilation affecting their ability to cough, putting them at risk of a chest infection.

Gastrointestinal problems

Impaired mobility can predispose to **constipation** as exercise stimulates digestion and the movement of the gastrointestinal system (Weaver 2005) and can also affect diet and fluid intake, further increasing the risk. Immobility may also cause weakening of the abdominal wall muscles, making straining and therefore defecation difficult (Kyle 2006). Immobility can impair **appetite**, and people with reduced mobility may find it difficult to pour out their own drinks or eat independently. Constipation not only causes discomfort but can also cause urinary tract infection, acute urinary retention or incontinence due to pressure of impacted faeces on the bladder (Pellatt 2007b).

Urinary problems

Urinary stasis may be caused by reduced mobility, which can cause **urinary tract infection** or **renal calculi** (stones). Stones caused by immobility consist of calcium and/or oxalate and uric acid (Pellatt 2007c; Steggall and Omara 2008). Patients with spinal cord injury are particularly at risk of developing upper urinary tract stones (Ramsey and McIlhenny 2011). People who are immobile rely on staff to take them to the toilet or provide bedpans, urinals or commodes. Impaired mobility may also cause difficulties removing or adjusting clothing, which could be an issue for all the people in this chapter's scenarios. Some people can experience incontinence due to inability to get to the toilet quickly because of impaired mobility. Having to be dependent on staff to assist with elimination can threaten dignity. Chapter 9 discusses how to assist people with going to the toilet, in a way that promotes safety and dignity.

Musculoskeletal problems

Disuse of muscles leads to atrophy and loss of muscle strength. It is estimated that 12% of muscle strength can be lost each week with atrophy occurring after only 72 hours of immobility, and after 3–5 weeks of bedrest, almost 50% of muscle strength is lost (Nigam et al. 2009). The lack of muscle activity causes degenerative changes involving the release of calcium from the bones (**osteoporosis**), with loss of bone density. A study of 10 healthy men found that deconditioning of the muscles and bone loss occurred after 5 weeks of bedrest and was not fully reversed after 4 weeks of active weight-bearing, which highlights the importance of exercise and early mobilisation (Berg et al. 2007).

If joints remain in one position for too long, the connective-tissue collagen fibres around the joint shorten, straighten and become tightly packed. This can occur after less than 1 day. If allowed to progress, the muscles, tendons, ligaments and joint capsule become involved causing a stiff joint that is limited in its use and range of movement. This combined process causes a contracture (Nigam et al. 2009). For patients with paralysed limbs, a range of positions should be adopted to discourage the development of abnormal tone and contractures (Gibbon 2002; Kneafsey 2007), but Marion already has some joint deformities. Joints particularly at risk are the shoulders, elbows, wrists, neck, fingers, hips, knees, ankles and toes. Diane has spasm in her legs, which leads to a restricted range of joint movement due to muscle shortening or contractures. Upper limb contractures reduce the ability to carry out activities of living such as showering, dressing and feeding. Lower limb contractures affect walking and increase the risk of falls, thus restricting mobility further (Clavet et al. 2008).

Immobility causes bone mineral density loss, and contracted joints put extra stress on long bones with the risk of spontaneous fracture (Takamoto et al. 2005). People with learning disabilities have a high risk of developing osteoporosis, and the prevalence of fractures is higher than that in the general population. This prevalence may be partly due to medication taken for epilepsy, and instability causing falls. There are also several other factors that contribute to this high risk, such as poor nutrition due to food spillage and low vitamin D levels due to lack of exposure to sunlight (Srikanth et al. 2011), which may apply to Marion.

Psychosocial problems

Loss of mobility can cause people to experience loss of self-esteem. Self-esteem and self-concept are made up of a person's body image, achievement, social functioning and self-identification. Nigam et al. (2009) suggest that loss of mobility affects three aspects of self:

- The achieving self – if they are unable to pursue their work or hobbies
- The social self – interactions with friends and family
- The private self – loss of independence and reliance on others

People with profound learning and multiple disabilities (like Marion) may experience frustration at having to rely on carers for moving and having to make needs known with limited communication ability.

Mobility problems can also contribute to depression and social isolation. John has had impaired mobility resulting from his accident for some time, and this could have contributed to his depression. In older people, cognitive performance may be affected (Zegelin 2008). People who live on their own or who have low social participation are more likely to experience functional disability (Nilsson et al. 2011). Diane may be frustrated that her mobility problems limit her ability to actively participate in activities with her family.

Learning outcome 2: Explain ways in which nurses can prevent complications of immobility

Roper et al. (2000) suggest that when planning care, the objective is to:

- prevent identified potential problems from becoming actual problems;
- solve actual problems;
- where possible alleviate problems that cannot be solved;
- prevent reoccurrence of problems that have been resolved;
- help the person to cope positively with those problems that cannot be alleviated or solved.

ACTIVITY

We have identified many potential and actual problems related to impaired mobility in our three patients/clients. Consider the nursing interventions that could be implemented to prevent or solve these problems.

A few points which you may have considered are discussed below.

Deep vein thrombosis/pulmonary embolus

Observations for signs and symptoms of DVT (painful, swollen calf) and of pulmonary embolus (chest pain, cough) are all part of ongoing nursing assessment.

Passive and active exercises

Passive exercises are where another person moves a client/patient's limb through a range of movements. Active exercises are when people carry out exercises by themselves.

NICE (2010) provides detailed guidelines for VTE prevention and advises for all patients, dehydration should be prevented and mobility should be encouraged. Nurses, in liaison with physiotherapists, can help people with **passive and active exercises** of the legs. These activities help to break the cycle of immobility and increase circulation (Van Wicklin et al. 2006).

Graduated compression stockings, intermittent pneumatic compression pumps and venous foot pumps are other preventive measures; these devices enhance venous return and blood flow. When using these devices, it is essential that the correct size is chosen and that they are applied correctly and are removed only for a short time each day (Mathias 2007). Anticoagulants such as heparin and/or oral anticoagulants may be prescribed for those at high risk (Nutescu 2007). The NICE (2010) guidelines for reducing the risk of VTE in patients who are admitted to hospital recommend that after following risk assessment for VTE, and an assessment of bleeding risk, a decision about pharmacological prophylaxis must be made, balancing risk of clotting with risk of bleeding.

Orthostatic hypotension

For Marion, orthostatic hypotension can be alleviated by gradually sitting her up in bed before she transfers into her chair. Marion's carers should be aware of the signs and symptoms of orthostatic hypotension as Marion may not be able to verbally communicate if she feels dizzy. It is also important to explain to Marion what is happening to reduce any anxiety relating to these symptoms.

Chest infection

Frequent repositioning and encouragement to do deep breathing exercises can help to prevent chest infection. The person can also be encouraged to cough to clear secretions and prevent them pooling in the lungs. Chapter 11 has a section on observation of sputum, which includes tips on how to encourage expectoration of sputum.

Loss of appetite and constipation

An adequate fluid and diet intake should be provided, taking individual preferences into account and ensuring that sufficient fibre is included. Patients' food and drinks should be positioned so that they can reach them. Patients with hemiplegia need to be provided with a non-slip mat to prevent the plate moving, a plate guard to help keep the food on the plate, and an appropriate cup for drinking from. John's dominant arm is in plaster, making it difficult to cut up his food, so he may need help. People with profound learning and multiple physical disabilities, like Marion, may have difficulty with eating and drinking; carers should aim to enhance the quality of their mealtime experience. Chapter 10 has more detail about these issues.

Urinary tract infection and incontinence

People who are at risk of urinary tract infection should be observed for signs such as cloudy, foul-smelling urine. Chapter 9 has a section on urinalysis and explains how urinary tract infection might be suspected and when a specimen of urine should be sent for microscopy, culture and sensitivity. Marion would require continence aids, but consideration must be given to body image, comfort and skin care and as to how continence can be promoted, rather than only contained. Patients with impaired mobility (e.g. after a stroke) should be positioned within a short walking distance from the toilet when they start to mobilise. People who are confused may need guidance with orientating to where the toilet is located. Diane will need to learn how to manage a suprapubic catheter as blockage, leakage and infection can be a problem. Chapter 9 explores these issues and will help you to develop your skills to assist people who need help with elimination.

Muscle wasting and contractures

As muscle contraction increases, joint movement becomes further limited, which is an issue for Marion and Diane. People with profound learning disabilities who are immobile are particularly at risk of developing deformities. Diane's spasms can be helped by careful positioning. Pillows, T-rolls or wedges positioned under the legs to put them in flexion can reduce extensor and adductor spasm (Pellatt 2007a). Splints may be prescribed, and physiotherapy and occupational therapy play an important role in preventing contractures.

Botulinum toxin can be used to reduce muscle tone and increase the range of movements in a joint. It can be targeted to individual muscles (Gibbon 2002). Antispasmodic drugs such as baclofen can be used to reduce spasm. However, some spasm can help to maintain blood circulation and aid transfers and walking, by acting as a splint to limbs, so treatment of spasticity should be selected carefully and regularly reviewed to maintain function (Jones 2004).

Loss of self-esteem, frustration, boredom and isolation

As discussed in Chapter 1, how nurses carry out care may affect how people feel about themselves. A caring and empathetic approach from nurses can assist in reducing the psychosocial effects of impaired mobility. Chapter 2 looks at the approach of nurses when carrying out practical skills and emphasises self-awareness. Family and friends have an important role in providing support too.

Pregnancy and birth: practice points – VTE risk and prevention

Although most are active and mobile, some pregnant or recently delivered women may have impaired mobility due to prolonged epidural anaesthesia, caesarian birth or coexisting debilitation, for example, pelvic girdle pain (PGP) or spinal injury. A significant risk for these women is VTE. If these factors are compounded by additional risks such as obesity, high maternal age, excessive blood loss/blood transfusion, multiple pregnancy or pre-eclampsia, then the risk increases significantly. All pregnant women with impaired mobility for whatever reason should have VTE prophylaxis, usually mechanical (antiembolic stockings) and pharmacological, with early ambulation too (NICE 2010).

For further reading about PGP, see www.pelvicpartnership.org.uk

Summary
- People who have reduced mobility are at risk of several physical and psychosocial complications.
- Nurses have an important role in identifying potential complications and implementing preventive care.

KEY PRINCIPLES OF MOVING AND HANDLING PEOPLE

Many patients require help with moving on an individual basis, which may change over the duration of their treatment and care. For example, Diane does not currently need help with moving, but if her condition deteriorates this situation may change. Patient handling practice is governed by legislation and NHS Trust policies. The principles of safe handling must be learned by all nurses. Smith's (2011) *Guide to the Handling of People* is a very useful resource for safe handling of patients and should be available in your organisation.

> **LEARNING OUTCOMES**
>
> By the end of this section, you will be able to:
> 1 conduct a moving and handling risk assessment;
> 2 identify appropriate equipment for individual patients' needs;
> 3 discuss the importance of communication in patient handling;
> 4 explain the legal implications of patient handling.

Learning outcome 1: Conduct a moving and handling risk assessment

ACTIVITY

Find out about the moving and handling assessment tools in use in your clinical area.

You will probably have seen moving and handling assessment tools being used in practice for carrying out and documenting a systematic assessment. They are likely to include sections relating to task, individual capability, load, environment and equipment (Chadwick 2010).
- **Task.** What exactly is the manoeuvre to be carried out? For example, the task might be to move Marion out of bed and into her wheelchair.
- **Individual capability.** Nurses need to assess their own ability, physical fitness and what they are capable of.
- **Load.** How much can the person do? A person who is fit and has no communication problems with support and training may eventually be able to transfer from bed to wheelchair using a lateral transfer board. Marion, although not particularly heavy, is unable to move and therefore needs a hoist to move her out of bed. If a person is in pain, they will be reluctant or unable to help, so pain

relief is vital before the manoeuvre is carried out and proper handling techniques will help to reduce pain.

- **Environment.** Is there enough room for you and the person to work in and to maintain a safe posture? Slippery floors are a danger for people like Diane and John who have difficulty walking or who are unsteady on their feet.
- **Equipment.** What is required and how and when should it be used

If people cannot move themselves, then equipment must be used. You will be able to practise using different equipment in your moving and handling sessions.

Learning outcome 2: Identify appropriate equipment for individual patient's needs

ACTIVITY What patient handling equipment is commonly in use in your clinical area?

If you are working in a clinical area that has very dependent patients/clients, you may have a wide range of equipment available. Hignett (2003) suggests that the minimum equipment list for a clinical environment where patient handling activities occur on a regular basis includes hoists, standaids, sliding sheets, lateral transfer boards, walking belts and height-adjustable beds and baths.

Nurses will need to use a hoist to move Marion from a height-adjustable bed to wheelchair and back, and in and out of a height-adjustable bath. They will also need to use a sliding sheet to move her around in bed. You may be working in an area where patient/clients are mostly independent – such as an acute mental health unit – but staff must have access to equipment if it becomes necessary and staff must keep their skills up to date. For example, if a patient like John falls and is unable to get himself up from the floor, a hoist will be needed.

Learning outcome 3: Discuss the importance of communication in patient handling

ACTIVITY Why is it important to communicate with your colleagues and patients involved in handling manoeuvres?

When moving and handling, both patient and carers are working as a team. It is vital that one person leads and coordinates the activity. Patients need to know exactly what to expect and how they can help when equipment is being used (Palmer 2004). The team leader must communicate the command to the team, and when everyone is ready give the command clearly (e.g. 'ready . . . brace . . . move') so that the manoeuvre is smooth and coordinated.

Learning outcome 4: Explain the legal implications of patient handling

ACTIVITY Identify some possible legal implications of patient handling.

Poor moving and handling practice has implications for patient safety. Moving patients in bed without using appropriate equipment can cause shear and friction to the skin. The 'drag lift' (whereby nurses hook their arms under the patient's armpits and drag them up the bed, or on to their feet from sitting) can cause bruising, fractures or dislocation of shoulders; this can be considered as abuse with associated legal consequences (Pellatt 2005).

Children: practice points – moving and handling

Key principles of assessment, use of correct techniques and selection of appropriate equipment should be applied when moving and handling children across the age range. There are paediatric sizes and child-friendly versions of the equipment available, for example, hoist slings and slide sheets. See Aylott's chapter below, which covers all aspects, including a developmental approach to risk, across the age range, lifting infants, transferring children and using a hoist with children:

Aylott, M. 2010. Manual handling for children's and young people's nursing. In: Glasper, A., Aylott, M. and Battrick, C. (eds.) *Developing Practical Skills for Nursing Children and Young People*. London: Hodder Arnold, 89–108.

Summary

- A risk assessment must be carried out before any moving and handling activity takes place.
- It is important that appropriate patient handling equipment is available for patients who need it.
- Patient handling requires teamwork which includes the person being moved.
- Using inappropriate handling techniques compromises patient safety and can have legal consequences.

ASSISTING WITH MOBILISATION AND PREVENTING FALLS

Assisting with mobility is an important role of nurses in many settings and involves overcoming barriers and working closely with the multidisciplinary team, particularly physiotherapists and occupational therapists.

LEARNING OUTCOMES

By the end of this section, you will be able to:

1 identify barriers to mobilisation;
2 examine ways of preventing falls;
3 discuss how people can be assisted with mobilisation.

Learning outcome 1: Identify barriers to mobilisation

ACTIVITY

What barriers could prevent a person from mobilising? How might these apply to the people in the scenarios?

A few possibilities are listed below, but you may well have thought of others.

- Pain or fear of pain may prevent a person from mobilising, and this is an important issue for John. Therefore, pain must be assessed and controlled (Kneafsey 2007). Read more about pain assessment and control in Chapter 12.

- Lack of motivation or reduced cognitive function, perhaps where people have depression or dementia, may lead to reluctance to mobilise (Swann 2006). John's depression could therefore present a further barrier to mobilisation.

- Foot problems such as in-growing toenails, fungal nail infections, calluses, corns and bunions can impede mobility by causing pain and discomfort. Neurological diseases and neuropathies such as multiple sclerosis can alter gait, causing calluses and corns to develop (Nazarko 2006; Chadwick 2010).

- Bunions and arthritic feet make it difficult to wear normal shoes, but unsuitable footwear makes mobilising difficult and dangerous. Slip-on shoes or slippers increase the tendency to shuffle (Woodrow et al. 2005). Shiny or plastic soles cause a frightened, small-step gait. Narrow shoes inhibit normal foot movement, reducing normal toe function and preventing normal toe 'push off', affecting gait pattern and weight transference. High heels put abnormal stress on knees, making the gait unstable (Godfrey 2006). Ill-fitting shoes can cause blisters, corns, calluses and bursae, which are painful and can lead to ulceration (Tyrrell 2002).

- Arthritic knees can cause instability and falls, which lead to loss of confidence.

- Shortening of one leg may occur after surgery for fractured neck of femur, making it difficult to put both feet on the ground together.

- Fear of falling is a common problem and can cause a fear of going outside, even leading to agoraphobia. When a person, like John, has already had one fall causing a significant injury, fear of another fall and a lack of confidence in mobilising are understandable.

- Fatigue is a common symptom of several medical conditions, one of which is multiple sclerosis (Swann 2006), and can be an overwhelming feeling of exhaustion in response to minor exertion. Diane is able to walk with sticks sometimes but needs a wheelchair when she becomes severely fatigued.

- Muscle damage can cause weakness, and increased muscle tone or spasticity due to multiple sclerosis, for example, can prevent a full range of movement (Swann 2006). This is a problem for Diane and Marion.

Learning outcome 2: Examine ways of preventing falls

The prevention of falls is focused on in *The National Service Framework Falls - Number 6* (DH 2008), and as falls in older people cost the NHS £2.3 billion a year, there is pressure to address the problem (Mitchell 2011). However, people in other age groups, like Diane and John, can be at risk of falling too. The effects of falls extend beyond physical injury and cost to the health services. Fear of subsequent falls can lead to restricted mobility and independence, contributing to functional decline and dependency, which in turn increases the risk of falling (McCarter-Bayer et al. 2005).

ACTIVITY

Consider people you have cared for in practice who were in hospital as the result of a fall, or perhaps fell while in hospital. List the reasons for their falls.

Parkinson's disease

There is a loss of dopamine-producing neurons within the brain, causing a chronic, progressive degenerative neurological disease with symptoms such as tremor, rigidity and bradykinesia (slow movement). It affects many activities including eating, with a risk of aspiration.

- *Physiological and psychosocial factors.* Physiological and psychosocial factors contribute to fear of falling. People may develop a morbid fear of falling (McCarter-Bayer et al. 2005). Fear increases with age and is more common in women; a previous fall is not necessary to trigger this fear (Halvarsson et al. 2011).
- *Poor vision.* Poor vision can be due to age-related deterioration or other visual problems (Lyons 2005). People may trip over objects in the dark, trip on carpets or uneven floors or miss stairs and fall.
- *Poor mobility with age-related changes in gait, posture and balance.* Neurological diseases cause motor and sensory impairment; for example, **Parkinson's disease** causes people to stoop, lean forward and develop a short-stepped, shuffling gait. Multiple sclerosis (Diane) causes gait problems due to spasm, and motor and sensory changes. Diabetic neuropathy may cause decreased sensation in legs and feet. Stroke affects mobility and balance (Lyons 2005).
- *Changes in the inner ear.* Inner ear changes can affect a person's sense of balance.
- *Loss of muscle strength and flexibility.* Loss of muscle strength and flexibility can cause difficulty in holding handrails or getting out of chairs and walking (Kneafsey 2007).
- *Medications and alcohol.* Medications and alcohol can cause dizziness, hypotension, blurred vision, weakness, poor balance and drowsiness (Jasniewski 2006). John's medication for his depression could have these effects. Diuretics and laxatives increase the number of trips to the toilet, often in a hurry. Taking more than four different medicines, particularly sedating or blood pressure lowering medicines, is a predisposing factor in falls (Anderson 2008).
- *Problems with bladder and bowels.* Falls can result from lack of bladder or bowel control, such as with urge incontinence (McCarter-Bayer et al. 2005).
- *Dementia.* Dementia causes cognitive impairment, memory loss and confusion, which may contribute to the danger of falling (Chaãbane 2007).

The *National Service Framework for Older People* (Standard 6: Falls) recommended that older people who have fallen should receive advice on prevention from a specialist falls service (DH 2001). NICE (2013) advise that there should be a multifactorial assessment, including discussion about falls history, checks on gait, balance, mobility and muscle weakness, assessment of osteoporosis risk, perceived functional ability and fear of falling, eyesight check, neurological and cognitive functioning examinations, discussion about continence and home hazards, cardiovascular examination and a review of medication.

All nurses should understand risk factors for falls and be aware of the falls service and how referrals are made.

| **ACTIVITY** | Think of how falls can be prevented for people who are identified as being at risk. |

The following interventions can be effective in preventing falls:

- Muscle strengthening, gait and balance training and exercise (Halvarsson et al. 2011).
- Home hazard assessment and modifications such as handles and rails to a person's home.
- Review and possible withdrawal of medications where appropriate (Anderson 2008).
- Cardiac pacing where appropriate (NICE 2013).
- Regular eye examinations and provision of correct prescription lenses, walking sticks or frames.
- Increasing exercise and physical activity.
- Continence management (Anderson 2008).
- Hip protectors may be provided to prevent hip fractures in older people who have a high risk of falling; research evidence to support this function is equivocal.

There is some evidence to suggest that Tai Chi exercises may help to prevent falls by improving balance and improve muscle and cardiorespiratory strength and fitness (Halvarsson et al. 2011). For detailed guidance on preventing falls, including falls in hospital, see NICE (2013).

Learning outcome 3: Discuss how people can be assisted with mobilisation

| **ACTIVITY** | Focus on the practice scenarios and identify strategies and equipment that might assist with mobilisation. |

You probably considered involvement of the multidisciplinary team and will have encountered mobility aids. Helping a person to mobilise requires a multidisciplinary approach. For example, the orthotist can supply walking sticks for Diane, and callipers, adapted shoes or knee braces, can overcome some of the barriers to mobility. Physiotherapists will assess people for mobility aids such as crutches, or walking frames, both standard or wheeled, for people who cannot lift a standard frame. Gutter frames can help people with arthritis.

People who are unable to walk (Marion), or whose walking ability fluctuates (Diane), will be supplied with wheelchairs. Transfer boards enable people with upper body balance stability to transfer independently or with minimal assistance from one seated position to another (Chadwick 2010). Special chairs with cushions that rise slowly can help people who have difficulty getting up from a chair (Swann 2006). For patients who have had a stroke, the physiotherapist will develop a plan for how the patient should be handled, moved and positioned to encourage upper extremity recovery and prevent shoulder pain (Zeferino and Aycock 2010). Aids and appliances must be cleaned and checked regularly as part of a regular maintenance programme to maintain patient safety (Swann 2007).

Restoring or minimising loss of mobility in people with dementia is challenging, but Logsdon et al. (2005) suggest an activity programme that uses both behavioural and exercise strategies. These strategies are enjoyable and help to improve physical and emotional health. When mobilising people with dementia, it is important that the nurse is calm and reassuring and gives clear step-by-step instructions (Varnham 2011). Box 6.4 provides suggestions for assisting a person with dementia to move from sitting to standing.

Dressing and undressing Marion, who has severe contractures, can be very difficult, and the occupational therapist can advise about techniques and suitable clothing. Splints and braces can help to maintain body and limb posture. If considered in her best interests, arm gaiters could help to minimise involuntary muscle action so that she might be able to use an adapted motorised wheelchair, thus increasing her independence in mobilising. However, careful assessment will be needed to ensure that she can operate the wheelchair safely (Swann 2007).

Safety

When helping a person to mobilise, the safety of both the individual and the nurse is a major consideration. As we have already discussed, some people may be unsteady on their feet or have lost confidence. Therefore, a risk assessment must be carried out before attempting to assist with mobilising. You will have looked at risk assessment within moving and handling training sessions and will be aware of the importance of documentation.

Box 6.4 Mobilising a person with dementia: sitting to standing

- Sound – Use a calm and reassuring tone, simple step-by-step instructions, and verbal cues and prompts.
- Physical – Guide patients' movement with one's own body movements. Touch and hand massage may reduce agitated behaviour.
- Visual – Make good eye contact, place mobility aids so that patients can see them, use other visual cues.
- Equipment and environment – Reduce background noise, have enough space and remove obstacles, ensure adequate lighting.

Source: Varnham, W. 2011. How to mobilise patients with dementia to a standing position. *Nursing Older People* 23(8): 31–6.

Assisting a person to walk

When assisting a person to walk, you stand beside them, facing forward so you both move the same way. The use of a handling belt around the person's waist gives you something to hold. For example, if someone has a slight weakness on the left side, you stand at their left side in a walk stance, with your right hand holding the belt around their waist, and their left hand placed on your left hand (Figure 6.4).

On the command 'ready ... brace ... stand', you both move forward as you transfer your weight from the back leg to the front. You can now use this hold to give the person confidence to walk. You will have the opportunity to practise these techniques under supervision in the classroom. A very important aspect is not to hurry the person, maintaining a slow steady pace. It is important that you have assessed how long the patient is able to stand, how far they can walk and if these abilities fluctuate (Chadwick 2010).

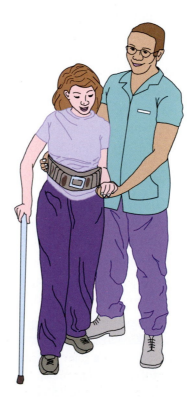

Figure 6.4: Helping a person to walk.

ACTIVITY

Reflect on situations where you have been caring for a person with dementia in hospital. Were there any issues related to their moving about the ward? If so, how have you dealt with these?

People with dementia: walking and moving about

Alzheimer's Society (2009) identified that nurses experienced difficulties regarding people with dementia walking and moving about in a hospital setting, for example, trying to leave the ward. In response Alzheimer's Society developed some 'Top tips'. Box 6.5 summarises these ways of dealing with such situations in a helpful way.

> ### Box 6.5 Moving and walking about for people with dementia: top tips for nurses
>
> - People with dementia can experience problems with orientation which are increased in unfamiliar environments such as hospital wards.
> - Try to understand why the person wishes to walk about so that you can find ways of meeting their needs. It is essential to help people with dementia maintain their independence.
> - Some people with dementia find it comforting to walk, so try to accommodate this comfort. Find out from the family or carers what support or supervision they usually need.
> - People often walk about if they are bored, so ensure the person has enough things to do. Involve the person in suitable activities on the ward, which will give a sense of purpose and self-worth.
> - Help the person find their way about the ward, for example, ensure they know where the toilet is and ask if they need to go there.
> - People often walk when in pain to try to ease discomfort. If the person cannot communicate they are in pain, investigate further.
> - If a person is feeling agitated or anxious, they may want to walk about. Try to encourage the person to tell you about their anxieties and reassure them.
> - Short-term memory loss can lead a person with dementia to start moving for a specific purpose but then forget where they were going and find themselves lost, which is very distressing.
> - They may set out to search for someone or something related to their past. Encourage them to talk about this and show them that you take their feelings seriously. Try to avoid correcting things that the person may say. It is important to focus on what the person feels rather than the factual accuracy of what they say.
> - People with dementia often become confused about the time. They may wake in the middle of the night and get dressed, ready for the next day. Try putting a clock, where they can see it, which shows the date, time, am and pm.
> - The person with dementia may walk because they feel they need to carry out a certain activity, which may be one they carried out in the past, for example, going to work. This action may be because they are feeling unfulfilled, so try to find them an activity that gives them a sense of purpose.
> - If the person is determined to leave, try not to confront them, as this could be upsetting. Instead, accompany them a little way and then divert their attention so that you both return.
>
> *Source*: Summarised from Alzheimer's Society, http://www.alzheimers.org.uk/site/scripts/documents_info.php?documentID=1211&pageNumber=6

As an example, in a study of students' experiences of caring for people with dementia in hospital, a student nurse explained how a man with dementia who was a former naval captain, kept packing his bags and attempting to leave the ward to 'go to sea' (Baillie et al. 2012). The student engaged him in conversation about the navy:

> *He started telling me about all the ports and places he'd been; what he had done during his service.*

The student found that he then calmly walked with her back to his bed to continue the conversation.

Summary

- Building people's confidence and self-esteem is an essential aspect of mobilisation.
- Nurses have an important role in the multidisciplinary team, managing and caring for people with problems of mobility.
- Nurses should be aware of barriers to mobilisation, so that these barriers can be addressed.
- Nurses should be aware of the people who are at risk of falling and implement interventions to prevent falls.
- When assisting with mobilising, risk assessment is essential and must be documented.
- Appropriate mobility aids should be provided for each individual. Nurses can give encouragement and support to people who are regaining mobility.
- Effective communication is key in relation to mobility, particularly when caring for people with dementia.

CHAPTER SUMMARY

There are many possible underlying reasons for impaired mobility, which can be temporary or permanent. The complications of impaired mobility can lead to much discomfort and further health problems, so nurses must take a proactive role to prevent these ill effects.

Pressure ulcers were discussed in depth as their incidence remains widespread even though they are largely preventable. This chapter has emphasised the importance of identifying potential problems, so that effective preventive strategies for each individual can be implemented.

Promoting mobility wherever possible is key to preventing many problems, and a multidisciplinary approach should be taken. Finally, when caring for people with impaired mobility, correct moving and handling techniques must be used to protect both patients and nurses. It was beyond the scope of the chapter to address this topic in depth. These techniques need to be learned under supervision, and attendance at moving and handling sessions is essential.

REFERENCES

Alzheimer's Society. 2009. *Counting the Cost: Caring for People with Dementia on Acute Hospital Wards.* London: Alzheimer's Society.

Anderson, C.M., Overend, T.J., Godwin, J., et al. 2009. Ambulation after deep vein thrombosis: A systematic review. *Physiotherapy Canada* 61(3): 133–40.

Anderson, K.E. 2008. Falls in the elderly. *Journal of Royal College of Physicians Edinburgh* 38(1): 38–43.

Anthony, D., Parboteeah, S., Saleh, M., et al. 2008. Norton, Waterlow and Braden scores: A review of the literature and a comparison between the scores and clinical judgement. *Journal of Clinical Nursing* 17(5): 646–53.

Anton, L. 2006. Pressure ulcer prevention in older people who sit for long periods. *Nursing Older People* 18(4): 29–36.

Baillie, L., Merritt, J. and Cox, J. 2012. Caring for older people with dementia in hospital: Part II: Strategies. *Nursing Older People* 24(9): 22–6.

Benbow, M. 2008. Pressure ulcer prevention and pressure-relieving surfaces. *British Journal of Nursing* 17(13): 830–5.

Bennett, G., Dealey, C. and Posnett, J. 2004. The cost of pressure ulcers in the UK. *Age and Ageing* 33: 230–5.

Berg, H., Eiken, O., Miklavic, L., et al. 2007. Hip, thigh and calf muscle atrophy and bone loss after 5-week bedrest inactivity. *European Journal of Applied Physiology* 99(3): 283–9.

Bergstrom, N., Braden, B.J., Laguzza, A., et al. 1987. The Braden scale for predicting pressure sore risk. *Nursing Research* 36: 205–10.

Black, J.M., Cuddigan, J.E., Walko, M.A., et al. 2010. Medical device related pressure ulcers in hospitalised patients. *International Wound Journal* 7(5): 358–65.

Bosch, M., Halfens, R.J.G., van der Weijden, T., et al. 2011. Organisational culture, team climate and quality management in an important patient safety Issue: Nosocomial pressure ulcers. *Worldviews on Evidence-Based Nursing* 8(1): 4–14.

Carter, K. 2009. Identifying and managing deep vein thrombosis. *Primary Health Care* 20(1): 30–9.

Chaâbane, F. 2007. Falls prevention for older people with dementia. *Nursing Standard* 2(6): 50–5.

Chadwick, M. 2010. Providing excellent service for those with mobility impairment. *Nursing and Residential Care* 12(6): 278–82.

Clark, M. 2002. Pressure ulcers and quality of life. *Nursing Standard* 16(22): 74–8, 80.

Clavet, H., Hébert, P.C., Fergusson, D., et al. 2008. Joint contracture following prolonged stay in the intensive care unit. *Canadian Medical Association Journal* 178(6): 691–7.

Clayden, V., Steeves, J. and Krassiovikou, A. 2006. Orthostatic hypotension following spinal cord injury: Understanding clinical pathology. *Spinal Cord* 44(6): 341–51.

Collins, F. 2002. Use of pressure reducing seats and cushions in a community setting. *British Journal of Community Nursing* 7(10): 15–22.

Cox, J. 2011. Predictors of pressure ulcers in adult critical care patients. *American Journal of Critical Care* 20(5): 364–74.

Department of Health (DH). 2001. Standard six: Falls. In: *National Service Framework for Older People.* London: DH. https://www.gov.uk/government/uploads/system/uploads/attachment_data/file/198033/National_Service_Framework_for_Older_People.pdf (accessed 27th October 2013)

Department of Health (DH). 2002. *Action for Health – Health Action Plans and Health Facilitation*. London: DH.

Department of Health (DH). 2009. *Health Action Planning and Health Facilitation for People with Learning Disabilities: Good Practice Guidance*. London: DH.

Department of Health (DH). 2010. *Essence of Care: Benchmarks for Prevention and Management of Pressure Ulcers*. Norwich: The Stationery Office.

Dinsdale, P. 2007. Under pressure. *Nursing Older People* 19(6): 18–24.

Disabled Living Foundation (DLF). 2006. *Choosing Pressure Relief Equipment*. London: DLF.

European Pressure Ulcer Advisory Panel and National Pressure Ulcer Advisory Panel (EPUAP and NPUAP). 2009. *Pressure Ulcer Prevention Quick Reference Guide*. Available from: http://www.npuap.org/wp-content/uploads/2012/02/Final_Quick_Prevention_for_web_2010.pdf (Accessed on 22 September 2013).

Fernandez, T. 2007. Preventing pressure ulcers: Selecting the right equipment. *International Journal of Therapy and Rehabilitation* 14(5): 235–9.

Finucane, C. 2006. A guide to dynamic and static pressure-distributing products. *International Journal of Therapy and Rehabilitation* 13(6): 283–6.

Gefen, A. 2009. Rewick and Rogers pressure-time curve for pressure ulcer risk. Part 1. *Nursing Standard* 23(45): 64–74.

Gibbon, B. 2002. Rehabilitation following stroke. *Nursing Standard* 16(29): 47–52, 54–5.

Godfrey, J. 2006. Toward optimal health: D. Casey Kerrigan, M.D., discusses the impact of footwear on the progression of osteoarthritis in women. *Journal of Women's Health* 15(8): 894–7.

Goldhill, D.R., Imhoff, M., McLean, B., et al. 2007. Rotational bed therapy to prevent and treat respiratory complications: A review and meta-analysis. *American Journal of Critical Care* 16(1): 50–62.

Gould, D., James, T., Tarpey, A., et al. 2000. Intervention studies to reduce the prevalence of pressure sores: A literature review. *Journal of Clinical Nursing* 9: 163–78.

Halvarsson, A., Olsson, E., Farén, E., et al. 2011. Effects of new, individually adjusted, progressive balance group training for elderly people with fear of falling and tend to fall: A randomised control trial. *Clinical Rehabilitation* 25(11):1021–31.

Hampton, S. 2003. The complexities of heel ulcers. *Nursing Standard* 17(31): 68, 70, 72, 74, 76, 79.

Hampton, S. and Collins, F. 2005. Reducing pressure ulcer incidence in a long-term setting. *British Journal of Nursing* 14(15): S6–12.

Hignett, S. 2003. Systematic review of patient handling activities in lying, sitting and standing positions. *Journal of Advanced Nursing* 41(6): 545–52.

Hignett, S. and Griffiths, P. 2009. Risk factors for moving and handling bariatric patients. *Nursing Standard* 24(11): 40–8.

Hopkins, A., Deeley, C., Bale, S., et al. 2006. Patient stories of living with a pressure ulcer. *Journal of Advanced Nursing* 56(4): 345–53.

Jasniewski, J. 2006. Putting a lid on medication-related falls. *Nursing* 36(6): 22–4.

Jaul, E. 2010. Assessment and management of pressure ulcers in the elderly. *Drugs Aging* 27(4): 311–25.

Jones, C. 2004. Multiple sclerosis update. *Primary Health Care* 14(2): 26–32.

Kelly, J. 2005. Inter-rater reliability and Waterlow's pressure ulcer risk assessment tool. *Nursing Standard* 19(32): 86–92.

Kelly, J. and Isted, M. 2011. Assessing nurses' ability to classify pressure ulcers correctly. *Nursing Standard* 26(7): 62–71.

Kneafsey, R. 2007. A systematic review of nursing contributions to mobility rehabilitation: Examining the quality and content of the evidence. *Journal of Clinical Nursing* 16(11c) 325–40.

Kyle, G. 2006. Assessment and treatment of older patients with constipation. *Nursing Standard* 21(8): 41–6.

Lindgren, M., Unosson, M., Fredrikson, M., et al. 2004. Immobility: A major risk factor for development of pressure ulcers among adult hospitalised patients – A prospective study. *Scandinavian Journal of Caring Sciences* 18(1): 57–64.

Liou, T., Pi-Sunyer, X. and Lafferrère, B. 2005. Physical disability and obesity. *Nutrition Reviews* 63(10): 321–31.

Lloyd Jones, M. 2012. Prevention and treatment of superficial pressure damage. *Nursing and Residential Care* 14(1): 14–20.

Logsdon, R., McCurry, S. and Terry, L. 2005. A home health care approach to exercise for people with Alzheimer's disease. *Care Management Journals* 6(2): 90–7.

Lyons, T. 2005. Fall prevention for older adults. *Journal of Gerontological Nursing* 32(11): 9–14.

Mathias, J. 2007. Preventing venous thromboembolism. *Supplement to OR Manager* 23(3): 23–6.

McCarter-Bayer, A., Bayer, F. and Hall, K. 2005. Preventing falls in acute care: An innovative approach. *Journal of Gerontological Nursing* 31(3): 25–33.

Mitchell, M. 2011. Falls prevention in the elderly: An update from Age UK. *British Journal of Community Nursing* 16(6): 300–1.

Moore, Z., Cowman, S. and Conroy, R.M. 2011. A randomised controlled clinical trial of repositioning, using the 30° tilt, for the prevention of pressure sores. *Journal of Clinical Nursing* 20(17/18): 2633–44.

National Institute for Health and Clinical Excellence (NICE). 2005. *The Prevention and Treatment of Pressure Ulcers*. Clinical Guidelines 29. London: NICE.

National Institute for Health and Clinical Excellence (NICE). 2008. *Physical Activity and the Environment*. Public Health Guidance 8. London: NICE. Available from: http://www.nice. org.uk

National Institute for Health and Clinical Excellence (NICE). 2010. *Venous Thromboembolism: Reducing the Risk Reducing the Risk of Venous Thromboembolism (Deep Vein Thrombosis and Pulmonary Embolism) in Patients Admitted to Hospital*. Clinical Guidelines 92. London: NICE. Available from: http://www.nice.org.uk (Accessed 27 August 2012).

National Institute for Health and Clinical Excellence (NICE). 2013. *The Assessment and Prevention of Falls in Older People*. Clinical Guidelines 161. Available from: http:// guidance.nice.org.uk/CG161 (Accessed 22 September 2013).

Nazarko, L. 2006. Helping older people to care for their feet. *Nursing and Residential Care* 8(3): 105–8.

NHS Institute for Innovation and Improvement. 2009. Your skin matters. Available from: http://www.institute.nhs.uk/building_capability/hia_supporting_info/your_skin_ matters.html (Accessed on 18 January 2013).

Nigam, Y., Knight, J. and Jones, A. 2009. Effects of bedrest 3: Musculoskeletal and immune systems, skin and self-perception. *Nursing Times* 105(23): 18–22.

Nilsson, C.J., Avlund, K. and Lund, R. 2011. Onset of mobility limitations in old age: The combined effect of socioeconomic position and social relations. *Age and Ageing* 50(5): 607–14.

Noble, M., Voegeli, D. and Clough, G. 2003. A comparison of cutaneous and vascular responses to transient pressure loading in smokers and non smokers. *Journal of Rehabilitation Research and Development* 40(3): 283–8.

Nursing and Midwifery Council (NMC). 2008. *The Code: Standards of Conduct and Performance and Ethics for Nurses and Midwives.* London: NMC.

Nutescu, E. 2007. Assessing, preventing and treating venous thromboembolism: Evidence-based approaches. *American Journal Health-System Pharmacists* 64(Suppl 7): S5–13.

Palmer, R. 2004. Moving and handling bariatric patients safely: A case study. *International Journal of Therapy and Rehabilitation* 11(1): 31–3.

Pancorbo-Hidalgo, P., Garcia-Fernandez, F.P., Lopez-Medina, I.M., et al. 2006. Risk assessment for pressure ulcer prevention: A systematic review. *Journal of Advanced Nursing* 54(1): 94–110.

Papanikolaou, P., Lyne, P. and Anthony, D. 2007. Risk assessment scales for pressure ulcers: A methodological review. *International Journal of Nursing Studies* 44(2): 285–96.

Pellatt, G. 2005. The safety and dignity of patients and nurses during patient handling. *British Journal of Nursing* 14(21): 1150–6.

Pellatt, G. 2007a. Clinical skills: Bed making and patient positioning. *British Journal of Nursing* 16(5): 302–5.

Pellatt, G. 2007b. Urinary elimination. Part 2: Retention, incontinence and catheterisation. *British Journal of Nursing* 16(8): 480–5.

Pellatt, G. 2007c. Anatomy and physiology of urinary elimination: Part 1. *British Journal of Nursing* 16(7): 406–10.

Persoon, A., Heinen, M., Carien, J.M., et al. 2004. Leg ulcers: A review of their impact on daily life. *Journal of Clinical Nursing* 13(3): 341–54.

Ramsey, S. and McIlhenny, C. 2011. Evidence-based management of upper tract urolithiasis in the spinal cord-injured patient. *Spinal Cord* 49(9): 948–54.

Reenalda, J., Geffen, P.G., Nederhand, M., et al. 2009. Analysis of healthy sitting behaviour: Interface pressure distribution and subcutaneous tissue oxygenation. *International Journal of Rehabilitation Research and Development* 46(5): 577–86.

Rinds, G. 2009. Exploring recent developments in manual handling. *Nursing and Residential Care* 11(6): 312–15.

Roper, N., Logan, W. and Tierney, A.J. 2000. *The Roper–Logan–Tierney Model of Nursing.* Edinburgh: Churchill Livingstone.

Smith, J. (ed.) 2011. *Guide to the Handling of People,* 6th edn. Teddington: BackCare.

Srikanth, R., Cassidy, G., Joiner, C., et al. 2011. Osteoporosis in people with intellectual disabilities: A review and a brief study of risk factors for osteoporosis in a community sample of people with intellectual disabilities. *Journal of Intellectual Disability Research* 55(1): 53–62.

Steggall, M.J. and Omara, M. 2008. Urinary tract stones: Types, nursing care and treatment options. *British Journal of Nursing* 17(9): S20–3.

Stephen-Haynes, J. 2006. Implementing the NICE pressure ulcer guideline. *Wound Care* 15(9): 516–18.

Swann, J. 2006. Keeping mobile: Part one. *Nursing and Residential Care* 8(12): 566–8.

Swann, J. 2007. Keeping mobile: Part 2. *Nursing and Residential Care* 9(1): 28–30.

Takamoto, S., Saeki, S., Yabumoto, Y., et al. 2005. Spontaneous fractures of long bones associated with joint contractures in bedridden elderly patients: Clinical features and outcome. *Journal of the American Geriatrics Society* 53(8): 1439.

Taylor, H. 2003. An exploration of the factors that affect nurses' record keeping. *British Journal of Nursing* 12(12): 751–8.

Thompson, M. 2011. Reducing pressure ulcers in hip fracture patients. *British Journal of Nursing* 20(15): S10–18.

Tyrrell, W. 2002. The causes and management of foot ulceration. *Nursing Standard* 16(30): 53, 54, 56, 58, 60, 62.

Vanderwee, K., Grypdonck, M. and Defloor, T. 2007. Non-blanching erythema as an indicator for the need for pressure ulcer prevention: A randomised controlled trial. *Journal of Clinical Nursing* 16(2): 325–35.

Vanderwee, K., Grypdonck, M. and Defloor, T. 2008. Alternating pressure air mattresses as prevention for pressure ulcers: A literature review. *International Journal of Nursing Studies* 45(5): 784–801.

Van Wicklin, S., Ward, K. and Cantrell, S. 2006. Implementing a research utilisation plan for prevention of deep vein thrombosis. *AORN Journal* 83(6): 1351–62.

Varnham, W. 2011. How to mobilise patients with dementia to a standing position. *Nursing Older People* 23(8): 31–6.

Vollman, K.M. 2010. Introduction to progressive mobility. *Critical Care Nurse* 30(2): S3–5.

Waterlow, J. 1985. Pressure sores: A risk assessment card. *Nursing Times* 81(48): 49, 51, 55.

Waterlow, J. 1988. The Waterlow card for the prevention and management of pressure sores: Toward a pocket policy. *Care – Science and Practice* 6(1): 8–12.

Waterlow, J. 2005. The Waterlow score card. Available from: http://www.judy-waterlow.co.uk (Accessed on 18 January 2013).

Weaver, D. 2005. Helping individuals to maintain mobility. *Nursing and Residential Care* 7(8): 343–8.

Weetman, C. and Allison, W. 2006. Use of epidural anaesthesia in post-operative pain management. *Nursing Standard* 20(44): 54–64.

Woodrow, P., Dickson, N. and Wright, P. 2005. Foot care for non-diabetic older people. *Nursing Older People* 17(8): 31–2.

Zeferino, S.I. and Aycock, D.M. 2010. Poststroke shoulder pain: Inevitable or preventable? *Rehabilitation Nursing* 35(4): 147–51.

Zegelin, A. 2008. 'Tied down' – The process of becoming bedridden through gradual local confinement. *Journal of Clinical Nursing* 17(17): 2294–301.

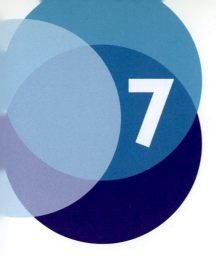

Principles of Wound Care

Janine Ashton

The maintenance of skin integrity and the retention of its protective barrier are major components of basic nursing care (Beldon 2012; Bryant 2007). Despite the emergence of new technologies and research into the field of acute and chronic wound management (Gray et al. 2004; McCluskey and McCarthy 2012; Timmons 2006), wound care continues to be described as a high-cost and unreliable healthcare activity. Inappropriate treatment leads to delayed healing, infection, preventable pain and a reduced quality of life (O'Brien et al. 2011).

It is estimated that in the United Kingdom (UK) approximately 200,000 patients have a chronic wound, with an estimated cost to the National Health Service (NHS) of £2.3–3.1 billion per annum (2005–2006 prices), and this cost will potentially increase over the next 20 years due to an ageing UK population (Posnett and Franks 2008). Wound dressings account for approximately £120 million of prescribing costs in primary care in England each year (Shorney and Ousey 2011). Posnett and Franks (2008) suggested that with proper diagnosis and treatment, this cost could be reduced while ensuring quality improvement.

The nurse's role in wound care encompasses the initial holistic assessment of the wound and the patient. The nurse needs to develop the ability to make the correct clinical and cost-effective decisions about treatment based on evidence-based practice (McCluskey and McCarthy 2012; Timmons 2006; Wounds UK 2008), while regularly evaluating and monitoring the progress of the wound. The care pathway should include the involvement of the patient in the decision-making process by setting small realistic goals; this approach will promote cooperation and compliance (Beldon 2012; DH 2010). This chapter aims to assist you to develop knowledge and understanding of the breadth of issues involved with wound healing physiology and to apply this understanding to your practice.

Wound management is a vast topic with an ever-expanding and developing knowledge base, to which whole books and journals are dedicated. Therefore, although this chapter provides a foundation, further reading is necessary, and you need to continually update your knowledge base. The Cochrane Library and the National Institute for Health and Clinical Excellence (NICE) – discussed in Chapter 1 – are good sources. When in the practice setting, there are specialist nurses (e.g. tissue viability, vascular and dermatology nurses) and other members of the multidisciplinary team (MDT) (e.g. podiatrists) who will be valuable resources for your learning.

This chapter includes the following topics:

- The phases of wound healing
- Classification of wounds and wound closure
- Factors affecting wound healing
- Wound assessment
- Wound management

Although you can study this chapter at any stage of your learning programme, you will find it most relevant to work through the sections when based in a setting where you have patients/clients with different wounds. There is no substitute for looking at real wounds and applying theory to practice. Chapter 3 is essential prior reading because when managing wounds, an understanding of how microorganisms are transmitted, and adherence to standard precautions and aseptic technique, is paramount.

Recommended biology reading:

The following questions will help you to focus on the biology underpinning this chapter's skills. Use your recommended textbook to find answers to the following:

- What characteristics must skin possess?
- What are the major layers of the skin?
- Which layer is avascular?
- What are the major functions of the skin? What role does skin play in homeostasis?
- How does the skin protect itself against damage and infection?
- What factors can lead to a breakdown in skin integrity? What would the consequences be?
- What is the goal of wound healing? What factors influence the degree of scarring?
- How does age alter the skin's characteristics? Consider the skin at birth, adolescence, young adulthood and old age.
- How does the appearance of skin change, during illness, injury or stress?
- What factors are necessary to maintain normal healthy skin?

An understanding of the physiology of wound healing is essential when assessing and managing wounds and is therefore included in this chapter.

PRACTICE SCENARIOS

The following practice scenarios illustrate different situations where wound care is required and are referred to throughout this chapter.

Adult

Mrs Warner is 78 years old and has a history of **type 2 diabetes**, which is managed with oral hypoglycaemic medication. Since her husband died 2 years ago, she has

Type 2 diabetes

Develops when the body makes insufficient insulin, or when the insulin that is produced does not work effectively (known as insulin resistance). See www. diabetes.org.uk.

lived alone with her two cats and has been treated for depression. After falling in her kitchen, she was unable to get off the floor and was found by a neighbour some hours later. After assessment in the emergency department, she was diagnosed with a stable fracture of her pelvis. She was also found to have an ulcer (open sore) on one of her toes, which had an offensive discharge. Her blood glucose was high. She was transferred to a ward for rehabilitation and pain management. A few days later, a large area of black necrotic (dead) tissue developed on her sacrum, and discoloured areas on both her elbows. These wounds appeared to have been caused by the period of prolonged pressure on the kitchen floor. Mrs Warner is keen to get home as soon as possible as she is worried about her cats. She normally smokes 10 cigarettes a day and is overweight. Her diet is high in fat and carbohydrates, and she rarely eats fruit or vegetables.

Learning disability

Susan is 32 years old and has a moderate learning disability. She lives in a small group home and was recently in hospital having her acutely inflamed appendix removed. She has been discharged home and has a small abdominal wound, which seems to be healing well. However, Susan is concerned about the wound and is worried about getting it wet when she showers, and drying and dressing afterward in case she harms the wound. She is due to have her sutures removed by the practice nurse. The community nurse for learning disability is visiting regularly to give some support in this situation. Susan's keyworker is her **health facilitator**.

Mental health

Colin is 28 years old and is being treated as an inpatient in the acute mental health unit, after deterioration in his mental health, which has affected his self-care ability. He has a diagnosis of substance abuse and schizophrenia, which is currently being treated with **clozapine**. Colin requires careful blood monitoring, as clozapine can affect white blood cell levels. While on the unit, he complained of pain in his left upper buttock. A large, hot, swollen area was found, which was diagnosed as being an **abscess**. Colin says that he has had several of these swollen areas before. Incision and drainage took place in theatre, and he has now returned to the unit, with a pack in situ in the wound. Antibiotics have been prescribed.

THE PHASES OF WOUND HEALING

A wound can be defined as (Lazarus et al. 1994)

> a disruption of normal anatomical structure and function which results from pathological processes beginning internally or externally to the involved organ.

This definition still remains relevant in 2012 and continues to be used in the literature.

Health facilitator

The role focuses on an individual's health outcomes and can be undertaken by a range of people, including support workers, family carers, friends and advocates as well as health professionals; see *Health Action Planning and Health Facilitation for People with Learning Disabilities: Good Practice Guidance* (DH 2009).

Clozapine

Clozapine is an atypical antipsychotic drug used to treat schizophrenia, which is claimed to have greater efficacy and to cause fewer movement disorders, but it carries a significant risk of serious blood disorders (Tuunainen and Wahlbeck 2010).

Abscess

A localised collection of pus. Pus is a thick fluid containing leucocytes, bacteria and cellular debris, and it indicates infection.

Different wounds do not necessarily follow the same pattern in the healing process. Doughty and Sparks-Defriese (2007) identify two ways in which wound repair occurs:

- Wounds confined to the epidermis and superficial dermal layers heal by regeneration.
- Wounds extending through the whole dermis heal by scar formation.

LEARNING OUTCOMES

By the end of this section, you will be able to:

1. distinguish the phases of healing and recognise tissue appearance at each stage;
2. appreciate that healing does not in reality occur in a simple linear manner.

Learning outcome 1: Distinguish the phases of healing and recognise tissue appearance at each stage

Wound healing is usually described in three distinct phases, but these descriptive models refer to the healing of acute wounds. Chronic wounds do not follow the normal sequence of events, so delays to the healing process are experienced (Timmons 2006). Some studies describe four or more phases/stages, but these variations are an expansion on the three phases described. You may also find different terminology being used to describe the phases. This chapter uses the approach that there are three interdependent phases during the wound healing process.

The inflammatory phase

The twofold inflammatory phase prepares the tissue for repair. After initial wounding, blood loss is controlled by a complex series of events, whereby the blood and lymphatic vessels undergo a short period of vasoconstriction, creating a haemostatic plug (Nguyen et al. 2009). This process is known as **haemostasis**. In addition to minimising the extent of the injury, this process initiates the inflammatory response through the release of growth factors, which in turn attract the migration of neutrophils, monocytes and macrophages to the wound bed (Timmons 2006). The primary function of these cells is to attract phagocytes to the inflamed area to kill bacteria and remove debris from dead and dying cells within the tissue spaces (Nguyen et al. 2009; Timmons 2006). This process is known as **phagocytosis**. The five cardinal signs of inflammation are heat, redness, pain, swelling and loss of function.

The proliferative phase

The proliferative phase rebuilds the tissue through three separate processes.

- **Granulation** leads to the formation of new blood vessels (angiogenesis), which deliver oxygen and nutrients to the healing tissues. Fibroblasts and endothelial cells are the primary cells in this phase. Fibroblasts from the surrounding tissue become activated by growth factors released in the inflammatory phase, enabling them to replicate and produce a collagen-rich matrix which builds elasticity and strength into the wound (Nguyen et al. 2009; Timmons 2006). Granulation tissue is characterised by a reddish velvety carpet in the base of the wound. Unhealthy granulation tissue may be dark in colour and bleed easily, indicating possible infection and poor vascular supply to the tissue (Timmons 2006).

- **Contraction** is the approximation of the wound edges believed to be caused by the 'push' and 'pull' effect of the myofibroblasts (Nguyen et al. 2009; Timmons 2006).
- **Epithelialisation** resurfaces the wound by regeneration of epithelial cells.

In full-thickness wounds, regeneration occurs from wound margins, whereas in partial-thickness wounds, remnants of partially ablated hair follicles also contribute to re-epithelialisation (Doughty and Sparks-Defriese 2007; Nguyen et al. 2009). Contraction and epithelialisation can be identified by a marginal zone of smooth tissue.

The maturation phase

The maturation phase involves remodelling the tissue to form a **scar**. This phase can take a year or more as cellular activity reduces and the number of blood vessels in the wound decreases (Nguyen et al. 2009).

ACTIVITY

Prepare notes on the phases of healing, which are outlined briefly above, from your recommended biology textbook. Focus your reading on the requirements for each phase of the healing process.

Your reading should have helped you to understand that the wound healing process is a complex interplay of events leading to complete healing.

ACTIVITY

Aim to observe an uncomplicated surgical wound, or a minor traumatic wound – this wound could even be a laceration on your own skin. Compare the appearance of the wound to the described criteria for different phases of healing. Discuss with a practitioner which phase of healing is predominant at present.

At different phases of wound healing, the tissue has a different appearance.

- When observed in the *inflammatory phase*, the wound appears swollen and red, and the surrounding tissue feels warm and can be painful. Recognising these signs (which occur due to local vasodilation) can be difficult at first. In the inflammatory phase, the wound is usually kept covered to prevent contamination.
- In the *proliferative phase*, signs of wound contraction commence. The appearance of tiny red buds is the first sign of primitive blood vessels emerging, acting as a transport system for nutrients, oxygen, cells and growth factors essential for connective tissue development (Nguyen et al. 2009; Timmons 2006). This friable tissue, which fills the deficit at the wound bed, is also referred to as

granulation tissue. New epithelial cells divide and, using a leapfrog action, migrate from wound edges and any remaining islands of epidermal cells that may encompass sebaceous glands and hair follicles.

- A wound in the *maturation phase* may remain in this phase for up to 2 years. It will appear smaller, and may be white and hard (scar tissue) and fixed to surrounding tissue, or similar in appearance to surrounding tissue, indicating a healed mature wound. The maximum tensile strength after injury is 70%–85% (Harrison et al. 2006).

Gray et al. (2004) summarise the implications of the different colours of wounds as follows:

- **Black:** necrotic (dead) tissue and therefore no healing has begun (Figure 7.1)
- **Yellow:** slough (made up of dead cells) – occurs near the end of the inflammatory stage (Figure 7.2)
- **Red:** granulation tissue (Figure 7.3)
- **Pink:** epithelialisation (Figure 7.4)

ACTIVITY

Consider how the community nurse for learning disabilities might reduce Susan's anxiety about her wound, and prepare her for suture removal.

The community nurse will need to have assessed Susan's cognitive and physical ability to care for her wound and would then be able to help Susan to understand the wound's healing and the care it requires. The nurse can use effective communication skills to ascertain Susan's understanding of the healing process, and her anxieties about this process. Photos and pictures might be helpful. The nurse could encourage Susan to look at the wound and point out the signs of healing, explaining about the sutures being removed when the wound is healed.

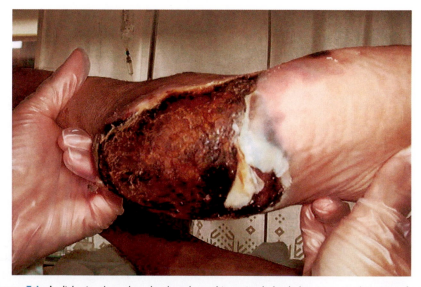

Figure 7.1: A diabetic ulcer that developed on this patient's heel due to a combination of poor circulation and unrelieved pressure. The tissue bed is covered in hard black necrotic tissue. The wound will not heal until this ulcer is removed. Unfortunately, this ulcer eventually led to amputation of the patient's lower leg and foot.

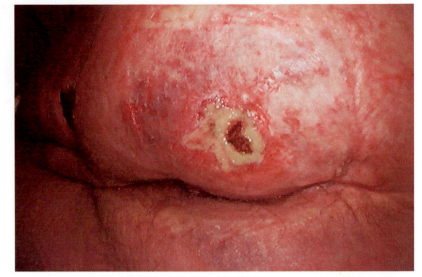

Figure 7.2: A pressure ulcer [European Pressure Ulcer Advisory Panel (EPUAP) category 3] that developed on the sacrum of a patient with multiple sclerosis. The wound bed is covered with yellow slough, except for a central necrotic area. Slough is soft necrotic tissue containing dead phagocytes, and the wound will not heal until this tissue is removed. Surrounding this ulcer are other areas of pressure damage, evidenced by discolouration (EPUAP category 1) and superficial ulceration (EPUAP category 2).

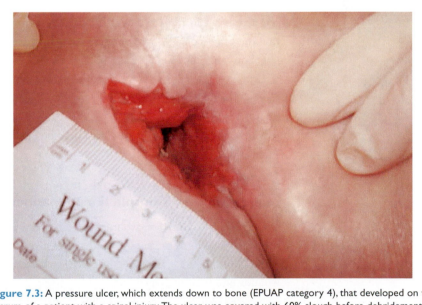

Figure 7.3: A pressure ulcer, which extends down to bone (EPUAP category 4), that developed on the sacrum of a patient with a spinal injury. The ulcer was covered with 60% slough before debridement by maggots. The wound is now almost filled with red granulation tissue. This photo also shows how a ruler placed by the side of a wound before the photo can provide a more accurate record of its dimensions.

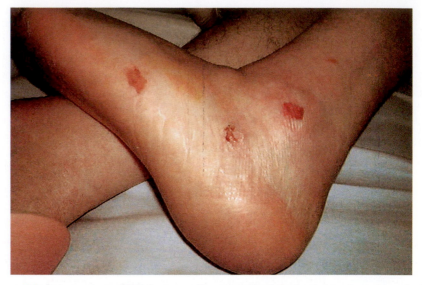

Figure 7.4: Pressure ulcers (EPUAP category 2) on the side of the foot/ankle of a patient who has multiple sclerosis. They are now almost healed, with tissue beds showing mainly pink epithelialising tissue.

Once Susan understands how the wound is healing, the nurse can then explain why she need not be afraid of showering and give her practical advice about drying herself without rubbing the wound itself and about wearing clothing that will not rub the wound. The nurse must similarly ensure that Susan's carers understand these issues, so they can reinforce the information and be consistent in their reassurance and explanation.

The nurse can prepare Susan for her suture removal and will be able to ensure that the practice nurse removing Susan's sutures knows how Susan communicates and how she has been prepared. If there is anyone who has a healed surgical wound, perhaps Susan could, with the person's permission, talk to them. Actually seeing a healed wound might help to allay her anxiety, if this viewing is possible to arrange.

All the above-mentioned aspects should be incorporated in Susan's **Health Action Plan**.

Learning outcome 2: Appreciate that healing does not in reality occur in a simple linear manner

Owing to several factors, wound healing is not always a straightforward process. A review of wounds caused by trauma, pressure or ulceration illustrates these issues. These wounds are considered in further detail in the section 'Classification of wounds and their management'.

> **Health Action Plan**
>
> A personal action plan developed for each individual with a learning disability, which details the actions needed to maintain and improve the person's health and any help needed to accomplish these; see *Action for Health – Health Action Plans and Health Facilitation* (DH 2002).

ACTIVITY

If possible, select a patient with a wound caused by trauma, pressure or ulceration, in discussion with your practice mentor. Try to find out about the history of the wound and its healing process to date. Compare your investigations with the discussion below.

Trauma

Traumatic wounds vary greatly in nature. Although minor wounds may heal in a straightforward manner, others involve extensive skin loss and contamination, which can affect the healing process and may require surgical intervention.

Pressure ulcers

Impaired circulation to the skin for even short periods is problematic in susceptible individuals, such as people who are frail, older or malnourished – consult Chapter 6 for a full discussion of pressure ulcers. Mrs Warner, as an older person, who also has diabetes, and had a period of immobility on a hard surface (the kitchen floor), is obviously a high-risk individual. The discoloured areas on Mrs Warner's elbows could potentially develop into necrotic ulcers similar to her sacral pressure ulcer.

Leg and foot ulceration

There are many causes of leg and foot ulceration, each having different distinguishing features, underlying pathology and treatment, but the majority are associated with circulatory problems (Nelson and Bradley 2007). For example,

- *diffusion* – problems arise when the distance between the capillary and tissue cells is increased (e.g. by oedema);
- *perfusion* – occurs when there is arterial or venous insufficiency.

Currently, there are three national guidelines for leg ulcer care, produced by the Royal College of Nursing (RCN 2006), the Clinical Resource Efficiency Support Team (CREST 1998) and the Scottish Intercollegiate Guidelines Network (SIGN 2010). The Leg Ulcer Forum (Whayman 2012) has further developed quality standards to ensure that patients receive the three quality domains of safety, clinical effectiveness and patient experience as outlined by the white paper Equity and Excellence: Liberating the NHS (DH 2010).

Leg ulcers are a common chronic wound and are often an extensive and long-standing problem (Anderson 2006). Figure 7.5 shows a large venous leg ulcer, which the patient has had for many years. The prevalence rates of leg ulcers in the UK is estimated to be 1.2%–3.2% of the population (Graham et al. 2003), representing 70,000–190,000 individuals (Norris et al. 2012). The total cost of leg ulcer management has been estimated to be £168–198 million per year (Posnett and Franks 2008); this figure does not include the personal cost to patients or take into account the impact on their quality of life (Moffatt et al. 2009), including pain, sleep disturbance, limited work and leisure, depression and a lack of self-esteem.

It is estimated that 70% of ulcers are venous in origin and 25% are arterial (Nelson and Bradley 2007), but the ulcer can be of mixed aetiology too. Useful overviews of lower leg ulceration can be found in Doughty and Holbrook (2007) and Anderson (2006, 2009). There are also many books devoted entirely to leg ulcers and their management.

Diabetic ulcers can occur on the feet of people with diabetes; these are complex wounds and cause unacceptably high levels of morbidity and mortality (Bilous and

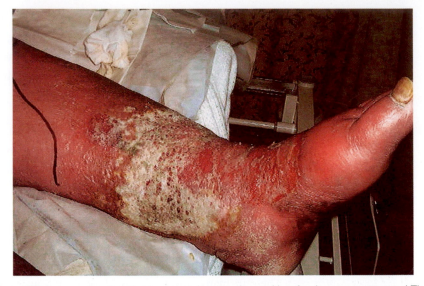

Figure 7.5: A venous leg ulcer that has been a long-standing problem for the patient concerned. There are large areas of yellow slough and areas of red granulation tissue covering the wound. The lower foot looks oedematous, and there is hard scaly skin (hyperkeratosis) present. The surrounding skin also looks red, suggesting cellulitis.

Donnelly 2010; McIntosh 2006). Figure 7.1 shows how severe these ulcers can potentially be. Diabetes care in the NHS costs approximately £9 billion, with up to 20% (£600 million) being used to treat diabetic foot ulcers (National Institute for Health and Clinical Excellence [NICE] 2011a). Common problems include infection, osteomyelitis, neuropathy, peripheral arterial disease, Charcot arthropathy and amputation (NICE 2011a). Education and patient empowerment are essential to ensure that foot ulceration is reduced in high-risk patients; this approach is being supported by the development of multidisciplinary care pathways within NHS acute care (NICE 2011a). However, Mrs Warner's depression could affect her ability to carry out this aspect of self-care (see Box 8.2).

You should now be aware that some wounds progress in a complicated manner owing to underlying health problems. These complex wounds often necessitate an MDT approach in diagnosis and management, with investigations performed to ensure accurate identification of the problem.

A scar is the end result of healing, but the formation of a mature scar can be a slow process. A scar is the product of many cells. However, specialist myofibroblast cells have a key role in healing, by shrinking the wound by contraction (Nguyen et al. 2009; Timmons 2006). Note that 75% of normal wound healing is by contraction, which results in a smaller, less visible scar. A scar initially consists of raised vascularised tissue – hence the red colour. Gradually, the redness disappears as the number of blood vessels reduces, and the colour changes to white. As noted, the new tissue will not be as strong as previously and may predispose an individual such as Mrs Warner to increased risk of pressure ulcer damage.

Some individuals have problems with **hypertrophic scars** and **keloids**. Although hypertrophic scars can regress, keloid scars do not. Management of both of these

Hypertrophic scar

A raised, healed red scar that is uncomfortable and tight. This is caused by an increased deposition of collagen within the area of the original wound (Aityeh et al. 2005).

Keloid

A firm mass of scar caused by excessive collagen deposition, but it extends outside the wound boundaries (Aityeh et al. 2005).

problems requires a specialist and MDT, for both the physical and the psychological problems that may accompany them.

Summary

- Wound healing is a complex process involving phases of healing through which the wound must pass to heal adequately.
- The process is theoretically sequential, but in reality parts of different phases occur concurrently.
- The end result is a scar of uncertain appearance and weakened structure in comparison to surrounding undamaged tissue.

CLASSIFICATION OF WOUNDS AND WOUND CLOSURE

Wounds are often divided into *acute* and *chronic*. Acute wounds result from surgery or trauma and usually heal relatively quickly with minimal need for external interventions, if no complications occur (Timmons 2006). Burns, due to the area of tissue damage, often behave more like chronic wounds (Timmons 2006). A wound is considered to be chronic when it has not healed in 4–6 weeks (Siddiqui and Bernstein 2010). Such wounds include leg ulcers, pressure ulcers, diabetic foot ulcers, malignant wounds and any non-healing acute wound. They are usually caused by underlying health problems, including age, heart disease, diabetes mellitus, peripheral arterial disease and neuropathy (Escandon et al. 2011; Siddiqui and Berstein 2010) and also social and psychological problems. Haemostasis may be absent from the process, and the individual's ability to heal is often impaired, with the inflammatory response being continually stimulated by the underlying disease process, resulting in a prolonged and excessive inflammatory phase of wound healing (Timmons 2006).

Learning to classify wounds will enable you to appreciate issues affecting their management, thus planning more effective care. There are a variety of ways of classifying wounds; this chapter uses a simple classification based on the cause.

LEARNING OUTCOMES

By the end of this section, you will be able to:
1 distinguish between acute and chronic wounds;
2 discuss the principles of wound closure for different types of acute and chronic wounds.

Learning outcome 1: Distinguish between acute and chronic wounds

ACTIVITY

Table 7.1 shows a classification of wounds, and Table 7.2 shows a classification of surgical wounds. Working from these tables, how would you classify the wounds of Mrs Warner, Susan and Colin?

Table 7.1: Wound classification

Classification	Types of wound	Causes and features
Acute	Penetrating wounds	Causative objects include missiles (e.g. bullets, explosion debris) or hand-held objects (e.g. knives, billiard cues, etc.). High infection risk.
Acute	Lacerations	Healing affected by the cause (whether it is a clean wound or is contaminated by dirt/debris), age of the wound and the individual. Wounds involving the eyes and joints are priorities.
Acute	Abrasions	Caused by the body being dragged against an abrasive surface, removing surface epithelium. Can be very painful and sensitive as nerve endings are exposed. If not meticulously cleaned, 'tattooing' results from dirt trapped in the dermis and epidermis, which is almost impossible to remove (Evans and Jones 1996).
Acute	Bites	Common cause of wounds; most are caused by dogs, but human bites are also common. High infection risk owing to the large number of microorganisms found in mouths.
Acute	Surgical	As these wounds are planned, risks (e.g. of infection) can be reduced to a minimum. Infection rates vary according to the type of surgery (see Table 7.2).
Acute	Burns	Can be thermal (caused by flame, hot fluid or radiation), chemical (acid or alkali) or electrical. Can damage the epidermis only (superficial), the epidermis and the dermis (partial thickness) or extend into deeper tissue (full thickness). The extent of the burn is very important to assess, as fluid resuscitation may be needed.
Chronic	Venous leg ulcers	Caused by damage to the venous system in the leg, especially the valves, causing pooling and distending of vessels; by-products of this process cause tissue death and ulcer formation. Risk factors include varicose veins and rheumatoid arthritis. Ulcers are usually shallow and situated in the gaiter area, with irregular edges (Doughty and Holbrook 2007). Pain may be severe, dull or aching.
Chronic	Arterial leg ulcers	Occur when impaired blood supply due to various causes leads to areas of skin death, as the blood vessel supplying the area becomes occluded. Ischaemic pain occurs and the ulcers tend to be small and deep with well-defined borders, situated at distal body locations (e.g. toes) (Doughty and Holbrook 2007).
Chronic	Diabetic neuropathic or neuroischaemic foot ulcers	Chronic hyperglycaemia causes impairment of the nerve supply to the foot and lower limb; the resulting loss of sensation can lead to pressure damage, repeated trauma and/or penetration by foreign bodies. These ulcers are neuropathic in origin. In neuroischaemic ulcers, the combination of neuropathy and arterial disease produces a very complex wound with a poor prognosis.
Chronic	Pressure ulcers	Prolonged pressure on the skin produces obstruction of small vessels, resulting in death of skin, and sometimes deeper tissues, owing to lack of blood supply. Shearing and friction also contribute to their development.
Chronic	Infection-induced	Opportunistic organisms gain access through the skin via a small wound, and produce an ulcer. Tropical ulcers are one of the most common forms.
Chronic	Ulcers caused by cancer	Referred to as fungating wounds, these can complicate cancers in various areas of the body. They present as a rapidly growing fungus or with a cauliflower-like appearance which may ulcerate (Goldberg and McGynn-Byer 2007).

Table 7.2: Classification of surgical wounds

Type	Features	Infection rate (%)
Clean	Surgery without infection present and no entry into hollow muscular organs	1.5
	Appendicectomy, cholecystectomy and hysterectomy are included in this category if there is no acute inflammation	
Clean contaminated	Hollow muscular organ penetrated, but minimal spillage of contents occurred	7.7
Contaminated	Hollow muscular organ opened with gross spillage of contents, or acute	15.2
	inflammation but no pus found	
	Traumatic wounds <4 hours of occurrence	
Dirty	Traumatic wound >4 hours old	40.0
	Surgery where there is presence of pus or a perforated viscus	

Source: Cruse, P. and Foord, R. 1980. The epidemiology of wound infection: A ten-year prospective study of 62,939 wounds. *Surgical Clinics of North America* 60: 27–40.

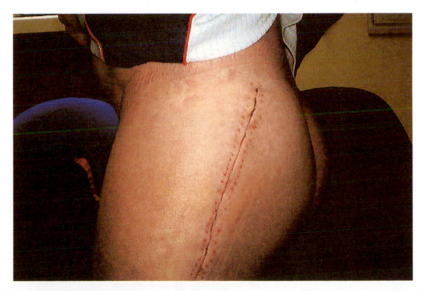

Figure 7.6: The hip wound of a man who had a total hip replacement, 10 days previously, and just had his skin closures (clips) removed. This is a good example of a clean surgical wound that has healed as planned by primary intention.

You should have identified that Mrs Warner's sacral wound is a chronic pressure ulcer and her toe wound is probably a chronic diabetic foot ulcer. Susan and Colin both have acute surgical wounds. However, although Susan's is a clean contaminated wound, Colin's is a dirty wound as it contained pus. Figure 7.6 shows the wound of a man who had a hip replacement 10 days previously and has now had his skin closures removed. This wound would be categorised as a clean surgical wound. Now, try using the table to classify wounds of patients/clients in the practice setting, in the following activity.

With reference to Tables 7.1 and 7.2, explore the nature and cause of wounds within your practice setting. Do all the wounds clearly fit into a category type? Are there any wounds that started as acute, and have ended up as chronic? If so, why?

Wounds are not always easy to categorise. Acute surgical wounds can break down and sometimes appear similar to pressure ulcers, thus starting as acute but becoming chronic. The underlying reasons are not always clearly understood but often relate to the person's physical health. Approximately 21,000 surgical wounds per year in England and Wales become difficult to heal (NICE 2001), and this difficulty can be related to surgical site infection (NICE 2008). Figure 7.7 shows an abdominal wound, 5 days after surgery. The distal part has broken down due to infection and the clips have had to be removed early.

Learning outcome 2: Discuss the principles of wound closure for different types of acute and chronic wounds

Gottrup (1999) identified that wounds may be closed through:

- primary closure;
- early (delayed primary) closure, that is, 4–6 days (performed before there is visible granulation tissue);
- late (secondary) closure, that is, 10–14 days;
- grafting using skin or artificial skin products;
- no closure (leaving the wound to heal by granulation).

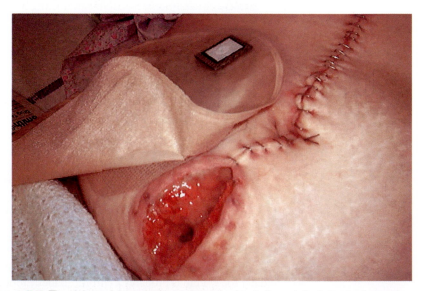

Figure 7.7: The abdominal wound of a woman who has had an abdominoperineal resection, with colostomy formation, for ulcerative colitis. The colostomy has been sited very close to the wound. The photo was taken on the fifth postoperative day. The wound had started to ooze pus from the distal part of the wound, and had dehisced. The clips from this area have been removed. Towards the top of the wound and the central area, there is slight inflammation. In the dehisced area, small patches of red granulating tissue can be seen, but other areas look unhealthy. There is a dark centre to this area, which was found to be a sinus.

When wounds are closed (i.e. the skin edges are brought together), the wound is said to be healing by **primary intention**. Figure 7.6 shows a good example of a surgical wound that has healed by primary intention. When wounds are left open, this is termed healing by **secondary intention**. Although the wound in Figure 7.7 was planned to heal by primary intention, the lower part may have to heal by secondary intention unless the wound is reclosed after the infection has cleared. **Tertiary intention** consists of wound closure via surgical reconstruction techniques. Dunn and Phillips (2004) provide a useful overview of wound closure.

ACTIVITY

Try to find out how and when wounds are closed by observing in practice and asking practitioners. Consider
- a surgical wound (such as Susan's abdominal wound);
- a traumatic wound;
- a chronic wound (such as Mrs Warner's pressure ulcer).

Also, find out how long closure materials (clips, staples or sutures), if present, are left in the wound before removal. Does the site of the wound have any effect on this?

Surgical wounds

Clean or clean–contaminated wounds are managed by primary closure, using sutures, staples or clips, at the end of surgery. The aim is to protect the wound from the bacteria circulating in a hospital environment (Chapter 3 has more information on preventing infection) and promote the best cosmetic result. Thus, Susan's wound will have been managed by primary closure at the end of her operation, as were the wounds shown in Figures 7.6 and 7.7.

With contaminated or dirty surgical wounds, delayed primary closure may be preferable. In some cases the wound may be left open, to heal by secondary intention. A dirty, infected wound, such as Colin's, will be left open to enable continuing drainage; closing the wound would allow buildup of pus and a further abscess.

Traumatic wounds

Management of traumatic wounds depends on the degree of contamination (taking into account where and how the wound occurred); the extent of skin damage/skin loss; the site of the wound; and how long ago the injury occurred. A clean incisional wound, with little tissue damage, that occurred less than 6 hours previously (caused by a knife, for example) can be irrigated, debrided and managed by primary closure. However, if the injury is more than 6 hours old, or is heavily contaminated, for example, by soil, then primary closure should be delayed (Leaper 2006; Morris 2006).

There may be differing priorities, though. Bites should usually be left to heal by secondary intention owing to their infection risk; exceptions are made where cosmetic effects are paramount, or restoring function takes priority (Mcheik et al. 2000). Facial wounds have an excellent blood supply and rarely become infected (White 2005).

Incised wounds and lacerations can be closed with tapes, sutures or tissue adhesive, the choice depending on factors such as size, depth and site. Tissue adhesive could be suitable for a small scalp wound, due to decreased procedure time and less pain, but should not be used for lacerations of the nostril, mouth or eye, where suturing is preferable to ensure accuracy of alignment (Leaper 2006).

If a person with a traumatic wound has delayed seeking attention, then prolonged bacterial access will have occurred. Usually, the wound will be cleansed with the aim of free drainage and/or detection of infection, followed by delayed primary closure by suturing at 4–6 days. Secondary closure should be used when a wound is heavily contaminated; although this leaves a broader scar than after primary (early or delayed) closure, it is still cosmetically preferable to that achieved through the healing of an open granulating wound (White 2005).

Chronic wounds

Chronic wounds are usually allowed to heal by secondary intention. Granulation tissue fills the defect, and new epidermis covers the surface. This process is slow and time-consuming and provides poor protection against risks such as repeated pressure and infection. It can, nevertheless, provide a successful outcome. Mrs Warner's pressure ulcer will need to heal by secondary intention. When surgical excision of necrotic tissue is performed, as might occur with a pressure ulcer, the aim is also for healing to occur by secondary intention. Attempts to directly close large defects by bringing the edges of the wound together have often been unsuccessful, since the tension on the suture line pulls the wound apart. An alternative is to use surgical techniques such as skin grafting and skin flaps, examples of tertiary intention. Beldon (2007) gives a brief overview of these techniques and their care.

When to remove skin closures

The decision on when to remove skin closures depends on various factors.
- Site can affect healing rate. The face heals fast – sutures are often removed in 5 days. The feet heal more slowly, so sutures may be left in situ for 7–10 days.
- Factors such as ageing and diabetes can affect the rate of healing (see the section 'Factors affecting wound healing').

Patients being discharged from hospital with skin closures in situ must be informed of exactly when and where the skin closures will be removed. Susan's sutures would probably be ready for removal at 7 days, and she can attend her local health centre for their removal by the practice nurse. Sometimes, it is necessary to arrange for the district nurse to visit a patient's home for skin closure removal, for example, if it is difficult for the person to leave the house due to poor general condition or lack of mobility. Adhesive glue has the advantage of not needing removal.

Summary
- Acute wounds usually heal uneventfully and quickly, but they can, in certain situations, become chronic.
- Chronic wounds frequently fail to heal in a timely and orderly manner.

- Different types of wound are managed in different ways. In general, clean surgical wounds heal by primary direct closure, contaminated traumatic wounds heal by delayed primary closure and chronic wounds heal by secondary intention healing.

FACTORS AFFECTING WOUND HEALING

There are a wide range of biological, psychological and sociological factors that influence wound healing. It is important to identify factors that may affect wound healing for individuals, as a perpetuating wound will result if underlying causes are not addressed (Morris 2006; Troxler et al. 2006). Gray et al. (2011a) have explored aspects of psychological and physical well-being and quality of life issues in relation to wound-healing outcomes. A multidisciplinary approach may be needed to address these factors. Patients with acute wounds that are healing by primary intention usually require less input, but each individual should be assessed.

> ### LEARNING OUTCOMES
> On completion of this section, you will be able to:
> 1 explore the range of factors that can affect wound healing;
> 2 examine how a multidisciplinary approach can address factors affecting wound healing;

Learning outcome 1: Explore the range of factors that can affect wound healing

Table 7.3 identifies general factors that can delay wound healing. When assessing a person with a wound, consider these questions:

- What underlying factors are interfering with wound healing?
- Does the patient have an underlying condition that is delaying wound healing?
- Does the wound require debridement?
- Is the wound infected?
- What needs to be changed to move the wound healing process forward?

The following exercise is based on this framework.

ACTIVITY

With the guidance of your practice mentor, identify a person who (like Mrs Warner) has a problematic wound. Carry out the activity below.
- Look at their assessment documentation. Identify any factors that could influence wound healing (Table 7.3 will give you clues). Remember to consider the person as a whole, as well as their wound.
- Then ask yourself, can these factors be altered/changed? What action could help?

Table 7.4 includes factors that might have been identified for Mrs Warner. Compare the list you prepared for your patient with this. You may well have identified a much wider range of issues, depending on your individual patient (also see Flanagan 2003; Thomas Hess 2011; Vowden 2011).

Table 7.3: General factors for delayed healing

Age	Immunosuppression
Anaemia	Microbes
Decreased oxygen	Necrotic tissue
Decreased perfusion	Nutrition (vitamins, minerals)
Dehydration	Oedema
Diabetes mellitus	Organ failure
Foreign body	Radiation
Malignancy	Smoking
Medication, such as corticosteroids, cytotoxics	Other wound-related factors

Source: Reproduced with kind permission from Troxler, M., Vowden, K. and Vowden, P. 2006. Integrating adjunctive therapy into practice: the importance of recognising 'hard to heal' wounds. *World Wide Wounds*. Available from: http://www.worldwidewounds.com (Accessed on 19 January 2013).

Table 7.4: Factors influencing Mrs Warner's wound healing

Factor	Rationale for identification	Can it be influenced?	Action required
Smoking	Serensen (2003) outlines effects of smoking. Smoking causes a compromised blood supply to the wound and impairs the cardiovascular system, delaying healing. It leads to inhibition of epithelialisation and a reduction in wound contraction.	Potentially	Reduction in smoking balanced against quality of life issues
Diabetes mellitus and elevated blood glucose level	People with diabetes have impaired wound healing (NICE 2011a). A wide range of underlying pathologies are responsible.	Yes	Blood glucose monitoring, medication and dietary considerations
Depression	Depression affects ability to self-care (Gray et al. 2011a), for example, to manage her diabetes, relieve pressure, and care for her feet.	Yes	Pharmacology and therapeutic approach
Poor nutritional intake	Adequate nutrients required for wound healing (see Table 7.5).	Yes	Promote nutritious and balanced diet
Ageing	The skin's ability to repair reduces with ageing (Miminas 2007; Pittman 2007). The disease processes that often accompany ageing may impair healing (Pittman 2007).	Indirectly by improving overall health	General health promotion
Stress and anxiety about being in hospital	Stress delays healing (Gray et al. 2011a; Jones 2003; Richardson and Upton 2011).	Potentially	Develop nurse–patient relationship, identify and address sources of anxiety
Infection in toe wound	Infection compromises healing, places stress on the body, and impairs diabetes stabilisation.	Yes	Investigations (e.g. x-ray to identify whether there is bone infection); wound management and antibiotics
Necrotic tissue in sacral ulcer	Necrotic tissue prevents wound healing.	Yes	Debride necrotic tissue using suitable method

You probably considered general health, age and nutrition. Other chronic conditions that affect wound healing include respiratory and cardiovascular disease, owing to their effect on tissue oxygenation (Flanagan 2003; Vowden 2011). Figure 7.8 shows how a lack of blood supply affects skin and deeper tissues. This patient had heart failure and a lack of circulation to her feet, causing necrosis. An adequate blood supply to the skin and underlying tissues is essential, both to prevent wounds and to promote wound healing.

Are you aware of the effect of steroids on wound healing? The anti-inflammatory response of steroids reduces the inflammatory response, and affects the function of the macrophages, thus slowing healing (Vowden 2011). Did you also identify stress and anxiety as a factor? These too can have a major influence on wound healing (Jones 2003; Richardson and Upton 2011); provision of information can contribute to effective healing (European Wound Management Association [EWMA] 2008). Colin has a long-standing mental health problem, and the discomfort associated with his wound may be a further source of stress. Susan, too, has been through a stressful experience. Now that she is back in her own environment with familiar staff members, it will be important to be supportive and reassuring. Thus nurses should aim to relieve their stress and anxieties and help them to relax (see Chapter 2).

Chapter 10 highlights the need for an increased nutritional intake for wound healing. However, many people with chronic wounds, such as pressure ulcers, have poor nutritional intake and risk factors for malnutrition (Johnston 2007). Every patient with a wound should be assessed nutritionally. Table 7.5 outlines the key nutrients required for wound healing and their role in the process. Stotts (2007) and Johnston (2007) extensively reviewed the literature linking nutrition and wound healing.

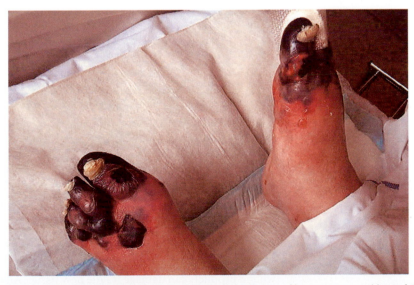

Figure 7.8: This patient, whose feet are shown here, had a history of heart surgery and heart failure. Over 2 weeks, she developed black necrotic toes, and the condition spread to the distal area of her feet owing to the lack of arterial circulation.

Table 7.5: Nutrients required for wound healing and their function

Nutrient	Function	Dietary sources
Fat	Energy source; involves in formation of inflammatory mediators and clotting components; fat-soluble vitamins are essential for the building of new cell membranes in wound repair.	Butter, margarine, other spreading fats, oils, cream, full fat milk, cheese
Carbohydrate	Energy source for increased cellular activity during wound healing; in the absence of sufficient dietary or stored energy, the body utilises protein as an energy source.	Complex: bread, pasta, rice, noodles, scones, pancakes, potatoes Simple: jam, sugar, biscuits, honey
Protein	Essential for building the new wound bed (collagen formation).	Meat, eggs, cheese, milk, yogurt, fish, poultry, pulses, nuts
Vitamin A	Enhances the immune response; antioxidant; promotes collagen synthesis and epithelialisation.	Butter, margarine, other spreading fats, oils, milk, cheese, carrots, red peppers, tomatoes, eggs
Vitamin B complex	Assists formation of collagen mesh which supports new blood vessels as they move into granulating tissue.	Whole grains, breakfast cereals, milk and milk products, meat, fish liver
Vitamin C	Assists formation of collagen mesh and angiogenesis; enhances iron absorption, promotes immune function.	Oranges, grapefruit, fruit juice, green vegetables, potatoes, strawberries
Vitamin E	With vitamin C, attacks damaging oxygen free radicals that are present in infected wounds and during the inflammatory phase of wound healing.	Vegetable oil, egg yolk, nuts, seeds
Vitamin K	Blood clotting.	Liver, green vegetables
Minerals: selenium, copper, manganese, zinc, iron	Fibroblast proliferation; collagen synthesis; improved oxygen delivery to tissue.	Selenium: brazil nuts, meat, vegetables, fish, cereals Copper: meat, vegetables, cereals, tea, coffee Manganese: tea, widely distributed in various foods Zinc: meat, milk, potatoes, bread Iron: red meat, liver, fortified breakfast cereals, eggs, pulses, green vegetables, sardines

Source: Adapted from Johnston, E. 2007. The role of nutrition in tissue viability. *Wound Essentials* 2: 10–21.

Finally, you may have identified factors to do with the condition of the wound and how it is being managed. Relevant factors include aspects to do with the wound itself, for example, the presence of necrotic (dead) tissue or infection – both factors relevant to Mrs Warner. How the wound is being managed is also relevant. For example, frequent and excessive exposure of the wound causes a drop in temperature at the wound bed, and inappropriate use of antiseptics or certain wound products can damage fragile new tissue. All these factors could delay healing and are considered later in this chapter in the section 'Wound management'.

Learning outcome 2: Examine how a multidisciplinary approach can address factors affecting wound healing

Addressing factors affecting healing requires MDT working, including relatives and the client, whose involvement is essential in the process of wound healing.

Look back at Table 7.4 and list members of the MDT who might be involved in addressing the factors affecting Mrs Warner's wound healing. Make a note of what their specific roles might be.

Mrs Warner, who has chronic wounds, would require considerable multidisciplinary teamwork to address the factors affecting her wound healing. Compare your list with Table 7.6, which gives some ideas; you may have thought of others. If psychological adjustment relating to a wound is problematic, a psychologist's input is sometimes necessary. Voluntary organisations can also help to support individuals – Diabetes UK in Mrs Warner's case.

Table 7.6: Addressing factors affecting wound healing: suggested MDT involvement for Mrs Warner

MDT member	Role
Ward nurse	Blood glucose monitoring; improving nutritional status; relieving stress/anxiety, etc.; mobilisation; pressure relieving strategies; wound assessment and appropriate wound care; education of patient/carer and health promotion; support and information giving; liaison with other nurses, relatives and MDT
Specialist nurses: infection control, diabetes, nutritional support, tissue viability, dermatology, discharge liaison	Specialist advice, education and support for patient and family, and ward team, to address the factors affecting wound healing and advise on appropriate strategies
Physiotherapist	Equipment provision and resources; promote mobility and correct positioning; education and advice
Occupational therapist	Positioning, mobility and dressing aids; seating; adaptations/equipment for home
Social worker	Discharge arrangements and support at home (e.g. home care, meals, day centre, financing of home adaptations/equipment)
Podiatrist	Foot care
Doctor	Blood glucose control, prescribing medication, surgical debridement of wounds (if needed), identifying and treating other health problems which may delay healing, liaison with general practitioner (GP)
Pharmacist	Advice on wound care products
Dietician	Assessment and advice on dietary supplements
Primary health care team: district nurse, health visitor, GP, practice nurse	Medical and nursing care in the community after discharge; Assessment of health needs in the community
Chaplain	Spiritual needs and support

Summary
- A range of factors can potentially interfere with the healing process of a wound. These factors relate to the individual's general health status, the condition of the wound and the care being received.
- Nurses should identify factors affecting wound healing in individuals and plan strategies to address them where possible, involving the MDT appropriately.

WOUND ASSESSMENT

As discussed in the previous section, when assessing a wound you must consider the whole person, so factors that could interfere with healing such as their psychological and nutritional status, pain and medication can be addressed wherever possible (International Consensus 2012). This section prepares you to assess the wound itself, based on your knowledge of the phases of wound healing, the ability to classify wounds and an awareness of wider issues that affect wound healing. All these aspects underpin the assessment process. Useful articles relating to wound assessment include Gray et al. (2004, 2009) and Ousey and Cook (2012).

LEARNING OUTCOMES

By the end of this section, you will be able to:
1 discuss the features of a wound assessment and how wound assessment tools/charts can be used;
2 record key information in a useful format that can be used to plan appropriate interventions.

Learning outcome 1: Discuss the features of a wound assessment and how wound assessment tools/charts can be used

Wound assessment tools provide information on the wound. For example, the *Pressure Ulcer Classification Guide* produced by European Pressure Ulcer Advisory Panel (EPUAP) is used to classify the degree of damage of pressure ulcers (see Box 7.1 and Figure 7.9 for illustrations). Charts may include a diagram of the body for marking the location of the wound(s). The Red–Yellow–Black (RYB) system (Gray et al. 2004) is based on assessing the condition of the tissue within the wound bed and has been incorporated in the wound assessment tool included in this chapter. Evaluating tissue type by a single variable such as colour has been described as limiting (Nix 2007), but it can be used as a basis for selecting a dressing. If you

Box 7.1 Pressure ulcer classification

- *Category 1*. Intact skin with non-blanching erythema of a localised area usually over a bony prominence. Discolouration of the skin, warmth, oedema, hardness or pain may also be present. Darkly pigmented skin may not have visible blanching.
- *Category 2*. Partial thickness loss of dermis presenting as a shallow open ulcer with a red pink wound bed, without slough. May also present as an intact or open/ruptured serum-filled or serosanguinous-filled blister.
- *Category 3*. Full thickness tissue loss. Subcutaneous fat may be visible but bone, tendon or muscle are *not* exposed. Some slough may be present. *May* include undermining and tunnelling.
- *Category 4*. Full thickness tissue loss with exposed bone, tendon or muscle. Slough or eschar may be present. Often include undermining and tunnelling.

Additional Categories for the United States
Unstageable/unclassified: Full thickness skin or tissue loss – depth unknown
Full thickness tissue loss in which actual depth of the ulcer is completely obscured by slough (yellow, tan, grey, green or brown) and/or eschar (tan, brown or black) in the wound bed.

Suspected deep tissue injury – depth unknown
Purple or maroon localised area of discoloured intact skin or blood-filled blister due to damage of underlying soft tissue from pressure and/or shear.

Source: European Pressure Ulcer Advisory Panel and National Pressure Ulcer Advisory Panel (EPUAP and NPUAP). 2009. *Treatment of Pressure Ulcers: Quick Reference Guide*. Washington, DC: NPUAP.

look at Figures 7.1 through 7.5, you can see how the colours in the RYB system could be applied to these wounds (e.g. Figure 7.1: black).

Figure 7.10 gives an example of a wound assessment chart, which incorporates elements of both the RYB and the EPUAP pressure ulcer classification systems. Its features are discussed below in relation to Mrs Warner's sacral pressure ulcer. Note that she would require a chart like this for each of her wounds as each must be assessed separately.

- *Wound site*. As stated, a body map can be used to indicate wound site as well as writing 'sacrum' at the top of the chart.
- *Wound category*. Wound category relates to the wound classification discussed earlier. Mrs Warner's sacral wound will be recorded as a pressure ulcer and then graded using the EPUAP pressure ulcer classification system (Box 7.1 and Figure 7.1).
- *Medication*. Mrs Warner could be taking medication that will affect wound healing.

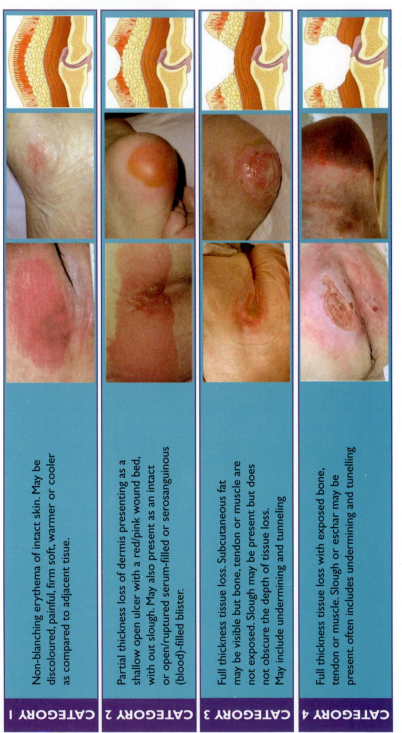

CATEGORY 1

Non-blanching erythema of intact skin. May be discoloured, painful, firm soft, warmer or cooler as compared to adjacent tissue.

CATEGORY 2

Partial thickness loss of dermis presenting as a shallow open ulcer with a red/pink wound bed, with out slough. May also present as an intact or open/ruptured serum-filled or serosanguinous (blood)-filled blister.

CATEGORY 3

Full thickness tissue loss. Subcutaneous fat may be visible but bone, tendon or muscle are not exposed. Slough may be present but does not obscure the depth of tissue loss. May include undermining and tunneling

CATEGORY 4

Full thickness tissue loss with exposed bone, tendon or muscle. Slough or eschar may be present. often includes undermining and tunelling

Figure 7.9: Pressure ulcer classification. (From European Pressure Ulcer Advisory Panel and National Pressure Ulcer Advisory Panel (EPUAP and NPUAP). 2009. *Treatment of Pressure Ulcers: Quick Reference Guide.* Washington, DC: NPUAP.)

Wound Assessment Record

WOUND SITE	

WOUND CATEGORY (please tick)	Patient Label
Surgical	
Traumatic	
Burn	
Fistula/sinus	
Pressure ulcer EPUAP 1 2 3 4	
Leg ulcer	
Diabetic foot ulcer	
Fungating lesion	**WARD**
Peg site	**CONSULTANT**
MEDICATION (anti-inflammatory, steroids, cytoxic, anticoagulants)	**ALLERGIES**

DATE OF ASSESSMENT			
PAIN -Site Intensity (circle score) Analgesics required?	1 2 3 4 5 6 7 8 9 10 Yes/ No	1 2 3 4 5 6 7 8 9 10 Yes/ No	1 2 3 4 5 6 7 8 9 10 Yes/ No
PHOTOGRAPH (consent obtained)			
MEASUREMENT (cm) Width Length			
DEPTH (cm) Partial/full thickness, tendon underlying structure exposed			
TYPE/COLOUR OF TISSUE (record%) Necrotic (black) Sloughy (yellow) Granulating (red) Epithelialising (pink) Infected (green)			
SIGNS OF INFECTION (redness, purulent, inflammation, pyrexia, patient unwell)			
MALODOUR	Yes/ No	Yes/ No	Yes/ No
SWAB TAKEN	Yes/ No	Yes/ No	Yes/ No
EXUDATE (High, medium, low)			
COLOUR OF EXUDATE			
SURROUNDING SKIN Healthy Macerated Erythema Eczema Cellulitis			
WOUND EDGES (shallow, rolled, punched out, undermined)			
DRESSING SELECTION			
FREQUENCY OF CHANGE			
ASSESSORS SIGNATURE			
DATE OF REASSESSMENT			

Figure 7.10: Example of a wound assessment chart. (Reproduced with kind permission from Buckinghamshire Healthcare NHS Trust.)

- *Allergies.* Mrs Warner could have a known allergy to a dressing product, which should be noted.
- *Pain.* Assessment of pain, using a number intensity scale where 1 is no pain and 10 is the worst pain imaginable, needs to occur before removing the dressing to establish whether Mrs Warner requires any analgesics and whether the current pain management strategy is effective. If the pain occurs only during dressing removal, a different product may be required. If the pain has increased and is associated with other signs and symptoms such as malodour, inflammation, increased exudate and delayed wound healing, a wound infection may be present (Kingsley et al. 2004; Ousey and Cook 2012).
- *Photograph.* Increasingly photos are used in wound assessment, but consent from the patient must be obtained in line with local policies (Ousey and Cook 2012). Often, a ruler is placed by the side of the wound when taking the photograph, showing the wound's size as well as its appearance (see Figure 7.3). Clearly, the sacral area would be a sensitive area to photograph and the reasons for doing so need careful explanation. However, the photos can be shown to Mrs Warner to help her to appreciate the nature of the wound, and how its healing is progressing.
- *Measurement.* The size is recorded in centimetres as width by length. Sometimes, a tracing is made, which creates a record of shape as well as size and this can be attached to the assessment tool (Ousey and Cook 2012).
- *Depth.* Depth is difficult to measure, but a wound probe or sterile wound swab can be used and then measured against a ruler. The depth of the wound can also be assessed through the identification of exposed structures such as tendon or bone.
- *Type/colour of tissue.* The type and colour of the tissue within the wound bed will assist in determining the treatment required to progress the wound. Black necrotic tissue (Mrs Warner's sacral pressure ulcer and Figure 7.1) and yellow sloughy tissue are considered to be non-viable tissue that require debridement. Red tissue is associated with a healthy granulating, well vascularised wound, with pink tissue indicating re-epithelialisation (Ousey and Cook 2012). Bright red granulation tissue, which is friable and exuberant and associated with new areas of slough, increased exudate and malodour, could be signs of infection in a chronic wound (World Union of Wound Healing Societies [WUWHS] 2008). The RYB system has been incorporated into the tool to assist in identifying the type of tissue within the wound bed.
  - Black: necrotic tissue
  - Yellow: sloughy tissue
  - Red: granulating tissue
  - Pink: epithelialisation
  - Green: infected tissue

The wound base may have several different types of tissue present. For example, Figure 7.5 shows a wound base that has both sloughy (yellow) areas and granulation tissue (red). Nurses assessing this wound would need to estimate the percentage of the wound bed covered with slough (yellow), and the percentage covered with granulation tissue (red) and record this on the chart. For Mrs Warner, the recording will be 100% necrotic (black), but in due course as the wound progresses there will be sloughy (yellow) areas, and then it is hoped some granulation tissue (red), and then areas that are epithelialising (pink).

- *Infection.* The presence of infection can delay wound healing. In an acute wound, infection maybe indicated by the presence of erythema (redness), swelling, localised heat and pain, purulent discharge and pyrexia (Ousey and Cook 2012). The identification of infection in chronic wounds is more challenging and frequently is associated with a general deterioration in the wound or the wound healing becoming stagnant. See the EWMA's (2005) position statement for identifying a wound infection.

- *Malodour.* A slight odour can occur due to wound occlusion and is associated with some types of dressing. However, an offensive odour is often a sign of infection. Necrotic wounds (Mrs Warner's sacral pressure ulcer) and fungating wounds are often malodorous. Assessing odour can help to identify infection, as one of a range of criteria, but also helps with dressing choice as some dressings are deodorising.

- *Swab taken.* Wound swabs taken should be recorded, but they have limitations. Chapter 3 discusses how and when to take wound swabs or preferably, collect a pus sample. The nurses must remember to check the results and discuss with the medical staff whether it is appropriate to treat the wound with antibiotics or with an antibacterial dressing containing substances such as iodine, silver or honey.

- *Exudate.* Exudate is fluid arising from the wound owing to increased permeability of capillaries. The WUWHS (2007) suggest that the exudate should be assessed for colour, consistency, odour and quantity. Estimating the amount of exudate (high, medium or low) is not easy, but a change in the volume or nature of the exudate could indicate an increasing bacterial load (Cook and Barker 2012). The presence and extent of exudate will influence your dressing choice.

- *Colour of exudate.* The colour of the exudate will also indicate if infection is present in the wound.

- *Condition of surrounding skin.* Condition of surrounding skin is important in considering the type of dressing to be used. For example, if the skin is moist/**macerated**, a more absorbent dressing may be needed. Also consider applying a barrier film such as Cavilon No-Sting Barrier Film beneath the dressing. If erythema (redness) or eczema is present, this could indicate an allergic reaction or that the dressing is being removed too frequently, causing trauma. Further information can be found in the excoriation tool developed by Health Improvement Scotland (2009). Cellulitis or spreading erythema needs to be reported if it is a new feature as it indicates infection is present and systemic antibiotics are needed.

- *Wound edges.* In large and/or deep wounds, the edge of the wound may be undermined, whereby it is possible to reach underneath the edges of the wound. As the wound progresses to the proliferative phase, a shallow white/pink almost transparent border appears. This new epidermal tissue is fragile and easily removed. Edges that are rolled in can delay healing time. In chronic wounds,

Macerated skin

Macerated skin is soft and breaking down due to prolonged contact with excessive amounts of fluid, such as wound exudate (Cutting 1999).

the edges can have a punched-out appearance, and small satellite wounds can be present. Wound edges that are hard and fibrous indicate a chronic wound.

As you can see in Figure 7.2, the wound chart includes spaces for recording wound care, which is planned on the basis of the assessment.

Assessing a wound might also include any of the following considerations:

- *Is the wound open or closed?* Remember from earlier in this chapter that an open wound is a wound healing by secondary intention; a closed wound is predominantly healing by primary intention. Thus, Susan's wound is healing by primary intention, but Mrs Warner's sacral wound is healing by secondary intention. A dehisced wound is a wound where tissue has become separated from deeper tissue owing to the presence of infection; this complicates some surgical wounds.
- *Extent of tissue involvement.* Does the wound involve epidermis, dermis, fat, fascia, muscle and/or bone?
- *Presence of foreign bodies.* Foreign bodies delay the healing process. Foreign bodies such as dirt or grit can also increase infection risk and lead to permanent marking (Leaper 2006).
- *Presence of a fistula or a sinus.* A fistula is an abnormal connection between two spaces such as skin surface and bowel. A sinus is a tract that ends in a blind cavity, and a sinus is frequently found in a deep pressure ulcer. A sinus should ideally heal from its base; if it heals first at the surface, fluid will accumulate within, promoting an abscess, which will subsequently break through to the surface. In Figure 7.7, the darkened central area of the dehisced part of the wound was found to be a sinus.
- *Wound drain and drain site.* Wound drains are inserted into some surgical wounds to promote the removal of fluid that would otherwise accumulate and form a potential growing medium for infection, or interfere with healing.

ACTIVITY

Find out whether there is a wound assessment tool/chart used in your local practice setting and try to access it. Otherwise, use a wound assessment tool/chart from the literature or from Figure 7.2. You also need a measuring instrument such as a ruler (disposable ones are available from wound product manufacturers) and good light. Under supervision, assess a patient's wound and document your assessment. After carrying out this exercise, consider the question: Should a wound assessment tool/chart be used for all wounds?

Minor straightforward wounds do not require a formal recorded assessment. If the wound is healing uneventfully, a record of this in the patient's notes will suffice. This record would have been adequate for Susan's surgical wound when she was in hospital, and for the wound shown in Figure 7.6, which is a straightforward clean surgical wound that healed without complication. Judging when to use a tool/chart involves issues such as a wound that is not healing as expected, possibly reverting to a previous stage, wounds with problems, or where required as a legal record, for example, after an assault or suspected neglect/abuse. The assessment of the patient's wound in

Figure 7.7 should be documented on a wound assessment chart as it is complicated by infection causing dehiscence. Mrs Warner's pressure ulcer and ulcerated toe (which could, as a diabetic ulcer, deteriorate) are both chronic and problematic wounds and so the use of assessment tools/charts would be advantageous.

Leg ulcer assessment

All patients presenting with a leg ulcer should be screened for arterial disease by Doppler ultrasound measurement of ankle brachial pressure index (ABPI) by staff trained to carry out this investigation (CREST 1998; RCN 2006; SIGN 2010), alongside a thorough clinical investigation. Often a specific leg ulcer assessment chart is used to record this assessment, which includes documenting assessment of factors affecting wound healing (e.g. smoking, nutritional status) as discussed earlier. The ABPI is calculated by dividing the brachial systolic blood pressure by the ankle systolic blood pressure. A normal ABPI reading is about 1 and if the reading is 0.8 or above, compression therapy can usually be applied (CREST 1998; RCN 2006; SIGN 2010). Compression therapy aims to provide graduated compression, with the highest pressure at the ankle and the lowest at the knee, thus returning blood from the lower limb and preventing pooling in distended lower leg veins. An arterial ulcer is caused by an inadequate arterial blood supply to the area, and a patient suspected of having an arterial ulcer may require vascular surgery. *Note:* Applying compression to a limb with an arterial ulcer will have catastrophic results for the ulcer and the patient, potentially leading to loss of the limb affected. Thus, accurate assessment is essential.

Learning outcome 2: Record key information in a useful format that can be used to plan appropriate interventions

ACTIVITY

Review the material that you recorded by using the wound assessment tool/chart earlier, and consider this question: Is it specific and comprehensive enough to help you to plan the wound's management, and to promote continuity of care?

- The tools used are generally very wound-specific. They have to be simple to use, yet all-encompassing, but not so inclusive as to waste valuable time and deter use.
- These are legal documents. Have you accurately described the wound environment? Have you avoided the use of colloquialisms, such as 'wound bed appears fine': what does 'fine' mean? Ensure that you use descriptive language that can be interpreted by anyone, not just yourself. This helps to promote continuity of care.
- A photograph of the wound can provide a more objective record of the wound's status, alleviating potential variation in the use of descriptive terms and their interpretation.
- Can the assessment help you to plan the wound management? Has it identified any problems with the current approach. For example, is the dressing allowing the wound to dry out, or the surrounding skin to become macerated? Was the dressing painful to remove?

Pregnancy and birth: practice points – wound infection risk and recognition

There is a significantly increased risk of postpartum septicaemia, wound problems and fever after lower segment caesarean section (LSCS). In the UK, there is an 8% risk of infection following LSCS, and antibiotic prophylaxis during the operation should be offered routinely (NICE 2011b). Prophylaxis reduces endometritis by 66%–75% and also reduces rate of wound infection (Smaill and Gyte 2010). If caring for a postnatal woman, for example, in intensive therapy unit (ITU) immediate referral to the obstetric team should be made if the following occur:

• Painful, red suture line
• Deep tenderness on palpation of abdomen
• Vaginal loss (lochia) pink/coloured, profuse and/or offensive smelling

Summary

● Wound assessment requires a holistic approach involving assessment of the whole person and the wound together.
● Wound assessment charts assist a systematic process and clear documentation of the wound's progress.
● Documentation is becoming increasingly important, for management as well as litigation reasons.
● Accuracy in recording assessment is an important skill to develop and does much to promote continuity of care, as well as a firm basis for planning interventions.

WOUND MANAGEMENT

You have already considered factors affecting wound healing and have identified that wound management must focus on both the wound and the patient as a whole. It is important to be aware of the psychosocial effects of wounds so that you can be supportive; this is relevant to both acute and chronic wounds. The effects on body image of acute wounds can result in a range of psychological reactions, including a grief response, anxiety and depression (International Consensus 2012). The skin is 'a major factor in a person's body image', with denial, anxiety, pain, immobility and altered body image experienced by people with chronic wounds. Being aware of this can help health professionals to be understanding, and effective assessment can promote helpful interventions, referrals and information provision (International Consensus 2012).

In this section, you focus on care of the wound itself, using a concept called **wound-bed preparation** (WBP). The focus of WBP denotes the importance of removing non-viable tissue (necrosis and slough) through cleansing/debridement, moisture balance, control of oedema and decreased bacterial burden (Fletcher 2003; Ousey and Cook 2012) to promote healing.

By the end of this section you will be able to:

1 discuss how wound dressings are performed;

2 explain methods of debridement and cleansing;

3 identify a range of wound dressings and explain how a dressing is selected for an individual;

4 discuss ways of reducing pain and discomfort associated with wounds.

Learning outcome 1: Discuss how wound dressings are performed

For information on aseptic technique, applied to wound dressings, see Chapter 3. A sterile technique has traditionally been used for wound care, but it may hold no advantage over a clean technique in chronic wounds. In essence, when using sterile technique, equipment, fluids and dressings are sterile, whereas with a clean technique, clean but non-sterile single-use gloves can be used, with tap water (that is safe enough to drink) used for cleansing (Fernandez et al. 2010).

ACTIVITY

How do you think you might identify when a sterile technique would be essential and when a clean technique might be sufficient?

A sterile technique must be used if the patient is immunocompromised or has undergone surgery, which carries a high infection risk. However, chronic wounds are likely to be colonised with bacteria, so a clean rather than sterile procedure may be sufficient.

Effective handwashing and gloving techniques are essential, whether a sterile or clean technique is used for wound care, and aprons should be worn too (see Chapter 3). Some dressings are difficult to apply using gloves – hand hygiene or a non-touch technique is then essential to prevent contamination of the dressing. Wound dressings must always be sterile. Use of dressings from an opened pack, even if for the same patient, could introduce contamination and thus delay healing.

Autolytic debridement

Describes the use of the body's own enzymes and moisture to rehydrate, soften and liquefy hard eschar and slough (Gray et al. 2011b).

Learning outcome 2: Explain methods of debridement and cleansing

Debridement

Debridement is the excision or wide removal of dead (necrotic) and damaged tissue (NICE 2008). The body can naturally carry out debridement via **autolytic debridement**, but if large quantities of debris are present, it delays healing and predisposes to infection (Gray et al. 2011b; Ousey and Cook 2012).

Box 7.2 Methods of debridement

Autolytic

- Involves the body's own mechanisms of selective liquefaction, separation and digestion of necrotic tissue that occurs in wounds due to phagocytosis (Gray et al. 2011b; Vowden and Vowden 2002).
- Enhanced through the presence of a moist wound environment, created by dressings such as hydrogels, hydrocolloids and hydrofiber.
- *Hydrogels* – designed to donate fluid to the wound bed through their high water content, which rehydrate the eschar and slough, promoting autolysis (Cowan 2012).
- *Hydrocolloids* – contain gel-forming agents combined with elastomers and an adhesive matrix, which in the presence of exudate forms a moist gel (Cowan 2012).
- *Hydrofiber* – highly absorbent non-woven sheets or ribbon composed entirely of hydrocolloid fibre, which in the presence of exudate converts to a soft moist gel (Cowan 2012).

Larval therapy

Larvae act by moving over the surface of a wound bed and secreting powerful enzymes that break down dead tissue into a liquefied solution, which they can then digest together with bacteria present in the wound (Thomas et al. 2002). Larval therapy is quicker than autolytic debridement and is most effective where the devitalised tissue is not dry; frequently autolytic treatment is required initially to soften and liquefy the devitalised tissue before application (Gray et al. 2011b). Larval therapy has also been demonstrated to reduce the bacterial burden of the wound bed and facilitate healing (Gray et al. 2011b).

Sharp debridement

The removal of dead or foreign material just above the level of viable tissue using a scalpel, performed without anaesthetic by a doctor or an experienced nurse (Gray et al. 2011b). It requires skill and knowledge of the anatomical structures and should be governed under strict local guidelines (Edwards 2000).

Surgical debridement

The excision or wide resection of necrotic tissue, often extending into the viable or healthy tissue. It is performed in the operating theatre by a surgeon (Fairbairn et al. 2002). It is most suitable for large areas or in wounds that contain contaminated tissue or sepsis where rapid removal is required (Gray et al. 2011b). This method of debridement can be costly, and risk of anaesthesia has to be considered (Gray et al. 2011b).

Wound debridement can lead to improved healing rates, reduced risk of infection and improved quality of life (Gray et al. 2011b). It was identified earlier that Mrs Warner's sacral wound requires debriding of its necrotic tissue. Debridement can be carried out in several ways (Box 7.2). NICE (2001) reviewed the evidence on debridement for difficult-to-heal surgical wounds, concluding that no particular method could be supported. So, the choice of debriding agent should be according to the individual and issues around comfort and odour control (Gray et al. 2011b).

Dressings promoting autolysis and biosurgical methods (sterile maggots) may be more acceptable to patients and less painful (NICE 2001). Gray et al. (2011b) provide an overview of the use and effectiveness of larval therapy. Figure 7.3 shows a deep sacral pressure ulcer the day after maggots had been removed after 3 days *in situ*. The ulcer, which was 60% covered with slough, is now about 85% granulation tissue. Vacuum-assisted closure uses negative pressure to remove slough and loosen necrotic tissue from the wound bed (Henderson et al. 2012). The use of honey in wound care is also gaining interest. It has been found to have a debriding action as well as many other beneficial effects, for example, antibacterial activity (Grothier and Cooper 2011; Morris 2006).

ACTIVITY

You have probably seen wound cleansing carried out in practice. Think about the following: Why are wounds cleansed? How are wounds cleansed? What are wounds cleansed with? Compare your thoughts with the points below.

Purpose of wound cleansing

Wound cleansing has sometimes been carried out ritualistically without sound rationale for practice. The aim of wound cleansing is to remove contaminated/foreign material from the wound bed, that is, slough, necrotic tissue, exudate and dressing debris. Nurses must decide whether this can be achieved by cleansing or debridement, as discussed earlier, is needed. Wound exudate is produced as a normal part of the healing process to prevent the wound bed from drying out, while facilitating the migration of cells and providing essential nutrients and growth factors. Cleansing is indicated if there are large quantities of exudate, as any leakage onto the surrounding skin (periwound) will cause maceration and make it susceptible to increased damage. In addition, enzymes in chronic wound exudate may cause skin stripping (excoriation) (Gouvela and Miguens 2007). Further reasons for wound cleansing are so that the wound can be assessed and to maintain hygiene and enhance well-being, particularly when there is excessive exudate and malodour (Gouvela and Miguens 2007; International Consensus 2012).

Cleansing methods

There are many documented methods for wound cleansing (Gouvela and Miguens 2007). We consider swabbing, irrigation and bathing/showering here.

- **Swabbing.** Swabbing of wounds, using gloves or forceps and gauze swabs, is a traditional method of wound cleansing, but it can lead to a redistribution of microorganisms.
- **Irrigation.** Irrigation of wounds is often considered preferable to swabbing. To irrigate you can use a syringe with a needle or quill, an aerosol spray, or a showerhead, or simply pour the fluid over the wound from a sachet. You need

to collect the fluid in a container such as a kidney bowl. The pressure of the irrigation may be difficult to measure or regulate, and there is a risk of contamination to the patient, nurse or the environment should the needle detach (Gouvela and Miguens 2007).

• **Bathing.** Patients with leg ulcers find it can be comforting, and psychologically enhancing, to bathe their legs in a bucket lined with a waterproof plastic bag, which can then be disposed of afterwards. The same principle can be used for a sacral pressure ulcer. If there is no wound infection present, cleaning of the bath with normal detergent is adequate but if the wound is infected, the bath should be cleaned with hypochlorite solution. This would be necessary, therefore, if Colin baths, which could well be a soothing method of wound cleansing for him.

Wound cleansing solutions

Although a wide selection of solutions have been used to cleanse wounds, normal saline is often considered the solution of choice, as it is isotonic and non-toxic to healing tissue (Gouvela and Miguens 2007). A review by Fernandez et al. (2010) supported the use of tap water for wound cleansing, noting that boiled and cooled water as well as distilled water can also be used as wound cleansing agents. The consensus on which cleaning agent is most effective remains debatable and requires further investigation (Cutting et al. 2007). Solutions used for cleansing/irrigating should be used at body temperature if possible, thus reducing the cooling of the wound bed which adversely affects healing. A review by Drosou et al. (2003) highlighted the clinical controversy surrounding use of antiseptics in open wounds, particularly in relation to:

• whether these solutions are toxic to healing tissue;
• whether they actually promote healing.

Wounds UK (2011) have published a Best Practice Statement reviewing the use of antiseptics and antimicrobials in wound healing. The main use of these products should be to treat wound infection, and their use should be avoided if no infection is present. Traumatic wounds are likely to be contaminated with bacteria, and it would be appropriate to use antiseptics/antimicrobials in these wounds.

Learning outcome 3: Identify a range of wound dressings and explain how a dressing is selected for an individual

Before considering which dressing to apply, see Table 7.7 for an overview of the requirements of the ideal dressing (Thomas 2008). The table details whether each requirement is purely attributed to design and construction of the product (design) or can be influenced by the nature and condition of the wound (wound related) – for example, contributes to autolytic debridement. Thomas (2008) points out that 'it is unlikely that a single dressing or dressing system will possess all of these attributes'.

Study Table 7.7 and relate it to the range of products you have access to in the practice setting and/or the skills laboratory. Which of the criteria do they meet? How might you select a dressing? Discuss with a practitioner how a specific dressing is chosen for an individual. There may be local clinical guidelines and, if so, try to locate them.

There are many dressings available in the UK, which can be categorised as in Table 7.8, with more emerging onto the market each day. Things to consider when deciding upon a dressing include the following:

- Does the wound require a dressing at all?
- What is the purpose of the dressing?
  - Promotion of autolytic debridement or granulation formation?
  - Absorption or rehydration?
  - Reducing the bacterial burden?
- Appropriate size of dressing
- Availability
- Ease of application and removal
- Comfort
- Frequency of dressing changes

Table 7.7: Performance requirements of the 'ideal dressing'

Primary requirements	Type of feature
Free of toxins or irritants	Design feature
Does not release particles or non-biodegradable fibres into the wound	Design feature
Forms an effective bacterial barrier (effectively contains exudate or cellular debris to prevent the transmission of microorganisms into or out of the wound)	Design feature
If self-adhesive, forms an effective water-resistant seal to the periwound skin, but is easily removable without causing trauma or skin stripping	Design feature
Maintains the wound and the surrounding skin in an optimum state of hydration (implies the ability to function effectively under compression)	Design/wound related
Requires minimal disturbance or replacement	Design/wound related
Provides protection to the periwound skin from potentially irritant wound exudate and excess moisture	Design/wound related
Produces minimal pain during application or removal as a result of adherence to the wound surface	Design/wound related
Maintains the wound at the optimum temperature and pH	Design/wound related
Secondary requirements	**Type of feature**
Possesses antimicrobial activity: capable of combating localised infection	Design feature
Has odour absorbing/combating properties	Design feature
Has ability to remove or inactivate proteolytic enzymes in chronic wound fluid	Design feature
Possesses haemostatic activity	Design feature
Exhibits effective wound cleansing (debriding) activity	Design/wound related

Source: Reproduced with kind permission from Thomas, S. 2008. The role of dressings in the treatment of moisture-related skin damage. *World Wide Wounds*. Available from: http://www.worldwidewounds.com (Accessed on 19 January 2013)

Table 7.8: Wound dressings

Dressing type	Examples	Description	Uses
Simple absorbent dressings (island dressings)	Cosmopor E Mepore Opsite Plus	Simple absorbent dressings consisting of an absorbent material that may be backed with an adhesive border. Suitable for low levels of thin exudate.	Wounds healing by primary intention (e.g. straightforward surgical wound).
Superabsorbent dressings	Cutisorb Ultra Eclypse Sorbion sachet S	These dressings are comprised of absorbent polymers that rapidly absorb and retain large volumes of exudate.	Venous leg ulcers, pressure ulcers, diabetic foot ulcers, abdominal wounds. Any highly exuding wounds.
Capillary action	Avadraw	Capillary action dressings draw wound fluid into the material. The denser the fluid, the lower the capillarity.	Venous leg ulcers, pressure ulcers, dehisced surgical wounds.
Impregnated gauzes	Jelonet Neotulle Paragauze	Open-weave cotton or rayon dressing impregnated with soft paraffin.	Minor burns or scalds. Donor and recipient skin graft sites. Lacerations and abrasions.
Alginates	ActivHeal alginate Kaltostat Sorbsan	Alginates are derived from brown seaweed (Phaeophyceae). They are available in sheet or rope form, and their primary function is absorption. Reacts with wound exudate to form a gel which aids autolytic debridement and granulation.	Moderately to heavily exudating wounds, including infected, sloughy, and granulating and epithelialising wounds. Can be used to loosely pack puncture and cavity wounds.
		Alginate dressings can absorb 15–20 times their own weight in fluid. The fluid handling capacity will be reduced under compression bandaging. Some alginates are licensed as haemostatic agents due to the release of calcium ions and activation of platelets.	Requires a secondary dressing. Not suitable for dry wounds.
Antimicrobials	Bactigras (Chlorhexidine) Acticoat, Aquacel Ag and Allevyn Ag adhesive (silver) Inadine, Iodosorb and Iodoflex (iodine) Coviden Kendall AMD Suprasorb X+PHMB (PHMB) Cutimed Sorbact (DACC)	These dressings are impregnated with antiseptics, the most common including chlorhexidine, silver, iodine, polyhexamethylene biguanide (PHMB), dialkylcarbamoyl chloride (DACC).	All chronic and acute wounds that are critically colonised or infected.
Film dressings	Bioclusive Hydrofilm Opsite	Transparent, vapour-permeable adhesive film dressing that acts as a barrier to bacteria and water. Allows bathing/showering. Allows observation of wound.	Primary wound closure (e.g. straightforward surgical wound). To protect skin susceptible to damage from shearing; superficial abrasions.

(Continued)

Table 7.8: (Continued)

Dressing type	Examples	Description	Uses
Foams	Allevyn Biatain Tielle Mepilex Border (soft silicone)	Absorbent dressings made from polyurethane or silicone. Mainly available as a flat dressing, with or without an adhesive border, the dressings are available in a variety of thicknesses. Trilaminate foam sheets have an outer transparent film, providing water repellent and barrier properties, while avoiding exudate strikethrough. In contrast the wound contact layer is hydrophilic, drawing fluid into the dressing. Soft silicone foams have been developed for sensitive/delicate skin. There are cavity versions available, which consist of foam chips enclosed in a low-adherent polymeric envelope.	Suitable for wounds with low-to-moderate exudate levels. They can be applied under compression therapy, although this is likely to adversely affect the absorbent capacity (Thomas et al. 2007).
Honey dressings	Activon Mesitran	Medical grade Manuka honey is a potent antibacterial agent with a broad spectrum of activity. It can be applied directly to the wound or be impregnated in a gauze or alginate dressing. Honey creates an environment that promotes autolytic debridement and supports granulation tissue formation, while reducing odour.	Indicated for a variety of wounds, including infected, acute and chronic wounds.
Hydrocolloids	Comfeel Plus Duoderm Granuflex Tegaderm hydrocolloid	Hydrocolloids are primarily made of carboxymethyl cellulose (CMC), a synthesised cellulose derivative. They are occlusive dressings, providing a moist wound healing environment, promoting autolytic debridement and granulation tissue formation and re-epithelialisation. Hydrocolloids are available in a variety of forms (sheets, paste, powder, fibrous) and thicknesses.	Suitable for clean, granulating wounds or sloughy/necrotic wounds. They are principally indicated for low to moderately exuding wounds.
Hydrogels	Intrasite Conformable (impregnated dressing) ActivHeal Hydrogel (gel) Hydrosorb (hydrogel sheet)	Hydrogels are comprised of polymers of starch compounds and CMC that donate moisture to the wound bed to rehydrate the tissue. They are available as gels or sheets, or as gels impregnated into a dressing material.	Hydrogels are suited to the management of dry wounds. Will usually require a secondary dressing.

(Continued)

Table 7.8: (Continued)

Dressing type	Examples	Description	Uses
Hydrofiber	Aquacel	Absorbent dressing comprised of sodium carboxymethyl cellulose that provides a moist wound healing environment, by transforming into a soft gel.	Moderately to heavily exudating wounds, including infected, sloughy and granulating wounds. Can be used to loosely pack puncture and cavity wounds. Requires a secondary dressing.
Odour Control	Carboflex Clinisorb	Activated charcoal dressings absorb toxins and reduce wound malodour.	Malodorous wounds, including fungating tumours.
Larval therapy	LarvE Biofoam	Medicinal quality larvae of the green bottle fly. Either applied directly to the wound or encased in a net pouch.	Debridement of slough and necrotic tissue in a wide variety of wounds.
Negative pressure wound therapy (NPWT)	KCI Vacuum Assisted Closure (VAC) Smith & Nephew Renasys Go	A non-invasive technology comprising a negative pressure pump connected by a tube to a dressing within a wound cavity. Negative pressure is exerted onto the wound bed removing excess fluid and bacteria, reduces soft-tissue oedema and promotes granulation tissue. There are two different types of dressing: Hydrophobic polyurethane foam dressing Gauze, plain or impregnated with an antimicrobial agent	NPWT is suitable for acute, chronic and traumatic wounds, as an adjunct to surgery, and for salvage procedures such as wound dehiscence.

Source: Adapted from Morris, C. 2006. Wound management and dressing selection. *Wound Essentials* 1: 178–83; Cowan, T. (ed.) 2012. *Wound Care Handbook 2012–2013*, 5th edn. Mark Allen Healthcare (except where stated).

Your choice of dressing should relate to your wound assessment, taking into account the attributes of an effective wound care product. Consider the stage of wound healing, type and colour of tissue, site of wound, pain relief and amount of exudate. Table 7.8 summarises key groups of dressings and their uses. Table 7.9 provides a wound dressing selection guide based on WBP and exudate level.

Gray et al. (2009) have further developed the concepts of WBP into Applied Wound Management (AWM) to provide a systematic and practical approach to wound management, assisting with establishing the immediate treatment goals. The concept utilises three different continuums each relating to a wound parameter, namely, viability of the tissue, presence of infection and levels of exudate. Focusing on these areas will help you to determine whether the dressing requires the properties to debride or promote healing, whether infection needs to be targeted and the level of absorbency that needs to be controlled. Always consult the manufacturer's instructions when applying dressings.

Table 7.9: Wound dressing selection guide[a]

	Low exudate	Medium exudate	High exudate
Necrotic (black)			
Primary	Hydrogel	Hydrogel or Hydrofiber	Hydrofiber
Secondary	Hydrocolloid	Hydrocolloid	Foam
Sloughy (yellow)			
Primary	Hydrogel	Hydrofiber	Hydrofiber
Secondary	Hydrocolloid	Foam	Foam
Granulating (red)			
Primary	Hydrocolloid	Hydrofiber	Hydrofiber
Secondary		Hydrocolloid	Foam
Epithelialising (pink)			
Primary	Hydrocolloid	Hydrocolloid or Foam	Hydrofiber
Secondary			Hydrocolloid Or Foam
Infected (green)			
Primary	Antimicrobial dressing	Antimicrobial dressing	Antimicrobial dressing
Secondary	Foam	Foam	Foam

Source: Reproduced with kind permission from Buckinghamshire Healthcare NHS Trust.

[a] The first-line treatment for diabetic foot ulcers is an antimicrobial or a low-adherent dressing.

NICE (2008) reviewed the evidence for postoperative dressings in preventing surgical site infection, concluding that it is generally accepted good clinical practice to cover the wound with an appropriate interactive dressing (a semipermeable film membrane with or without an absorbent island) for a period of 48 hours, unless there is excess wound leakage or haemorrhage. Susan's wound dressing could, therefore, have been removed after 48 hours and the wound left open, but it is important to understand how Susan feels and to determine whether she would feel more comfortable and less worried with a film dressing left in place.

Orthopaedic surgery, such as hip and knee replacements, tends to be complicated by inflammation, fluid collection and blister formation. The Molndal dressing technique has become standard practice in the majority of orthopaedic centres in Sweden (Folestad 2002) and has been adopted across many centres throughout the UK. The technique uses a hydrofiber dressing called AQUACEL covered with a film or thin hydrocolloid dressing. A new dressing combining the two products is now available called AQUACEL SURGICAL.

Dressings for diabetic foot ulcers must be chosen with particular care as excess moisture and occlusive environments can cause bacteria to multiply quickly, and spread infection. People with diabetes do not display the classic signs of infection, and their circulation can be affected by peripheral arterial disease. Historically, hydrocolloid dressings have been avoided in people with diabetes, favouring antiseptic products such as iodine and honey. McIntosh (2006) has reviewed their use and suggests that they can be used on appropriate wounds after a thorough patient assessment, but they need to be regularly reviewed.

As noted at the start of this chapter, there are constantly new products being developed. This chapter has incorporated available systematic reviews, clinical guidelines and Best Practice Statements, but there are many more in progress; check the Cochrane Library, NICE, Wounds International and Wounds UK for their latest publications.

All patients/clients need education about their wound care and dressings. Such education has already been discussed a little in relation to Susan and her wound.

ACTIVITY

If you were being discharged home with a dressing in situ, or had had a dressing applied by the community nurse, what sort of things would you want to know?

You would probably want to know some of the following:
- Can I get the dressing wet? If not, how can I manage activities such as washing?
- When should the dressing be redone, and by whom?
- What should I do if the dressing becomes loose, uncomfortable, too tight, falls off or soaks through?
- What should I expect of the wound? For example, when will it heal?
- Will the wound be painful? If so, how can I deal with this?
- How will I know if the wound is becoming infected?
- Are there any special instructions I should follow?

Education should involve relatives and carers as applicable. For Susan, her carers should have been educated before her discharge, and explanations given to Susan using appropriate communication methods. This information is also important to people receiving inpatient care to allay anxiety, build confidence and promote self-care. Written information can back up verbal instructions; it is difficult for people to retain a lot of new information, particularly when under stress. Written patient information should be readable, understandable and culturally relevant to be effective in promoting self-care and relieving anxiety (International Consensus 2012).

Leg ulcer bandaging

The standard treatment for venous diseases including oedema, venous leg ulcers and lymphoedema, is appropriate wound management in combination with compression therapy from toe to knee. Compression therapy supports the veins and valves to push the venous blood up the leg towards the heart, reducing congestion in the capillaries and veins. In conjunction, the extra fluid from the tissue is squeezed back into the veins, reducing oedema. The increased blood velocity ensures that more nutrients reach the tissues to improve the skin condition, reduce dryness and restore elasticity. The compression is applied so that the pressure at the ankle is higher than the pressure at the knee, that is, graduated. There are many different types of compression therapy:

- Elastic bandages
  - Multilayer
  - Long stretch
- Inelastic bandages
  - Short stretch (only suitable for mobile patients as the treatment relies on calf muscle movement)
- Intermittent pneumatic compression therapy
  - Boot producing wavelike motion
- Compression hosiery
  - Stocking/sock

The required amount of pressure applied to the limb to achieve therapeutic levels is determined by the patient's underlying pathologies and the patient's ability to tolerate the compression as it can be extremely painful (WUWHS 2008). Before selecting a compression bandage, each patient should be individually assessed and their lifestyle considered. RCN guidelines (2006) state that leg ulcer bandaging should be applied by a trained practitioner, have adequate padding and be capable of sustaining compression for at least a week. The recommended standards are mild (<20 mmHg), moderate (≥20–40 mmHg), strong (≥40–60 mmHg) and very strong (>60 mmHg). The standard for venous leg ulcers is ≥40 mmHg (Partsch et al. 2008). However, compression should be used only in the absence of significant arterial disease, so as discussed earlier in this chapter, arterial blood supply must first be assessed.

In addition to the previously mentioned guidelines (CREST 1998; RCN 2006; SIGN 2010), three useful documents that discuss compression therapy are available from EWMA (2003), WUWHS (2008) and Wounds UK (2012). Treatment needs to be continued after healing, as without compression, the underlying problem – venous hypertension – will return, and a leg ulcer will form once more (EWMA 2003; Wounds UK 2012; WUWHS 2008). Therefore, patient education and involvement are essential.

You should get the opportunity to observe leg ulcer bandaging in practice, possibly at a clinic, or with the district nurse. Try to find out about a local leg ulcer clinic, and arrange a visit.

Learning outcome 4: Discuss ways of reducing pain and discomfort associated with wounds

Unfortunately, patients often associate their wounds with pain; this pain can be based on physical or psychological reasons. Any care relating to wounds can cause fear and distress, be this removal of a surgical drain, a dressing change or removal of skin-closing devices such as staples, clips or sutures. A person with a traumatic wound experienced pain when the injury occurred, so the thought of having a wound dressing could be distressing. A pain assessment should be completed for each patient; a numerical analogue scale is incorporated into the wound assessment tool (Figure 7.2). Wounds UK (2004) have developed a Best Practice Statement related to minimising pain associated with wound management. Table 7.10 provides a summary of factors contributing to pain associated with wounds, and possible solutions. Taylor (2010) examines the principles of wound pain assessment, and Chapter 12 considers assessment and management of pain in detail.

Analgesia before dressing changes may be required. Opiates are necessary if the pain is severe; otherwise, non-steroidal anti-inflammatory drugs or simple analgesics are suitable. Sufficient time should be allowed for them to take effect

Table 7.10: Causes of wound pain and measures to minimise pain and trauma to the tissues and the surrounding skin

Cause of wound pain	Issues to consider and ways of minimising pain
Wound cleansing and debridement	• Gentle irrigation of the wound with warm normal saline or tap water • Restrict the use of antiseptics to contaminated traumatic wounds • Plan and organise dressing changes to reduce prolonged exposure to air • Avoid wiping gauze or cotton across the wound bed
Wound management products: areas to consider	Select the correct dressing for the conditions at the wound bed, related to tissue type and level of exudate present. Does the dressing need to absorb exudate or donate fluid? • Hydrogels and hydrocolloids will cause maceration to the periwound area if used on heavily exudating wounds, extending tissue damage and increasing pain levels • Alginates and hydrofiber will adhere to wounds with low exudate, causing pain and trauma upon removal • Avoid adhesive dressings on patients with very fragile skin, an excoriated periwound area or those on long-term steroid treatment • Some dressings such as honey products can create an osmotic pull on the wound bed, which some patients find extremely painful • Antibacterial dressings containing iodine and silver can cause increased pain • Refrain from changing the dressing too frequently if not indicated • Always remove dressings as per the manufacturer's instructions
Treatments	• Compression therapy can be extremely painful • Negative pressure wound therapy (NPWT) can increase pain and can cause tissue trauma upon removal • Larval therapy can increase pain
Emotional and social aspects	• Increased pain may be related to how the patient perceives their wound and the effect it has upon their lives, so nurses should empathise and help to alleviate their anxieties • Malodour may contribute to these negative feelings
Disease processes	• Identify and treat clinical wound infection as this may cause the pain at the wound bed • Associated diseases may contribute to the pain, such as peripheral vascular disease, ischaemia, rheumatoid arthritis, osteoarthritis, diabetic neuropathy, phantom limb pain, oedema, cellulitis, cancer, eczema

Source: Adapted from Hollinworth, H. 2005. The management of patients' pain in wound care. *Nursing Standard* 20(7): 65–70.

before removing the dressing and commencing any treatments. Nitrous oxide (Entonox) also can help some people. Other pain reduction strategies include use of relaxation and distraction (Wounds UK 2004).

Drawing on the material in this section, identify possible strategies for wound care for Mrs Warner, Colin and Susan. Remember to consider debridement, cleansing, wound dressing choice and pain management.

Table 7.11 presents points that you might have identified.

Table 7.11: A possible wound management strategy for Colin, Mrs Warner and Susan

	Colin	Mrs Warner	Susan
Wound type	Dirty surgical wound on buttock	1. Necrotic sacral pressure ulcer 2. Infected diabetic neuropathic ulcer on toe	Clean contaminated surgical wound on abdomen
Debridement needed?	Surgical debridement performed	1. Yes, identify an appropriate option for this individual (see Box 7.2)	Not required
Cleansing?	Yes, bathing, showering or irrigation with warm saline	1. Could bath or shower, or the wounds could be irrigated with warm saline when the dressings are renewed 2. Consider use of antiseptic for infected toe ulcer (Wounds UK 2011)	Not required Can bath or shower as she wishes
Which dressing?	Pack wound with alginate or hydrofiber and cover with a foam dressing	1. Sacrum: Dress with a hydrogel covered with a hydrocolloid to initiate autolytic debridement. Once the tissue has liquefied, apply larval therapy. 2. Toe: Dress with an antimicrobial dressing with foam as a secondary dressing	Not necessary after first 48 hours (NICE 2008), but Susan may find it more comfortable or acceptable if her wound is covered with a film dressing until her sutures are removed
Pain management	Assess pain Information giving and explanations Regular analgesics (e.g. non-steroidal anti-inflammatory drugs) The alginate or hydrofiber dressing should be comfortable to wear and painless to remove	Assess pain Information giving and explanations Hydrogel, hydrocolloid and foam dressings are all comfortable to wear and should be painless to remove if the manufacturers' recommendations are followed Regular analgesics if needed (neuropathic ulcers are usually painless)	Assess pain Information giving and explanations Regular analgesics may be needed Remove film dressing with care, following manufacturers' recommendations Removal of skin closures will need careful preparation, reassurance and support

Children: practice points – wound dressing application

Children can find the process of a wound dressing distressing; fear and pain are potential problems. The type of dressing used should be carefully chosen, to minimise pain on removal; dressings with silicone adhesive facilitate a non-traumatic removal. Nilsson and Renning (2012) provide useful information about pharmacological and non-pharmacological methods of managing pain associated with wound care; suggestions include music, films, games and distraction.

For further information and guidance, see

Macqueen, S. Bruce, E.A. Gibson, F. 2012. *The Great Ormond Street Hospital Manual of Children's Nursing Practices*. Chichester: Wiley-Blackwell, Chapter 1 'Assessment pp. 1–37, and Chapter 6 'Burns and Scalds' pp. 108–111 (specifically on wound care management).

Summary

- Wound assessment must precede effective wound management, which requires the application of suitable cleansing methods, the most appropriate dressing to cover the wound and pain-relieving strategies.
- Application of these skills in the care of each individual is the product of knowledge and experience.

CHAPTER SUMMARY

This chapter has aimed to introduce an understanding of how wounds heal, with an emphasis on the systemic nature of wound healing, and the range of factors that may impair wound healing. An awareness of how wounds can be assessed and managed, taking into account their underlying causes, has also been promoted. The chapter emphasised an individualistic and holistic approach to wound care and discussed different options available for managing wounds.

You have been encouraged to take the opportunity to apply knowledge to practice and to start to gain experience in observing wounds and identifying their stage of healing. Involving patients/clients and their families, working with the multidisciplinary team, accessing expert knowledge and being aware of the need to continually update have all been addressed. This chapter did not attempt to include specialist knowledge – further in-depth reading in relation to individual topics such as leg ulcers and burns should be undertaken where applicable.

To conclude, an understanding of wound care is important for all nurses. This chapter has aimed to introduce key principles to act as a foundation for future learning.

REFERENCES

Aityeh, B.S., Costagliola, M. and Hayek, S.N. 2005. Keloid or hypertrophic scar: the controversy: Review of the literature. *Annals of Plastic Surgery* 54(6): 676–80.

Anderson, I. 2006. Aetiology, assessment and management of leg ulcers. *Wound Essentials* 1: 20–37.

Anderson, I. 2009. What is a venous leg ulcer? *Wound Essentials* 4: 36–44.

Beldon, P. 2007. What you need to know about skin grafts and donor site wounds. *Wound Essentials UK* 2: 149–55.

Beldon, P. 2012. Editorial: Welcome to the new look wound essentials. *Wound Essentials* 7(1): 5.

Bilous, R. and Donnelly, R. 2010. *Handbook of Diabetes*. Oxford, UK: Wiley-Blackwell.

Bryant, R.A. 2007. Preface. In: Bryant, R.A. and Nix, D. (eds.) *Acute and Chronic Wounds: Current Management Options,* 3rd edn. St. Louis, MO: Mosby Elsevier, vii–ix.

Clinical Resource Efficiency Support Team (CREST). 1998. *Guidelines for the Assessment and Management of Leg Ulceration.* Northern Ireland: CREST.

Cook, L. and Barker, C. 2012. Exudate: Understand it, assess it, manage it. *Nursing Residential Care* 14(5): 234–8.

Cowan, T. (ed.) 2012. *Wound Care Handbook 2012–2013,* 5th edn. Mark Allen Healthcare.

Cruse, P. and Foord, R. 1980. The epidemiology of wound infection: A ten-year prospective study of 62,939 wounds. *Surgical Clinics of North America* 60: 27–40.

Cutting, K., White, R., Wilson, M., et al. 2007. Is it time to re-evaluate the preferred cleansing solution for use on chronic wounds? *Wounds UK* 3(3): 89–91.

Cutting, K.F. 1999. The causes and prevention of maceration of the skin. *Journal of Wound Care* 8: 200–1.

Department of Health (DH). 2002. *Action for Health – Health Action Plans and Health Facilitation.* London: DH

Department of Health (DH). 2009. *Health Action Planning and Health Facilitation for People with Learning Disabilities: Good Practice Guidance.* London: DH.

Department of Health (DH). 2010. White paper: equity and excellence, liberating the NHS. London: DH.

Doughty, D.B. and Holbrook, R. 2007. Lower-extremity ulcers of vascular etiology. In: Bryant, R.A. and Nix, D.P. (eds.) *Acute and Chronic Wounds: Nursing Management,* 3rd edn. St. Louis, MO: Mosby, 258–306.

Doughty, D.B. and Sparks-Defriese, B. 2007. Wound-healing physiology. In: Bryant, R.A. and Nix, D.P. (eds.) *Acute and Chronic Wounds: Nursing Management,* 3rd edn. St. Louis, MO: Mosby, 56–81.

Drosou, A., Falabella, A. and Kirsner, R.S. 2003. Antiseptics on wounds: An area of controversy (part one). *Wounds* 15(5): 149–66.

Dunn, D.L. and Phillips, J. 2004. *Ethicon Wound Closure Manual.* Somerville, NJ: Ethicon.

Edwards, J. 2000. Sharp debridement of wounds. *Journal of Community Nursing* 14: 1.

Escandon, J., Vivas, A.C., Tang, J., et al. 2011. High mortality with patients with chronic wounds. *Wound Repair and Regeneration* 19(4): 526–8.

European Pressure Ulcer Advisory Panel and National Pressure Ulcer Advisory Panel (EPUAP and NPUAP). 2009. *Treatment of Pressure Ulcers: Quick Reference Guide.* Washington, DC: NPUAP.

European Wound Management Association (EWMA). 2003. Position document: Understanding compression therapy. London: MEP.

European Wound Management Association (EWMA). 2005. Position paper: Identifying criteria for wound infection. London: MEP.

European Wound Management Association (EWMA). 2008. Position document: Hard-to-heal wounds: A holistic approach. London: MEP.

Evans, R.C. and Jones, N.L. 1996. The management of abrasions and bruises. *Journal of Wound Care* 5: 465–8.

Fairbairn, K., Grier, J., Hunter, C., et al. 2002. A sharp debridement procedure devised by specialist nurses. *Journal of Wound Care* 11(10): 371–5.

Fernandez, R., Griffiths, R. and Ussia, C. 2010. Water for wound cleansing. *Cochrane Database of Systematic Reviews* (2). Art. No.: CD003861. DOI: 10.1002/14651858.CD003861.pub3.

Flanagan, M. 2003. *The Philosophy of Wound Bed Preparation in Clinical Practice*. Hull, England: Smith and Nephew.

Fletcher, J. 2003. The benefits of applying wound bed preparation into practice. *Journal of Wound Care* 12(9): 347–9.

Folestad, A. 2002. The management of wounds following orthopaedic surgery: The Molndal dressing. *European Orthopaedic Product News,* March/April, 33.

Goldberg, M.T. and McGynn-Byer, M. 2007. Oncology-related skin damage. In: Bryant, R.A. and Nix, D.P. (eds.) *Acute and Chronic Wounds: Nursing Management,* 3rd edn. St. Louis, MO: Mosby, 471–89.

Gottrup, F. 1999. Wound closure techniques. *Journal of Wound Care* 8: 397–400.

Gouvela, J.C. and Miguens, C. 2007. Is it safe to use saline solution to clean wounds. *EWMA Journal* 7(2): 7–12.

Graham, I.D., Harrison, M.B., Nelson, E.A., et al. 2003. Prevalence of lower-limb ulceration: A systematic review of prevalence studies. *Advances in Skin and Wound Care* 16(6): 305–16.

Gray, D., Acton, C., Chadwick, P., et al. 2011a. Consensus guidance for the use of debridement techniques in the UK. *Wounds UK* 7(1): 77–84.

Gray, D., Boyd, J., Carville, K., et al. 2011b. Effective wound management and wellbeing for clinicians, organisations and industry. *Wounds International* 2(2). Available from: http://www.woundsinternational.com.

Gray, D., White, R., Cooper, P., et al. 2004. The wound healing continuum, an aid to clinical decision making and clinical audit. Applied Wound Management Supplement. *Wounds UK* 1(1): 9–12.

Gray, D., White, R., Cooper, P., et al. 2009. An introduction to applied wound management and its use in the assessment of wounds. *Wounds UK* 5(4): 4–9.

Grothier, L. and Cooper, R. 2011. Medihoney dressings made easy – Products for practice. Wounds UK 6(2). Available from: http://www.wounds-uk.com (Accessed on 19 January 2013).

Harrison, C.A., Gossiel, F., Layton, C.M., et al. 2006. Use of an in vitro model tissue-engineered human skin to investigate the mechanism of skin graft contraction. *Tissue Engineering* 12(11): 3119–33.

Health Improvement Scotland. 2009. Excoriation tool. Available from: http://tiny.cc/xnx0ew (Accessed on 19 January 2013).

Henderson, V., Timmons, J., Hurd, T., et al. 2012. NWPT in everyday practice made easy. *Wounds International* 1(5). Available from: http://www.woundsinternational.com (Accessed 19 January 2013).

Hess, C.T. 2011. Checklist for factors affecting wound healing. *Advances in Skin and Wound Care* 24(4): 192.

Hollinworth, H. 2005. The management of patients' pain in wound care. *Nursing Standard* 20(7): 65–70.

International Consensus. 2012. Optimising wellbeing in people living with a wound. *Wounds International*. Available from: http://www.woundsinternational.com (Accessed on 19 January 2013).

Johnston, E. 2007. The role of nutrition in tissue viability. *Wound Essentials* 2: 10–21.

Jones, J. 2003. Stress responses, pressure ulcer development and adaptation. *British Journal of Nursing* 12(Suppl 11): S17–22.

Kingsley, A., White, R. and Gray, D. 2004. The wound infection continuum: A revised perspective. Applied Wound Management Supplement. *Wounds UK* 1(1): 13–18.

Lazarus, G.S., Cooper, D.M., Knighton, D.R., et al. 1994. Definitions and guidelines for assessment of wounds and evaluation of healing. *Archives of Dermatology* 130: 489–93.

Leaper, D.J. 2006. ABC of wound healing: Traumatic and surgical wounds. *British Medical Journal* 332: 532–5.

McCluskey, P. and McCarthy, G. 2012. Nurses' knowledge and competence in wound management. *Wounds UK* 8(2): 37–47.

Mcheik, J.N., Vergniss, P. and Bondonny, J.M. 2000. Treatment of facial dog bite injuries in children: A retrospective study. *Journal of Paediatric Surgery* 35: 580–3.

McIntosh, C. 2006. Diabetic foot ulcers: What is the best practice in the UK? *Wound Essentials* 2: 162–9.

Miminas, D.A. 2007. Ageing and its influence on wound healing. *Wounds UK* 3(1): 42–50.

Moffat, C., Franks, P., Doherty, D., et al. 2009. Psychological factors in leg ulceration: A case control study. *British Journal of Dermatology* 161: 750–6.

Morris, C. 2006. Wound management and dressing selection. *Wound Essentials* 1: 178–83.

National Institute for Health and Clinical Excellence (NICE). 2001. *Guidance on the Use of Debriding Agents and Specialist Wound Care Clinics for Difficult to Heal Surgical Wounds*. London: NICE.

National Institute for Health and Clinical Excellence (NICE). 2008. *Surgical Site Infection: Prevention and Treatment of Surgical Site Infection*. Clinical Guidelines 74. London: NICE.

National Institute for Health and Clinical Excellence (NICE). 2011a. *Diabetic Foot Problems: Inpatient Management of Diabetic Foot Problems*. Clinical Guidelines 119. London: NICE.

National Institute for Health and Clinical Excellence (NICE). 2011b. *Caesarian Section Guidelines*. London: NICE.

Nelson, E.A. and Bradley, M.D. 2007. Dressings and topical agents for arterial leg ulcers. *Cochrane Database of Systematic Reviews* (1). Art. No.: CD001836. DOI: 10.1002/14651858. CD001836.pub2.

Nguyen, D.T., Orgill, D.P. and Murphy, G.F. 2009. The pathophysiologic basis for wound healing and cutaneous regeneration. In: Orgill, D.P. and Murphy, G.F. (eds.) *Biomaterials for Treating Skin Loss*. Cambridge: Woodhead Publishing, 25–57.

Nilsson, S. and Renning, A-C. 2012. Pain management during wound dressing in children. *Nursing Standard* 26(32): 50–5.

Nix, D.P. 2007. Patient assessment and evaluation of wound healing. In: Bryant, R.A. and Nix, D.P. (eds.) *Acute and Chronic Wounds: Nursing Management,* 3rd edn. St. Louis, MO: Mosby, 130–48.

Norris, R., Staines, K. and Vogwill, V. 2012. Reducing the cost of lower limb wound management through industry partnership and staff education. *Journal of Wound Care* 21(5): 216–22.

O'Brien, M., Lawton, J.F., Conn, C.R., et al. 2011. Best practice wound care. *International Wound Journal* 8(2): 145–54.

Ousey, K. and Cook, L. 2012. Wound assessment made easy. *Wounds UK* 8(2). Available from: http://www.wounds-uk.com/made-easy (Accessed on 19 January 2013).

Partsch, H., Clark, M., Mosti, G., et al. 2008. Classification of compression bandages: Practical aspects. *Dermatology Surgery* 34(5): 600–9.

Pittman, J. 2007. Effect of aging on wound healing: Current concepts. *Wound Ostomy Continence Nursing* 34(4): 412–15.

Posnett, J. and Franks, P.J. 2008. The burden of chronic wounds in the UK. *Nursing Times* 104(3): 44–5.

Richardson, C. and Upton, D. 2011. Managing pain and stress in wound care. *Wounds UK* 7(4): 100–7.

Royal College of Nursing (RCN). 2006. *The Nursing Management of Patients with Venous Leg Ulcers*. London: RCN.

Scottish Intercollegiate Guidelines Network (SIGN). 2010. *Management of Chronic Venous Leg Ulcers: A National Guideline*. Edinburgh: SIGN.

Serensen, L.T. 2003. Smoking and wound healing. *European Wound Management Association Journal* 3(1): 13–15.

Shorney, R.H. and Ousey, K. 2011. Tissue viability: The QIPP challenge. *The Clinical Services Journal* 26–9.

Siddiqui, A.R. and Bernstein, J.M. 2010. Chronic wound infection: Facts and controversies. *Clinics in Dermatology* 28: 519–26.

Smaill, F.M. and Gyte, G.M.L. 2010. Antibiotic prophylaxis versus no prophylaxis for preventing infection after cesarean section. *Cochrane Database Systematic Reviews* (1). Art. No: CD007482. DOI: 10.1002/14651858.CD007482.pub2.

Stotts, N.A. 2007. Nutritional support and assessment. In: Bryant, R.A. and Nix, D.P. (eds.) *Acute and Chronic Wounds: Nursing Management,* 2nd edn. St. Louis, MO: Mosby, 149–60.

Taylor, A. 2010. Principles of pain assessment. *Wound Essentials* 5: 104–10.

Thomas, S. 2008. The role of dressings in the treatment of moisture-related skin damage. *World Wide Wounds*. Available from: http://www.worldwidewounds.com (Accessed on 19 January 2013).

Thomas, S., Fram, P. and Phillips, P. 2007. The importance of compression on dressing performance. *World Wide Wounds*. Available from: http://www.worldwidewounds.com (Accessed on 19 January 2013).

Thomas, S., Wynn, K., Fowler, T., et al. 2002. The effect of containment on the properties of sterile maggots. *British Journal of Nursing* 11(12): 21–8.

Timmons, J. 2006. Skin function and wound healing physiology. *Wound Essentials* 1: 8–17.

Troxler, M., Vowden, K. and Vowden, P. 2006. Integrating adjunctive therapy into practice: the importance of recognising 'hard to heal' wounds. *World Wide Wounds*. Available from: http://www.worldwidewounds.com (Accessed on 19 January 2013).

Tuunainen, A. and Wahlbeck, K. 2010. Newer atypical antipsychotic medication versus clozapine for schizophrenia. *Cochrane Database of Systematic Reviews* (2). Art. No.: CD000966. DOI: 10.1002/14651858.CD000966.

Vowden, K. and Vowden, P. 2002. Wound bed preparation. *World Wide Wounds*. Available from: http://www.worldwidewounds.com (Accessed on 19 January 2013).

Vowden, P. 2011. Hard-to-heal wounds made easy. *Wounds International* 2(4). Available from: http://www.woundsinternational.com

Whayman, N. 2012. Nursing standards and outcomes developed by the Leg Ulcer Forum. *Wounds UK* 8(1): 59–61.

White, R. 2005. *Skin Care in Wound Management: Assessment, Prevention and Treatment.* Aberdeen: Wounds UK.

World Union of Wound Healing Societies (WUWHS). 2007. *Wound Exudate and the Role of Dressings. A Consensus Document.* London: MEP. Available from: http://www. woundsinternational.com (Accessed on 19 January 2013).

World Union of Wound Healing Societies (WUWHS). 2008. *Principles of Best Practice: Compression in Venous Leg Ulcers. A Consensus Document.* London: MEP. Available from: http://www.woundsinternational.com (Accessed on 19 January 2013).

Wounds UK. 2004. Best practice statement: Minimising trauma and pain in wound management. Available from: http://www.wounds-uk.com/best-practice-statements (Accessed on 19 January 2013).

Wounds UK. 2008. Best practice statement: Optimising wound care. London: Wounds UK. Available from: http://www.wounds-uk.com/best-practice-statements (Accessed on 19 January 2013).

Wounds UK. 2011. Best practice statement: The use of topical antiseptic/antimicrobial agents in wound management. Available from: http://www.wounds-uk.com/best-practice-statements (Accessed on 19 January 2013).

Wounds UK. 2012. Best practice statement: Compression hosiery. Available from: http://www. wounds-uk.com/best-practice-statements (Accessed on 19 January 2013).

USEFUL WEBSITES

World Wide Wounds: www.worldwidewounds.com

Wounds UK: www.wounds-uk.com

Wounds Research: www.woundsresearch.com

Wounds International: www.woundsinternational.com

European Wound Management Association: www.ewma.org

European Pressure Ulcer Advisory Panel: www.epuap.org

8 Meeting Personal Hygiene Needs

Moira Walker

Assisting people to meet their fundamental hygiene needs has always been at the forefront of nursing care. The importance of personal hygiene is reinforced by its inclusion in the Department of Health's (DH 2010) *Essence of Care 2010* benchmarks. The Chief Nursing Officer's review of mental health nursing, *From Values to Action*, also highlighted personal and physical care as being important skills for mental health nurses (DH 2006).

The ability to maintain one's own personal hygiene is a skill learnt early in life and affects a person's self-esteem, confidence and health. However, sometimes disability and/or physical and mental health problems lead to people needing assistance on either a temporary or a permanent basis. Meeting hygiene needs greatly contributes to comfort and well-being, provides the opportunity to build up a trusting relationship and is the basis for therapeutic care (Cowdell 2010). As with any other skill/procedure, hygiene must be discussed fully with the person beforehand and verbal consent must be obtained, so it is tailored to individual's needs. As this chapter focuses on the care of the body, care of the body after death also is included.

The principles of care (e.g. observation, comfort, communication, safety and prevention of cross-infection) discussed in this chapter are generally relevant to everyone, but how they are carried out for each individual varies, with privacy and dignity being at the forefront of that care. It is also important to consider the religious and cultural needs of individuals when meeting hygiene needs.

This chapter includes the following topics:

- Rationale for meeting hygiene needs and potential hazards
- Bathing a person in bed
- Bathing and showering in the bathroom
- Facial shaving
- Oral hygiene
- Care of the body after death

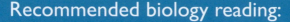

Recommended biology reading:

You should revise the layers of the skin. In addition, these questions will help you to understand the biology underpinning this chapter's skills. Use your recommended textbook to find out the following:

- The skin and oral cavity host a range of microorganisms. Which of these are potentially pathogenic?
- What is saliva composed of? Where is it produced, and what is its role in maintaining a healthy mouth?
- What protective mechanisms do eyes have that prevent them from infection?
- Distinguish between transient and resident bacteria found on the skin. Which of these bacteria cannot be removed by handwashing? Chapter 3 will help you with this answer.
- How does skin maintain its waterproof properties?
- Why does the skin of the palms of the hands and soles of the feet wrinkle when soaked in water?
- How does ageing affect the skin?
- What part does nutrition play in maintaining a healthy skin, hair and nails?
- Why do we sweat and what does sweat contain?
- Why does stale sweat smell?
- What is the 'acid mantle' and how can it be destroyed?

PRACTICE SCENARIOS

The following practice scenarios are referred to throughout this chapter in relation to meeting hygiene needs.

Adult

Metastases

Secondary deposits of cancer that have spread from the primary site, either directly or via blood or lymph.

William Newton, who likes to be called 'Bill', is a retired accountant aged 73. He is terminally ill with a history of oesophageal cancer and **metastases** in his lungs. He is cared for by his wife at home with the support of community nurses and the Macmillan nurse. He is taking regular oral morphine for pain control. He has a very low haemoglobin and has been admitted for a blood transfusion. He is weak, breathless and his general condition is poor. He has a **body mass index (BMI)** of 16. He can swallow only very small amounts of liquidised food and drink. He has some of his own teeth but also a partial denture, which he likes to wear, although it is now ill-fitting. His tongue appears coated and his mouth is dry.

Body mass index (BMI)

BMI is explained in Chapter 10 in the section 'Nutritional screening'. A BMI of 16 indicates a person is underweight.

Learning disability

Ellen Grey is a 47-year-old woman with a learning disability. She lives in sheltered accommodation in her own flat. There is a communal lounge. She has always managed her own personal hygiene adequately. However, recently she has developed an unpleasant smell, and other residents have begun to avoid her because of this smell. The community nurse for learning disabilities has been asked to assess the situation and find out what has changed. She identifies that the reason Ellen's personal hygiene has become compromised is because of the recent development of nocturnal incontinence. As well as her bed linen being wet, the situation has disrupted Ellen's usual hygiene routine.

Mental health

Miss Smith, aged 83 years, was admitted to an inpatient assessment unit for older people after concerns from her social worker and general practitioner (GP) about her inability to cope at home due to severe depression. She lives on her own with only her pet dog for company. As she can no longer climb her stairs, she has been sleeping in an armchair downstairs. Her poor mobility also prevented her from reaching the bathroom. Although Miss Smith is in reasonable physical health, her clothing has obviously not been changed for many months and is encrusted with dirt and excrement. Her hair is badly knotted and matted, and her skin is in poor condition. She also has poor oral hygiene, which she has obviously neglected for some time. Miss Smith was initially distrusting of staff and resisted all attempts to help her have a bath and clean clothes. Eventually, she agreed to do this but remained hostile towards staff, accusing them of stealing her dog and her house. However, nurses explained that her dog had been taken to the local RSPCA kennels and was in good health. Gradually, Miss Smith became more accepting of her new surroundings and began to engage nurses in conversation without her previous hostility or suspicion.

RATIONALE FOR MEETING HYGIENE NEEDS AND POTENTIAL HAZARDS

LEARNING OUTCOMES

By the end of this section, you will be able to:

1 explain why facilitating people to meet their hygiene needs is a beneficial nursing action;
2 discuss possible hazards and problems associated with meeting hygiene needs.

Learning outcome 1: Explain why facilitating people to meet their hygiene needs is a beneficial nursing action

ACTIVITY

Why is it important for nurses to assist with hygiene needs? Consider how you might feel if you were incapacitated mentally or physically and unable to meet your hygiene needs.

- Feeling clean and comfortable is an important social need for most people; to feel well groomed and not offensive to others can help to maintain self-esteem. Thus, for Ellen to be aware that she has an unpleasant odour which others are discussing could cause her some distress. Miss Smith's poor mobility has prevented her maintaining her hygiene, and this is probably upsetting for her. Being unkempt can at times also mask the deterioration of an illness (Gústafsdóttir 2011) either physical or mental, so it is important to understand the reasons behind the decline.

- Cleanliness is important within culture and religion (see later discussion). For example, for Muslims, cleanliness has both a spiritual and physical dimension (Rassool 2000). A study of older South Asian people's experiences of culturally sensitive care highlighted that maintaining their hygiene was essential for dignity (Clegg 2003).

- The act of assisting people with personal hygiene needs allows nurses to build up a trusting relationship (Winkworth 2003). It is a private time where communication may be facilitated. Brawley (2002) points out that for people living in care homes, bath time may be one of the only opportunities for individual attention.

- Valuable observations can be made, for example, the condition of the skin (Cowdell 2010). This will be important for all the people in this chapter's scenarios.

- Cleansing the skin removes potentially harmful microorganisms and also sweat, dead skin cells and the bacteria which produce body odour. This is especially important with regard to the genitalia of both men and woman, particularly if there is urinary or faecal incontinence.

- Washing stimulates the circulation; the movement associated with washing and the effect of warm water on the skin are beneficial, both physiologically and psychologically (Sloane et al. 1995).

- Bathing has been described as one of the 'great pleasures in life' (Brawley 2002).

For some people, being washed or bathed by others can be humiliating, so nurses must protect self-esteem and dignity as far as possible by adhering to individual wishes (DH 2010). As identified above, observant nurses can learn a great deal about people when assisting with their hygiene needs.

ACTIVITY

What could you observe while assisting a person with hygiene? Looking at the scenarios may give you some clues.

Oedematous

Swelling caused by the accumulation of fluid in the interstitial spaces.

- **Condition of the skin.** Is there redness or bruising, and are there breaks in the skin? Is there any skin infection? Are there any old scars? This is important for Bill because of advancing disease, but it is also relevant to Ellen and Miss Smith.

- **Hydration and nutrition.** Does the skin feel dry, loose or **oedematous**? Any of the people in this chapter's scenarios could become dehydrated due to poor fluid intake and their skin could become dry.

- **Mental state.** Is the person anxious, calm, restless, depressed, demotivated, cheerful, lethargic or confused?

- **Physical ability.** How much can the person do? Do they require prompting? With Ellen, the nurse will be able to assess how much she can do for herself, what aspects she requires assistance with and what aids she might require. Does the activity cause breathlessness or fatigue? These issues will affect Bill's ability to care for himself.

- **Condition of wounds, drains, intravenous (IV) sites (IV).** These could apply to Bill, for example, inflammation of his IV site.

Learning outcome 2: Discuss the possible hazards and problems associated with meeting hygiene needs

As discussed above, meeting a person's hygiene needs should be a therapeutic intervention, yet there are several potential complications or difficulties.

ACTIVITY | What hazards or problems could be associated with meeting hygiene needs?

Review the points below and reflect on the questions raised:
- **Access.** The person might be unable to get into a bathroom or the shower owing to mobility issues. *Can you think what those mobility issues might be?*
- **Environment.** People can become cold if left exposed for too long. There are health and safety aspects in relation to wet floors, and water being too hot/cold. *How does skin exposure affect the temperature control of a child/adult/older person who is unwell?*
- **Cross-infection.** Some studies have shown that there were more bacteria on a person's skin after a bed bath than before (Parker 2004). *Can you think of the possible cause for the increase of the bacteria on the skin and how this could be minimised?*
- **Damage to skin.** The person might have allergies to particular soaps, or overwashing may remove essential oils. *What other factors could impact on the skin, while meeting hygiene needs?*
- **Fatigue.** For example, meeting Bill's hygiene needs could exhaust him. *What is it about Bill's illness that might have an impact on his energy levels?*
- **Embarrassment.** People may have a fear of their bodies being seen naked by others. Cultural or religious beliefs need to be considered. *What might you do to help maintain the dignity of the individual you are helping?*

ACTIVITY | Consider further the cultural and religious beliefs of the people you care for. What particular aspects are you aware of?

The list that follows gives some examples but take care not to make assumptions and find out about individuals' wishes.
- *African–Caribbean.* Hair type requires regular moisturising. The hair and scalp should be moistened every other day at least and the skin moistened once or twice a day (Christmas 2002).
- *Rastafarian.* The person might wear hair natural and uncut in obedience to God, who told the Nazarenes (a group of ancient Israelites) to do so. Some Rastafarians

keep their hair covered. Modesty in dress is important. Hospital gowns may be viewed as immodest for women (Baxter 2002).

- *Sikhism*. Personal hygiene is very important. Hands and face must be washed and teeth brushed before eating. Showering is preferred to bathing (Gill 2002).
- *Islam*. A very high standard of hygiene is required (Rassool 2000). Muslims must wash before they pray (Holland and Hogg 2010).
- *Hinduism*. Handwashing is essential before and after eating. Washing in running water is very important for Hindus (Holland and Hogg 2010).

Assessment and discussion with people on how they would like their hygiene needs met are key for this procedure to be therapeutic and will ensure any individual cultural/religious needs are met. The *Essence of Care* (DH 2010) emphasises the need for assessment and re-assessment to maintain their optimum levels of hygiene.

Summary

- Assisting people to meet their hygiene needs can greatly increase comfort and provide an excellent opportunity for observation and assessment.
- Nurses must remember that not all people will enjoy the experience of being washed. They should therefore consider the key principles of dignity and comfort, so care is delivered therapeutically.

BATHING A PERSON IN BED

Bathing a person in bed is necessary when people are unable to get out of bed for medical reasons (e.g. after certain surgery or injuries), or when they are too unwell or weak to be able to get out of bed. Bill may need this option at present. The procedure described in this section – bed bathing – involves washing a person's body while they are in bed, using a bowl of water and cloths or alternatives such as emollients.

Although this section focuses on bathing in bed, some people who are unable to wash in the bathroom can sit out in a chair to wash, using a bowl. Nurses need to give assistance according to individual needs, based on assessment; the principles discussed in this section can be adapted to each situation.

LEARNING OUTCOMES

By the end of this section, you will be able to:

1 discuss ways of maintaining dignity and enhancing comfort when bathing a person in bed;

2 describe the procedure for carrying out bed bathing and hair washing in bed.

Learning outcome 1: Discuss ways of maintaining dignity and enhancing comfort when bathing a person in bed

ACTIVITY

How might you maintain a person's dignity and comfort while undertaking a bed bath?

Points you may have considered include the following:

- Ensuring that you have all necessary equipment before starting, to avoid leaving the person during the procedure
- Ensuring privacy by drawing the curtains and informing other members of staff of what you are doing to limit interruptions
- Ensuring windows are closed to avoid draughts
- Encouraging the person to do as much as possible, and allowing them the time to do so
- Asking the person how they normally wash, and what they use for cleaning
- Covering the person with a towel, thereby only exposing areas of the body when necessary
- Using your communication skills – the atmosphere and relationship the nurse builds with the person will do much to promote dignity
- Being aware that clothing may have special significance within some religions (Holland and Hogg 2010)

Learning outcome 2: Describe the procedure for carrying out bed bathing and hair washing in bed

Before commencing the bathing of a person in bed, you must assess the individual.

ACTIVITY

Using one of the scenarios as a guide, what items should you include in your assessment? Compare your list with the following.

- What is the person's normal hygiene routine? When do they normally wash/bathe? Can that be facilitated while they are in hospital?
- What toiletries do they use? Are they available?
- How does the person feel today? Do they want a full wash or the bare minimum? This may change on a daily basis depending on how the person is feeling.
- Does any care need to be given before the wash? For example, if the person is due to have an enema, it would be preferable to administer the enema before the wash.
- Does the person require any analgesia before the bed bath to ensure comfort when moving and turning?
- How much assistance is required? How much can the person do? Does the nurse need to be present to prompt and guide, or does the person want to be left alone to undertake some aspects?
- Does the person want a family member to be involved in providing care? If yes, have they been asked? What is that person willing to do?

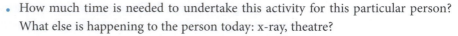
- How much time is needed to undertake this activity for this particular person? What else is happening to the person today: x-ray, theatre?
- How many staff are needed to undertake this activity for a particular person?
- Are other healthcare professionals involved in the person's care: occupational therapist, physiotherapist? Do they need to be involved to make a needs assessment?

Equipment

It is important to gather everything required before starting, to avoid having to leave the person unattended; this preparedness will enhance privacy, dignity and comfort. Box 8.1 lists the equipment that you are likely to need, but always consider the person's own individual requirements.

Procedure

Listed below is a suggested procedure for bathing a person in bed that is likely to maintain comfort and prevent the person from becoming cold. A sensitive and empathetic approach should be maintained throughout. It is also important that the nurse does not impose their idea of what is cleanliness but respects what the person feels is a level of hygiene that is appropriate for them (Downey and Lloyd 2008). Ensure that you have introduced yourself to the person and that you use the bed-bath as an opportunity to build further rapport. People may be pleased to engage in conversation or they may feel too weak and wish for a minimum of interaction, so be sensitive to non-verbal cues.

- Wash your hands and put on the plastic apron (and gloves if needed – see Chapter 3).
- Fill the bowl with comfortably warm water.
- Remove the top bedclothes, leaving the person covered by a blanket, sheet or towels.
- Remove the pyjama jacket or nightdress. If the person has a weak arm or has an intravenous infusion attached (as has Bill), remove this arm from the clothing last.

Box 8.1 Preparing to bath a person in bed: equipment required

- Person's own washing bowl
- Soap, skin cleanser
- Person's own flannel or disposable flannel
- Towels
- Comb and/or brush
- Toiletries as required (e.g. shaving foam, razor, antiperspirant, moisturiser)
- Clean bed linen and bed clothes
- Linen bags and waste bag
- Plastic apron and disposable gloves

ACTIVITY Practise with a friend or colleague, removing a jacket or cardigan from each other, while pretending that one arm's mobility is impaired. Now try replacing it, inserting the affected arm first.

- Can the person wash their own face? Even quite unwell people often like to do this for themselves. Otherwise, wash the person's face, using soap if wanted. Never poke inside ears. Rinse off soap, if used, and pat dry carefully. With eyes, take care to wash from the inner to outer corner of the eye, thus reducing the risk of contamination. Make sure there is little or no soap on the cloth as soap can be extremely painful if it gets into the eyes. Always approach any care relating to eyes with gentleness and cleanliness to avoid risk of trauma or cross-infection.

ACTIVITY With a friend or colleague, practise washing and drying each other's face. How did it feel? Is there a difference in feeling of being pat dried or rubbed dry?

People with sensitive skin such as babies, toddlers or those who have had radiation treatment for cancer might find rubbing of the skin extremely uncomfortable. Can you think of who else might have sensitive skin?

People who are unconscious or semiconscious are at risk of their eyes becoming dry. Eyes need to be assessed regularly for signs of irritation, corneal drying, abrasions and oedema (Geraghty 2005).

ACTIVITY Find out about the eye care policy in your current care setting.

Having completed your person's face wash, the bathing procedure should continue:
- Place a towel under the arm furthest away from you, and wash from the hand to the axilla. Rinse off the soap and pat dry thoroughly, taking care not to dislodge any cannulae or dressings. Repeat with the other arm.
- Uncover the chest and abdomen and wash and dry this area in the same way, again taking care not to dislodge dressings or attachments. Work gently but quickly to prevent the person from becoming chilled. Pay special attention to skin folds and under the breasts, as these areas may be moist through sweat and therefore heavily colonised with microorganisms. When cleaning under the breasts use the back of your hand gently to lift. Cover the chest and abdomen once this is completed. Toiletries such as antiperspirant or body spray can be applied as wished by the person. If a person is sweating excessively putting gauze under the breasts or between the folds can help to prevent heat rash and help to keep the area dry. The areas must be closely monitored for any abrasions or rashes.
- Change the water at this point, or at any time if it feels cool or becomes excessively soiled. If water is not changed and the same washcloth is used for the whole body,

the water can become full of bacteria and be a potential hazard to people with breaks in their skin (Ayliffe et al. 2001).

- Now remove any lower body clothing including antiembolism stockings, cover the leg nearest you, and place the towel under the opposite leg. Wash the leg from toes to groin, rinse and dry. Apply moisturising lotion if the skin appears dry over the shins or feet. Repeat with the other leg.

ACTIVITY

What observations should you be making while washing arms, body and legs?

Your observations should include condition of the skin, checking for dryness, colour, bruises, abrasions, rashes, swelling or oedema. Nurses should apply skin moisturisers as needed. You should also note any tenderness in the limbs, particularly the calves, which might indicate a deep vein thrombosis (see Chapter 6).

For some people, attention to foot care is particularly important. People at risk of foot problems include older people and people with diabetes, peripheral vascular disease or peripheral neuropathy (Thompson 1999). Foot problems in people with diabetes are discussed in detail elsewhere (e.g. Howell and Thirlaway 2004; NICE 2004, 2011); also see Chapter 7. A systematic review indicated that patient education about foot care may reduce foot ulceration and amputations, especially in high-risk people (Dorresteijn et al. 2010). When people are unable to self-care, nurses must carry out the foot care and observation required and report any concerns immediately. In some circumstances, nurses can use this opportunity to educate people about foot care. Box 8.2 outlines the key principles. Some people find it comforting to soak their feet in warm water for a while. Soaking can be done easily by sitting them in the chair (if they are able) and putting their feet into a bowl of warm water. Make sure that when you dry the feet you pay particular attention to drying in between the toes as this area can often harbour bacteria and fungi.

The bathing procedure should continue as follows.

- Using a disposable washcloth and wearing gloves, wash the genitals and perineal area, working from front to back to prevent contamination of the urethra and/or vagina with faecal matter. Catheter care may be required at this point (see Chapter 9, section on 'Caring for people who have urinary catheters'). Change the water now – remember the rationale for this change (see learning outcome 2).
  Note: when cleaning the penis, the foreskin needs to be drawn back from the glans and the area gently cleaned. It is essential that the foreskin is then brought back over the glans after cleaning otherwise a **phimosis** or **paraphimosis** can develop. In boys up to the age of 17–19 years, the foreskin is still attached and should not be forced down the glans as this could cause pain and damage (Wilson et al. 2009)
- When cleaning the labia in women, it is important that the soap is properly rinsed from the area as any soap residue can cause extreme irritation and itching.
  Note: Cleaning the genital area must be conducted with sensitivity as this particular area is extremely private and the person could feel very embarrassed.

Phimosis

Tight foreskin which will not retract over the glans of the penis.

Paraphimosis

Once retracted, a tight foreskin gets stuck behind the glans.

Box 8.2 Advice about foot care for people with diabetes

- Wash feet daily, drying them carefully and thoroughly, particularly between the toes.
- Examine feet daily for problems (colour change, swelling, breaks in skin, pain or numbness). If they occur, report them to a healthcare professional. People with a foot care emergency (new ulceration, swelling, discolouration) should be seen by a multidisciplinary foot care team within 24 hours. Check the top of the foot, the sole of the foot (people can be taught to use a mirror to do this), between the toes and pressure areas, that is, tips of toes and heels.
- Check for signs of redness around nail areas, and ensure nails do not cut into adjacent toes. Cut immediately after bathing when nails are soft, following the shape of the toe and not down into tissue. If nails are thick and brittle, **do not** attempt to cut – refer to podiatrist. *Note:* Follow local policies regarding nail-cutting.
- Make sure that shoes and hosiery fit well.
- Ensure that feet are assessed at least annually by trained personnel.

In addition, people at increased or high risk of foot ulcers (neuropathy, and/or absent pulses or other risk factor) should be aware of the following:

- Have feet reviewed by a foot protection team 3–6 monthly.
- Never walk barefoot.
- Realise that any break in the skin is potentially serious.
- Check bath temperatures carefully (numb feet cannot assess temperature).
- Avoid hot waterbottles, electric blankets, foot spas and sitting with feet too close to fires.
- Get help to deal with calluses and corns (avoid over-the-counter remedies).
- Regularly inspect footwear for rough areas, ripped linings, and other signs of damage.

Source: Adapted from National Institute for Health and Clinical Excellence (NICE). 2004. *Type 2 Diabetes: Prevention and Management of Foot Problems.* Clinical Guidelines 10. London: NICE.

Be sure to ask permission and if possible encourage the person to do much of the care themselves to reduce their feelings of vulnerability, although some people will be too physically or mentally impaired. Although Bill is weak, he might be able to do this for himself with some help.

- At this point, you need to assess how you can wash the person's back. You can either sit the person forward or lie them on their side. Sitting Bill forward to wash his back would be best as he might become breathless if lying on his side for long, You can ask/assist him to lean forward, wash, rinse and dry his back, using a clean washcloth. The pillowcases can be changed, and he can be assisted into a clean pyjama jacket. For a woman, a clean nightdress can be put on at this point.

- To wash a person's back if they cannot sit forward, and to wash a person's buttocks, you need to turn them on their side; you may require assistance to do this. The bottom sheet can be changed at this time. You can insert a slide sheet to assist with turning and then moving the person up the bed after completing the wash. If you feel assistance is not required, you need to raise the opposite bed rail to provide security for the person when rolling on to their side. Assist the person to roll over, using the log roll method and putting a pillow under their top knee to make it more comfortable and prevent them going onto their front. Roll up the soiled bottom sheet lengthways, close to the person. Place a towel along the person's back, wash, rinse and dry the back and buttocks, noting any skin problems as previously outlined.

ACTIVITY | Which areas of skin do you think you should pay most attention to while the person is on their side?

You should observe the areas most at risk from pressure damage. These include the sacrum, trochanters, elbows and shoulder tips, base of the skull and heels. See Chapter 6 section on 'Pressure ulcer risk assessment' for details. Box 6.1 outlines how to inspect skin for signs of early pressure damage.

- Now assist with putting on pyjama trousers or adjusting a nightdress. Some people prefer to wear underwear in bed, so then ensure you help them with this. Replace the antiembolism stockings if worn and change the bottom sheet. To do this, roll or concertina fold a clean sheet close to the person, taking care not to contaminate the clean sheet with the soiled one. Assist the person to roll back towards you, and support them while your assistant removes the soiled sheet, pulls though the clean one and secures it.

ACTIVITY | What might be the infection control issues when disposing of the soiled sheet?

Look back to the principles of preventing cross-infection outlined in Chapter 3. Used linen (soiled and foul) should be disposed of in white or off-white bags. Infected linen should be placed into a water-soluble bag and then into a red bag (or according to local policy).

ACTIVITY | You will need two friends/colleagues for this exercise, and access to a bed in the skills laboratory. Practise changing the bottom sheet, taking it in turns to be the 'patient'. Consider whether you felt vulnerable during this. What reassured you?

- Using safe moving and handling methods, assist the person into an appropriate and comfortable position, according to their condition and care plan.
- Brush or comb the person's hair into their preferred style. Carry out any other hair care needed at this stage – check the person's personal requirements and what assistance they need.

- Assist with makeup if required and with oral hygiene (see later section).
- Place the locker and call bell within reach.
- Wash and dry the bowl, and dispose of soiled equipment appropriately (see Chapter 3, section on 'Waste disposal'). Washbowls should be stored upside down to reduce colonisation by microorganisms, which prefer horizontal surfaces. Also, if washbowls are not dried properly and are stacked together, bacteria multiply in the moisture trapped between the bowls; contaminated washbowls have been implicated in infection outbreaks, Gram-negative bacteria being most likely to be found (Ayliffe et al. 2001).
- People's own washcloths need to be washed thoroughly after use and stored so that they can dry. They should not be wrapped around the soap (Parker 2004).
- Document any observations made, and the care given, in the care plan or nursing notes.

Hair washing in bed

People whose health condition requires them to stay in bed for more than a few days are likely to need their hair washed while in bed, to promote their comfort and well-being. Box 8.3 summarises equipment and procedure used.

Box 8.3 Washing hair in bed: equipment and procedure

Equipment

Large jug or bowl of hand-hot water, empty bowl, shampoo guard if available, plastic sheeting if available, small jug, shampoo and conditioner (according to the person's wishes), towels and flannel, brush/comb and hairdryer, plastic apron.

Procedure

- Remove the head of the bed and assist the person to lie flat. For people who cannot lie flat, hair can be washed over a bowl on a bed table.
- Place the empty bowl on a chair/bed table at the head of the bed, at a lower level. Arrange the plastic sheet to protect the mattress and a towel to protect the person's shoulders.
- Move the person, using a slide sheet, so that their head is over the bowl.
- Check the water temperature and wet the hair using the small jug. The person may like to protect their eyes with a clean flannel.
- Apply shampoo, massage gently into the scalp, and rinse off, repeat if desired, and then apply conditioner and rinse until the hair feels clean. Empty the bowl at intervals, before it gets too full.
- Wrap the person's hair in a clean towel and move the bowl out of the way.
- Slide the person back on to the bed, and remove the plastic sheet. Check the bottom sheet is not damp; replace if necessary.
- Replace the head of the bed, and assist the person to sit up if able, using a safe moving and handling technique.
- Empty the bowl of water, once the person is comfortable. Wash and dry the bowls and jug, and dispose of all equipment safely.
- Towel the hair dry, and style the hair as desired, using a hairdryer if necessary. Take care with the hairdryer: ensure that it not too hot and avoid trailing flexes.
- Leave the person comfortable, with bed table, locker and call bell within reach. Document the care given in the care plan or nursing notes.

Children: practice points – meeting hygiene needs

Meeting the hygiene needs of the child is negotiated with the parents/carers and nurses in partnership as parents will naturally want to be involved, but it cannot be assumed that they will undertake all care. It is important however that the nurse teaches the parents what they need to look out for with regards to skin integrity and other factors relevant to their condition. Depending on the child's condition, they may also need help with moving and handling. For detailed discussion of caring for personal hygiene needs in infants and children, including 'topping and tailing' infants and umbilical cord care, see

Himsworth, J. 2010. Caring for personal hygiene needs. In: Glasper, A., Aylott, M. and Battrick, C. (eds.) *Developing Practical Skills for Nursing Children and Young People*. London: Hodder Arnold, 188–202.

Macqueen, S., Bruce, E.A. and Gibson, F. 2012. Personal hygiene and pressure ulcer prevention. In: *The Great Ormond Street Hospital Manual of Children's Nursing Practices*. Chichester: Wiley-Blackwell, 167–220.

Pregnancy and birth: practice points – hygiene after birth

After childbirth, irrespective of the type of delivery, women will have a vaginal blood loss known as **lochia** and this can sometimes last until the end of the pueperium (6 weeks post delivery). The colour, odour and amount can change and sometimes indicates signs of illness or infection. When caring for a critically ill mother, close observation and reporting changes to the midwife or obstetric team, as well as strict vulval hygiene, are vital for the early detection and prevention of infection. It is also important to ensure that the mother's breasts are kept clean and dry, always supporting milk expression from the breast using a mechanical pump if the mother wants to breast feed. This can help to prevent **engorgement** (swollen, tender and hard breasts) or **mastitis** (painful, inflamed breast, maybe due to infection).

Summary

- It is important to assess the suitability of a bed bath for the individual person and to negotiate involvement by the person and their family, as desired.
- Respect for the individual's privacy and dignity, and maintenance of comfort, should be promoted.
- Adherence to infection control procedures and safe moving and handling techniques is vital.

BATHING AND SHOWERING IN THE BATHROOM

If people are able to visit the bathroom to meet their personal hygiene needs, this is usually preferable for various reasons. For some people, actually going in the bath or shower may not be possible, but they may be able to at least sit and wash at the sink, which is usually preferable to washing in, or by, the bed. It is important to remember to attend to the feet and lower legs, as they are often overlooked when people are taken to the sink for a wash.

LEARNING OUTCOMES

On completion of this section, you will be able to:

1. explain the particular benefits and possible problems of meeting hygiene needs in the bathroom rather than at the bedside;
2. discuss the procedure for assisting with bathing/showering in the bathroom, including health and safety issues.

Learning outcome 1: Explain the particular benefits and possible problems of meeting hygiene needs in the bathroom rather than at the bedside

ACTIVITY

Which of the people in this chapter's scenarios may be able to visit the bathroom to meet their hygiene needs?

Health Action Plan

A personal action plan developed for each individual with a learning disability, which details the actions needed to maintain and improve the person's health and any help needed to accomplish these; see *Action for Health – Health Action Plans and Health Facilitation* (DH 2002).

All should be able to at some stage, but as previously mentioned, Bill may be too weak, tired or in pain to do so at present. Miss Smith will be able to visit the bathroom but will require mobility aids. Ellen will carry out her hygiene care in her own bathroom, but the nurse must revisit her knowledge and skills and reinforce the importance of good hygiene and a bathing routine. Underlying causes of her incontinence must be investigated using a specific tool which addresses physical, psychological and environmental dimensions. The nurse can support Ellen in accessing the necessary services (e.g. continence advisor). The aim should be for Ellen to regain continence and her ability to maintain her hygiene so her **Health Action Plan** should be amended to address these issues. The nurse should broach the subject sensitively; it is important to ensure that this short-term problem does not impact on her social integration and relationships in the longer term. Perhaps a carer could visit in the mornings and evenings, to help Ellen structure her day and ensure that her hygiene needs are being met.

Ellen will probably not require physical assistance in the bathroom, but she needs prompting, encouragement and praise for success in meeting her hygiene needs plan. As she re-establishes her skills, support can reduce until Ellen is self-caring once more.

The presence of a surgical wound is not a contraindication to a shower or bath, as long as the skin edges of the wound are sealed (Briggs 1997). However, a shower is preferable to a bath for a person with a wound as there is less risk of cross-infection from a previous user (Gilchrist 1990). People with chronic wounds can bath or shower according to preference. If there is no wound infection present, cleaning of the bath with normal detergent is adequate, but if the wound is infected, the bath should be cleaned with hypochlorite solution (see Chapter 7).

ACTIVITY

Why might it be preferable for hygiene needs to be met in the bathroom if possible, rather than at the bedside?

- The bathroom is a more familiar environment for hygiene, which is important for someone who is confused, or who is preparing for discharge home. Ellen's teaching programme to meet her hygiene needs will be more effective if carried out in her own familiar bathroom. The bathroom is the most appropriate environment for Miss Smith to re-establish a routine of hygiene care.
- Privacy can be more easily maintained in a bathroom than behind curtains at the bedside.
- There is a continuous supply of water which may be desirable for cultural and/or religious reasons. For example, in Hinduism, washing in running water, as a shower or by pouring water from a jug, is very important (Holland and Hogg 2010). This is easier to achieve in the bathroom.
- For older people, going into a bath is a familiar activity. Some people, for example, those with muscle spasm, find a bath relaxing and enjoyable.

ACTIVITY

Although there are good reasons why people can better carry out hygiene in the bathroom, you may be able to think of some possible problems. List these problems.

- People can become chilled if a suitable temperature cannot be maintained. It can also be exhausting for people with few reserves of strength, like Bill. There are various health and safety hazards; these are discussed later.
- A bathroom may cause problems for a person whose condition is unstable – physically and mentally. Unless a nurse stays with them, observation is more difficult in bathrooms than when they are behind curtains in the ward.
- Brawley (2002) points out that for a person with dementia, particularly if they have a visual or hearing impairment, bathrooms can be noisy and disorientating, causing fear and confusion. However, these problems can be minimised; see later discussion and Box 8.4.

The *Essence of Care* (DH 2010) emphasised the importance of providing an appropriate environment for hygiene needs to be met in the benchmark of best practice. People with impaired mobility, like Miss Smith, have special moving and handling requirements and need suitable equipment to enable them to access baths or showers. Nurses must maintain sound moving and handling practices within bathrooms to prevent injury to patients/residents and themselves. Occupational therapists can advise on equipment. There are shower trolleys available, which can be useful for people with spinal injuries or other neurological conditions such as cerebral palsy. There is a wide range of other equipment available to assist with bathing and showering.

Learning outcome 2: Discuss the procedure for assisting with bathing/showering in the bathroom, including health and safety issues

As with washing a person in bed, you should introduce yourself and build a rapport before assisting with personal care. Miss Smith was initially resistant to going to the bathroom, but as a relationship with the staff was established she became more accepting of their help. Nurses should be patient and understanding in such situations. Assisting with hygiene in the bathroom provides opportunities to further the relationship with the person, as it involves one-to-one interaction in a private environment.

The carers of some adults might wish to continue to be involved in bathing. A person with dementia, for example, may be more comfortable if their usual carer assists. This involvement in care should be negotiated by nurses and not taken for granted, as some informal carers may be exhausted and might appreciate a break. Involving families in bathing can be important preparation for discharge, particularly where a person has a new disability. Nurses can teach families about use of equipment and skin observation and care, for example.

Equipment

As always, it is important to plan ahead, gathering all equipment likely to be needed. Having to leave the bathroom to fetch items when the person is undressed could lead to chilling and exposure; if a person is unsafe to leave, the nurse would have to ring the call bell and wait for help to arrive. The toiletries required vary between individuals, so always ask about preferences, which some people may indicate through non-verbal rather than verbal communication. You are likely to need towels, soap/shower gel or other cleansing agent, shampoo/conditioner (if hair washing is to be carried out), clean clothing (of the person's choice), brush/comb, toothbrush and toothpaste and flannel/disposable washcloths. Some people are prescribed specific skin care agents for use in the bath or afterwards.

Preparing the bathroom

After assembling the equipment, check that the bathroom is free and warm and has been cleaned after any previous user.

ACTIVITY

Why is it necessary to check the bathroom prior to taking a person there?

Apart from any physical soiling, you should consider cross-infection risk. As mentioned earlier, normal detergent can be used to clean baths/showers but apply hypochlorite solution after use by a person with an infection or adhere to local infection control policy. You should also check that the floor is not wet or slippery and that any extra equipment, such as a hoist or shower stool, is available and in safe working order. Also check the temperature of the bathroom, as some people are susceptible to the cold, particularly if underweight like Bill or older people like Miss Smith. Warm the bathroom first, if necessary.

Bathing or showering procedure

The following steps provide a suggested procedure that will maintain comfort and safety. As with bed bathing, nurses must be sensitive and respectful when assisting with hygiene in the bathroom.

- If bathing, fill the bath with warm water, using your elbow or a bath thermometer to check the temperature.
- Assist the person to the bathroom, offering them the opportunity to use the toilet first.
- Give consideration to people who have sensory impairment. People with visual impairment can find bathrooms difficult as there are often white walls and white bathroom suite, making it difficult to locate the sink or bath. Therefore, always take time to orientate them to the environment, showing them where everything is.
- Assist with undressing, maintaining dignity and comfort and avoiding unnecessary exposure by using towels.
- If the person has a urinary catheter in situ, a shower is preferable. However, if a bath is used, then the catheter should be clamped if the catheter has to be lifted above bladder level (e.g. when assisting the person in and out of the bath), to prevent reflux of urine back into the bladder (Pratt et al. 2007).
- If bathing, check the bathwater temperature again and allow the person to check for themselves if they are able. *Remember*: some people have impaired sensation in their feet and will not be able to feel the temperature accurately.
- Using suitable equipment if necessary, help the person into the bath, or on to the shower chair. If the shower is being used, check the temperature before use.
- Promote independence by supporting/enabling people to wash themselves as far as possible. Miss Smith's independence should be encouraged to rebuild her confidence in meeting her hygiene needs. Ellen will need gentle prompting without being patronising.
- As with bathing in bed, particular attention should be given to skin creases, and areas susceptible to becoming sore – for example, under breasts, palms of hands which are fixed in tonic flexion. Remember from the earlier section 'Bathing a person in bed', the importance of foot care for some people, particularly those with diabetes. Check Box 8.2, to remind yourself of the essential observations and care. Miss Smith's feet could be in a poor condition as she might not have been able to reach them for some time. She may need to be referred to a podiatrist.
- You should only leave a person alone in the bath or shower if you have assessed that it is safe to do so. For example, people who have epilepsy should not be left alone and neither should people who are confused. Always check with the registered nurse, if unsure. If it is safe to leave a person, ensure that the call bell is within reach, and working, before leaving.
- Remember, skin condition can be specifically observed, as well as psychological and physical conditions – for example, any pain or breathlessness on movement, level of motivation to assist. These will all be important observations when assisting Miss Smith.

- If hair washing is required, as for Miss Smith, use clean water in a washbasin or bowl, and a jug, or shower attachment. Wet the hair, allowing the person to protect their eyes with a flannel. Apply shampoo, and massage gently into the scalp. Rinse and repeat, if necessary, and apply conditioner, as needed. Rinse again, and dry with a clean towel.

- Before assisting the person out of the bath, it may be easier to let some water out, and dry the upper body to minimise the time for the person to become chilled. Assist the person out of the bath or shower, using equipment as necessary, and assist with drying as needed, again thinking about maintaining comfort and dignity by avoiding unnecessary exposure. Toiletries can be applied at this point.

- Assist the person to dress in clean clothes, to clean teeth (see oral hygiene section), and to brush/style hair as desired. Once again, assess the person's ability to participate in these activities. Both Miss Smith and Ellen may need verbal encouragement and reinforcement. A structured, behavioural approach may be needed.

- Dispose of used equipment in accordance with waste disposal policy and leave the bathroom clean and ready for the next user.

- Document the care given in the care plan or nursing notes.

Alzheimer's Society (2009) identified that nurses and carers reported concerns related to washing and bathing of people with dementia. In response, Alzheimer's Society developed some 'Top tips'. Box 8.4 includes some of these additional points.

Box 8.4 Washing and bathing for people with dementia: top tips for nurses

- Talk to the person about how they would prefer you to do things or ask their carer about preferences. Ask about their normal routine and encourage them to continue with these routines by providing support as needed.
- Some people may be worried by deep water. You can reassure them by making sure the bath water is shallow or set up a bath seat for their use.
- People with dementia sometimes lose the ability to judge temperature, so check the water temperature is not too hot or too cold.
- An overhead shower's rush of water can be frightening or disorientating, particularly when hitting the head. It may be preferable to use a hand held shower or a bath.
- Whereas most people like having their hair washed regularly, others do not enjoy this process. If hair washing is distressing for the person with dementia, stop.
- Give gentle reminders about washing but think about the timing of your request and how you phrase it.
- Use the time to chat and reassure the person with dementia, explaining what you are doing or about to do.
- Make the experience as pleasant and stress-free as possible, using pleasant toiletries, relaxing music or singing.

Source: Summarised from Alzheimer's Society, http://www.alzheimers.org.uk/site/scripts/documents_info.php?documentID=1211&pageNumber=4

Summary
- Meeting hygiene needs in the bathroom is preferable for many reasons, for example, privacy and the availability of running water.
- When assisting with hygiene in the bathroom, always assemble all equipment beforehand, to avoid leaving people alone.
- The bathroom is potentially hazardous. It is important to take active steps to avoid accidents, such as falls or scalding, and only leave people alone if you have assessed that it is safe to do so.
- Maintain privacy and dignity throughout, and promote independence.

LEARNING OUTCOMES

On completion of this section, you will be able to:
1 discuss the rationale for shaving people who are unable to do this for themselves;
2 identify the equipment needed and describe the procedure for shaving.

FACIAL SHAVING

Learning outcome 1: Discuss the rationale for shaving people who are unable to do this for themselves

Facial hair has important social and cultural meanings. In some religions, for example, Sikhism, neither facial nor hair on the head may be cut. In many Western European cultures, a wide variety of facial hair is socially acceptable and contributes to maintaining self-esteem. Although facial shaving is usually associated with men, some females (particularly older women) have unwanted facial hair which they prefer to remove. This is important to their body image. If a woman requests assistance with shaving or using tweezers, always approach this sensitively and matter-of-factly. Some younger women might also want their underarms and legs shaved as this is an important part of their own body image.

ACTIVITY

Talk to a male relative or friend who is usually clean shaven. Ask him how he would feel if unable to shave himself.

For many men, being clean shaven is important, and being unable to self-care in this way would be distressing. In addition, families visiting can be upset to find the person unshaven if they are usually clean shaven and would view such a lack of care as neglectful, leading to a loss of confidence in staff. For some people shaving may be hazardous. For example, individuals receiving anticoagulant medication can be at risk of bleeding from minor cuts, so it is safer to use an electric razor rather than carrying out a wet shave.

Learning outcome 2: Identify the equipment needed and describe the procedure for shaving

Equipment

You need

- either a razor, with shaving soap/foam and shaving brush, or the person's own electric razor (communal razors pose a high risk of cross-infection);
- towel and flannel/disposable washcloth;
- bowl of hand-hot water;
- aftershave, if desired.

Procedure

Assemble the equipment and assist the person to sit up if possible. Protect the person's chest with a towel. Assess to what extent the person can assist. For some men, careful positioning, provision of a shaving mirror and having all equipment to hand may enable them to be independent with shaving. Shaving requires very fine motor control, so it is important to assess the person's capability. The individual's care plan should clarify this and any particular precautions needed.

Wet shaving

- Wet the brush and apply the soap to the face, or use the foam, working up a good lather.
- Work in the direction of the hair growth, starting with the cheeks and moving on to the neck and around the mouth.
- Hold the skin taut and avoid any sores or moles. The person may be able to help by tightening his facial muscles. However, this would not be possible for all men, for example, if facial weakness is present.
- For some men the facial skin can be hypersensitive and therefore take great care.
- Rinse the razor after each stroke.
- When you have finished, rinse the face with clean water and dry, apply aftershave if used. Dispose of used equipment safely. Document your care in the care plan or nursing notes.

Dry shaving

- The skin should be clean and dry; a little talcum powder may help. Work with circular strokes, keeping the skin taut as for wet shaving.
- Assist the person to rinse his face when finished, apply aftershave if desired and clean the razor ready for the next occasion. Document your care in the care plan or nursing notes.

ACTIVITY

Find a willing male friend, relative or colleague and practise both a wet shave and a dry shave. Even if you shave yourself, you may find this more difficult than you expect. Ask your 'patient' to comment on your technique.

Summary
- Facial shaving is important to many people. Nurses should assist if people are unable to self-care, thus maintaining self-esteem.
- A gentle and careful technique should be used, using the person's preferred equipment.

ORAL HYGIENE

Maintaining oral hygiene is an important aspect of nursing care, which can do much to enhance quality of life and promote health. A high standard of oral hygiene should also be promoted in people who can self-care. The *Essence of Care 2010* (DH 2010) benchmark on 'Personal hygiene' explicitly includes mouth hygiene which it defines as 'the effective removal of plaque and debris to ensure the structures and tissues of the mouth are kept in a healthy condition' (p. 7). NHS Quality Improvement Scotland (NHS QIS 2005) presents best practice statements for good oral health for older people, which are a useful reference guide.

LEARNING OUTCOMES

By the end of this section, you will be able to:
1 reflect on the rationale for maintaining good oral hygiene;
2 explain factors that increase vulnerability to poor oral hygiene and consider how those at risk can be identified;
3 discuss how oral hygiene can be carried out safely and based on best evidence.

Learning outcome 1: Reflect on the rationale for maintaining good oral hygiene

Oral hygiene aims to maintain a healthy oral mucosa, teeth, gums and lips, by using toothpaste, brush or other cleansing agents.

ACTIVITY

What problems may arise if oral hygiene is poor, as in Miss Smith's case?

You may have considered the following:
- Poor oral function/hygiene and chronic oral problems can lead to systemic ill health and can be life-threatening if not treated properly (Paju and Scannapieco 2007).

- Mouth and gum infections may develop, such as candidiasis (thrush), which is a fungal infection.
- Inability to eat may result, leading to malnutrition (NHS QIS 2005).
- Halitosis may develop, leading to social withdrawal.
- Infection risk increases, particularly in people who are immunocompromised.
- Low self-esteem may result (Huff et al. 2006).
- Discomfort and distress may develop.

NHS QIS (2005) also highlights a link between pneumonia and poor oral health in older people.

Learning outcome 2: Explain factors that increase vulnerability to poor oral hygiene and consider how those at risk can be identified

ACTIVITY

You already know that Miss Smith's oral hygiene is poor. What might be the reasons for this? Now consider the other people in this chapter's scenarios. Do you think any of them are at risk of poor oral hygiene too?

Miss Smith's poor mobility has affected her ability to carry out her usual hygiene care as she cannot get to the bathroom. Although she could clean her teeth at the kitchen sink, she might not have been able to adapt her routine in this way, perhaps because of her depression. She may not have been able to access a dentist or buy the necessary equipment to carry out oral hygiene. Her poor oral hygiene might have led to poor oral intake of food and fluids, thus worsening her mouth condition.

Bill is at risk of oral hygiene problems. He has an ill-fitting denture, he can drink only small amounts and he is generally debilitated and thus at risk of developing an oral *Candida* infection.

Ellen may be maintaining good oral hygiene, but the community nurse for learning disabilities could check that she is coping with her oral hygiene. Some people with learning disabilities can have oral hypersensitivity, making it uncomfortable to clean their teeth. The Royal College of Nursing (RCN 2011) highlights that people with learning disabilities are more likely to have various mouth and dental problems, including tooth decay, loose teeth and gum disease, which may be due to poor diet, poor dental hygiene or a lack of access to oral health promotion. The **health facilitator** should provide support in overcoming these problems and regular visits to the dentist must be included in Ellen's Health Action Plan. Tooth decay would adversely affect her quality of life, leading to pain, the need for dental treatment and poor food intake.

There are many factors that can lead to poor oral hygiene (Table 8.1). Looking at this table might prompt you to identify further risk factors for the people in the scenarios; for example, Bill is taking morphine, which causes mouth dryness. The Alzheimer's Society (2011) explains how dementia can affect oral health at different stages of dementia and provides a detailed factsheet with useful advice.

Health facilitator

The role focuses on an individual's health outcomes and can be undertaken by a range of people including support workers, family carers, friends and advocates as well as health professionals; see *Health Action Planning and Health Facilitation for People with Learning Disabilities: Good Practice Guidance* (DH 2009).

Table 8.1: Factors predisposing to mouth problems

Drugs	• Cytotoxic drugs (reduce autoimmune response)
	• Corticosteroids (affect tissue healing)
	• Antibiotics (alters oral bacterial balance, allowing infection by *Candida albicans*)
	• Antihistamines, antispasmodics, anticholinergics, psychotropics, antidepressants and tranquillisers (reduce salivary production)
	• Diuretics (increase fluid loss)
	• Morphine (causes mouth dryness)
Treatments	• Radiotherapy of head/neck (causes localised inflammation, affects ability to eat/drink normally)
	• Oxygen therapy, particularly if given unhumidified at high flow rates (dries oral mucosa)
	• Suction (can damage oral mucosa)
	• Restricted oral intake, such as 'nil by mouth' pre- or post-operatively (potential for dehydration and dry mouth)
Mental or physical health problems or disability	• Diseases: diabetes, thyroid dysfunction, oral disease/trauma, cerebrovascular disease, swallow dysfunction
	• Mental health problems: confusion, depression
	• Terminal illness
	• Acute/chronic breathing problems
	• Unconsciousness
	• Lack of manual dexterity

Source: Adapted from Thurgood, G. 1994. Nurse maintenance of oral hygiene. *British Journal of Nursing* 3(7): 351–3.

People's ability to self-care for oral hygiene can change quickly, so nurses should regularly reassess this and other risk factors.

ACTIVITY — What aspects would you consider when assessing oral hygiene needs?

You may have thought of the following:

- Condition of the teeth – plaque, cavities
- Condition of the tongue – coated, clean
- Condition of the lips
- Ability to undertake oral care
- Ability to eat
- Whether people have their own teeth or plates/dentures

Doing an initial Oral Health Risk Assessment (OHRA) can help you to understand whether there are any problems with the person's oral cavity such as dry mouth/tongue, infections, any sores, broken teeth or broken or ill-fitting dentures (British Society of Gerodontology 2010). Assessment tools can be helpful for assessing the need for, and frequency of, mouth care. They incorporate scoring systems indicating levels of risk; see examples in Dickinson et al. (2001) and British

Society of Gerodontology (2010). Factors commonly included are current mouth condition, nutritional status and special risk factors, such as those in Table 8.1 (e.g. certain medication, oxygen therapy).

ACTIVITY

Find out whether an oral assessment tool is used in your current clinical area and, if so, look at the aspects included and ensure you understand any scoring systems used.

Learning outcome 3: Discuss how oral hygiene can be carried out safely and based on best evidence

As with any other nursing practice, best available evidence should be used for oral hygiene. A variety of equipment may be needed, depending on the care identified as appropriate for the individual. Possible items are listed in Box 8.5.

Rationale for choice of equipment

A small, soft-bristled toothbrush is the most effective agent for removing plaque and debris from the mouth, teeth and tongue (British Society of Gerodontology 2010). A trial comparing the ability of foam swabs and toothbrushes in removing plaque confirmed that toothbrushes perform substantially better (Pearson and Hutton 2002). Fluoridated toothpaste should be used (NHS QIS 2005), and with people with swallow reflex problems, a low foam toothpaste is recommended (British Society of Gerodontology 2010).

Jones (1998) advised that toothpaste has a generally drying effect so it should be used sparingly – about the size of a pea. Most antiseptic mouthwashes have a very transient effect, so they are of limited value (Jones 1998). However, those containing chlorhexidine gluconate, for example, Corsodyl, if used for 1 minute, can reduce bacterial counts by up to 80% (Schiott et al. 1970, cited by Jones 1998). Its use is therefore worthwhile in very vulnerable people, for example, immunocompromised,

---

Box 8.5 Equipment for oral care

- Spatula and pen torch (to inspect the oral cavity)
- Small, soft-bristled toothbrush (for teeth cleaning)
- Mouthwash, for example, chlorhexidine (to prevent dental plaque) or water (for teeth cleaning)
- Toothpaste – if poor swallow reflex, use low-foaming toothpaste to limit aspiration
- Container for dentures, if needed
- Lip lubricant, for example, non-petroleum-based (especially if on oxygen), to prevent dry lips
- Beaker and receiver (for mouth rinsing)
- Disposable gloves and plastic apron
- Towel, tissues

very sick or frail older people. Mouthwash is also useful in areas that are hard to reach (Xavier 2000).

Jones (1998) advised that, for cleansing and moistening oral mucosa, pH-balanced swabsticks are preferable; but if foam swab sticks are used, they are best when coated with Corsodyl gel, which is gentler to the delicate oral mucosa. Avoid using a foam mouth swab if the person might bite down on it as if the foam head detaches, it can be a choking hazard (Medicine and Healthcare products Regulatory Agency [MHRA] 2012). If foam mouth swabs are used, always check that the foam head is firmly attached to the stick before using and do not soak it before use as this can reduce the strength of the attachment (MHRA 2012). There are also saliva substitutes available for people with dry mouths. It has been shown in diabetes research that the use of saliva substitutes actually helps in maintaining the immune defence (Montaldo et al. 2010).

ACTIVITY

Drawing on your practice experience, how could nurses approach promoting oral hygiene for each of the people in this chapter's scenarios?

Bill may be able to carry out his own oral hygiene if equipment is placed within his reach. Perhaps he could sit at a sink to carry out his oral care, which will include cleaning his teeth and dentures. Due to his mouth's current poor condition, and if his condition worsens, he may need regular oral hygiene carried out in between teeth cleaning. This is discussed later.

Ellen can be verbally encouraged and supported in carrying out her own oral hygiene in the bathroom. For Miss Smith, equipment for oral hygiene will need to be provided, and nurses should support her and encourage her to re-establish teeth cleaning, which can be done in the bathroom at the sink. She should be approached sensitively about visiting a dentist.

Teeth cleaning should be carried out twice daily (British Dental Health Foundation; see www.dentalhealth.org.uk). Cleaning of dentures should be carried out at least daily but ideally after meals too. If people are unable to carry this out independently, nurses must provide the necessary equipment and assistance. Some people, who are more dependent and debilitated, require nurses to carry out oral hygiene on a regular basis by the bedside. The frequency of oral care should be determined on an individual basis. This care, which may be necessary for Bill, is described below.

Oral hygiene procedure: key points

- After explaining the procedure and gaining consent, the person should be assisted into a sitting position or, if unconscious, on their side to prevent inhalation of solutions or secretions.
- Protect the person's chest with a towel, or the bed with the waterproof sheet. Provide a receiver for spitting into.
- Assemble the equipment. Any mouthwash solution should be freshly prepared, and renewed after 24 hours.

- Wash your hands and put on gloves and apron, if required. Ayliffe et al. (2001) recommend that gloves should be worn as some infectious agents (e.g. herpes, hepatitis B) can be present in the mouth or saliva. However, oral hygiene is a hygienic procedure rather than an aseptic procedure; it does not breach body defences but instead enhances them (Ayliffe et al. 2001). Therefore, gloves need not be sterile.
- Lip crusting can be removed by gently sponging with warm water (Jones 1998). Observe for any breaks in the skin or signs of herpes simplex (cold sore), which would require treatment with acyclovir cream.
- Remove the person's dentures, if worn. They should be brushed well to remove debris using denture paste – ordinary toothpaste is too abrasive – and rinsed well. Box 8.6 lists key points for effective denture care.

If the person has their own teeth, they should be brushed using the toothbrush and paste. Box 8.7 explains how teeth cleaning should be carried out, and Figure 8.1 illustrates teeth cleaning. If people can clean their own teeth, it is better to facilitate this self-cleaning.

- Assist the person to rinse the mouth thoroughly with the chosen mouthwash solution, or use a rinsed toothbrush to do this if they are unable. Suction can be used to remove excess fluid from the mouth if they are unconscious, or have dysphagia (swallowing difficulty), as it is essential to prevent choking or aspiration of fluid (Jones 1998). A conscious person who is nursed flat, for example, after a spinal injury, can use a straw to suck fluid into the mouth to rinse and to spit through afterward.
- Replace any dentures, top set first. Some people use denture fixative.
- Apply lip lubricant, if lips are dry. Use tissues to blot any excess water or lubricant.

Box 8.6 Denture care

- Wash hands and wear gloves.
- Remove dentures (noting any damage) into a container and rinse to remove loose debris.
- Use the person's special denture brush, scrubbing all surfaces, using denture paste or a little soap, to remove all debris.
- Rinse thoroughly.
- When dentures are not being worn, store in a marked container filled with clean water.
- Soaking plastic dentures 2–3 times per week in dilute sodium hypochlorite will help to prevent oral candidiasis. Always rinse thoroughly before replacing in the mouth.
- Dentures with a metal portion should be soaked in dilute hypochlorite for only about 20 minutes, because of the danger of corrosion.

Source: Adapted from Jones, C.V. 1998. The importance of oral hygiene in nutritional support. *British Journal of Nursing* 7: 74, 76–8, 80–3.

Box 8.7 Teeth cleaning

- Explain the procedure and gain consent.
- Wash hands, wear gloves and maintain privacy.
- It may be best to work at the side of the person, cradling the head.
- Remove any partial dentures into a bowl.
- Start at the front of the mouth in the upper jaw.
- Use a soft brush with a small amount of toothpaste pressed into the surface (to avoid it dislodging into the mouth and possible aspiration). Use toothpaste that has limited foam.
- Place the brush sideways against the teeth overlaying the gum edges with bristles pointing towards the teeth roots.
- Use a side-to-side motion, moving the brush head just a fraction of an inch at a time, using light pressure to squeeze the gum tissue against the teeth.
- Move around the upper teeth, replacing the brush section by section against the teeth.
- Try to use the same action inside the upper jaw.
- Repeat for the outer and inner surfaces of the lower jaw.
- Finally, scrub the chewing surfaces of the upper and lower teeth with a forward and backward motion.
- Teeth should be cleaned for a minimum of 90 seconds.
- Ask the person to rinse the mouth with warm water to remove debris, paste, etc., or use foam sticks moistened with water to gently sweep away the debris and toothpaste.
- Wash toothbrush well and leave it to dry in the air. Do not store in a sponge bag or container. Toothbrushes should be replaced every 6–12 weeks.

Source: Adapted from Jones, C.V. 1998. The importance of oral hygiene in nutritional support. *British Journal of Nursing* 7: 74, 76–8, 80–3.

- Leave the person comfortable, and dispose of equipment according to waste disposal policy. Document the care given in the care plan or nursing notes. The British Dental Health Foundation's website (www.dentalhealth.org) covers all aspects of oral hygiene and is a useful source.

ACTIVITY

With a friend or colleague, take turns to clean each other's teeth, using your own toothbrushes and the instructions in Box 8.7 and Figure 8.1.

Children: practice points – oral hygiene

For information about children's teeth and dental care, see

http://www.dentalhealth.org/tell-me-about/topic/children-s-teeth/children-s-teeth

For oral hygiene for children, see

Himsworth, J. 2010. Caring for personal hygiene needs. In: Glasper, A., Aylott, M. and Battrick, C. (eds.) *Developing Practical Skills for Nursing Children and Young People.* London: Hodder Arnold, 196–7.

Macqueen, S., Bruce, E.A. and Gibson, F. 2012. Personal hygiene and pressure ulcer prevention. In: *The Great Ormond Street Hospital Manual of Children's Nursing Practices.* Chichester: Wiley-Blackwell, 167–220.

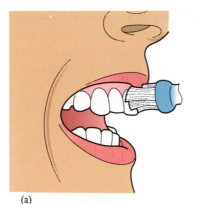
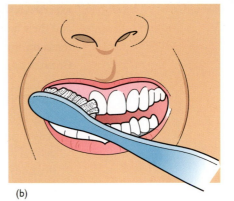

(a)

(b)

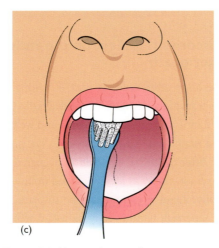
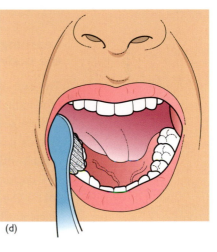

(c)

(d)

Figure 8.1: How to clean teeth.

Summary

- Effective oral care makes an important contribution to people's physical, psychological and social well-being.
- Nurses should ensure that best evidence is used as a basis for assessing and implementing oral care.

CARE OF THE BODY AFTER DEATH

This section explains the care of the body after death. The term 'last offices' (thought to be derived from military/religious practices) does not encompass the multicultural society that we live in today and does not cover the differing nursing tasks involved (National End of Life Care Programme [NEoLCP] and National Nurse Consultant Group (Palliative Care) [NNCG(PC) 2011]) so the term 'care of the body after death' is more appropriate. There are a variety of points to consider when assessing the extent of the care required. The practice of preparing the body of a person who has died for removal to the mortuary or undertaker is the last caring act that nurses can perform for their patients, and it may be regarded as an expression of holistic care and respect. The management of people who are dying and their families is beyond the scope of this section; there are many textbooks that focus on this topic; also see the NHS NEoLCP (http://www.endoflifecare.nhs.uk/). Chapter 12 addresses managing pain and comfort.

> ### LEARNING OUTCOMES
>
> By the end of this section, you will be able to:
> 1 reflect on the rationale for the care of the body after death;
> 2 discuss religious and cultural factors affecting the performance of the care of the body after death;
> 3 explain the procedure for care of the body after death, with attention to safety and dignity.

Learning outcome 1: Reflect on the rationale for the care of the body after death

The care of the body after death is part of a long human tradition in the ritual of marking the transition between life and death (Quested and Rudge 2003). For families, seeing their loved one looking clean and well cared for may help the grieving process. It is also important that the body does not pose a risk to staff who come into contact with it. After death has apparently occurred, it must be confirmed, usually by a doctor, or senior nurse, as locally agreed policy permits (NEoLCP/NNCG(PC) 2011). The family, if not present, must be informed as soon as possible. In cases where death is expected, families may be asked whether they wish to be informed immediately if the death occurs at night or would prefer to wait until morning.

Places where people die

Bill is terminally ill and can be expected to die in the near future, perhaps in the acute setting where he is currently cared for. However, depending on his condition after his blood transfusion, and on how he and his wife feel about him continuing to be cared for at home, he might be discharged with appropriate support. Alternatively, he may be cared for in a hospice for his final days. The place where Bill would prefer to die should have been discussed with him and his family so that staff can assist in facilitating this choice.

ACTIVITY

> What difference might the care setting and the circumstances of a death make to what happens to the body after death?

If Bill dies in an acute care setting, care of the body after death will be carried out by nursing staff; his body will initially be moved to the hospital mortuary by porters and at a later stage collected by an undertaker. However, if he dies at home, care of his body after his death may be minimal before his body being removed by an undertaker. After death in a non-acute care setting, for example, a care home or hospice, local policies affect procedures, but again the body is likely to be removed by an undertaker. In some instances, legal constraints dictate what care may be given.

For example, after an unexpected death or a death that takes place within 24 hours of an operation, in England the coroner's office must be informed and a post-mortem may be required (NEoLCP/NNCG(PC) 2011).

ACTIVITY

What hazards may a body present to those who handle it after death?

There may be leakage of body fluids or sharp objects such as cannulae attached to the body (also see Chapter 3 on preventing cross-infection). There will also be moving and handling issues. Therefore, staff caring for a body after death should take appropriate measures to prevent problems arising.

Learning outcome 2: Discuss religious and cultural factors affecting the performance of care of the body after death

Regardless of the deceased person's cultural and religious background, privacy and dignity must be maintained for them and their family. Drawing the curtains around the bed in an open ward is the least requirement. Where possible, the body may be moved to a side room for greater privacy, and to minimise distress to other patients.

The person's religious and cultural background must be considered at this point. Many of the world's major religions have specific rules and rituals concerned with death, for example, about who can touch the body. However, it is important not to assume that the person or their families will wish these rules to be followed to the letter (Pattison 2008; NEoLCP/NNCG(PC) 2011). As with all human activities, there are many shades of opinion and belief. Ascertaining these beliefs in advance, if possible, is part of sensitive, holistic care. The person was once alive and must be treated with dignity, and it is important that the environment, actions and behaviour of the staff convey respect (NEoLCP/NNCG(PC) 2011).

ACTIVITY

Find out the differing needs of cultures and religions in relation to the care of the body after death.

You will find that there are particular practices associated with different religions and cultures. Nurses should familiarise themselves with these practices so that all interventions are spiritually and culturally acceptable and do not cause offence. It is important to find out what the person's preferences and wishes are before death, and these should always take priority (Pattison 2008).

ACTIVITY

Have you been present when a patient, or care home/unit resident, has died? Did the other patients/residents show awareness of what had occurred? What comments did they make? How can you respond?

In most settings other than the person's own home, there will be other patients or residents around. At least some of them will be aware of the event and may ask, directly or indirectly, about the deceased person. It is important to answer questions sensitively and honestly, but without revealing confidential details.

ACTIVITY

Regarding Bill, who can be expected to die fairly soon, what would you expect his religious/cultural background to be?

From his name, you might assume that he will have a Western/Christian background, but such assumptions can be dangerous; always ask and do not assume. Among Christian religions too, there are variations, with different religious practices around the time of death.

ACTIVITY

Do you know how to contact the local chaplain, rabbi, imam or other religious leaders, so that you can gain advice about any special requirements at the time of death and when carrying out care of the body after death?

Nurses need to be aware of how to contact local religious leaders, as referring to, and liaising with, them is an important contribution to people's spiritual support. You may find there is a folder produced by the hospital chaplaincy with contact details and information regarding different religions. In many instances, if they follow a particular religion, patients and their families will have their own contacts.

Learning outcome 3: Explain the procedure for care of the body after death, with attention to safety and dignity

Immediate care after death

In whatever setting, a death takes place there are a few actions that should be carried out very soon afterward, within 2–4 hours to preserve their appearance, condition and dignity (NEoLCP/NNCG(PC) 2011).

- Close the eyes by gently applying pressure to the eyelids for about 30 seconds.
- Lay the person down flat, leaving one pillow, and straighten the body and limbs into neutral positions as soon as possible.
- Insert dentures, if usually worn (e.g. with Bill, we know he likes to wear his denture).
- Close the mouth and support the jaw with a pillow, to ensure it remains closed.

The body starts to become rigid soon after death and all these actions become more difficult to perform later.

In a hospital setting, it is usual to leave the body for about an hour before full care after death is carried out. During this period, the family may visit and sit with the person, holding their hand if they wish. Therefore, immediately after death the surrounding environment should be tidied up, equipment removed and the bed linen attended to so that the person looks peaceful and comfortable. Families need to be given time and support and will, before they leave, need written information about what to do next (e.g. when and how to collect property, register the death, arrange the funeral) (NEoLCP/NNCG(PC) 2011).

Care of the body after death procedure

Before commencing the procedure, you should gather the equipment required, including items for washing the person (Box 8.1) and for cleaning the mouth (Box 8.5).

ACTIVITY

What other items do you think might be needed in addition to those in Boxes 8.1 and 8.5?

- If the person is not to wear their own nightclothes, a shroud (long white gown) might be required. Local hospital policies vary on this issue, however; sometimes, hospital nightclothes are used if a person's own are not available as some people consider shrouds, which were traditionally used, to be upsetting to families.
- The person's property should be listed and packed ready for collection by the family, so the appropriate documentation (Property Book) will be needed. If the person has a wound, a waterproof dressing is required. If there are tubes to be left in, spigots will be needed to plug these. Additional name bands and identity labels may be necessary according to the setting and local policy. A disposable receiver may also be required.

The procedure described below includes usual practice, but must always be guided by local policy, people's individual circumstances and particular religious and cultural requirements. Sometimes, a family member of the deceased may wish to be involved, perhaps helping with washing or hair brushing. Ensure privacy as previously described. Two nurses are usually required for this procedure due to moving and handling needs but also for the emotional support.

- Protect yourself against possible infection by using plastic apron and gloves (see Chapter 3 on preventing cross-infection). For people with communicable diseases, the existing infection control measures should continue.
- Wash the person as described in 'Bathing a person in bed', as culturally appropriate.
- Cover any wounds with waterproof dressings. Check local policy relating to removal of drains, tubes, cannulae or catheters. If a post-mortem is to take place, these materials should be left in unless advised otherwise but can be spigotted. If no post-mortem is going to be performed, these tubes can usually be removed, but always check if unsure.
- If leakage from any orifice seems likely to continue, insert packing, according to local policy, or an incontinence pad can be applied.
- Manually express the urinary bladder into a disposable receiver, if necessary and as per local policy.
- Place a clean sheet under the person, using safe moving and handling techniques.
- Remove and/or record the whereabouts of any jewellery, as previously discussed, with family (or the person). Recording should always be done in the presence of a witness. Jewellery left on the body should be secured with tape to prevent it being lost.

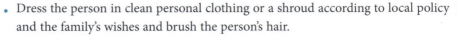

- Dress the person in clean personal clothing or a shroud according to local policy and the family's wishes and brush the person's hair.
- Shaving a deceased person while they are still warm can cause bruising and marking which will show up days later. Usually, the funeral director will attend to shaving (NEoLCP/NNCG(PC) 2011).
- Clean the mouth and replace any dentures.
- If the family have not yet viewed the body, this could be an appropriate point for them to do so.
- Attach identification labels to the person according to local policy.
- Wrap the body in a clean sheet, securing it with tape but not too tight to prevent leaving marks.
- A body bag may be necessary if there are infection control issues. Consult the local infection control policy or contact the infection control nurse for advice.
- Dispose of the used equipment according to infection control principles and wash your hands.
- Make a list of, and store, property and jewellery according to local policy, in the presence of a witness. When packing soiled clothing, ask sensitively if the family would like them included or disposed of safely.
- Arrange for the porters to collect the body, or the undertaker in a residential setting.

ACTIVITY

Find and compare the local policy on care of the body after death with what you have read above.

As with any other clinical practices, there will be a local policy, probably developed by a multidisciplinary group including the hospital chaplaincy, which takes the local situation into account.

 ## Children: practice points – end of life care

For all aspects of end of life care for children, including care after death, see

Bennett, H. and Hopper, L. 2010. End of life care. In: Glasper, A., Aylott, A. and Battrick, C. (eds.) *Developing Practical Skills for Nursing Children and Young People*. London: Hodder Arnold, 616–23.

Macqueen, S., Bruce, E.A. and Gibson, F. 2012. Palliative care. In: *The Great Ormond Street Hospital Manual of Children's Nursing Practices*. Chichester: Wiley-Blackwell, 585–97.

Also see the 'Together for short lives' website at http://www.togetherforshortlives.org.uk/.

Summary

- Meeting the hygiene needs of a person who has died in a safe and culturally sensitive way is an essential part of nursing care.
- The extent to which care of the body after death is carried out may vary according to the setting and will be influenced by local policy and the individual family.

CHAPTER SUMMARY

Giving personal care, with attention to the individual's dignity, privacy and personal needs, is a fundamental and essential skill for nurses, and this care extends to the care of a person's body after death. Further key principles include cultural sensitivity and prevention of cross-infection. It is important to assess carefully how hygiene needs can be met for each individual, maintaining and promoting independence where possible. People with physical and mental health problems may be able to regain self-care skills with appropriate aids, encouragement and support. Teaching people to manage personal hygiene and dressing can be an important part of rehabilitation and should involve the multidisciplinary team and an individualised approach.

ACKNOWLEDGEMENT

The author acknowledges the contribution of Jenni Randall to this chapter in the third edition of this book.

REFERENCES

Alzheimer's Society. 2009. *Counting the Cost: Caring for People with Dementia on Acute Hospital Wards*. London: Alzheimer's Society.

Alzheimer's Society. 2011. Dental care and dementia. Factsheet 448. Available from: http://www.alzheimers.org.uk/site/scripts/documents_info.php?documentID = 138 (Accessed on 6 January 2013).

Ayliffe, G.A.J., Babb, J.R. and Taylor, L.J. 2001. *Hospital-Acquired Infection: Principles and Prevention*, 3rd edn. London: Arnold.

Baxter, C. 2002. Nursing with dignity. Part 5: Rastafarianism. *Nursing Times* 98(13): 42–3.

Brawley, E.C. 2002. Bathing environments: How to improve the bathing experience. *Alzheimer's Care Quarterly* 3: 38–41.

Briggs, M. 1997. Principles of closed wound care. *Journal of Wound Care* 6: 288–92.

British Society of Gerodontology. 2010. Guidelines for the oral healthcare of stroke survivors. Available from: http://www.gerodontology.com/forms/stroke_guidelines.pdf (Accessed on 6 January 2013).

Christmas, M. 2002. Nursing with dignity. Part 3: Christianity 1. *Nursing Times* 98(11): 37–9.

Clegg, A. 2003. Older South Asian patient and carer perceptions of culturally sensitive care in a community hospital setting. *Journal of Clinical Nursing* 12: 283–90.

Cowdell, F. 2010. Promoting skin health in older people. *Nursing Older People* 22(10): 21–6.

Department of Health (DH). 2002. *Action for Health – Health Action Plans and Health Facilitation*. London: DH.

Department of Health (DH). 2006. *From Values to Action: The Chief Nursing Officer's Review of Mental Health Nursing*. Gateway Reference 6140. London: DH.

Department of Health (DH). 2009. *Health Action Planning and Health Facilitation for People with Learning Disability – Good Practice Guidance*. Gateway Reference 11238. London: DH.

Department of Health (DH). 2010. *Essence of Care 2010 Benchmarks for Personal Hygiene*. Gateway Reference 14641. London: DH.

Dickinson, H., Watkins, C. and Leathley, M. 2001. The development of THROAT: The holistic and reliable oral assessment tool. *Clinical Effectiveness in Nursing* 5: 104–10.

Dorresteijn, J.A.N., Kriegsman, D.M.W., Assendelft, W.J.J., et al. 2010. Patient education for preventing diabetic foot ulceration. *Cochrane Database of Systematic Reviews* (5). Art. No.: CD001488. DOI: 10.1002/14651858.CD001488.pub3.

Downey, L. and Lloyd, D.L. 2008. Bed bathing patients in hospital. *Nursing Standard* 22(34): 35–40.

Geraghty, M. 2005. Nursing the unconscious patient. *Nursing Standard* 20(1): 54–64.

Gilchrist, B. 1990. Washing and dressing after surgery. *Nursing Times* 86(50): 71.

Gill, B.K. 2002. Nursing with dignity. Part 6: Sikhism. *Nursing Times* 98(14): 39–41.

Gústafsdóttir, M. 2011. Keeping up health promotion in specialized day care units for people with dementia. *American Journal of Alzheimer's Disease and Other Dementias* 26(6): 437–42.

Holland, K. and Hogg, C. 2010. *Cultural Awareness in Nursing and Health Care,* 2nd edn. London: Arnold.

Howell, M. and Thirlaway, S. 2004. Integrating foot care into the everyday clinical practice of nurses. *British Journal of Nursing* 13(8): 470–3.

Huff, M., Kinion, E., Kendra, M.A., et al. 2006. Self-esteem: A hidden concern in oral health. *Journal of Community Health Nursing* 23(4): 245–55.

Jones, C.V. 1998. The importance of oral hygiene in nutritional support. *British Journal of Nursing* 7: 74, 76–8, 80–3.

Medicine and Healthcare Products Regulatory Agency (MHRA). 2012. *Medical Device Alert*: *Oral Swabs with a Foam Head, All Manufacturers* (MDA/2012/020). Available from: http://www.mhra.gov.uk/Publications/Safetywarnings/MedicalDeviceAlerts/CON149697 (Accessed on 6 January 2013).

Montaldo, L., Montaldo, P., Papat, A., et al. 2010. Effects of saliva substitutes on oral status in patients with Type 2 diabetes. Original article: treatment. *Diabetic Medicine: A Journal of the British Diabetic Association* 27(11): 1280–3.

National End of Life Care Programme (NEoLCP) and National Nurse Consultant Group (Palliative Care) (NNCG(PC)). 2011. *Guidance for Staff Responsible for Care after Death.* Available from: http://www.endoflifecare.nhs.uk/search-resources/resources-search/publications.aspx (Accessed on 6 January 2012).

National Institute for Health and Clinical Excellence (NICE). 2004. *Type 2 Diabetes: Prevention and Management of Foot Problems.* Clinical Guidelines 10. London: NICE.

National Institute for Health and Clinical Excellence (NICE). 2011. *Diabetic Foot Problems: Inpatient Management of Diabetic Foot Problems.* Clinical Guidelines 119. London: NICE.

NHS Quality Improvement Scotland (NHS QIS). 2005. *Working with Dependent Older People to Achieve Good Oral Health.* Edinburgh: NHS QIS.

Paju, S. and Scannapieco, F. 2007. Oral bio films, periodontitis, and pulmonary infections. *Oral Diseases* 13(6): 508–12.

Parker, L. 2004. Infection control: Maintaining the personal hygiene of patients and staff. *British Journal of Nursing* 13(8): 474–8.

Pattison, N. 2008. Care of patients who have died. *Nursing Standard* 22(28): 42–8.

Pearson, L.S. and Hutton, J.L. 2002. A controlled trial to compare the ability of foam swabs and toothbrushes to remove dental plaque. *Journal of Advanced Nursing* 39: 480–9.

Pratt, R.J., Pellowe, C., Wilson, J.A., et al. 2007. National evidence-based guidelines for preventing healthcare-associated infections in NHS England. *Journal of Hospital Infection* 65(Suppl 1): S1–64.

Quested, B. and Rudge, T. 2003. Nursing care of dead bodies: A discursive analysis of last offices. *Journal of Advanced Nursing* 41: 553–60.

Rassool, G.H. 2000. The crescent and Islam: Healing, nursing and the spiritual dimension. Some considerations towards an understanding of the Islamic perspectives on caring. *Journal of Advanced Nursing* 32: 1476–84.

Royal College of Nursing (RCN). 2011. *Meeting the Health Needs of People with Learning Disabilities.* London: RCN.

Sloane, P., Rader, J., Barrick, A., et al. 1995. Bathing persons with dementia. *Gerontologist* 35: 672–8.

Thompson, J. 1999. Foot problems and care of feet. Part 2: Common disorders. *Community Practitioner* 72: 178–9.

Thurgood, G. 1994. Nurse maintenance of oral hygiene. *British Journal of Nursing* 3(7): 351–3.

Wilson, N.J., Cumella, S., Paramenter, T.R., et al. 2009. Penile hygiene: puberty, paraphimosis and personal care for men and boys with an intellectual disability. *Journal of Intellectual Disability Research* 53(2): 106–14.

Winkworth, J. 2003. Bathing is an intimate and valuable aspect of care. *Nursing Standard* 17(21): 30.

Xavier, G. 2000. The importance of mouth care in preventing infection. *Nursing Standard* 14(18): 47–51.

9 Meeting Elimination Needs

Lesley Baillie and Rachel Busuttil Leaver

Elimination of urine and faeces is an essential bodily function that we usually become independent in within the first few years of life, continence being an important milestone in a child's development (Slater-Smith 2010). Elimination is then usually a private function, but disability or physical or mental health problems often affect independence in elimination, and nurses then play an important role in preventing problems and maintaining comfort. Wherever possible, the aim will be to return to independent elimination, although some patients will need ongoing support with elimination, particularly where long-term, progressive conditions affect elimination. Promoting dignity and privacy is integral to meeting people's elimination needs; it requires great skill and sensitivity to carry out this care while preserving patients' self-esteem. Many other chapters in this book are relevant to care related to elimination, particularly Chapter 2, which focuses on communication, and Chapter 3, which focuses on preventing cross-infection. The Department of Health's (DH 2010) *Essence of Care Benchmarks* includes benchmarks for 'bladder, bowel and continence care', which are recommended as a resource.

This chapter includes the following topics:

- Assisting with elimination: Helping people to use the toilet, bedpans, urinals and commodes
- Urinalysis
- Collecting urine and stool specimens
- Caring for people who have urinary catheters
- Preventing and managing constipation
- Stoma care
- Promoting continence and managing incontinence

Recommended biology reading:

The following questions will help you to focus on the biology underpinning this chapter's skills. Use your recommended textbook to find out:

- What are the components of the urinary system?
- Within the kidney, blood is filtered. What forces are involved in filtration?
- Where does filtration occur? Which substances are not filtered out and why?
- What is the role of the juxtaglomerular apparatus?

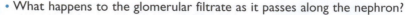

- What happens to the glomerular filtrate as it passes along the nephron?
- How and why does the concentration of urine vary?
- What factors affect renal function?
- Urine is stored in the bladder. How does the bladder expand as it fills up?
- What is micturition and how does it occur?
- What is cystitis? Why is it generally more common in females than in males?
- How can urinalysis be used to assess health?
- What factors can increase the risk of urinary tract infection (UTI)?
- What are the signs of UTI?
- What are the different regions of the digestive tract and their functions?
- How does food move through the digestive tract?
- How are peristalsis and segmentation distinguished?
- What is the consequence of increased gut motility? When might this occur?
- What is the gastro colic reflex?
- What do stools/faeces consist of?
- How do we defaecate?
- What is constipation?
- What factors increase the risk of constipation?
- How does the digestive tract respond to local infection or irritation?
- How does stress affect the digestive tract?

Rheumatoid arthritis

A chronic, progressive and disabling autoimmune disease that can affect any joint causing pain, swelling and disability. It is a systemic disease and can affect the whole body, including the lungs, heart and eyes.

Stoma

An artificial permanent opening on the body such as those made in the abdominal wall during a surgical procedure to form a colostomy, ileostomy or urinary conduit.

Ileostomy

The end of the small intestine, the ileum, is surgically brought out through an opening (stoma) in the abdomen.

PRACTICE SCENARIOS

The following scenarios illustrate situations where assistance with elimination is needed, and this chapter will refer to these scenarios throughout.

Adult

Jean is a 68-year-old woman who was diagnosed with cancer in the large bowel. Jean has **rheumatoid arthritis** and she has difficulty mobilising. She uses a motorised wheelchair and is cared for by her husband who is 75 years. He is well but has problems with his sight as he has cataracts. They live in a ground-floor council flat which has been adapted to enable her to be as independent as possible. Jean is able to transfer unaided. Jean has been admitted for surgery to have the tumour removed and a **stoma** formed. She is distressed that she has cancer and is concerned about undergoing surgery. She is worried that she will not cope afterwards and does not want to be 'more of a burden' on her husband.

The stoma care specialist spends time with Jean to reassure her and answer her questions. The nurse also marks the site on Jean's abdomen for stoma placement. Jean has a total large bowel resection with formation of an **ileostomy**. On return to the ward, Jean has a stoma bag over the newly formed stoma and a urinary catheter in her bladder. The discomfort from the abdominal wound means that Jean has trouble moving and is incapable of transferring herself independently. Due to her lack of mobility, it is decided that the catheter should be left in the bladder until she regains the ability to transfer to the toilet. She develops a urinary tract infection (UTI), which is treated with antibiotics.

Once she has recovered from surgery, Jean and her husband start to learn how to care for her stoma. She will not be discharged until she is able to do this, but she is finding it difficult to get used to the change and her progress is slow.

Learning disability

Mark is 28 years old and has a syndrome that includes a learning disability, impaired renal function and deteriorating sight. He eats with some assistance and walks short distances. He has very limited verbal communication, and he also has frequent UTIs and bowel disturbances – both constipation and diarrhoea. He is cared for by his mother, who manages his physical health needs. Mark is usually continent but requires prompting and support, due to his visual impairment. When he is ill or in new surroundings, he can become incontinent of both urine and faeces and wears continence pads at these times. His mother, who is Mark's **health facilitator**, has contacted the community learning disability nurse (CLDN) as she has noticed blood in his urine, which he is infrequently passing even though she is encouraging fluids. Mark is also not eating, has a raised temperature and his mother believes he is in pain. The nurse arranges to take samples of both urine and faeces, liaises with the general practitioner (GP) and Renal Consultant, who decide to admit Mark to hospital for further investigations. Mark's mother completes a 'passport' with him, which includes essential information to help hospital staff care for him.

Mental health

Bob is 58 years old. He has a long history of psychosis. During an acute psychotic episode, while admitted to an acute psychiatric ward, he was prescribed an atypical antipsychotic drug, clozapine, which is licensed for treatment of resistant schizophrenia only, due to its known side effects. These include effects on white blood cell levels, causing vulnerability to infection. After six weeks, there was a marked improvement in Bob's mental state, but he developed urinary incontinence at night (nocturnal enuresis). He found this extremely embarrassing and distressing, never having been incontinent before. Unfortunately, urinary incontinence is known to be another side effect of clozapine, the exact reasons for which are unknown. A urinalysis performed on admission had shown no abnormalities.

ASSISTING WITH ELIMINATION: HELPING PEOPLE TO USE THE TOILET, BEDPANS, URINALS AND COMMODES

> ### LEARNING OUTCOMES
>
> By the end of this section, you will be able to:
> 1 identify why a person might need help with elimination and what equipment you could use to give assistance;
> 2 discuss important principles for assisting with elimination.

Health facilitator

The role focuses on an individual's health outcomes and can be undertaken by a range of people including support workers, family carers, friends and advocates as well as health professionals, see *Health Action Planning and Health Facilitation for people with learning disabilities: good practice guidance* (DH 2009).

Learning outcome 1: Identify why a person might need help with elimination and what equipment you could use to give assistance

Reflect back on your practice experiences and write down all the reasons as to why a person might need help with elimination.

There are many situations where a person might need help with elimination. A patient's assessment should include elimination issues and assistance needed. For example, patients who are temporarily confined to bed following orthopaedic surgery, or people who are very weak or confused need help with elimination. Mark will need assistance as the hospital is an unfamiliar environment and he has impaired eyesight.

Whenever possible, a person should be helped to reach the toilet and so sufficient and accessible toilets should be available. The toilet is a more familiar environment for elimination (helpful for people with dementia, or who are disorientated or, like Mark, have a learning disability). The toilet is also more private; to eliminate in a ward, behind closed curtains, may not feel very private as noise and smell may be obvious. This potential embarrassment can lead to patients ignoring the need to defaecate, leading to constipation. You might need to accompany the person, sometimes with sticks, a walking frame or crutches (see Chapter 6, section on 'Assisting with mobilisation and preventing falls'). If patients are unable to walk, you could take them to the toilet in a wheelchair.

If the person cannot leave the bedside, you can use equipment to help them.

What equipment could assist with elimination? There may be examples of equipment in the skills laboratory or within your practice setting.

The commode

If a patient is very ill or weak, or has a great deal of invasive equipment attached to them, it may be safer to eliminate by the bedside. When making these decisions, check their care plan and seek advice if you are unsure. If a patient can get out of bed, a commode is preferable to a bedpan, as it promotes a more conducive, comfortable position for elimination. A commode has a pan underneath, which is removed after use and either macerated (if disposable) or cleaned in the washer–disinfector, if reusable.

Bedpans/urinals

Some people must stay in bed for medical reasons, so they require bedpans or urinals. There are standard bedpans, which patients sit up on, and flat 'slipper' pans, which patients roll on to – suitable when someone has to remain flat. There are both male and female urinals. Male patients sometimes find it difficult to urinate in sitting or lying positions, so they may need assistance to stand, if their medical condition allows. Female urinals are useful for women lying flat (e.g. following back surgery) or where changing position is difficult, perhaps due to pain.

Learning outcome 2: Discuss important principles for assisting with elimination

ACTIVITY

If you are assisting someone with elimination, what do you think would be important principles of care?

Box 9.1 lists the principles which you could have identified; these are discussed next.

Approachability and communication

> ### Frequency
>
> Passing urine more frequently than about seven times in 24 hours. A common symptom arising from conditions such as enlarged prostate and UTI.

People needing help with elimination often describe this as embarrassing and even distressing. The authors have known patients who admit to reducing their fluid intake, thus increasing their risk of complications such as a UTI, so that they need not ask for help so often. Some people have urinary symptoms such as **frequency** and others have urgency – where they cannot 'hold on' for very long. Elstad et al. (2010) identified a stigma associated with urgency and frequency with people experiencing embarrassment and shame, and Wareing (2005) found that men who experienced severe urgency described how 'having to hold on' was accompanied by panic and embarrassment. If a nurse does not appear approachable, then people may not feel comfortable asking for help and may experience emotional and physical discomfort, incontinence, retention of urine or constipation.

If people have communication difficulties, nurses must observe for non-verbal cues (e.g. restlessness or agitation). Sometimes a picture board (with a picture of a toilet) can be used to help communicate. Mark's passport should include information about how Mark communicates that he needs to go to the toilet, which may be through a signing system, including gestures. If the nurses ask Mark whether he needs to go to the toilet, they should give him enough time to answer, as processing information may take longer for people with learning disabilities. While assisting patients with elimination, nurses can build their relationship through conversation, which should help put the person at ease. Nurses should speak privately and quietly when assisting with elimination; using non-verbal communication may reduce the verbal communication needed, with less risk of other patients overhearing.

Box 9.1 Principles to follow when assisting with elimination

- Approachability and communication
- Privacy and dignity
- Promptness
- Prevention of cross-infection
- Observation
- Prevention of accidents
- Promotion of independence
- Promotion of hygiene and comfort

Privacy and dignity

If privacy and dignity are not addressed, people may feel embarrassed, degraded and experience a loss of self-esteem. Always ensure that bedside curtains are pulled, shut properly, or the toilet door closed, and that patients are covered up while on the bedpan or commode. The British Geriatrics Society's (2007) campaign to ensure that vulnerable people can use the toilet in private in hospitals and care homes has produced a best practice toolkit. The standards addressed accessibility, timeliness, equipment, safety, choice, privacy, cleanliness, hygiene and respectful language. Nurses should be person-centred and approach each person as an individual, being sensitive and aware of the effect of cultural norms and religious beliefs (Heath 2009). For example, some patients may prefer a nurse of the same sex to help them, and modesty within South Asian cultures is particularly important (Holland and Hogg 2010).

Promptness

People with certain types of incontinence (urge incontinence) will not be able to wait to pass urine (see later section 'Promoting continence and managing incontinence'). Ransack et al. (2006) found that care home staff contributed to residents' incontinence by not attending to them quickly enough. Clearly, such a situation is unacceptable as incontinence is distressing for people. If patients cannot attempt to open their bowels when they feel the need, faeces are pushed back into the sigmoid colon or remain in the rectum, where water continues to be reabsorbed. Thus, faeces become harder, more painful and difficult to pass, which may lead to constipation. Nurses should prioritise meeting elimination needs as patients are in a powerless position, dependent for help with this basic need. When patients have finished eliminating, nurses should respond promptly, to avoid discomfort and maintain safety. Patients should be given their call bell and shown how to use it.

Prevention of cross-infection

Patients in hospital are often particularly vulnerable to infection owing to their medical conditions (see Chapter 3 for more information), so measures to prevent cross-infection must be scrupulously applied. These include careful hand washing and application of personal protective equipment – non-sterile gloves and aprons – to prevent hands and uniform being contaminated (Pratt et al. 2007). Hands must be decontaminated after glove removal (National Institute for Health and Clinical Excellence [NICE] 2012a). Equipment used to assist with elimination must be cleaned effectively. Disposable bedpans and urinals are disposed of in macerators. Non-disposable urinals and bedpans should be disinfected by thermal disinfection (exposure to hot water or steam), and supports for disposable bedpans should be washed after use, with a chlorine-releasing agent, if contaminated with faeces (Fraise and Bradley 2009). The seat and frame of commodes should be cleaned after use with particular attention to the arms, and if the seat is soiled, or used by a patient with an enteric infection, it should be disinfected with a chlorine-releasing agent, rinsed and dried (Fraise and Bradley 2009). However, Bucior and Cochrane (2010) found that commodes were not always cleaned adequately.

Urine is normally sterile, but it is often contaminated while voiding, by bacteria present around the urethral opening (Gould 1994). Urine provides an excellent medium for bacterial growth, especially Gram-negative bacteria (*Pseudomonas, Klebsiella, Escherichia coli, Proteus*), which can survive only when water and inorganic ions are present (Gould 1994). Urine passed into a bedpan or urinal should therefore be disposed of quickly, as standing at room temperature allows any bacteria present to divide rapidly, doubling approximately every 30 minutes (Gould 1994), thus becoming a reservoir of infection.

When a patient has diarrhoea that could be infective, cross-infection measures needed are prompt and careful disposal of the faeces, use of non-sterile gloves and aprons, scrupulous hand washing and source isolation (see Chapter 3). When caring for people with diarrhoea caused by *Clostridium difficile*, alcohol hand rub is ineffective against the spores produced, so wearing non-sterile gloves, with hand washing following glove removal, is essential.

Observation

There are many useful observations you can make when assisting with elimination, such as assessing the person's ability to move, or about the condition of their skin (see Table 9.1). If the person's urine output is measured, the jug used must be disposed of or cleaned in the bedpan washer, and a fluid chart will be used to record fluid balance. Chapter 10 provides a detailed description of fluid balance measurement. The Bristol stool chart can be used to record stool type (see Figure 9.1).

ACTIVITY

When next in placement, look at any charts used for monitoring urine output and stools. What are the types of fluids listed for input and output? Does the stool chart incorporate the Bristol stool chart, as shown in Figure 9.1?

Prevention of accidents

Highlighting the hazardous nature of elimination, Thompson's (2007) falls and continence audit found that 36.8% of falls were related to toileting or incontinence. A moving and handling risk assessment should be carried out (see Chapter 6 for more information), and the moving and handling care plan should specify the equipment needed and the number of staff required. If patients are using bedpans in bed, you must ensure that they do not topple over. Balancing on a bedpan can be difficult so it may be safer to raise the bed or trolley rails for support. The National Patient Safety Agency (NPSA 2007) recommended that organisations should have a policy about bedrail use – a risk assessment form may be required as they can be hazardous. You must be sure about your reasons for using them (i.e. not using them as a form of restraint).

Using the commode by the bedside is potentially hazardous. You should ensure that brakes are secure and that there are no fluids or slippery substances on

Table 9.1: Observations to make when assisting with elimination

Observation	Explanation/examples
Emotional well-being	The person's mood and ability to cope with a situation.
Cognitive functioning	The person's memory of what to do, ability to retain information and follow instructions.
Mobility	The patient's ability to move on to a bedpan, to transfer on to a commode or toilet, or stand to use a urinal.
	Whether any apparent discomfort/pain, breathlessness or weakness when moving.
Skin condition	Redness or broken areas on sacrum or buttocks; soreness of groins, perineum, penis or vulva.
Self-care ability	Physical/mental ability to remove or adapt clothing, before and after elimination, and to carry out hygiene afterwards.
Amount and frequency of urine output	A fluid input/output chart may be maintained if there are concerns about fluid balance.
	Urine will be measured in a jug and recorded in millilitres. Pads can be weighed: 1 g = 1 mL.
	Poor urine output (oliguria) could occur in dehydration or shock.
	No urinary output (anuria) could mean retention of urine.
	Frequent small amounts of urine might indicate a urinary tract infection (UTI).
	Monitoring of frequency and amount may be part of a bladder re-education programme.
Appearance of urine	See Urinalysis, next section.
	Very dark, concentrated urine might indicate dehydration, and smoky, offensive urine might indicate UTI.
	Presence of blood may be due to kidney trauma or disease.
Appearance of stools	Consistency and frequency of stools; hard and infrequent stools could indicate constipation, or frequent and loose stools could indicate diarrhoea, which could be infected.
	A stool chart to record frequency, appearance and consistency might be maintained: the Bristol stool chart is often used so that descriptions of stools are reliable (see Fig. 9.1).
	If infection is suspected, a stool specimen will be collected and sent.

the floor. You must assess whether the person is safe to leave: are they confused and likely to try to stand up alone and fall? Privacy is a very important principle when assisting people with elimination but has to be balanced against safety. A falls risk assessment scale can help to identify people who are at risk of falls (see Chapter 6).

Promotion of independence

While assisting with elimination, you should assess ability and promote independence while also maintaining hygiene and safety. Learning how to use the toilet unaided, after a **stroke,** for example, may take some time, and both short- and long-term goals may be necessary. The study by Clark and Rugg (2005) highlighted the importance of gaining independence in using the toilet for people following stroke to prevent decreased self-esteem. Nurses can liaise with occupational therapists to facilitate a return to people's normal methods and if that is not possible, how to assist patients to adjust. Education could include teaching people how to manage transfers safely (e.g. from wheelchair to toilet), how to remove clothing or how to walk to the toilet on crutches.

> **Stroke**
>
> Cerebral damage caused either by decreased blood flow or by haemorrhage. Effects vary, but a stroke often causes paralysis down one side of the body (hemiplegia), speech and swallowing difficulty, and elimination difficulties.

Type 1		Separate hard lumps, like nuts (hard to pass)
Type 2		Sausage-shaped but lumpy
Type 3		Like a sausage but with cracks on its surface
Type 4		Like a sausage or snake, smooth and soft
Type 5		Soft blobs with clear-cut edges (passed easily)
Type 6		Fluffy pieces with ragged edges, a mushy stool
Type 7		Watery, no solid pieces, entirely liquid

Figure 9.1: Bristol stool chart. [Reproduced with kind permission from Taylor & Francis Ltd. (www.tandf.co.uk/journals). From Lewis, S.J. and Heaton, K.W. 1997. Stool form scale as a useful guide to intestinal track time. *Scandinavian Journal of Gastroenterology*, 32, 920–4.]

To promote independence for people with learning disabilities, orientate them to their environment well, showing them where the toilet is and take them to the same toilet by the same route each time. These steps could also be helpful for people who have dementia. Ideally, Mark's bed would be situated near the toilet. The ward nurses could show Mark where the toilet is and how the facilities work. For example, Mark may be used to a toilet with a pull handle and separate taps, while the ward might have a toilet with a button to press for flushing and a mixer tap. Mark's mother will know the best way of explaining this to him. A toilet door which is a different colour to the wall, with a picture of a toilet on, will help people with visual impairments and those with dementia.

Promotion of hygiene and comfort

For people whose elimination needs are met by their bedside, you must assist with hygiene. Within some cultures, which emphasise cleanliness, people are required to cleanse the perineal area with running water after using the toilet (Heath 2009). When you take people to the toilet, ensure that they can wash their hands at the sink afterwards. Always ensure access to toilet tissue, and if people cannot wipe themselves, then do it for them, or give assistance to people who are learning or relearning this skill. With female patients, always wipe the vulval area from front to back to prevent transmission of bowel bacterial flora (such as *E. coli*) from the anal area to the urethra. Females have a short urethra (4 cm), which can easily become contaminated by such bacteria. In Asia, the left hand is traditionally reserved for washing underneath after using the toilet, the right hand being used for eating and other activities (Holland and Hogg 2010). Make sure that the patient does not become cold during elimination, by covering their legs with a blanket. Ensure that anyone using a bedpan is comfortably supported with pillows. You will promote psychological comfort by your attitude and communication (see Chapter 2 for more information).

Children: practice points – nappy changing

Infants and small children normally wear nappies until they are toilet-trained, usually by 3 years of age. Some children who have not yet reached successful toilet training or who have developmental delay may require nappies. Nappy-changing practice is described in detail in:

Himsworth, J. 2010. Caring for personal hygiene needs. In: Glasper, A., Aylott, M. and Battrick, C. (eds.) *Developing Practical Skills for Nursing Children and Young People.* London: Hodder Arnold, 188–202.

Macqueen, S., Bruce, E.A. and Gibson, F. 2012. Personal hygiene and pressure ulcer prevention. In: *The Great Ormond Street Hospital Manual of Children's Nursing Practices.* Chichester: Wiley-Blackwell, 167–220.

Summary

- Many health problems lead to people needing help with elimination.
- Various items of equipment are available to assist people who are unable to get to the toilet. Nurses must assess which is appropriate for each individual.
- There are important principles that must be followed when helping people with elimination to ensure that care is dignified, effective and safe.

URINALYSIS

Urinalysis is the testing of urine for the presence of various substances. This simple, non-intrusive test provides useful information about an individual's renal and urinary function (Beynon and Nicholls 2004).

You should be able to access urinalysis equipment either in the skills laboratory or in your practice setting.

LEARNING OUTCOMES

By the end of this section, you will be able to:

1 understand the process of urinalysis;
2 show insight into the meaning of urinalysis results and what action to take if abnormal results are obtained;
3 identify in what situations urinalysis should be performed.

Learning outcome 1: Understand the process of urinalysis

ACTIVITY

Look at the reagent strips that are used to test urine in the skills laboratory or in a practice placement. Find the expiry date and note the substances that are tested for and the timings for reading the results on the side of the bottle.

Reagent strips must be in date, and stored and used properly, otherwise results may not be accurate. The Medicines and Healthcare Products Regulatory Agency (MHRA 2011) advises that the strip container lid must be closed immediately after removing a strip so that the remaining strips do not deteriorate. The full range of substances which can be tested in a urinalysis are leucocytes, nitrite, urobilinogen, protein, pH, blood, specific gravity, ketones, bilirubin and glucose. The reagent strips that you looked at may include this full range, but there are also strips available that test for only a selection or even just one substance, such as blood.

Conducting a urinalysis

Figure 9.2 summarises key points for conducting a urinalysis, with some additional explanatory notes and rationale given below.

Urine for analysis should be collected in a clean, dry, preservative-free container, and infection control aspects should be adhered to throughout the procedure (MHRA 2011). First-voided morning urine is best for a urinalysis as it is most concentrated. Ideally, the urine should be tested immediately or within 4 hours. Otherwise, you can refrigerate the specimen, but you must let it return to room temperature before testing. It is particularly important to use fresh urine when testing for bilirubin and urobilinogen as these compounds are relatively unstable when exposed to room temperature and light. When testing for nitrite, use a first morning sample if possible so that the urine will have been in contact with bacteria, if present, for at least 3 hours.

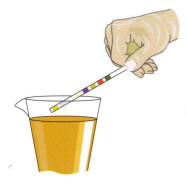

Requirements
- Reagent strip and bottle
- Freshly voided urine in a clean (preferably sterile) container

Procedure
- Observe urine for colour, consistency and smell
- Immerse all reagent areas in fresh urine and remove immediately
- Run the edge along the rim of the container to remove excess urine
- Hold the strip horizontally to prevent mixing of the chemicals from adjacent areas and prevent soiling of hands with urine
- Compare the test areas with the corresponding colour chart at the specified time or analyse in electronic reader following reader's instructions

Figure 9.2: Conducting a urinalysis: key points.

> ### Jaundice
>
> A condition characterised by yellowness of skin, whites of eyes, mucous membranes and body fluids due to the presence of bile pigment resulting from excess bilirubin in the blood.

When testing urine, always observe the appearance of the urine sample first. Normal fresh urine is pale to dark yellow or amber in colour, and clear. If the urine is red or red–brown, this could be from a food dye, eating beetroot, a drug or the presence of haemoglobin. If there are many red blood cells present, the urine will be cloudy as well. A strongly yellow sample could indicate **jaundice**.

The smell of the urine should also be noted; freshly voided, non-infected urine should be virtually odourless, but if infected, urine may smell offensive.

The strips must be read accurately as per the timings given on the bottle. Nurses on a busy ward may not wait the correct amount of time before reading the result, and lighting and colour vision may affect readings. The MHRA (2011) advises that coloured charts used for reading results must be stored away from direct sunlight to prevent fading, and the strip must be read at the correct time in good light. There are electronic readers available which can help to minimise reader error, leading to greater uniformity and consistency in readings. These readers also print the results, include the time and date, and indicate abnormal readings. The MHRA (2011) advises that the readers should be maintained and cleaned correctly and checked regularly; only strips validated for use with this device should be used.

Learning outcome 2: Show insight into the meaning of urinalysis results and what action to take if abnormal results are obtained

If you look on the side of the urinary reagent bottle, you will find the key as to what each colour is testing for, the normal results, and abnormal results, which should be reported. Table 9.2 indicates the significance of abnormalities and suggests some possible actions. A nursing dictionary will help you with some of the technical terms included.

When to collect a urine specimen for microscopy and culture

A urinalysis can help in determining whether to send a urine specimen for microscopy, culture and sensitivity (MC&S). In this laboratory test, the urine is

Table 9.2: Clinical significance of test results

Significance of positive results	Commonest causes of abnormalities and possible action to be taken
Glucose	
Not normally detectable in urine	• In people with raised blood glucose concentration: diabetes mellitus or glucose infusion
Found when its concentration exceeds the renal threshold	• In people without raised blood glucose concentration: pregnancy or renal glycosuria
	Action: If positive, a blood glucose measurement should be performed, and further action may follow
Bilirubin	
Presence in urine indicates an excess of conjugated bilirubin in plasma	• Liver cell injury: e.g. viral or drug-induced hepatitis, paracetamol overdose, late-stage cirrhosis
Note that stale urine may give a false-negative result	• Biliary tract obstruction: e.g. by gall stones, carcinoma of the head of pancreas
	Action: Should always be reported as further investigations will be needed
Ketones	
Indicates accumulation of acetoacetate secondary to excessive breakdown of body fat	• Fasting, particularly with fever and/or vomiting
Some drugs (e.g. L-dopa) may give a false-positive result	• Diabetic ketoacidosis
	Action: Urgent action is needed if the person is known or suspected to have diabetes
Specific gravity	
A measure of total solute concentration in urine	• High values found in dehydration, or in impaired kidney function (e.g. chronic renal failure)
In health, varies widely according to the need to excrete water and solutes	• Low values found in people with intact renal function and high fluid intake, diabetes insipidus, chronic renal failure, hypercalcaemia, hypokalaemia
	Action: Depends on likely cause and results of other investigations
Blood	
May be haematuria (intact blood cells) or haemoglobinuria (free haemoglobin, excreted from plasma or liberated from red cells in the urine)	*Haematuria:* • Due to kidney disorders (e.g. glomerulonephritis, polycystic kidneys, tumour) • Due to urinary tract disorders (e.g. stones, tumour, infection, benign prostatic enlargement) *Haemoglobinuria:* • Severe haemolysis (e.g. sickle cell disease crisis) • Breakdown of red cells in urine (especially when urine is dilute and testing is delayed) *Action:* Should be reported; follow-up will depend on other tests and the clinical picture

(Continued)

Table 9.2: (Continued)

Significance of positive results	Commonest causes of abnormalities and possible action to be taken
pH	
In health, the pH of uncontaminated urine ranges from 4.5 to 8.0	• Low values found in acidaemia as in diabetic ketoacidosis; also starvation or potassium depletion
A high pH will be found if testing stale urine, so *such specimens should not be used*	• High values found in stale urine, alkalaemia (except when due to potassium depletion), for example, due to vomiting and consumption of large amounts of antacids, renal tubular acidosis, urinary tract infection with ammonia-forming organisms
	Action: Depends on other test results
Protein	
A range of proteins can be detected but the reagent is most sensitive to albumin, so a negative result does not rule out presence of other proteins	• Albuminuria may be found in acute and chronic glomerulonephritis, urinary tract infection, glomerular involvement in systemic lupus erythematosus, nephrotic syndrome, pre-eclampsia, fever, heart failure and postural (orthostatic) proteinuria
	Action: Transient results are seldom important but persistent positive results need investigating for underlying cause
	Other test results and clinical picture should be considered
Urobilinogen	*Increased secretion:*
Urinary excretion of urobilinogen reflects the combined effects of conversion of bilirubin to urobilinogen in the gut and reabsorption into the bloodstream	• May be due to increased production (e.g. in red blood cell disorders such as sickle cell disease), or due to decreased uptake by the liver (e.g. in viral hepatitis and cirrhosis)
Note that false-negatives are found in stale urine	*Decreased secretion:*
	• May be due to biliary tract obstruction (e.g. gallstones, carcinoma of pancreas), or due to sterilisation of the colon by unabsorbable antibiotics (e.g. neomycin), which prevents bacterial conversion of bilirubin to urobilinogen
	Action: Urgent investigation is needed
Nitrite	
Most organisms which infect the urinary tract contain an enzyme system that catalyses the conversion of dietary nitrate, which is normally present in urine, to nitrite, which is not found in urine unless there is a urinary tract infection	• Presence indicates urinary tract infection due to nitrite-producing organisms
	• However, absence does not exclude infection, as some organisms are unable to convert dietary nitrate to nitrite
	• False-negatives are also found if there is insufficient dietary nitrate, or urine has not been in the bladder long enough (4 hours is ideal) for the conversion to take place
	Action: Specimen should be sent for microscopy and culture
Leucocytes	
Will be present when some of the leucocytes that have entered inflamed tissue from the blood are shed in the urine	Indicates a urinary tract infection, especially when it is accompanied by acute inflammation of the urinary tract
	Action: Specimen should be sent for microscopy and culture

Source: Adapted from Bayer. 1997. *Urine Analysis: The Essential Information.* Newbury: Bayer; Bayer. 1998. *A Practical Guide to Urine Analysis.* Newbury: Bayer.

examined under the microscope, and the urine is cultured to see whether bacteria grow and what antibiotics the bacteria are sensitive to. The presence of nitrite in urine is particularly indicative of UTI as over 90% of urinary pathogens can reduce urinary nitrate to nitrite if they are in contact with urine in the bladder for a minimum of 3 hours (Panagamuwa et al. 2004). A positive test for leucocyte esterase (an enzyme within white blood cells) can also indicate infection.

The British Infection Association (BIA) and Health Protection Agency (HPA) (2011) provide a detailed and evidence-based flow chart for diagnosing UTI and when to send urine for culture. They recommend that with older people who have a positive urinalysis but are asymptomatic of a UTI, urine should not be sent for culture routinely, and that two or more UTI symptoms (especially dysuria, pyrexia over 38 degrees or new incontinence) should be present before sending off urine for culture. Older people, especially women and people with urinary catheters, may have bacteria present in their urine (termed 'bacteriuria') without an infection being present (Nazarko 2009). For people aged under 65 years who have mild UTI symptoms and cloudy urine, a urinalysis should be performed and if nitrite is present, a UTI is likely. However, if urine is negative to nitrite but positive to leucocytes, a UTI diagnosis is possible though not definite and sending urine for culture is appropriate to assist diagnosis (BIA and HPA 2011).

The National Institute for Health and Clinical Excellence (NICE 2006) recommends that all women with urinary incontinence should have a urinalysis performed, and if it is positive to leucocytes and nitrites, and symptomatic of UTI, a mid-stream specimen (see the next section) should be sent for MC&S. It is worth noting that typical symptoms of UTI, such as pain on micturition (dysuria), frequency, fever and sometimes loin or suprapubic pain may not be present in older people (Midthun et al. 2004; Woodford and George 2009).

Learning outcome 3: Identify in what situations urinalysis should be performed

ACTIVITY

For each person in the scenarios at the start of the chapter, identify why a urinalysis would be appropriate.

A urinalysis gives many clues about a person's health and well-being, so a nursing assessment of a newly referred or admitted person should always include a urinalysis. Urinalysis is also performed for other people at risk of developing health problems that can be indicated through a urinalysis, for example, after an abdominal injury (to screen for blood which might indicate renal damage).

When Bob was first admitted, a urinalysis could have been performed as part of a general health screen. He should have been reassured that it is routine and there is nothing to be worried about and given a clean container in which to collect urine the morning after admission. When he developed urinary incontinence, he should have been asked for a further morning specimen to rule out UTI, which can predispose to, or compound, urinary incontinence. Remember that taking clozapine has rendered him more vulnerable to infection.

Mark is known to have a renal impairment and frequent UTIs. The CLDN has already collected a urine specimen. On admission to the ward, a urinalysis will give immediate information about his renal function and indicate whether he could have a UTI. Jean's urine would have been tested on admission to hospital as part of her general health assessment, including the likelihood of a UTI preoperatively. Postoperatively, Jean has a urinary catheter which is accompanied by a risk of UTI, which the scenario states did occur. If Jean was symptomatic of a UTI, a catheter specimen of urine (CSU) (see Box 9.3) would be obtained to test her urine initially before sending a sample for culture.

Children: practice points – urinalysis

UTI symptoms in infants and small children are often non-specific, so NICE (2007a) guidelines advise conducting a urinalysis for those with an unexplained temperature of 38 degrees or higher, as well as for children and infants with UTI symptoms.

Pregnancy and birth: practice points – urinalysis

Pregnant women must have their urine tested at each antenatal assessment. Protein in the urine, in conjunction with oedema or hypertension, could indicate pre-eclampsia, a potentially serious complication of pregnancy or infection. Glucose in the urine could indicate gestational diabetes, a type of diabetes which affects women in pregnancy. See www.nice.org.uk/CG063

Summary

- Urinalysis is a non-invasive and frequently performed practical skill that can provide very useful information about people's health status.
- To obtain an accurate result, the steps in a urinalysis must be carried out carefully with an appropriately collected specimen.
- It is important to understand the significance of abnormal results and the subsequent plan of action.

COLLECTING URINE AND STOOL SPECIMENS

In this section, common types of urine specimen and the collection of a stool (faeces) specimen are discussed. It is often necessary to obtain specimens such as these from patients/clients as they can provide important diagnostic information, which impacts on management and care. General principles of specimen collection are considered in Chapter 3, but key points can be found in Box 9.2.

LEARNING OUTCOMES

By the end of this section, you will be able to discuss the collection of:
1 a catheter specimen of urine (CSU);
2 a mid-stream specimen of urine (MSU);
3 a 24-hour specimen of urine;
4 a stoma urine specimen;
5 a stool specimen.

Learning outcome 1: Discuss the collection of a catheter specimen of urine (CSU)

A CSU is often taken for bacteriological examination to find out if treatment is required when symptoms of a UTI are present in a person who is catheterised. However, a person with a catheter may not display these symptoms, and in an older and/or confused person the symptoms can be still less apparent. As discussed earlier in the chapter, a CSU may have to be collected from Jean if a UTI is suspected. The risk of infection increases by 5–8% each day of catheterisation (Maki and Tambyah 2001), so the longer the catheter is left in place, the more likely the patient will have bacteriuria. Bacteria prefer to live on surfaces rather than in a solution such as urine. A catheter provides this surface and bacteria can coat it and form what is called a **biofilm**. Bacteria that live in a biofilm are more resistant to treatment, so that even if eliminated in urine by using antibiotics, the ones on the catheter will persist and recontaminate the urine (Saye 2007).

Box 9.2 Collection of specimens: Key points

- Adherence to infection control standard principles (hand hygiene, personal protective equipment)
- Clear explanations
- Maintenance of patient/client privacy, dignity and comfort
- Avoidance of contamination of the specimen
- Prompt transportation to the laboratory, or retention in a designated specimen refrigerator for up to 24 hours
- Clear labelling
- Correct and comprehensive accompanying information
- Documentation in patient/client notes of the date and time of the specimen collection

It is important to distinguish between bacteriuria and a 'clinical infection'. Bacteria can colonise the urinary tract without invading the surrounding tissues (bacteriuria), often not causing clinical symptoms, and not being susceptible to treatment. However, clinical infection involving invasion of surrounding tissues, often producing symptoms in infected people, requires treatment.

Whatever the classification of the infection, if a specimen is considered necessary, then nurses must use aseptic technique and sterile equipment. This is to reduce the risk of further contaminating the specimen and potentially introducing different bacteria to those from the patient. This is particularly important since the treatment is based on the results of the bacteriological examination of the urine.

Urine should be obtained from the special sampling port on the drainage system; the catheter and drainage system should never be disconnected to take a specimen. You should adhere to manufacturers' instructions concerning the number of times the port may be punctured safely. Urine should never be taken from the catheter bag because the bag acts as a reservoir where microorganisms can multiply. It is thus likely to contain greater numbers of microorganisms than urine accessed via the port. The bag can also be heavily contaminated from environmental sources. Box 9.3 outlines the key principles to follow when taking a CSU.

Learning outcome 2: Discuss the collection of a mid-stream specimen of urine (MSU)

The MSU is collected if a UTI is suspected in a non-catheterised patient, and it is obtained using a clean procedure. It is a useful aid in diagnosis and the aim is to collect the mid-stream specimen, which is not contaminated by microorganisms outside the urinary tract.

How MSUs should be collected has been the subject of much research but the evidence base for best practice remains unclear. People have often been asked to undertake perineal cleansing with sterile swabs and saline prior to giving an MSU to prevent contamination. However, a Canadian study concluded that contamination of urine specimens from women with acute dysuria who cleaned the perineal area prior to collection did not differ from those who did not (Blake and Doherty 2006). A study on toilet-trained children, however, found that those who did not clean their genital area did have a higher contamination rate than those who did (Vaillancourt et al. 2007). However, it is debatable whether results on children are transferable to adults. The Health Protection Agency (2012) recommends thorough peri-urethral cleaning but also states that the need for this has been questioned in both men and women. It is therefore good practice to assess the patient's level of personal hygiene and follow local guidelines regarding peri-urthral cleaning when obtaining an MSU. It is theorised that the first part of the stream flushes away microorganisms from the first part of the urethra, and that the urine does not flow over the perineum as long as there is sufficient urine in the bladder to produce a good stream. If there is insufficient urine in the bladder, the specimen should be collected later. The equipment required and key points of the procedure are listed in Box 9.4.

Box 9.3 Collection of a catheter specimen of urine: equipment and key points

Equipment
- Alcohol swab, receiver, specimen pot, request form, syringe (20 mL). A needle (21 g bore) if the sampling port is not needleless.
- A gate clamp may be required.

Key points
- Adhere to general points outlined in Box 9.2.
- Locate the sample port on the catheter bag tubing. Needleless sampling ports are preferable but some drainage bags have a latex port which requires a needle and syringe to aspirate the urine.
- If there is no urine present in the catheter tubing, clamp the tubing below the sample port until sufficient urine collects. Never clamp the actual catheter, as this could damage it.
- Swab the sample port with alcohol swab and allow the port to dry.
- If using a needleless port, attach a syringe directly to the port to withdraw the urine.

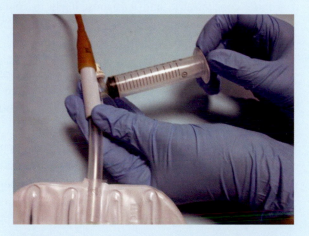

- If the sampling port is not needleless, insert the needle into the port at an angle of 45 degrees to prevent going straight through the tubing.

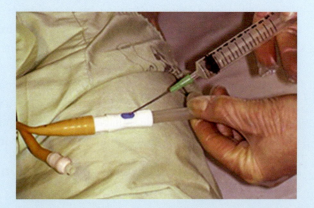

- Withdraw the required amount of urine, remove the top from the specimen pot and fill the pot with urine. Dispose of the syringe (and needle if used) into a sharps box immediately. Replace the cap on the pot.

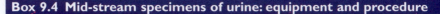

> **Box 9.4 Mid-stream specimens of urine: equipment and procedure**
>
> **Equipment**
> A toilet/commode/bedpan/urinal as appropriate, specimen pot and request form, disposable gloves
>
> **Procedure**
> - Adhere to key points in Box 9.2.
> - Follow local policy as regards meatal cleansing.
> - Ask the person to start passing urine as usual, then catch some urine (about 20 mL: about 2.5 cm up the pot) in the specimen pot, and then finish voiding into the toilet or commode. Wear gloves and assist the person, if necessary.

If a urine specimen is being collected because of suspected tuberculosis (TB) or cancer of the urinary tract, then an early-morning specimen is preferable because it is more concentrated, and it is most likely to contain the tubercle bacillus or malignant cells (Beynon and Nicholls 2004). Usually, three consecutive early-morning specimens are required.

ACTIVITY

Read through Box 9.4. As you can see, the person's cooperation and understanding would be needed. Look at the practice scenarios: to what extent might you achieve understanding and consent from Bob and Mark?

You are more likely to gain informed consent and cooperation from anyone if you explain the procedure and its importance carefully and confidentially. You should respect the person's right to privacy and dignity throughout the whole episode of care. Remember that what may be a simple and routine procedure in your eyes may feel quite different to the person concerned. It is likely that Bob would be able to produce the specimen with little assistance. Mark may have become used to giving urine samples at his GP's surgery because of his frequent urine infections. One approach would be for his mother or a nurse to take him to the toilet about 30 minutes after a drink (assuming he is not being kept 'nil by mouth') and try to collect the specimen in a clean receptacle in the toilet or, if possible, catch the mid-stream in a pot for him, while wearing gloves. This approach can also be used for people who are confused.

It can be difficult to produce an MSU, especially if patients are confined to bed. Adaptations will need to be made, for example, placing a waterproof pad beneath the patient to soak up any possible spillage, helping to diminish fears of wetting the bed. Allowing people plenty of time and not rushing is also important.

Learning outcome 3: Discuss the collection of a 24-hour specimen of urine

Sometimes, it is necessary to collect the total volume of urine passed within a 24-hour period. This is then analysed within the laboratory so that the 24-hour excretion of a variety of key metabolites (e.g. protein, creatinine) can be assessed (Beynon and Nicholls 2004). Box 9.5 outlines the equipment needed and the procedure.

Box 9.5 Twenty-four-hour urine collection: equipment and key points

Equipment

A jug, a 24-hour urine collection container, gloves

Procedure

• Assess the person's ability to participate in the collection. When the person next passes urine, it is discarded. This marks the beginning of the 24-hour period for collection.

• Label the container with the person's details (name, ward and hospital number) and the time and date the collection started.

• Put a sign on the bed or door of the room belonging to the person indicating that a 24-hour urine collection is in place, the date and time it started and when it will finish.

• Every time the person passes urine, it is collected and poured into the container. The person may be able to do this independently or may need assistance. Check their understanding and ability.

• Ask the person to empty their bladder just before the end of the 24-hour collection period.

• Advise that this ends the collection period.

• Remove the sign from the door or bed.

• Clean or discard the jug used.

• Record the completion time and ensure that the urine collection and laboratory request forms are dispatched correctly as soon as possible.

Note: If one sample of urine becomes contaminated or is accidentally discarded, the test must be discontinued and restarted.

Learning outcome 4: Discuss the collection of a stoma urine specimen

In learning outcome 1, the importance of not obtaining a CSU from the drainage bag was stated. The same rationale applies to patients who have had an ileal conduit (i.e. urinary stoma) formed (see section on stoma care later). If taken from the stoma bag, the urine will have multiple bacteria and may be contaminated.

The correct method of collecting a stoma urine is by passing a small intermittent catheter into the stoma (see Box 9.6). This is a sterile procedure. The catheter is introduced into the opening of the stoma and gently pushed in (2.5–5 cm deep only) until urine starts to flow down the catheter into the waiting collection pot (Fillingham and Fell 2004). Occasionally, this may be difficult as the stoma may be narrow or very long, or the patient may not be able to tolerate a catheter being used. In these instances, a non-touch technique can be used with a sterile collecting pot held under the stoma, making sure that the rim does not touch the stoma or the surrounding skin. Urine should start to drip out of the stoma and into the pot. This may take a few minutes but should ensure the specimen is not contaminated. Alternatively, a clean new bag can be put onto the abdomen over the stoma and the urine collected within a few minutes. The bag

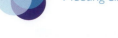

> **Box 9.6 Collection of a stoma urine specimen: equipment and key points**
>
> ### Equipment
> Sterile pack containing gloves and sterile gauze, sterile single-use catheter (8–14 Ch), sterile specimen pot, disposable plastic apron, water or normal saline, clean stoma appliance (if required), disposal bag, incontinence pad or paper towel.
>
> ### Procedure
> - Adhere to general points in Box 9.2.
> - Prepare a new stoma bag, if this needs to be replaced after the procedure.
> - Position an incontinence pad or paper towel under the patient.
> - Remove the stoma bag and dispose of it.
> - Cover stoma with sterile gauze.
> - Wash and dry hands.
> - Open sterile pack and prepare sterile field. Put on sterile gloves. Open sterile catheter and place on sterile field.
> - Clean around stoma with sterile water or saline and gauze using strokes from the centre outwards. Dry the area.
> - Insert the catheter tip into the stoma opening and gently push it in to a depth of 2.5–5 cm only. Wait for urine to start to drain out into the sterile container. A minimum of 2–5 mL is sufficient, though more is preferable.
> - Remove catheter and seal specimen container.
> - Clean around stoma again, if needed. Make sure skin is dry. Reapply stoma bag.
> - Dispose of equipment as per local policy.

is not sterile, but it will be clean and therefore there is less risk of contamination or multiple bacteria.

Learning outcome 5: Discuss the collection of a stool specimen

ACTIVITY

When do you think it might be necessary to collect a stool specimen? Thinking about a 'normal' stool will help you begin to answer this question.

You may have identified that a stool specimen is collected if a person has complained of abnormal stools, or you have observed an abnormality (e.g. diarrhoea), which may be caused by gastrointestinal infection. Infection is particularly likely if the stool is offensive and has an abnormal colour such as green. In these instances, the stool is sent for MC&S, to detect the causative microorganism and identify any antibiotics to which it is sensitive.

Normal frequency of passing stools varies from person to person, but if frequency is altered, it can be a reason to collect a specimen. Altered consistency might also be a reason. For example, lots of mucus can indicate disease such as **ulcerative colitis**, whereas fatty, offensive-smelling and floating stools sometimes indicate gall bladder disease.

> **Ulcerative colitis**
> Ulceration of the mucosa of the colon, causing offensive, watery stools with mucus and pus. Can cause haemorrhage and perforation.

Stool specimens are sent for examination for occult (hidden) blood, if rectal bleeding is suspected but not obvious. If the colour of a stool is different from that normally seen, that too can be suggestive of disease, indicating that a specimen should be taken. Bright red, fresh blood must be reported and may indicate the presence of **haemorrhoids** or other diseases. Stools that are black and tarry in consistency can indicate digested blood from the alimentary tract (termed malaena). Sometimes, stool specimens are sent for examination for parasites. In addition, if a person experiences pain or discomfort associated with defaecation, or flatus is a problem, then a stool specimen might be taken.

See Box 9.7 for key points on collecting a stool specimen. There are stool specimen collectors available that have a spoon attached to the lid. Although these are easy to use when collecting the specimen, they can be difficult for laboratory staff to handle without getting contaminated. Also, pots should not be overfilled as the contents may ferment and build up sufficient pressure to force off even a tight-fitting lid.

> **Haemorrhoids**
>
> Dilated blood vessels in the rectal mucosa. The common term is 'piles'.

Children: practice points – urine and stool specimens

To obtain a urine sample from a child who is not toilet-trained, NICE (2007a) recommends collecting a 'clean catch' sample (catching the urine in a clean container, that is, a potty washed in hot water – 60 degrees with washing up liquid). If a clean catch specimen is unobtainable, other non-invasive methods such as urine collection pads should be used, though they are less accurate. NICE (2007a) outlines criteria for sending urine off for culture, and UTI treatment, in children. Stool specimens can be collected from nappies in children not yet toilet-trained.

For further information, see

Macqueen, S., Bruce, E.A., Gibson, F. 2012. *The Great Ormond Street Hospital Manual of Children's Nursing Practices.* Chichester: Wiley-Blackwell, Chapter 5 'Bowel Care' 87–101 and Chapter 14 'Investigations.' 353–4.

Willock, 2010. Elimination: Collecting, measuring and testing urine. In: Glasper, A., Aylott, M. and Battrick, C. (eds.) *Developing Practical Skills for Nursing Children and Young People.* London: Hodder Arnold, 259–76.

Summary

- Explaining the procedure and its importance carefully, while maintaining dignity, privacy and respect for people, is of prime importance when collecting specimens.
- It is essential to be certain about the purpose of collecting the specimen so that it is collected appropriately.
- Great care should be taken when collecting urine and stool specimens to prevent their contamination, which would in turn invalidate results.
- Precautions to prevent cross-infection must be adhered to when collecting urine and stool specimens.
- It is essential to label specimens accurately and to document their collection in patients' notes.

Box 9.7 Collection of a stool specimen: equipment and key points

Equipment

Bedpan, gloves, apron, sterile stool specimen pot or sterile specimen pot and spatula, specimen bag, laboratory request form.

Procedure
- Adhere to general points in Box 9.2.
- If possible, the patient should be helped to a toilet rather than use a commode. A disposable bedpan can be placed under the toilet lid. Otherwise, a bedpan or commode is used to catch the specimen.
- When the stool is available, take the bedpan to the sluice, open the sterile container and using a spatula fill the container about a third full with faeces and then secure the lid.
- Place the specimen in a dedicated specimen refrigerator if it cannot go to the laboratory immediately. In infections, such as amoebiasis, the stool must be fresh and warm (Mead 1998), thus special arrangements for collection must be made with the laboratory.
- Remember to complete the stool chart if a record is being kept.

CARING FOR PEOPLE WITH URINARY CATHETERS

Urinary catheterisation involves the insertion of a hollow tube into the bladder for evacuating or instilling fluids. The catheter may be inserted intermittently, or left *in situ* (termed 'in-dwelling'), and emptied intermittently via a catheter valve. In these instances, the bladder then retains its function as a reservoir. In many cases, an in-dwelling catheter continuously drains the bladder within a closed system into a bag, in which case only a small volume of urine will be present at the base of the bladder. This method was used as a temporary measure for Jean immediately after surgery.

Some people are taught to self-catheterise intermittently, termed 'intermittent self-catheterisation', often to manage incontinence or incomplete emptying in those with neurological disorders such as multiple sclerosis. Teaching a person to self-catheterise requires specific skills and knowledge (Getliffe and Fader 2007).

Urinary catheters are usually passed along the urethra, but sometimes a suprapubic catheter is passed directly through the mid-suprapubic region of the anterior abdominal wall into the bladder. This is a surgical procedure, performed under anaesthesia, and may be used for people who need a long-term urinary catheter or after certain surgical procedures and in pelvic/urethral trauma or disease. The principles of catheter care for patients who have suprapubic catheters are the same as for those with urethral catheters (Colpman and Welford 2004). However, as the catheter is inserted into a tract into the skin, this can result in infection, bleeding and encrustation around the catheter site. Any secretions that form around the catheter site can be removed with soap and water. Most patients

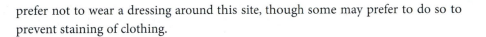

prefer not to wear a dressing around this site, though some may prefer to do so to prevent staining of clothing.

LEARNING OUTCOMES

By the end of this section you will be able to:

1 identify the main indications for urinary catheterisation;

2 show awareness of equipment commonly used for catheterisation;

3 state the main complications associated with urinary catheterisation;

4 understand the principles underpinning urethral catheterisation;

5 discuss the care required for people who have an in-dwelling urinary catheter.

You may be able to access a urinary catheter in the skills laboratory. An opened one would be particularly useful. If not, see if you can look at equipment in your practice setting.

Learning outcome 1: Identify the main indications for urinary catheterisation

It has been estimated that up to 25% of people in hospital have an in-dwelling catheter (Schumm and Lam 2010), with up to 28% of patients residing in care homes and 4% in the community having long-term in-dwelling catheters (McNulty et al. 2003).

ACTIVITY

Make a list of the reasons why people are catheterised. Thinking back to your practice experience will give you some clues.

> **Neurogenic bladder**
>
> Commonly results from lesions of the central nervous system (e.g. spinal injury, multiple sclerosis). Effects include urinary retention, overactive, underactive or uncoordinated detrusor activity.

You may have identified the following reasons:

- To relieve retention of urine (e.g. because of enlarged prostate or **neurogenic bladder**).
- Before pelvic surgery and certain investigations, to minimise the risk of damage to the bladder.
- To measure urine output accurately postoperatively and in very ill patients (e.g. major trauma, shock) – Jean's urethral catheter was originally inserted for this reason.
- To empty the bladder during labour.
- To introduce fluids into the bladder for irrigation purposes.
- To introduce drugs as direct therapy (e.g. **cytotoxic drugs**).
- To facilitate bladder healing.
- following certain pelvic, urethral or bladder neck surgery.

> **Cytotoxic drugs**
>
> Drugs that have a destructive effect on cells and are used to treat cancer.

Incontinence is not given as a primary reason for catheterisation above because long-term catheterisation is rarely free of complications and should, therefore, only be considered when other options have failed, or are no longer appropriate. The major complications of catheterisation are considered in more detail later in this section.

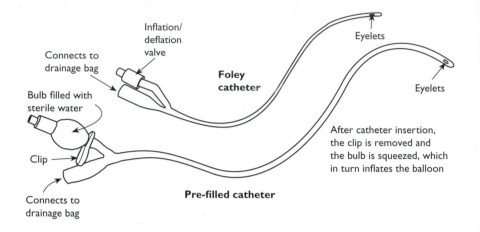

Figure 9.3: Examples of urinary catheters.

Learning outcome 2: Show awareness of equipment commonly used for catheterisation

In the skills laboratory, there may be a sterile or non-sterile (for demonstration purposes) urinary catheter complete with packaging material. See Figure 9.3 for examples. Take note of the following:

- The manner in which it is packaged, batch number, expiry date
- Size
- Length
- Balloon capacity
- The catheter material

If you have access to a non-sterile catheter, try inflating and deflating the balloon using a syringe and water. Some catheters are manufactured pre-filled with water for inflation. Now read through the following points and relate them to your observations.

Packaging

Catheters are packaged to enable ease of insertion into the bladder. With the exception of self-catheterisation, a strict aseptic technique is employed. The way in which the catheter is packaged, including double wrapping, assists in maintaining sterility. There is a batch number and expiry date on the packaging which must be entered into patients' documentation. Many packets have removable sticky labels printed with these details that are put on the patient's notes for future reference.

Catheter size

The catheter size is measured according to its external diameter and is measured in Charrière (Ch) or French gauge units (Fg). One Ch unit equals 0.3 mm, and the catheters range in size from 6–8 (for paediatric use) to 30Ch. A size 12Ch catheter is 4 mm in diameter and is usually adequate for urine drainage for both men and women. The key general rule to follow is that the smallest size catheter that will allow free urinary outflow should be used (Pratt et al. 2007). Large catheters are associated with complications including urethral irritation, urethral trauma, bladder spasm, urinary bypassing, pressure necrosis and increased risk of infection (Wilson 2012).

Catheter length

Catheters are usually manufactured in three lengths: standard catheters (sometimes referred to as 'male-length'), 40–44 cm in length; female catheters, 30–40 cm in length; and paediatric catheters, 30 cm in length (Wilson 2011). The standard catheter is often used for women, particularly if obese, because it allows easier access to the junction of the catheter and the drainage bag (Colpman and Welford 2004). Female catheters must never be used urethrally in males as they are too short for the male urethra and would not reach the bladder. If inflated in the urethra, the balloon may cause this to rupture and haemorrhage and may lead to severe trauma (Getliffe and Fader 2007).

Balloon

The Foley catheter is the design most frequently used for in-dwelling urethral catheterisation (Getliffe and Fader 2007). It has a rounded tip with two drainage eyes and an integral balloon, which, when inflated, holds the catheter *in situ*. There are two channels, one for drainage and the other for inflating the balloon. The balloon sits at the sensitive base of the bladder and can potentially cause irritation, spasm and mechanical damage to the bladder. Retention balloons come in various sizes: 10 mL is recommended for adults, but larger 30 mL balloons are sometimes used after some urological procedures (Pratt et al. 2007). Inflation valves are colour-coded according to the Charrière size (Yates 2012).

Catheters for intermittent use are usually a simple tube design and do not have an inflatable balloon as there is no requirement for them to be retained in the bladder. Some suprapubic catheters do not have a balloon, but are secured by a flange and held in place by skin sutures.

Material

Catheters are available in various materials. The choice of which type to use depends on the clinical experience of the practitioner, patient assessment and the length of time it is envisaged the catheter will remain *in situ* (Pratt et al. 2007).

For short-term use, plastic, latex (up to 7–10 days) and Teflon-coated latex (up to 28 days) are commonly used; these materials are considerably cheaper than long-term catheter materials. Some patients are allergic to latex, and screening is advisable if latex is to be used (Newman 2012; Wilson 2012). Plastic catheters have been found to exert low toxicity because of the inert nature of plastic. Also, the rate at which this material absorbs water is low and so the catheter retains the widest internal diameter, making these catheters a common choice for drainage of postoperative blood clots and debris. However, plastic catheters can remain rigid at body temperature and have been associated with bladder spasm, pain and leakage of urine (Wilson 2012). The DH (2003) recommends that in-dwelling catheters used for long-term use should have low allergenicity. Silicone, silicone-elastomer-coated latex and hydrogel-coated catheters are suitable products (Newman 2012; Wilson 2012; Yates 2012).

Recent research has focused on developing catheters with properties specifically intended to reducing infection incidence. These tend to have special coatings such as silver ions or aloe vera along their length. The aim is to either stop or limit formation of biofilms (Godfrey and Fraczyk 2005). These substances have been found to have anti-infection properties. However, a review found that very few trials have compared different types of catheter for long-term use and most were carried out on small numbers of patients (Jahn et al. 2007). The reviewers concluded that the evidence was too weak to provide reliable evidence about which type of catheter is best for which patients. The cost of the catheter should not be the primary factor in the selection process, but nurses should be aware of the different costs when selecting.

Urine drainage bags and catheter valves

In-dwelling catheters are normally used in conjunction with an attached collection bag to allow periodic emptying. This is known as a **closed system.** Figure 9.4 shows a catheter attached to a leg bag, which would be secured to the patient's leg with straps. Figure 9.5 shows a urinary catheter attached to a urine drainage bag supported on a stand, which is suitable for overnight use or for a person who has to remain in bed. A catheter valve (see Figure 9.6) may provide an alternative for some patients but an adequate bladder capacity is required. Unless a committed carer is available, the user requires good manual dexterity for manipulating the valve, and sufficient cognitive function to understand the need to release the valve regularly to prevent overdistension (Gibney 2010; Yates 2012). Catheter valves are also unlikely to be suitable if the person has uncontrolled detrusor overactivity, ureteric reflux or renal impairment (Gibney 2010).

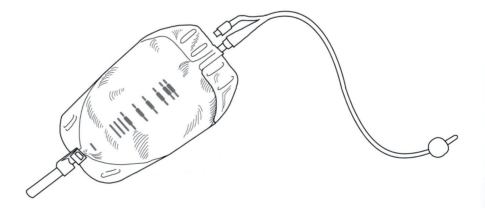

Figure 9.4: A urinary catheter attached to a leg bag.

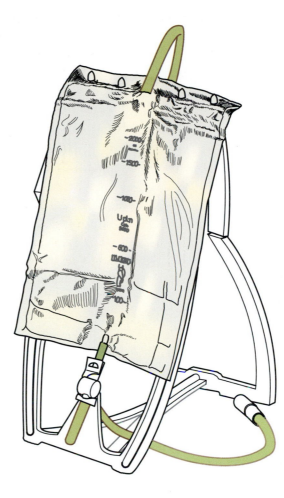

Figure 9.5: A urine drainage bag on a stand.

When selecting a bag, factors to consider are capacity, length of inlet tube and type of outlet tap for emptying. Bags vary in capacity from 350 to 750 mL and up to 2 L for use overnight or postoperatively. Some bags are specially designed for wheelchair users. Outlet taps are usually of a lever-type design or push-across mechanism, but other designs are also available. The manual dexterity of patients and carers needs to be considered. There are catheter supports available for people with restricted mobility which aim to provide firm support to prevent tugging, without restricting movement or impeding drainage.

Whatever equipment is used, you must document details of the catheter and drainage system used in the patient's records carefully. You should also provide the person with adequate information about the rationale for insertion, the insertion itself, and the maintenance and removal of catheter.

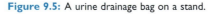

ACTIVITY　　　What sort of drainage bag might be suitable for Jean?

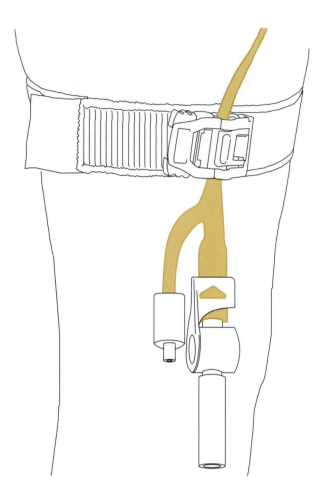

Figure 9.6: A urinary catheter strapped to the leg, with a valve in place, for emptying.

Following discussion with Jean, you may decide to use a leg bag. The length of the inlet tube selected would depend on whether Jean found it most comfortable to position the bag on her thigh, knee or calf. At night, the nurses will be able to attach a night bag on a stand, directly to the leg bag. For most patients, body-worn bags are preferable because their attachment to the person's leg or suspended from the waist allows maximum freedom and at the same time can be concealed beneath clothing. This reduces discomfort and promotes dignity for people like Jean who find themselves in the difficult and sometimes embarrassing situation of needing a urinary catheter *in situ*. A body-worn bag will help Jean as she begins to mobilise as she will not have to contend with carrying the bag or long trailing drainage tubes. Once she is comfortable moving and fully mobile, the catheter can be removed.

Did you know?

Prior to the use of closed drainage systems, almost all patients developed UTIs within 96 hours (Kass 1957, cited by Macauley 1997). As closed drainage systems have been shown to reduce this rate of infection, they are now accepted as good practice (Wilson 2011). However, many healthcare-associated infections are related to urinary catheterisation, causing significant morbidity and even mortality. Therefore, care for people with catheters must aim to prevent infection, as well as promote comfort and understanding.

ACTIVITY

Figure 9.7 shows a diagram of a closed urinary drainage system. Where do you think bacteria could enter into the system?

The following are the potential ports of entry:
- The catheter tip during catheterisation
- The urethral meatus around the catheter
- The junction between the catheter and the tubing to the catheter bag
- The specimen sampling port
- The drainage outlet

Bacteria are also believed to enter the bladder at the time of catheterisation via the peri-urethral space. Coagulase-negative staphylococci or micrococci can normally be found in the anterior urethra, and these are a common cause of infection immediately following catheterisation (Tlaskalová-Hogenová et al. 2004).

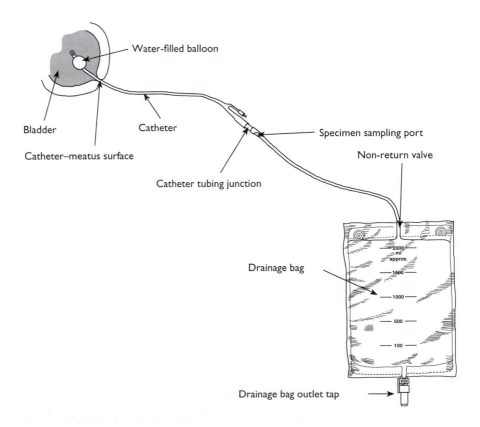

Figure 9.7: A closed urinary drainage system.

Some systems now have a tamper-evident seal at the junction between the catheter and the connection tube aimed at preventing bacteria from entering here.

Learning outcome 3: State the main complications associated with urinary catheterisation

ACTIVITY

Look back over this section and see whether you can name one major complication associated with catheterisation. Try to identify some other complications.

You probably identified that infection is a major complication of catheterisation. Encrustation and eventual blockage are also problems associated with urinary catheterisation (Wilson 2012). Other complications include urethral strictures, pressure necrosis, spasm, discomfort and pain (Yates 2012).

With a catheter *in situ*, the bladder's normal closing mechanism is obstructed and the natural flushing mechanism of micturition is lost. In addition, the close proximity of the catheter to the bowel presents a risk of infection, because bacteria can be mechanically transferred across skin surfaces from anus to urethral meatus (Tlaskalová-Hogenová et al. 2004). As discussed earlier, bacteria having entered the urinary system may cling to the surface of the catheter, which creates a living biofilm that is almost impossible to remove and one that is highly resistant to antibiotics (Getliffe 2002). The bacteria can cause the urine to become more alkaline than usual leading to encrustation on the catheter surface, which can lead to blockage and then to retention of urine or to leakage and pain. These outcomes are distressing for patients and can result in loss of comfort and dignity (Stickler 2008).

When tissue is invaded by bacteria, problems include local infection, which may result in foul-smelling urine, or systemic infection leading to pyrexia (raised body temperature). Catheterising patients places them in significant danger of acquiring a UTI, and the longer a catheter is in place, the greater the danger. Of patients with a catheter-associated UTI, 1–4% develop bacteraemia and of these, 13–30% die (Pratt et al. 2007). Therefore, catheterisation is best avoided, if at all possible (Pratt et al. 2007), and catheters should be removed as soon as possible, if no longer needed.

Learning outcome 4: Understand the principles underpinning urethral catheterisation

Catheterisation is a skilled aseptic procedure and should be carried out only by healthcare personnel who are trained and competent to carry it out (Pratt et al. 2007). Catheterisation is an invasive procedure and the effects on patients may be many: physical, psychological and social.

ACTIVITY

Before reading the following section, refer to Chapter 3 for an explanation of the aseptic technique. These principles underpin the procedure of urinary catheterisation.

Appropriate and effective communication and sensitivity are essential when catheterisation takes place (see Chapter 2 for more information). Care should be taken to explain where the catheter is inserted, and why the procedure is necessary, ensuring that verbal consent is gained. This could be difficult with a person who is confused. Also, catheters should not be changed unnecessarily or as part of routine practice.

Box 9.8 outlines the equipment needed and the key points to be adhered to while undertaking female urethral catheterisation. In many NHS Trusts, additional training must be undertaken by trained nurses to perform male urethral catheterisation. However, many of the principles are synonymous with female urethral catheterisation. Suprapubic catheterisation is usually a medical procedure and is not considered here.

Once the catheter has been inserted, dietary advice, including fluid intake and avoidance of constipation, is an important part of patient education (European Association of Urological Nurses [EAUN] 2012). Further explanations and instructions concerning why and how the catheter has been inserted, its maintenance requirements and discussion of removal will be required if the person goes home with a urinary catheter *in situ*. Patients and carers should also be educated about techniques to prevent infection (NICE 2012a). The district nurse will probably be involved.

Learning outcome 5: Discuss the care required for people who have an in-dwelling urinary catheter

ACTIVITY

What specific care might be needed in relation to catheter care for Jean?

You may have thought of:
- maintaining hygiene;
- emptying the catheter bag;
- appropriate positioning of the catheter bag;
- adequate fluid intake.

These pertinent issues will now be discussed.

Maintaining hygiene

The main aim of cleansing is to remove secretions and encrustation and prevent infection. Where possible, patients should be encouraged to attend to their own meatal and perineal hygiene needs, thus reducing the risk of cross-infection while promoting self-care and dignity. Maintaining routine daily hygiene is all that is needed, with the meatus being washed with soap and water (Wilson 2011). However, for people unable to maintain their own hygiene, nurses should carry this out, wearing gloves, in a gentle and sensitive manner. Vigorous cleansing may increase the risk of infection (Pratt et al. 2007).

Cleansing of the perineum and the area surrounding the catheter–meatus junction is essential after faecal incontinence and should be carried out using clean wipes.

Box 9.8 Female urethral catheterisation: equipment and procedure

Equipment

- A catheterisation pack, if available, or a dressing pack and sterile receiver, sterile gloves, an appropriate catheter, sterile sodium chloride, catheter bag and stand or holder, sterile single-patient-use lubricant or anaesthetic gel, syringe and sterile water of appropriate size to inflate the balloon (often included with catheter), disposable waterproof absorbent pad, specimen pot, if required, and a good light source

Note: A second nurse may be needed to help position the patient, who needs to be preferably flat with legs apart to allow good access and visibility.

Procedure

- Aseptic technique should be strictly adhered to throughout (see Chapter 3 sections on 'Hand hygiene' and 'Aseptic technique').
- Explain the procedure and ensure consent.
- Maintain privacy and reassure the patient throughout.
- Place the disposable pad under the patient's buttocks.
- Open the catheter bag and arrange at the side of the bed, ensuring the attachment tip remains sterile.
- Open the catheterisation or dressing pack, and open the catheter on to the sterile field but do not remove it from its internal wrapping.
- Draw up the sterile water to inflate the balloon (unless pre-filled syringe is supplied or catheter is pre-filled).
- Pour sodium chloride into the gallipot.
- Open sterile gloves, wash hands and apply gloves.
- Place sterile towels over patient's thighs and between legs.
- Cleanse the perineal area with the sodium chloride, and then using non-dominant hand, separate labia minora and cleanse the meatus.
- Carefully locate the urethra and insert single-patient-use lubricant gel to minimise urethral trauma and infection (NICE 2012a). Some gels contain anaesthetic too. Inserting the gel directly into the urethra opens up and lubricates the length of the urethra. Lubricating the tip of the catheter only is ineffective as the lubricant is quickly wiped away on insertion. Wait for the time recommended by the manufacturer, usually 5 minutes.
- Place a receiver with the catheter on the sterile towel between the patient's legs.
- Expose the tip of the catheter by pulling open the wrapper at the serrations.
- Hold the catheter so that the distal end remains in the receiver and gradually advance it out of its wrapper as you insert it into the meatus in an upward and backward direction along the line of the urethra.
- Advance the catheter 5–7 cm or until urine flows out of the catheter.
- Advance the catheter a further 5 cm. Never force the catheter. If resistance is encountered, stop and seek medical advice.
- Inflate the balloon with the correct amount of sterile water, generally 10 mL for adults (NICE 2012a). Incorrectly filled balloons can inflate irregularly and irritate the bladder mucosa.
- Attach the urinary drainage bag, and make the patient comfortable.
- Send a urine specimen, if indicated, and measure and record the urine collected.
- Document the catheterisation in the patient's notes, including date of insertion, catheter size and amount of water used to inflate the balloon. The catheter packaging may have an adhesive label with the catheter's details which can be used.

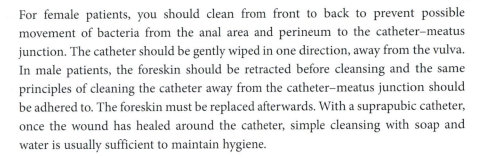

For female patients, you should clean from front to back to prevent possible movement of bacteria from the anal area and perineum to the catheter–meatus junction. The catheter should be gently wiped in one direction, away from the vulva. In male patients, the foreskin should be retracted before cleansing and the same principles of cleaning the catheter away from the catheter–meatus junction should be adhered to. The foreskin must be replaced afterwards. With a suprapubic catheter, once the wound has healed around the catheter, simple cleansing with soap and water is usually sufficient to maintain hygiene.

Emptying the catheter bag

ACTIVITY

You may recall that microorganisms can be introduced into the drainage system at the junction between the catheter and the bag or via the drainage tap. Bearing this in mind, work out the equipment you would need, and how you would use it, to safely empty a catheter bag. Compare your answer with Box 9.9.

Unless hands are thoroughly washed between patients and a clean container is used to collect the urine, microorganisms are readily transferred to the next patient. Although disinfection of hands with 70% alcohol is rapid and effective, hands that are visibly soiled or potentially grossly contaminated with dirt or organic material must be washed with soap and water (see Chapter 3, section on 'Hand hygiene').

The urinary drainage bag should be emptied frequently enough to maintain urine flow and prevent reflux, and to prevent it from becoming so heavy that its weight pulls on the catheter and causes urethral trauma. There is no evidence that bags need

---

Box 9.9 Emptying a catheter bag: equipment and procedure

Equipment
Non-sterile gloves and apron, a heat-disinfected or disposable container, for example, a urinal or jug, paper towel to cover, alcohol swabs.

Procedure
- Explain the procedure to the patient and ensure privacy.
- Wash hands and put on apron and gloves.
- If the drainage bag is on a stand, it may not need removing. If it is hanging on the bed, you may need to access it by removing the bag and placing it over the jug.
- Clean the outlet port with alcohol swab and allow it to dry.
- Open the port and drain the urine into the receptacle, ensuring that the port does not touch the side of the receptacle.
- Close the port and wipe with alcohol swab.
- Reposition bag.
- Cover the container and take to sluice for disposal. Measure the urine first if a fluid balance chart is being kept.
- The container should be disinfected, or macerated, if disposable.
- Remove gloves and apron and wash hands.

to be changed at specific intervals though they should be changed when damaged or blocked with deposits. Bags should be changed when clinically indicated and/or in line with the manufacturers' recommendations (Pratt et al. 2007). But the key principle – and the way to prevent bacteria or other harmful organisms entering the system – is to leave the closed system alone as much as you can. NICE (2012a) recommends that the connection between the catheter and the drainage system should not be broken except for sound clinical reasons.

Jean has a leg drainage bag attached to her catheter which can remain unchanged for up to a week as per the manufacturer's advice. A night drainage bag can be attached to the open tap of the leg bag for overnight drainage. This can be removed and discarded during the day as Jean goes back to draining into her leg bag. This process ensures that the closed drainage system is not broken. Disconnection of the catheter from the drainage bag significantly increases the risk of introducing bacteria into the system and should therefore be avoided, if possible (Wilson 2006). Patients with a catheter on drainage who live at home where the risks of cross-infection are low can reuse the night drainage bag for up to one week, if rinsed with water and allowed to dry between use. However, in hospital and other institutional settings, patients should have a new night drainage bag each time as the risk for cross-contamination and infection is too great to allow reuse. Adding antiseptic or antimicrobial solutions into drainage bags is not recommended (Pratt et al. 2007).

Appropriate positioning of the catheter bag

Catheter bags should be positioned to avoid reflux and facilitate the use of gravity, and positioned clear of floors or other sources of contamination (NICE 2012a). Drainage bags should always be positioned below the level of the bladder with the catheter and the inlet tubing secured in a downward position (Colpman and Welford 2004). This is because reflux urine is associated with infection, so bags must be positioned to prevent backflow of urine. When it is difficult to maintain the level of the bag below the bladder, for example, when moving the patient, the drainage bag tube should be clamped and the clamp removed only on resumption of dependent drainage (Pratt et al. 2007). The catheter itself should never be clamped as this can easily be damaged.

The catheter should be secured to prevent movement of the catheter within the urethra, which may introduce infection (EAUN 2012). A variety of straps, 'net' sleeves, holsters and sporrans are available to suspend the drainage bag. Securing the catheter also ensures that it does not pull on the urethra and cause ulceration or cleaving where pressure from the tube can split the urethra. In extreme cases, the whole urethra may be split open and require surgical repair (Colpman and Welford 2004; EAUN 2012).

Adequate fluid intake

If the patient's condition allows, encourage oral fluids. This has traditionally been believed to result in dilute urine containing fewer nutrients, thus discouraging the growth of bacteria in the drainage bag and encrustation of components. It is believed that the larger volume of urine maintains a constant flow through the drainage system, making it more difficult for bacteria to multiply in the drainage bag (Wilson 2006).

Getliffe and Fader (2007) identified that although there is no clear evidence that drinking large quantities of fluid will prevent infection, in practice it is sensible to promote good fluid intake to prevent dehydration and constipation.

Catheter removal

ACTIVITY

Think about how you would prepare Jean, or any other patient, for catheter removal.

A clear explanation should be given, emphasising that the procedure is not normally painful but that there may be a feeling of discomfort. Box 9.10 outlines equipment and key points for removing a catheter.

You should ensure that urine is passed satisfactorily after catheter removal and observe for problems such as incontinence, frequency and retention. A person who is

---

Box 9.10 Removal of a urethral catheter: equipment and procedure

Equipment
- Non-sterile gloves and apron, syringe of sufficient volume to remove the water from the balloon, disposable absorbent pad, receiver and waste bag. If a CSU is required: specimen pot, 20 mL syringe, needle and alcohol swab.

Procedure
- Give explanation, ensure privacy and position the person comfortably. For a female, the knees and hips should be slightly flexed and apart.
- Wash and dry hands and apply gloves and apron.
- Obtain a specimen of urine from the sampling port, if indicated (see Box 9.3).
- Place the disposable pad under the patient's buttocks and then place the receiver between the thighs.
- Check the balloon volume and attach an appropriately sized syringe to the balloon port of the catheter. Withdraw the water from the balloon via the syringe.
- Ask the patient to breathe in and out, and as they exhale, the catheter is gently withdrawn and placed in the receiver. If problems are encountered, stop and seek medical advice.
- Remove gloves and apron and wash hands.
- The patient should be made comfortable and because frequency may be experienced, the nurse should ensure that a toilet or commode is close by. If the patient needs help with mobility, ensure a call bell is nearby.
- Document the date and time of catheter removal in the clinical notes and record the amount of urine in the catheter bag.
- The patient may be encouraged to increase fluid intake to 'flush' out the bladder.
- Monitor whether the person is passing urine satisfactorily. A chart may be kept so that frequency and amount can be monitored. Also, ask the patient to inform a nurse if any unusual symptoms are experienced, for example, dysuria (pain when passing urine).

confused may need prompting to pass urine (see section on promoting continence). Some people, particularly men who have had prostate surgery, should perform pelvic floor exercises to help them regain control (see the later section). People with long-term catheters for specific medical reasons will require periodic changing of the catheter depending on clinical need, such as any problems experienced, and/or in line with manufacturers' recommendations (Pratt et al. 2007).

Children: practice points – catheterisation

To read about urethral catheterisation for children and related care, see

Macqueen, S., Bruce, E.A. and Gibson, F. 2012. Urinary catheter care. In: *The Great Ormond Street Hospital Manual of Children's Nursing Practices*. Chichester: Wiley-Blackwell, 718–32.

Willock, 2010. Elimination: Collecting, measuring and testing urine. In: Glasper, A., Aylott, M. and Battrick, C. (eds.) *Developing Practical Skills for Nursing Children and Young People*. London: Hodder Arnold, 259–76.

Summary

- Urinary catheterisation is experienced by many patients/clients and may be a short-term or long-term measure.
- Catheterisation is an invasive procedure and there are many complications associated with it, infection being particularly common. Therefore, catheterisation should be performed only if there is a clear indication.
- Strict asepsis should be maintained, and the catheter should be removed as soon as possible, using the correct technique.
- Nurses should be aware of the different types of equipment available, and make appropriate choices regarding types of catheter and drainage bag.
- The closed system should not be broken except for good clinical reasons.
- Care should be taken to reduce physical and psychological discomfort for people with urinary catheters.

Getliffe and Fader (2007) cover catheterisation in depth, so further reading from that source is recommended.

PREVENTING AND MANAGING CONSTIPATION

Constipation is a common condition with multifactoral causes. People with constipation can experience various uncomfortable symptoms including headache, bloatedness, loss of appetite, nausea and vomiting (Kyle 2011a). Chronic constipation with **faecal impaction** is the most important cause of faecal incontinence in frail, older people as the bowel produces mucus to try to soften the hard mass of faeces causing overflow (Kyle 2010).

For some people constipation can be dangerous; Pellatt (2007) explains that if patients with spinal cord injury above the sixth thoracic vertebra develop bowel

Faecal Impaction

In very severe constipation, a large mass of faeces which cannot be passed accumulates in the rectum and can back up in the sigmoid colon or even higher (Kyle 2010).

distension due to constipation or impaction, they can develop autonomic dysreflexia (severe hypertension) which may lead to cerebral haemorrhage, seizures or cardiac arrest. Risk of constipation should be assessed so that preventative measures can be implemented, rather than waiting until constipation has developed. If constipation occurs, it should be managed effectively to relieve discomfort and prevent complications. Enemas and suppositories may be required to treat constipation, but they are also a means of medicine administration via the rectal route. Therefore, principles of medicine administration should be followed (see Chapter 5).

LEARNING OUTCOMES

By the end of this section, you will be able to:

1 identify how to assess risk of constipation;
2 discuss how to prevent and manage constipation;
3 understand key principles of administering suppositories and enemas.

Learning outcome 1: Identify how to assess risk of constipation

ACTIVITY

What are the likely risk factors for constipation? Think back to patients/clients you encountered in placement. Who was at risk of constipation?

There are many risk factors for constipation (see Kyle 2007a; Richmond and Wright 2004); some examples of people likely to become constipated will be discussed here. Candy et al. (2011) identified that constipation is common in palliative care and can generate considerable suffering due to the unpleasant physical symptoms. Constipation is more common in people with learning disabilities than the general population (Marsh et al. 2010), particularly if they are less mobile, have inadequate nutrition and fluid intake or are taking long-term medication that has constipation as a side effect (RCN 2011). Patients who are in hospital often experience reduced exercise alongside a changed diet, increasing their risk of constipation. Psychological and environmental factors can also contribute to constipation in hospital. Constipation is a side effect of many medicines, including antipsychotic medication (de Hert et al. 2011). Constipation is not an inevitable result of ageing (Holman et al. 2010), but it is common in older people (Gallagher et al. 2008; Kyle 2010; Woodward 2012).

Kyle (2007a, 2009) presents the Norgine risk assessment tool for constipation (see Figure 9.8). The tool includes the main risk factors for constipation. The assessor ticks and adds up all that apply; the higher the score, the greater the risk. The tool is designed to be used with adult patients on admission, and alerts nurses to patients' risk of constipation – leading to proactive preventative measures (Kyle 2007a).

ACTIVITY

Look back at Mark's scenario and, using the Norgine risk assessment tool in Figure 9.8, assess his risk.

Norgine® Risk Assessment Tool for Constipation

NORGINE

PATIENT'S NAME	
PATIENT'S DATE OF BIRTH	
PATIENT'S NHS NUMBER	

Medical Condition	
Cancer	
Clinical depression	
Diabetes	
Haemorrhoids, anal fissure, rectocele, local anal or rectal pathology	
History of constipation	
Impaired cognition/dementia	
Multiple sclerosis	
Parkinson's disease	
Postoperative	
Rheumatoid arthritis	
Spinal cord conditions (injury, disease or congenital)	
Stroke	

Current Medication	✓
Aluminium antacids	
Anticholinergics	
Anti-Parkinson drugs	
Antipsychotic drugs	
Calcium channel blockers	
Calcium supplements	
Diuretics	
Iron supplements	
Non-steroidal anti-inflammatory drugs (NSAIDs)	
Opioids	
Tricyclic antidepressants	
Polypharmacy (more than 5 drugs including ones not on this list)	

Toileting Facilities	✓
Bedpan	
Commode by bed in hospital/care home/home	
Supervised use of lavatory/commode	
Commode/raised toilet seat at home (without foot stool)	

Mobility	✓
Restricted to bed	
Restricted to wheelchair/chair	
Walks with aids/assistance	
Walks short distances but less than 1/3 mile (0.5km)	

Nutritional Intake	✓
At nutritional risk as identified by local nutritional screening tool	
Fibre intake 6 g or less per day	
Difficulty in swallowing/chewing	
Needs assistance to eat	

Daily Fluid Intake (see below for calculation table)	✓
Minimum fluids not achieved	

Fluid Requirement Calculation
30 mL fluid per 1kg of body weight

Patients minimum fluid intake should be:

Weight in kg= _____ × 30 mL= _____

Patients actual fluid intake is:

INSTRUCTIONS

1. Tick all relevant categories in each table.
2. There may be more than one tick in a table.
3. Add all the ticks together.
4. Fill in the number of ticks in the box below.
5. Date and sign.

DATE	TOTAL NO. OF TICKS	SIGNATURE

Figure 9.8: Norgine risk assessment tool for constipation. (Reproduced with kind permission from Gaye Kyle, Senior Lecturer, Thames Valley University; Phil Prynn, Continence Services Manager, Berkshire West PCT; and Terri Dunbar, Advanced Nurse Practitioner, Berkshire West PCT. © 2006 Norgine Pharmaceuticals Ltd.)

> ## Box 9.11 Action to take when risk of constipation is identified
>
> - Complete full bowel assessment using locally approved care pathway.
> - Monitor and record bowel movements daily using the Bristol stool chart (see Figure 9.1) and bowel record chart.
> - For stool type 1 or type 2 on the Bristol stool chart, prescribe appropriate laxative therapy.
> - Advise on toileting position.
> - Review medication, including over-the-counter medicines.
> - Advise on ways to improve mobility.
> - Encourage patients to achieve at least minimum fluid intake.
> - Improve nutrition according to nutritional intake score.
>
> *Source:* Reproduced with kind permission from Gaye Kyle, Senior Lecturer, Thames Valley University; Phil Prynn, Continence Services Manager, Berkshire West PCT; and Terri Dunbar, Advanced Nurse Practitioner, Berkshire West PCT. © 2006 Norgine Pharmaceuticals Ltd.

You will have found that the tool is quick and easy to use. Mark's score is 5. Under 'Medical condition' you should have ticked 'History of constipation' and 'Impaired cognition'. For 'Toileting facilities', you should have ticked 'Supervised use of lavatory/commode', and for 'Mobility', you should have identified 'Walks with aids/assistance'. For 'Nutritional intake', Mark 'Needs assistance to eat'. If Mark is prescribed any of the medications listed, these would add to his risk. If Mark's fluid intake is inadequate, his risk increases further.

Patients who, like Mark, score more than 4 on the Norgine risk assessment tool should have further assessment leading to appropriate actions (see Box 9.11).

Learning outcome 2: Discuss how to prevent and manage constipation

The first section in this chapter included many aspects relevant to preventing constipation in hospital: ensuring that people felt able to ask for assistance, encouraging them to go to the toilet when the 'call to stool' occurs (often early in the morning or about 30 minutes after a meal), attending to them promptly giving assistance to go out to the toilet when required, ensuring that they are comfortable and well-supported, and giving them unhurried time and privacy.

As regards the correct position to open the bowels, you should advise patients to:

- sit with the knees higher than the hips;
- lean forward with elbows on knees;
- bulge out the abdomen and straighten the spine.

A footstool may be needed to assist patients into this position. Any patient who can use the toilet or commode can be advised to use this position, unless there are contraindications owing to their medical condition.

Adequate fluid intake is important and dietary fibre should be increased gradually alongside increased fluid intake to prevent bloating. Intake of high-fibre foods, fruits and vegetables should be encouraged according to people's preference. For example, if Mark likes biscuits, he could be encouraged to eat flapjacks, oatcakes, digestive biscuits or fig rolls. Depending on the risk factors, referrals to other health professionals and specialists may be helpful (e.g. doctor, continence advisor, dietician, dentist, physiotherapist, occupational therapist, speech and language therapist and pharmacist). The community nurse for learning disabilities can work with Mark and his mother to ensure that Mark has appropriate multidisciplinary support.

NICE (2007b) advised that people with faecal loading need rectally administered treatment to clear the bowel – which may need to be repeated daily for a few days. If these do not work satisfactorily, oral laxatives should be given and a plan developed to prevent recurrence. The main groups of laxatives are bulking agents (e.g. Isogel, regulan), stimulants (e.g. senna, bisocodyl), stool softeners and lubricants (liquid paraffin, ducoset sodium) and osmotic agents (e.g. lactulose); see the British National Formulary for more details (www.bnf.org). Although laxatives may be necessary to prevent and manage constipation, they are preferable only as a short-term measure. The Royal College of Nursing (RCN 2011) identified that, for people with learning disabilities, there has been an over reliance on laxatives rather than promoting adequate nutrition and fluid intake. Where feasible, medicines that predispose to constipation should be avoided particularly in those who are at risk. Exercise should be increased, if possible.

A digital rectal examination (DRE) might be carried out to check for faecal impaction, and for abnormalities such as blood, pain or obstruction. DRE involves observing the perianal area and inserting a gloved and lubricated finger into the rectum (Kyle 2007b). You will also see DREs carried out during abdominal examinations of patients and for screening for rectal or prostate cancer, or prostate enlargement (Steggall 2008). Digital removal of faeces (DRF) (using a lubricated, gloved finger) is an invasive procedure only conducted after individual assessment, but it can be part of the bowel management regime for some patients, for example those with spinal cord injuries (RCN 2012). DRE and DRF can be carried out only by registered nurses who can demonstrate competence in these skills, but they can also delegate these procedures to carers or patients if their competence has been assessed (RCN 2012). These procedures are invasive and require consent of the patients; the RCN (2012) discusses these procedures and consent issues. There are contraindications to these procedures and potential risks, and many organisations have developed their own policies. Steggall and Cox (2009) explain the DRE procedure in detail.

In some instances, suppositories or enemas may be needed to treat constipation – these are considered in learning outcome 3.

Learning outcome 3: Understand key principles of administering suppositories and enemas

An enema is a liquid that is inserted into the rectum, whereas a suppository is a medicated solid formulation, usually torpedo-shaped, that is inserted into the rectum, where it dissolves at body temperature. An enema that should be retained following administration is termed a 'retention enema' and is primarily used for its local effect. For example, a steroid enema may be administered to people with ulcerative colitis for its anti-inflammatory effect. An 'evacuant enema' is given to initiate bowel emptying and is used for constipation or to empty the bowel prior to surgery or investigations of the gastrointestinal tract. Suppositories are often administered for evacuant purposes, but they are also often used to administer medication and may be administered as a local treatment, as for haemorrhoids.

ACTIVITY

Drugs commonly prescribed rectally include paracetamol (for its analgesic and/or antipyretic effect) and anticonvulsants. What are the advantages and disadvantages of this route of drug administration?

You might have thought of the following advantages:

- The rectum is an alternative route for when people cannot take oral medication because they are vomiting, unable to swallow or are 'nil by mouth' (e.g. preoperatively).
- Drugs administered rectally are absorbed into the bloodstream and bypass the liver (Greenstein 2009). For example, a person who is having a seizure cannot take oral medication, and rectal administration is safer and more rapid than intramuscular injections. As faecal impaction can inhibit rectal drug absorption, constipation should be prevented in people who might require emergency rectal medication.

Disadvantages include:

- Suppository and enema administration is more invasive and embarrassing than oral administration and involves some discomfort, undressing and moving into the correct position.
- Traumatic and even fatal side effects of enemas, including inflammation, electrolyte imbalance and perforation of the colonic mucosa have been reported (Schmelzer and Wright 1996). Newer, small, pre-packaged enemas aim to prevent such problems. However, enemas should only be used if there is no other alternative.

ACTIVITY

Can you think of any physical problems that might be contraindications?

Anal fissure

A painful crack in the mucous membrane of the anus, generally caused by hard faeces.

Rectal prolapse

A protrusion of rectal mucosa through the anus.

Prior to administering an enema or suppository, the nurse should carefully assess the appropriateness of this route.

Contraindications might include recent colorectal or gynaecological surgery, malignancy or other pathology of the perineal area, and a low platelet count, as this predisposes to bleeding. Thus, the nurse should check with both the patient and the case notes for any previous anorectal surgery or abnormalities. Further visual inspection should also be made immediately before administration. The perianal region should be checked for abnormalities, including haemorrhoids, **anal fissure** and **rectal prolapse**.

ACTIVITY

Find out what types of enemas and suppositories are available to evacuate the bowel. There may be examples in the skills laboratory, or you can look at them in your practice setting.

When giving an enema or suppositories for evacuation purposes, there can be a choice of products.

Suppositories may be of the type that will simply soften the stools, or they may have a stimulant effect. Greenstein (2009) recommends that glycerol suppositories are satisfactory and other types offer no advantage. There are microenemas available containing only 5 mL of solution which act as a colon stimulant. For more vigorous bowel cleansing (e.g. prior to a bowel investigation), a larger phosphate enema may be used. Phosphate enemas work through osmosis – by extracting water from the bowel to draw into faeces, thus increasing the faecal mass (Bowers 2006). Bowers asserts that there is a lack of evidence to support use of phosphate enemas for constipation above other products, but that they are an effective way of clearing the colon prior to **flexible sigmoidoscopy**. Complications of phosphate enemas are rare but can be serious. Patients with severe constipation often have other underlying conditions that may make them more at risk of complications. It is important to check the manufacturer's instructions when administering a phosphate enema. There are a number of contraindications, and Addison et al. (2000) advise that they are unsuitable for older or debilitated patients. The systematic review of sodium phosphate enema administration by Mendoza et al. (2007) identified that side effects (mainly water and electrolyte disturbances) were rare, mainly occurring in the very young (under 5 years) or people older than 65 years. Patients suffering side effects often had conditions such as neurological, gastrointestinal or renal disorders.

Box 9.12 provides guidance for safe administration of suppositories/enemas based on the evidence available.

Flexible sigmoidoscopy

The sigmoid colon is examined with a lighted scope, usually for bleeding, non-cancerous growths (polyps) or colorectal cancer.

Children: practice points – constipation

Constipation within childhood is a very common problem (Gordon et al 2011) and NICE (2010a) have produced detailed guidelines. For further reading, see

Macqueen, S., Bruce, E.A. and Gibson, F. 2012. Bowel care. *The Great Ormond Street Hospital Manual of Children's Nursing Practices*. Chichester: Wiley-Blackwell, 87–101.

Slater-Smith, S. 2010. Promoting children's continence B) Childhood constipation. In: Glasper, A., Aylott, M. and Battrick, C. (eds.) *Developing Practical Skills for Nursing Children and Young People*. London: Hodder Arnold, 229–41.

Box 9.12 Administration of enemas and suppositories: equipment and procedure

Equipment

An absorbent under pad, tissues, lubricating gel, the enema or suppository/ies, gloves and apron.

Ensure that a good light source is available and that privacy can be maintained.

Procedure

- Local medicine policy should be followed (see Chapter 5). Check the expiry date of suppositories/enema.
- Explain the procedure and gain consent. If the person is known to regularly require rectal anticonvulsants, consent should be obtained in advance and documented.
- Some people can insert a suppository themselves; if so, carefully explain the procedure.
- Ensure privacy, dignity and sensitivity throughout the procedure.
- Maintain infection control procedures throughout: hand hygiene, use of gloves and aprons, correct waste disposal (see Chapter 3).
- Give explanations, encouragement and reassurance.
- Some enemas should be warmed before administration – check the manufacturer's instructions. Warm by placing the enema in a jug of warm water. The temperature should be slightly higher than body temperature, feeling warm to the wrist (Schmelzer and Wright 1996).
- Position the person on the left side to allow easy flow of the fluid into the rectum by following the patient's anatomy. Place the under-pad under the patient's buttocks, and ask them to lie at the edge of the bed with knees flexed, and covered by a blanket. This position aids the passage of the nozzle of the enema through the anal canal. This position may need adapting for someone with a physical disability.
- Examine the area around the anus (see discussion on contraindications).
- **Enemas**: Remove the enema cap, expel any air from the enema container (if introduced into the colon this can cause distension and discomfort). Lubricate the nozzle of the enema (some enemas have a pre-lubricated tip). Part the buttocks and gently insert into the anal canal. Squeeze the fluid gently into the rectum from the base of the container to prevent backflow. Some enemas include one-way valves which prevent backflow. Then slowly withdraw the container nozzle to avoid reflux emptying of the rectum. Clean the perianal area and make the patient comfortable.
- **Suppositories**: Lubricate the end of the suppository with the gel. There is conflicting evidence about which end should be inserted first (Bradshaw et al. 2009). Abd-el-Maeboud et al. (1991) suggested that inserting the blunt end first allowed the contracting sphincter to close tightly around the anus, aiding retention. However, most manufacturers suggest the pointed end is inserted first; follow the manufacturer's advice unless local policy advises otherwise. If there is stool present in the rectum, introduce the suppository around the side of the stool, so that it is in contact with the bowel mucosa; avoid embedding it in the stool which will be ineffective (Bradshaw et al. 2009). Wipe the patient's perianal area.
- If the enema or suppository/ies were given to empty the bowel, ask the patient to retain it inside for as long as possible (Schmelzer and Wright 1996). The patient may find it more comfortable to remain lying down. However, an enema can be very difficult to hold on to for long as the effect is likely to be rapid. The person should be assisted to the toilet or other receptacle as necessary.
- Medication administered as a suppository should be retained by the patient. With a retention enema, the patient should remain lying down for the amount of time prescribed on the manufacturer's instructions. A call bell must be near at hand.
- Document that the enema/suppository/ies have been administered in the nursing notes or prescription chart if a medication.
- If the enema or suppositories were given to empty the bowel, you will need to note the result using the Bristol stool chart (see Figure 9.1).

Summary

- Constipation is a common condition that can cause considerable discomfort. The causes are multifactoral and a risk assessment tool can help nurses to identify people at risk.
- Prevention of constipation involves adequate fibre and fluid intake, exercise and avoiding constipation-inducing medicines, if possible. Laxatives can be used but should be a short-term measure.
- Suppositories or enemas may be given to administer medication or to evacuate the bowel. Careful assessment should precede administration as there are contraindications.
- Preparation of the patient/client should include explanation and gaining consent, correct choice of enema/suppositories and other equipment, maintenance of dignity and privacy, and correct positioning of the person to prevent damage to the wall of the rectum.

STOMA CARE

Some patients have to cope with major changes to the way they empty their bladder or bowels. In some cases, the only remedy is the removal of the malfunctioning or diseased bladder or intestine. A stoma is formed (see example, Figure 9.9), and the patient wears an appliance that attaches to the abdomen to collect and dispose of the elimination products.

There are three main types of stoma:

- *Ileal conduit* – formed to drain urine into the stoma bag, if the bladder is removed or bypassed.
- *Ileostomy* – formed when the whole of the large bowel is removed (liquid stool is collected by the stoma bag).
- *Colostomy* – formed when only part of the large bowel is removed (faeces are usually more formed and solid or semi-solid).

Colostomies are the most common types of stoma with more than 11 000 formed a year, compared to approximately 6500 ileostomies and just over 2000 ileal conduits (Coloplast 2010).

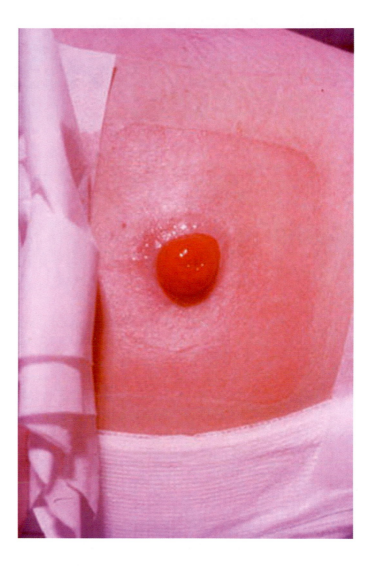

Figure 9.9: An example of a stoma.

This surgery requires careful planning and major inputs by stoma care nurses and other members of the multidisciplinary team. Their roles are meant to ensure that the individual is able to recover and reintegrate into society and the family and cope with everyday life (Parascandolo and Doughty 2001). Not all surgery can be planned, and sometimes a stoma is formed after emergency surgery. These patients therefore have no preparation or stoma nurse involvement prior to surgery, making it more difficult for them to come to terms with the changes and learn to look after their stoma (Erwin-Toth 2003; Richbourg et al. 2007). Whether planned or not, caring for this group of patients is always a challenge (Erwin-Toth 2003). This section focuses on key aspects of nursing care. Other specialist textbooks should be consulted for further details.

Learning outcome 1: Identify the main indications for stoma formation

ACTIVITY

Make a list of some diseases that may lead to someone's bladder or small or large bowel having to be removed or bypassed, resulting in stoma formation.

Different types of stoma and the reasons for their formation are discussed below.

Ileal conduit

This is formed when the patient's lower urinary tract is malfunctioning. The most common cause is bladder cancer, where the bladder is removed. However, ileal conduits are also an option for patients with intractable incontinence or post-pelvic trauma. The ureters are attached to a segment of small bowel (ileum), which is brought to the surface of the body forming a stoma, and draining into a urostomy bag. It is usually sited in the right iliac fossa or, though rarely, on the left.

Ileostomy

This can be formed for cancer of the bowel but most commonly for individuals with inflammatory bowel disease such as ulcerative colitis. When the disease progresses to the point when the pain and diarrhoea and urgency becomes debilitating and interferes with quality of life, then sometimes an ileostomy is recommended. The stoma is usually in the right iliac fossa. The stoma is made of the small bowel. Nowadays, some patients opt to have an ileoanal pouch formed instead of having a permanent ileostomy. In this case, a temporary ileostomy is usually formed first. An ileoanal pouch is an internal reservoir made of bowel in which faecal matter collects and is emptied out by a catheter inserted into a continent stoma. The ileostomy is formed to allow the pouch to heal before being reversed and allowing faecal matter to move into the pouch (Black 2012).

Colostomy

Partial resection of the large intestine means that the stoma is formed of the patient's large bowel. Colon cancer may result in partial bowel resection and stoma formation. Unlike the ileostomy or the ileal conduit, this stoma can be positioned in different parts of the abdomen, depending on the part of the colon that is being removed. The stoma can be placed in either the sigmoid, descending, ascending or transverse colon. This can be a permanent stoma (called a 'permanent end-colostomy') or a temporary one. A temporary colostomy is used when the bowel is not being resected but may need time to heal. Collecting faeces in the stoma bag rather than allowing it to move down the colon promotes this healing. The bowel is partially opened and both ends are brought through the stoma still attached on one side. A plastic 'bridge' is fixed in place under the bowel stoma to stop it slipping back into the abdomen. The stoma is reversed when the two sections of bowel are reattached to each other and pushed back into the abdomen before closing the wound.

Learning outcome 2: Show awareness of the range of equipment commonly used for the different types of stoma

ACTIVITY

In the skills laboratory, there may be sterile or non-sterile (for demonstration purposes) stoma appliances complete with packaging material. See Figure 9.10 for examples. If you can access 'real' equipment, take note of the following:
* The manner in which it is packaged, batch number, expiry date
* The difference between one- and two-piece bags and emptying devices
* The different materials forming the base-plate and how these affect the flexibility of the appliance

There are a huge number of appliances available for patients to choose from. Most bags are made specifically to cope with the output of a particular type of stoma. They come in one- or two-piece format:

- The **one piece** (Figure 9.10a and d) has the bag and flange or base-plate (i.e. the flat part that sticks to the patient's abdomen) attached to each other. To change the bag, the whole appliance is peeled off the abdomen and replaced by a new one.

- The **two piece** (Figure 9.10b and c) has a separate bag which clicks on to the base-plate (similar to a Tupperware lid) (Figure 9.10e). In some products, a locking system can be activated to ensure greater security. If the bag needs changing, it can simply be clicked off and replaced by a new one. As the base-plate remains in place rather than being peeled off the skin each time, it is kinder to the skin. If a patient has to change bags more than once a day (e.g. for religious reasons), then a two-piece appliance allows them to do this without compromising the skin by having to change the base-plate each time.

The base-plate is usually made of a hydrocolloid (natural or artificial) with an integral adhesive area. This can have an extra taped area surrounding it for extra

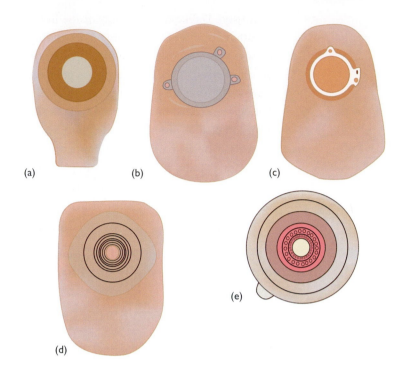

Figure 9.10: Types of stoma appliances. (a) One-piece drainage bag; (b) two-piece drainage bag; (c) two-piece non-drainable bag; (d) one-piece non-drainable bag; (e) flange/base-plate for fitting with two-piece systems, for example, (b) and (c).

security. This taped area is also more flexible than the hydrocolloid area and can fit to the body's contours more easily (Black 2012). The bags can be clear plastic or flesh coloured.

Bags may be drainable or non-drainable:

- **Drainable bags** (Figure 9.10a and b). As ileal conduit and ileostomy stomas produce constant liquid output, bags are used which can be emptied via a tap (if urine) or via an opening device like a clip (if stool; see Figure 9.10a and b). This means patients do not need to change their bags each time, especially if they choose to wear a one-piece bag. Bags should be able to hold a reasonable capacity to avoid patients constantly having to empty the bags. Bags come in different sizes – from paediatric (holding as little as 100 mL) to adult (holding anything up to 750 mL). If the colostomy is in the ascending or hepatic flexure of the transverse colon, then the output is semi-solid and a drainable bag should be used.

- **Non-drainable bags** (Figure 9.10c and d). These are used for the more formed output of colostomies sited in the descending or sigmoid colon. Patients simply change the bag once they have had their bowels open and dispose of it with its contents. Some companies now produce biodegradable colostomy bags that can be flushed down the toilet. Many patients can anticipate when they are going to have their bowels open because, if regular, most people have them open at a certain time of day (e.g. morning, before or after breakfast) and usually only once a day. Thus, bags need not be large or bulky as the patient can anticipate when a larger bag is warranted.

Some patients prefer not to wear a colostomy bag. They wear a small pouch or cap to cover the stoma. To ensure they do not have their bowels open unexpectedly they opt to perform a washout or irrigation of the bowel. This is similar to a rectal washout but performed via the stoma instead. Ensuring the bowel is clean in this way means that elimination is predictable and most patients achieve complete continence in between washouts. The whole procedure can take 30–60 minutes, though experienced patients can complete it in 15 minutes (Collett 2002; Karadag et al. 2005).

Use of suppositories or enemas with stomas

If a patient becomes constipated then suppositories or an enema can be inserted down the stoma to either lubricate or stimulate the bowel to pass a motion (Collett 2002). However, specific techniques are required as there are no sphincters to control motions in stomas (see Williams 2012). Suppositories should not be inserted into ileostomies as these do not become constipated and lack of output is likely to be a blockage (Williams 2012).

Learning outcome 3: Discuss the care required for people who have a stoma

ACTIVITY

Try to put yourself in the place of a patient who has to have stoma surgery. What feelings or fears do you have? What skills do you think you will have to learn to be able to care for yourself once you recover?

Preoperative preparation

Effective preoperative preparation is essential and patients should therefore be referred to a stoma care nurse specialist well in advance. There may be psychological issues such as coping with a change in body image. Meeting a patient who has already had a stoma can help patients to see what living life with an appliance is really like. Bowel preparation is necessary only if the patient is impacted with faeces which cannot be cleared by restricting food intake and only allowing fluids to drink.

Siting the stoma is an extremely important consideration. The stoma care nurse specialist will address both physical and social aspects during assessment, ensuring that the bag will not hinder the patient's daily activities. It is also important to ensure the patient is not allergic to the adhesive or hydrocolloid in the base-plate, the plastic material or cover of the drainage bag, so a patch test should be carried out.

Postoperative care

The most vital part of the postoperative care is to ensure that the stoma is viable and healing well. Besides the usual postoperative care after major abdominal surgery, the stoma should be checked to ensure it is pink and warm and it should adhere to the abdominal wall. The stoma should not look blue or black, or feel cold as this means that the circulation is compromised and if allowed to deteriorate the stoma may become sloughed, black and necrotic. The output should be checked; if it is an ileal conduit, then the output should be urine; if it is a colostomy, then there may be flatus though not necessarily stool; and an ileostomy should have some liquid faecal matter.

Sometimes, there is a delay in the stoma becoming active and producing faeces. Any prolonged delay should be reported as the patient may need more surgery. Diet following stoma formation needs consideration, both postoperatively and in the long term (see Floruta 2001).

Teaching self-care

Ideally, patients are discharged from hospital only when they have learnt how to care for their stoma. Usually, patients are ready to start learning how to empty and change the bags after the first week following surgery. The patient must also learn what a normal stoma looks like, how it should function and what complications to look out for, as well as how to clean the stoma area and how to safely dispose of the output and the appliances. Ideally, the patient should have the support of district nurses or community stoma care nurses on returning home to help adjust to living with a stoma in a non-hospital environment (Richbourg et al. 2007).

Managing the appliance

The stoma is usually swollen postoperatively, but it slowly shrinks to a more normal size as the patient recovers. The base-plates which adhere to the abdomen need a central aperture cut out to fit around the stoma. These base-plates are usually all one size but are made such that the hydrocolloid area varies in size, allowing it to be cut to fit all sizes of stoma. The nurse specialist will provide a template of the correct size which the patient can use to cut out a hole in the centre of the base-plates. This must fit snugly around the stoma without being too tight or cutting off circulation to the stoma. Correct fitting ensures that the skin under the base-plate is protected from the effluent produced by the stoma which otherwise may cause excoriation and leakage and result in the bag not adhering securely and falling off. As the stoma shrinks, this template may have to be altered.

Stoma appliances are available on prescription and are provided free of cost to stoma patients in the United Kingdom. They can be obtained from pharmacies, though many patients prefer to use supply companies who deliver the appliances in discreet packages directly to their homes. Delivery in most cases is within 24 hours of placing an order, and many companies provide extras such as cleaning wipes and disposal bags at no extra cost. If patients find it difficult to cut the template openings, then these companies also provide a cutting service using a personalised template which the patient can send in or which the nurse specialist can fax to the company.

ACTIVITY — What equipment do you think you will need to change an appliance?

The materials needed to change a stoma appliance are as follows:
- A new appliance
- Wipes for cleaning and drying skin
- Warm water
- A waste disposal bag (at home the patient may use a nappy sac)
- Scissors (if the base-plate is not pre-cut)
- Measuring guide, to measure the size of stoma and cut out correct size in template for base-plate
- Gloves and apron

Once the old base-plate and bag are removed, the skin and stoma are cleaned using warm water and a soft wipe. The skin around the stoma is dried thoroughly to ensure the new base-plate sticks to the abdominal skin securely. Applying gentle but firm pressure over the base-plate helps this process. If the base-plate cannot lie flat on the abdomen, then there are products (e.g. stoma paste) and appliances that can help – the stoma care nurse specialist can advise.

Patients with ileal conduits may wish to clip a larger drainage bag to the tap at the bottom of the stoma bag at night. Once the tap is open, urine will drain out of the stoma bag into the larger drainage bag. This ensures that the stoma bag will not leak or come off if it becomes too full of urine when the patient is in bed.

Colostomy bags come with built-in flatus outlets to let gas out as it builds up in the bag. This allows the bag to lie flat under clothes and not come off or leak because of the build-up.

ACTIVITY — What steps would you follow to teach Jean to empty her stoma bag?

Jean should be encouraged to do this by herself as soon as possible following recovery from the effects of surgery. She should be supervised as she goes through the following steps:
- Encourage her to find the best position, such as sitting on the toilet or kneeling or standing beside it.
- Put toilet paper in the toilet bowl to avoid splashback.
- Open the tap/clip/velcro end of the bag and drain into the toilet bowl.
- Squeeze out all the contents.
- Close and clean the tap/clip/velcro on the outside to avoid staining clothing.
- Flush the toilet and wash her hands (Stoma Care 2007).

ACTIVITY — How should you dispose of used stoma equipment in a hospital? How would Jean dispose of used stoma equipment at home?

In hospital, hand hygiene and use of gloves and apron are necessary (see Chapter 3), and the equipment should be disposed of in the infective waste bag unless local policy advises otherwise. The DH (2006) advised that, in the community, stoma care waste can be disposed of in the black-bag waste stream. Accordingly, Stoma Care (2007) advises that disposal at home does not require any special arrangements and suggests that, after emptying, the appliance can be wrapped in newspaper, put in a nappy sac and disposed of in normal household refuse. However, if when at home Jean developed any type of gastrointestinal infection or the site became infected, her bag must be disposed of as infectious waste – the community nurse should advise her about this.

Most bags can stay on for up to 3 days as long as the patient is comfortable. Some patients may prefer to change the bags daily, so regimes must be tailored to individuals (Erwin-Toth 2003). If the skin becomes sensitive there are specially developed non-greasy lotions to sooth it and protect it from the adhesive. There are also lotions or wipes that dry on application to the skin forming a plastic barrier layer to protect the skin under the base-plate.

Teaching patients how to change bags and care for the stoma can be time-consuming. Patients with learning disabilities or physical problems with dexterity or eyesight may need a lot of time and input from nurses and carers. If Jean, the patient in our scenario, cannot change the bag and care for the stoma herself, her husband may have to do it instead. Even if Jean is successful, she will need his help and support as someone will have to take over this part of her care should she become ill and unable to cope. This may be problematic for her husband who has problems with his sight. It is imperative, therefore, that Jean learns how to care for this herself no matter how much time it takes for her to become confident and competent. Patients should not be rushed; support and continued teaching should ideally continue after discharge.

All stomas present similar management problems for patients. Patients should be followed up regularly by the stoma nurse to continue supporting the patient and to identify and deal with any problems. Richbourg et al. (2007) found that patients who had been counselled by nurses both before and after surgery suffered fewer complications – or at least found they coped with them more effectively. Patients who had their stoma sites marked preoperatively and were assessed by a stoma nurse also suffered fewer problems with sore skin and badly fitting appliances (Parascandolo and Doughty 2001; Ratliff et al. 2005). However, complications such as stenosis, prolapse, incisional or bowel hernias or disease progression could not be predicted or avoided by nursing intervention.

Nurses should be aware of other complications which often occur, including sexual dysfunction (e.g. after cystectomy for bladder cancer), problems with body image, decrease in social activities and interaction, isolation, anxiety and depression (Ratliff et al. 2005), and have strategies in place to help patients cope. This may include counselling or regular visits to nurse clinics to reinforce teaching and offer support. The likelihood of long-term complications (e.g. upper urinary tract changes in ileal conduit patients) increases the longer the patient has a stoma (Madersbacher et al. 2003).

Caring for patients with a stoma who have dementia

There are different types of dementia which produce similar symptoms though may progress and be treated differently (Nazarko 2011). One of the main problems for people with dementia is memory loss, which can occur early at the onset of the disease and has significant impact on the ability to learn and retain new information or experiences (Milwain 2010). Learning how to care for a stoma has a huge impact on anyone and for someone with dementia this may be even more challenging. Many stoma care patients with dementia do not acknowledge that they even have a stoma, so teaching them to care for it presents challenges for healthcare professionals and carers alike, for example, inappropriate disposal of stoma bags.

People with dementia need more time to acclimatise to the ward environment before surgery, and their discharge should be delayed until they are able to take care of themselves (Black 2011). Nurses teaching these patients should take the time to get to know the patient and identify their specific needs such as what causes them anxiety or triggers challenging behaviour. Any care should be tailored to the needs of patients and carers (Scottish Intercollegiate Guidelines Network [SIGN] 2006). Black (2011) advocates individualised learning programmes which take into consideration the patient's memory, communication and understanding problems. She also advises that how and where the patient is taught may also impact on the eventual outcome, for example, teaching self-care in small steps and in an environment that is quiet and has few distractions. Using repetition and ensuring continuity also help.

However, being completely independent in caring for the stoma may be beyond some patients' abilities no matter how much time and care is invested. Ultimately, having a stoma may result in patients with dementia going into residential care because relatives and carers cannot cope with the extra stress of a stoma (Black 2011). Healthcare professionals therefore face an ethical dilemma when it comes to performing this surgery in patients with dementia as it can have far reaching impact on the quality of life of both the patients and their carers.

Caring for young people with a stoma

If possible, young patients should be offered alternative surgery to avoid them having a permanent stoma. However, this may not always be appropriate or feasible. Nurses who care for patients of this age group need to have an understanding of adolescent physical and cognitive development and what young people want from the hospital experience and those who care for them. Ideally, they should be cared for in special units which have specific facilities and staff trained to support young people.

During adolescence, the young person is developing both physically and cognitively, and it is during this period that they address issues around their sexual development, self-esteem and body image. So, having stoma care surgery at this time could impact greatly on normal development and their ability to build relationships and reach maturity (Busuttil Leaver and Leach 2004). Communication is key to building a rapport. Nurses should develop active listening skills, be non-judgemental, straightforward in approach, use clear language and ensure privacy

(Deering and Cody 2002). Nurses should be prepared to offer alternatives and allow for compromise when setting limits. The way a young person copes with illness, hospitalisation, disability and the family dynamics should also be assessed especially in long-term illness. Physical and psychological care should go hand in hand in order to help the young person cope.

Summary

- Having stoma surgery is life-changing and can have serious psychological consequences for patients, such as problems with body image.
- Planned, individualised preoperative preparation, and postoperative care and teaching, minimise complications and help patients cope and achieve self-care.
- Understanding these problems and having a good knowledge of stoma appliances and accessory products will help nurses to offer acceptable solutions to patients and in some cases avoid further surgery.
- However, complications cannot always be anticipated and tend to increase the longer a patient has a stoma.
- Continued support of the patient and/or carer and long-term follow-up will help ensure the patient continues to have a good quality of life and ultimate survival.
- Special consideration should be given to supporting people with dementia or young people who have stomas formed, and how adjustment and self-care can be facilitated.

PROMOTING CONTINENCE AND MANAGING INCONTINENCE

The DH (2010) defines continence as: 'people's control of their bladder and bowel function' (p. 7). Urinary incontinence is the inability to control the leakage of urine and is a common and distressing problem (Wallace et al. 2009). Faecal incontinence is defined as the involuntary passage of faecal material through the anal canal (Deutekom and Dobben 2012). This section focuses on understanding the causes and effects of incontinence and practical issues of management, but not specialist interventions. Continence is a huge topic to which whole books are devoted; for example, Getliffe and Dolman (2007) cover all aspects in detail.

LEARNING OUTCOMES

By the end of this section, you will be able to:

1 discuss the causes and effects of urinary and faecal incontinence;
2 explain principles of assessment relating to incontinence;
3 identify interventions for promoting urinary continence;
4 discuss appropriate nursing interventions for promoting faecal continence and managing faecal incontinence;
5 explain the nursing management of incontinence.

Learning outcome 1: Discuss the causes and effects of urinary and faecal incontinence

Continence is a complex skill and relies on being able to recognise the need to eliminate faeces and/or urine, identify an appropriate place in which to eliminate and being able to wait until arriving there. When any of these fail, incontinence occurs.

ACTIVITY

> Reflect back on patients/clients you have been in contact with and consider what causes urinary and faecal incontinence?

Urinary incontinence

Causes are diverse and varied and you may see different classifications in different texts. The main types are as follows:

Urge incontinence: leakage of urine when a person is unable to control the strong desire to pass urine (void) (Wallace et al. 2009) as a result of over activity of the detrusor (bladder) muscle (overactive bladder syndrome) (Pellatt 2012).

Stress urinary incontinence: the involuntary leakage of urine on effort or exertion, for example, on sneezing or coughing, presumably due to raised abdominal pressure; contributing factors include: obesity, high impact sport and severe constipation (Billington 2010).

Mixed urinary incontinence: where there is involuntary urine leakage associated with both urgency and exertion, effort, sneezing or coughing (NICE 2006).

Functional incontinence: the inability to get to the toilet in time due to mobility or other functional difficulties such as dexterity.

Although urinary incontinence can be an isolated condition, it also occurs in the context of other health problems, particularly those which affect activity (Chiarelli and Weatherall 2010). Some medicines can contribute to incontinence; Bob's incontinence was probably caused by clozapine. Studies have indicated an association between urinary incontinence and diabetes (Jackson et al. 2005; Lewis et al. 2005). As the central and peripheral nervous systems regulate bladder function, neurological conditions, such as multiple sclerosis, often affect continence (see NICE 2012b for a detailed consideration). Bar and Sowney (2007) identified that incontinence rates are often higher among people with learning disabilities due to accompanying physical disabilities and impaired mobility. People with learning as well as a physical disability may not be able to communicate that they need to be taken to the toilet, especially if staff are not familiar with their method of communicating this need, which may be through signing or symbols. People with dementia may develop functional incontinence due to difficulties in finding the toilet, memory problems, poor manual dexterity, impaired cognition or reduced mobility (Hägglund 2010). The unfamiliarity of the hospital environment may increase these difficulties. For prevalence of urinary incontinence, see Box 9.13.

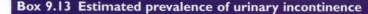
> ### Box 9.13 Estimated prevalence of urinary incontinence
>
> **Women living at home**
>
> 15–44 years: between 1 in 20 and 1 in 14
>
> 45–64 years: between 1 in 13 and 1 in 7
>
> Aged 65 years plus: between 1 in 10 and 1 in 5
>
> **Men living at home**
>
> 15–64 years: over 1 in 33
>
> Aged 65 years plus: between 1 in 14 and 1 in 10
>
> **Both sexes living in institutions**
>
> One-third of those in residential homes
>
> Nearly two-thirds of those in nursing homes
>
> One-half to two-thirds in wards for older people, or older people with mental health problems
>
> *Source:* Department of Health (DH). 2000. *Good Practice in Continence Services.* London: DH.

Faecal incontinence

NICE (2007b) identifies that faecal incontinence is a sign or symptom, not a disease. High-risk groups for faecal incontinence include: people who are old and frail, have loose stools/diarrhoea from any cause, have a neurological or spinal disease/injury, have severe cognitive impairment, urinary incontinence, pelvic organ prolapse or rectal prolapse following colonic resection or anal surgery, people with learning disabilities and women following obstetric injury in childbirth (NICE 2007b). NICE (2007b) asserted that faecal incontinence is largely a hidden problem due to its social stigma but estimates that up to 10% of adults are affected by faecal incontinence and between 0.5 and 1% of adults have regular faecal incontinence affecting their quality of life.

Establishing accurate prevalence figures for incontinence in the population can be problematic as people do not always seek help for continence issues.

ACTIVITY

Consider: why might people not seek help for continence problems?

There are two main reasons for non-reporting of incontinence: embarrassment, and the belief that nothing can be done to help. MacDonald and Butler (2007) identified the isolation of women with incontinence who did not talk to anyone about it as they felt it was not a socially acceptable topic of conversation and that it was untreatable. Wells and Wagg (2007) found that Bangladeshi women saw bladder weakness as a loss of self-control and a personal problem rather than a medical problem, so they did not seek professional help. People's definitions of incontinence vary, so they may not interpret their problem as incontinence. Studies have found that older people with urinary incontinence consider it to be an inevitable part of ageing (Avery et al. 2006; Palmer and Newman 2006) and even some nursing staff share this view with patients and relatives (Kristiansen et al. 2011). However, urinary incontinence is not a disease or a normal result of ageing, but a symptom of an underlying condition.

You read in the scenario that Bob was distressed and embarrassed about his urinary incontinence.

ACTIVITY	How might incontinence affect people: physically, psychologically and socially?

The many possible effects include physical (e.g. increased falls, skin problems, dependency), social (e.g. impact on relationships, sexuality, employment and leisure) and psychological (e.g. embarrassment, lack of self-esteem). Kristiansen et al. (2011) identified that urinary incontinence led to increased vulnerability, loss of independence and a feeling of being a burden. Faecal incontinence is a particularly distressing condition with significant medical, social and economic implications (Norton and Cody 2012). Faecal incontinence is also a common reason for older people to need nursing home care (Brown et al. 2013).

To accurately assess the underlying cause and suggest possible ways of managing incontinence, a thorough assessment is necessary (see learning outcome 2).

Learning outcome 2: Explain principles of assessment relating to incontinence

As people are often too embarrassed to report incontinence to health professionals, staff should provide opportunities for people to discuss any concerns about their bladder or bowel functions during consultations and offer an initial bladder and bowel continence assessment, as indicated (DH 2010). As discussed under learning outcome 1, there are many possible underlying causes of incontinence. Temporary causes of urinary incontinence, such as UTI, confusion, medication, faecal impaction, impaired mobility and depression, should be identified. In Bob's case, staff investigated further the side effects of clozapine and discovered that incontinence was a recognised side effect, but it was also important that their assessment included a urinalysis.

ACTIVITY	Assessment includes interviewing, observation and measurement. Keeping these in mind, consider how a nurse might initially assess a patient's urinary incontinence.

Box 9.14 identifies some key points, and these are expanded on below.

When using interviewing skills to assess incontinence, approach and terminology used need careful consideration. Stewart (2010) suggests that assessment needs to be undertaken by an empathetic, sensitive practitioner who uses easily understandable language and avoids technical medical jargon. For example, when assessing nocturia, the patient should be asked, 'how many times do you get up to go to the toilet

> **Box 9.14 Assessment of urinary incontinence: key points**
>
> Interviewing
> • Sensitive, empathetic approach
> • Careful and appropriate use of language
> • Involvement of carers
>
> Observation
> • Physical factors, for example, obstructive symptoms, hesitancy, intermittent stream, dribbling after voiding and straining to void, urgency, difficulty in undressing
> • Psychological factors, for example, confusion, fear
> • Environmental factors, for example, access to the toilet
>
> Measurement
> • Urinalysis
> • Charting frequency and amount
>
> NB: Referral to a continence advisor may be required. Use of an assessment tool will promote a systematic approach.

at night?' rather than 'do you suffer from nocturia?' Similarly, a patient can be asked how often they pass water rather than being asked if they have frequency. Palmer and Newman (2006) identified that questions should be worded carefully (e.g. 'Do you lose water when you don't want to?') rather than asking if they are incontinent. Rassin et al. (2007) found that women often did not perceive they had incontinence but described 'leaking'. If a person has a cognitive impairment, involvement of the carer to obtain a history is particularly important. Likewise, observation while assisting the person to go to the toilet will be very helpful (see Box 9.14). As regards measurement, NICE (2006) recommends bladder diaries should be completed for a minimum of 3 days to more accurately assess urinary frequency and incontinence episodes.

NICE (2007b) recommends that healthcare professionals should ask people in high-risk groups for faecal incontinence sensitively about symptoms. Smith (2010) suggests that nurses should initially seek to identify each patient's risk factors for developing faecal incontinence during the initial assessment process, as some will be modifiable. These risk factors range from reduced dietary and fluid intake to the complex symptoms associated with long-term conditions. NICE (2007b) recommends that a baseline assessment for people with faecal incontinence should comprise relevant medical history, a general examination, an anorectal examination and a cognitive assessment, if appropriate.

The RCN (2011) warn that incontinence may be attributed to a person's learning disabilities rather than other causes, including ill-health. This is termed **diagnostic overshadowing**, where signs and symptoms are attributed to the learning disability rather than investigating for other causes. Bar and Sowney (2007) recommend that when assessing a person with a learning disability, the nurse should observe what the person is able to do, and ask questions such as 'How do you get on with using the toilet?', or ask a carer 'How does he manage with the toilet?' Closed negative questions asking whether the person is incontinent should be avoided. People with a physical disability and a communication difficulty may know when they want to go to the toilet, but carers will not be able to recognise this need if a method of communication has not been established.

Some people with urinary and/or faecal incontinence require a more specialised assessment and should be referred to the continence service, to see a continence specialist nurse, for example. Specialist investigations are sometimes necessary.

ACTIVITY

When next in practice:
1 Find out how referrals are made to a continence advisor in your area of practice.
2 Investigate whether any specific assessment documents are used in practice for assessment of incontinence.

Many practice settings have a specific continence assessment tool that will help to identify both the cause and possible management of incontinence. The DH (2010) advises that assessment tools are evidence-based and adapted for specific groups.

For people with neurological conditions, NICE (2012b) outlines a detailed and evidence-based assessment.

Mark's CLDN should work with him and his mother to empower him to access continence services and could carry out a joint assessment with a continence advisor. Mark's continence should be addressed in his health action plan. Smith and Smith (2007) examine continence training for people with learning disabilities in detail.

Learning outcome 3: Identify interventions for promoting urinary continence

How urinary continence is promoted obviously depends on the underlying cause, which is why an understanding of causes and careful assessment is important.

ACTIVITY

Think back to patients you have encountered who had urinary continence problems. What methods have you seen being used to promote continence for people in practice settings?

The methods you have seen should have been chosen to address the type of incontinence, based on the person's assessment. You might have seen lifestyle advice (e.g., fluid intake, weight loss) being given, pelvic floor muscle (PFM) training being taught (for stress or mixed incontinence), or have assisted with bladder training (for urge or overactive bladder syndrome) or voiding programmes. Following a systematic review, Chirarelli et al. (2009) recommended addressing inter-related factors associated with both falls and incontinence. Risk factors that could be modified include: mobility and transfer impairments, visual impairment, cognitive decline, poly-pharmacy, environmental hazards, and orthostatic hypotension (Chirarelli et al. 2009). To reduce functional incontinence, physiotherapists can help with mobility and balance, enabling quicker transfers; and occupational therapists help in making

Box 9.15 Promoting continence for people with dementia: top tips for nurses

1 Check whether the person with dementia can get to the toilet without any problems. They may want to use the toilet but be unable to find it.
2 Make sure the person knows where the toilet is by showing them. A picture of a toilet on the door can act as a visual reminder. Make the image bright and easy to see by positioning it at eye level.
3 Remove any obstacles in the way such as awkwardly placed furniture or doors that are hard to open.
4 Remind the person to go to the toilet, or take them there, at regular intervals (see sections on prompted voiding and timed voiding).
5 Observe for signs that the person wants to go to the toilet such as fidgeting, getting up and down or pulling at their clothes.
6 Encourage other patients to keep the toilet door open when not in use so it is obvious when the toilet is vacant. However, ensure that the door is fully closed when in use.
7 A coloured toilet that contrasts with the pan can make it easier to see as bathroom facilities that are all the same colour can be disorientating to people with dementia.
8 Ensure that clothing can be quickly removed and unfastened. For example, velcro fastenings may be easier to use than zips or buttons.

Source: Summarised from Alzheimer's Society, http://www.alzheimers.org.uk/site/scripts/documents_info.php?documentID=1211&pageNumber=5

the environment and dressing and undressing easier, for example, with clothing adaptations. Vickerman (2003) asserts that many people are rendered incontinent by a poorly adapted environment and advises that the heights of chairs, beds and toilets should be assessed and adjusted, as well as considering lighting, signs, floor coverings, grab rails and provision of commodes and hand-held urinals. You may also have seen medical interventions which can include pharmacology (Rigby 2007) or surgery (when conservative measures have failed). According to Alzheimer's Society (2009), nurses and carers identified concerns related to continence of people with dementia. In response, Alzheimer's Society developed some 'Top tips'. Box 9.15 includes some of these additional points.

NICE (2006) recommends that, at initial assessment of women, urinary incontinence should be categorised as either 'stress urinary incontinence', 'mixed urinary incontinence' or 'urge/overactive bladder syndrome', so that appropriate interventions can be planned. NICE (2006) provides algorithms for each type of incontinence.

Some of the measures for promoting urinary continence will be explained in more detail.

PFM training

PFM training involves the PFMs being squeezed and lifted, then relaxed, several times in a row, up to three times a day (Herderschee et al. 2011). The exercises can help strengthen the muscles and improve their endurance and coordination, so that the muscle squeezes hardest when the risk of leaking is greatest (e.g. with a cough) (Herderschee et al. 2011).

PFM training is the most commonly used physical therapy for women with stress urinary incontinence and is sometimes advised for mixed and, less commonly, for urge urinary incontinence (Hay-Smith et al. 2011). NICE (2006) suggests a trial of supervised PFM training for at least three months as the first-line treatment for women with stress or mixed urinary incontinence, which should involve at least eight contractions performed three times a day. Women receiving regular (e.g. weekly) supervision are more likely to report improvement than women doing PFM training with little or no supervision (Hay-Smith et al. 2011). Weighted vaginal cones can be inserted into the vagina and the pelvic floor is contracted to prevent them from slipping out (Herbison and Dean 2009). Biofeedback can be used to teach contraction of the correct muscles and when and how to contract the muscle to prevent leakage (Herderschee et al. 2011). Biofeedback uses a vaginal or anal device to measure the muscle squeeze pressure or the electrical activity in the muscle and gives feedback as a sound or visual display (Herderschee et al. 2011).

In men, stress incontinence may occur following prostatectomy, for whom NICE (2010b) advises PFM training for at least 3 months before considering other options. Dorey (2007) details exercises that can be taught to men to perform at home in different situations and positions, but states that they should be taught by a specialist to ensure that they are performed correctly.

Bladder re-education

Bladder re-education involves re-educating the bladder to an improved pattern of voiding and has several variations, suitable for different client groups. All staff should be fully aware and motivated towards these programmes, so that they are implemented consistently. Roe et al. (2006) explained that bladder training is used for cognitively and physically able adults, while prompted voiding, habit retraining and timed voiding – collectively known as voiding programmes – are generally used for people with cognitive or physical impairments in institutional settings. NICE (2012b) recommends that for people with neurogenic lower urinary tract dysfunction, a behavioural management programme (e.g., timed voiding, bladder retraining or habit retraining) can be used but only after assessment by a healthcare professional trained in the assessment of people with neurogenic lower urinary tract dysfunction and combined with education about the lower urinary tract function for the person and/or their carers.

Bladder training

Based on limited evidence, bladder training may be helpful for the treatment of urinary incontinence (Wallace et al. 2009). Bladder training aims to increase the interval between voids so that continence might be regained and is widely used for the treatment of urinary incontinence (Wallace et al. 2009). For example, the person might initially be asked to go to the toilet every hour. This is then gradually extended by half an hour at a time. NICE (2006) recommends that, for women with overactive bladders, with or without urge incontinence, bladder training for a minimum of six weeks should be offered. Education of patients and carers, use of a continence chart and continuous encouragement are all important elements. Carers need to praise to build up confidence and reinforce behaviour and they should be patient and understanding.

Voiding programmes

Timed voiding

Timed voiding is also referred to as scheduled, fixed, routine or regular toileting/voiding. The main feature is voiding to a fixed time pattern; for example, 2-, 3- or 4-hourly. Timed voiding is promoted for people with urinary incontinence who cannot participate in independent toileting and is commonly assumed to represent current practice in residential care settings for older people (Ostaszkiewicz et al. 2011). It is often used for people with a neurogenic bladder, such as those with spinal cord lesions, and for people with a physical or mental disability. It can include techniques to trigger voiding, such as tapping over the suprapubic region or running water. However, there is currently little evidence about the effects of timed voiding on the management of urinary incontinence (Ostaszkiewicz et al. 2011).

Habit retraining

Habit retraining involves the identification of a person's natural voiding pattern and the development of an individualised toileting schedule, which pre-empts involuntary bladder emptying (Ostaszkiewicz et al. 2010). A record of voiding and incontinent episodes is kept so that the schedule can be adjusted, with voiding intervals lengthened if the person is dry, and reduced if incontinence occurs. NICE (2012b) recommends that habit retraining is particularly suitable for people with cognitive impairment.

Prompted voiding

Prompted voiding is a behavioural therapy, which aims to improve bladder control for people with or without dementia using verbal prompts and positive reinforcement (Eustice et al. 2009). Prompted voiding programmes have been recommended for women who have urinary incontinence and cognitive impairment (NICE 2006) and other people with cognitive impairment (NICE 2012b). Prompted voiding has been used with people with learning disabilities too and could be an appropriate strategy for Mark, in our scenarios. Ostaszkiewicz (2006) found that prompted voiding was more sustainable than habit retraining or timed voiding, but it needed more resources to implement. Although there is evidence of short-term benefits of prompted voiding, it is not known if these persist (Eustice et al. 2009).

Learning outcome 4: Identify appropriate nursing interventions for promoting faecal continence and managing faecal incontinence

Faecal incontinence is a distressing disorder with high social stigma (Deutekom and Dobben 2012). NICE (2007b) includes a comprehensive flow chart for managing faecal incontinence in adults. Underlying conditions should be addressed and, if faecal incontinence continues, people should be referred for specialised management. Anal sphincter exercises (PFM training) and biofeedback therapy have been used to treat the symptoms of people with faecal incontinence (Norton and Cody 2012). Other measures include PFM training, bowel retraining, specialist dietary assessment and management, and electrical stimulation or rectal irrigation. Some interventions recommended are discussed below.

Diet

There should be a balanced nutrient intake and at least 1.5 L of fluid intake daily for people with hard stools or those who are dehydrated (unless contraindicated). Hansen et al. (2006) found that diet modification was central to managing faecal incontinence: restricting foods that exacerbated faecal incontinence, avoiding gas-producing foods, and limiting portion or meal size.

Bowel habit

Predictable bowel emptying should be promoted by encouraging bowel emptying after a meal, ensuring toilet facilities are private, comfortable and safe, allowing sufficient time, encouraging people to adopt a sitting/squatting position and avoiding straining. Akpan et al. (2006) highlighted that many older people, especially those who were dependent, lacked privacy during bowel movements.

Toilet access

Staff can help the person to access the toilet by ensuring that the location is clear to them, provide equipment to assist access, and advise them about easily removable clothing. A home/mobility assessment may be necessary.

Medication

Alternatives to those contributing to faecal incontinence should be considered. Anti-diarrhoeal drugs (e.g. loperamide) may be appropriate.

Coping strategies

These include continence products (disposable body-worn pads, bed pads, anal plugs and faecal collectors), skin care, odour control, laundry advice and support. Learning outcome 5 addresses incontinence pads and skin care. Anal plugs aim to block the loss of stool (Deutekom and Dobben 2012). Though they can be difficult to tolerate, they can be effective; they are available in different designs and sizes and plug selection can affect performance (Deutekom and Dobben 2012). Palmieri et al. (2005) studied the use of a bag to collect stools in faecal incontinence and found no adverse reactions. The bag was well tolerated and it was not painful to remove or apply. The 'Flexi-Seal faecal management system' is a temporary containment device, consisting of a soft, flexible silicone catheter with a low-pressure balloon that is filled with water or saline to aid retention. The device is inserted into the patient's rectum and attached to a catheter bag. It can collect liquid or semi-liquid stools and is most suitable for bed-bound patients, for example, in critical care. In the evaluation of this system by Padmanabhan et al. (2007), skin condition was maintained or improved in most patients. Along with diverting faeces from the skin, the system also assists with infection control and allows more accurate fluid balance monitoring.

Education and support

Targeted patient/carer education improved bowel dysfunction symptoms in the study by Harari et al. (2004). Chelvanayagam and Stern (2007) found that group therapy facilitated by experienced therapists improved both physical and psychological well-being of people with faecal incontinence.

Learning outcome 5: Explain the nursing management of incontinence

Incontinence should be managed in a manner that is unobtrusive, reliable and comfortable. If incontinence cannot be prevented, then a suitable containment method is needed, for example, pads, or, for a man with urinary incontinence, possibly a penile sheath. As mentioned in the previous section, for faecal incontinence there are also anal pugs, faecal collection bags and systems. Incontinence aids should preserve hygiene, dignity, psychological and social comfort.

Urethral catheterisation is rarely appropriate for managing urinary incontinence as it may lead to catheter-related problems such as UTI (see section 'Caring for people with urinary catheters'). However, NICE (2006) recommends that catheterisation should be considered for women with persistent urinary retention that causes incontinence, symptomatic infections or renal dysfunction that cannot be corrected. NICE (2006) suggests that the risks and benefits should be discussed considering urine contamination of skin wounds, pressure ulcers, irritation, distress and disruption caused by bed and clothing changes, and women's preferences. Intermittent urethral catheterisation is another option that can be taught to the person or their carer.

NICE (2006) recommends that absorbent products (pads) should not be considered a treatment option for urinary incontinence in women and should only be used to help patients who are waiting for treatment, as an adjunct to other therapies, and for long-term management, if other treatments have failed. Similarly for men, NICE (2010a) recommends use of temporary containment products (for example, pads or collecting devices) to achieve social continence until a diagnosis and management plan have been established.

ACTIVITY

If you find that a person has been incontinent, what would your priorities of care be?

Priorities are to assist the person quickly, to prevent skin damage, relieve discomfort and restore dignity. Many of the principles discussed earlier related to dealing with a person's elimination needs are relevant, in particular: approachability and communication, privacy and dignity, promptness, prevention of cross-infection, observation, hygiene and comfort. The nurse's approach when dealing with incontinence is crucial to the level of distress experienced. Nurses dealing with Bob's urinary incontinence should be discreet and matter-of-fact in changing his bed while reassuring him that the cause would be investigated. In faecal incontinence, in particular, prompt changing of soiled pads or clothing is essential to help to prevent odours and skin excoriation, and reduce the risk of cross-infection.

Skin care

Ersser et al. (2005) identified that urinary incontinence is an important cause of skin vulnerability and that older people are a high-risk group for skin damage as their skin is more permeable, enabling external moisture to infiltrate epidermal layers and increasing the friction coefficient at the skin's surface. Incontinence-associated dermatitis can develop, which is an inflammatory condition of the skin that is associated with faecal or urinary incontinence (Wolfman 2010). Ersser et al. (2005) explained that incontinence leads to skin problems because:

- wetness of the skin encourages maceration, disrupting the skin barrier leading to breakdown;
- decomposition of the urinary urea by microorganisms releases ammonia, forming the alkali ammonium hydroxide, thus altering the skin's pH (the pH of normal skin ranges from 5.4 to 5.9, providing an acid mantle);
- chemical irritation of the skin arises from urine, the rise in alkalinity and bacterial proliferation;
- the presence of faecal urease results in breakdown of the urinary urea causing increase in pH, increasing activities of faecal proteases and lipases.

Candida albicans is the most common fungus found on the skin, and as it prefers a moist environment, this fungus can proliferate in people with incontinence leading to fungal infection and skin breakdown (Beldon 2012).

Skin care following incontinence is very important; see Box 9.16 for some key points.

ACTIVITY

Compare Box 9.16 to skin care following incontinence that you have seen in practice.

Box 9.16 Skin care after incontinence: key points

- Ensure prompt action, with privacy, dignity and sensitivity.
- Observe infection control: hand hygiene, gloves and apron, correct waste disposal.
- Use skin cleanser rather than soap (Bale et al. 2004; Nix and Ermer-Seltun 2004; Bliss et al. 2006; Hodgkinson et al. 2007). Wash gently, avoiding friction.
- Cleanse from front to back, and least soiled area to most soiled area.
- Start with the labia with females, and the tip of the penis with men.
- Cleanse the anal area last.
- Observe the skin condition.
- Dry skin carefully to avoid maceration and undue cooling, maintain comfort and permit dressing. Pat rather than rub to reduce friction (Ersser et al. 2005).
- Apply barrier cream, or for moderate/severe incontinence dermatitis, barrier film (Bale et al. 2004; Baatenburg de Jong and Admiraal 2004; Beldon 2012).

Soap and water is not advised for skin cleansing following incontinence; soap removes the skin's natural oils, causing dryness and could alter the pH from its natural acid state (Ananathapadmanabhan et al. 2004). Skin cleansers have evaluated well in several small studies (Bale et al. 2004; Bliss et al. 2006). Barrier creams can help prevent skin damage caused by incontinence. Barrier creams are protective products, designed to form an occlusive barrier between the skin and noxious substances, not to be confused with emollients which moisturise the skin (Voegeli 2008). Beeckman et al. (2010) recommend that optimal **skin** care should be provided according to a structured perineal **skin** care programme, including a skin cleanser, moisturiser and **skin** protectant. A barrier cream that contains dimethicone can provide an almost invisible barrier, and it will not affect the absorbency of body-worn continence pads (Beldon 2012).

Containment of incontinence: Pads

Super-absorbent pads aim to prevent mixing of urine and faeces by keeping skin dry. Pads are produced for all situations, ranging from light to severe and night-time use. Light urinary incontinence is defined as urine loss that can be contained within a small absorbent pad (Fader et al. 2009a). A practical definition of moderate–heavy incontinence is urine or faecal loss that requires a large absorbent pad (typically with a total absorbent capacity of 2000–3000 g) for containment (Fader et al. 2009b).

ACTIVITY	Find out what incontinence pads are available in your practice setting.

There is a wide range of incontinence pads available: all-in-one body-worn products, pads worn with elasticated pants or insert pads. Under-pads are also available but should be used only as a procedure pad when a clean (not sterile) field is needed, for extra chair/bed protection, for example, after administration of an enema, or where a body-worn pad is not practical or possible as with a very obese person, or for persistent diarrhoea in bed which cannot be contained with alternative methods (e.g. faecal collector). The systematic review by Hodgkinson et al. (2007) identified that disposable body-worn pads may prevent deterioration of skin condition better than non-disposable under-pads or body-worns. Box 9.17 summarises key points in the choice and use of incontinence pads.

Kristiansen et al. (2011) found that patients, close relatives and nursing staff all expressed that a good urinary incontinence aid had good absorption capacity, shape and comfort level, and suited the individual. Differently shaped pads are available for men and women. It is important to read the manufacturers' instructions as correct fitting of pads is essential to contain urine and faeces, and it will reduce skin contact with excreta to the minimum. As urine is broken down into its constituents – ammonia and urea – on contact with air, close-fitting pads

> **Box 9.17 Choice and use of incontinence pads: key points**
>
> **Choice of pad**
> - Disposable, super-absorbent pads are preferable.
> - Body-worn pads (either all-in-ones, or pad and pants) should be used rather than under-pads.
> - Choose the correct pad for the individual person, considering gender, size, and extent and frequency of incontinence.
>
> **Fitting**
> Always follow the manufacturer's instructions for fitting, but the following general principles normally apply:
>
> - Maintain privacy, dignity and prevention of cross-infection during pad changes.
> - If using pants, ensure the seams are on the outside and pull up to mid-thigh.
> - Fold the pad lengthways and create a cupped shape.
> - Place the pad from front to back with largest area at the back.
> - Ensure pad is smoothed out both front and back, and fitted into the groin well.
> - If using pants, pull up; or if all-in-ones, seal the tapes firmly. Lower tapes should be sealed first.
> - Check if the pad is as close to the body as possible.

ensure that urine and air are not mixed. Kristiansen et al. (2011) evaluated the use of an alarmed pad at night and found that patients, close relatives and nursing staff all viewed the alarmed pad system as a good complement to ordinary care as it improved the quality of patients' nightly rest as staff did not have to wake them to check if it was necessary to change their pad. However, there were some concerns that the design needed improvement, that there should not be over-reliance on the alarm and that the alarm's sound might be confusing for people with dementia.

When changing a pad, **never** refer to it as a 'nappy', which is demeaning. Nurses should take care not to show annoyance or embarrass patients and should use discreet communication (see Chapter 2). It is important to ensure that people have a clean pad at mealtimes and before going out anywhere. When changing the pad, maintain privacy by shutting curtains, and change any wet or soiled clothing. To prevent cross-infection, use of gloves and aprons; hand hygiene and correct waste disposal are essential (see Chapter 3).

Fader et al. (2004) found that incontinence pads had an adverse effect on pressure redistribution properties on mattresses, with pad folds contributing to this effect. Thus, patients who are incontinent and wearing pads may be at increased risk of pressure damage, but smoothing out the folds reduced interface pressures.

Getliffe and Fader (2007) address absorbent products for containment in detail, fully illustrated; further reading from that source is recommended. A detailed

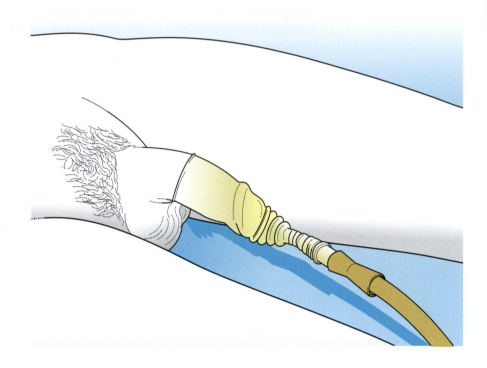

Figure 9.11: Penile sheath.

evaluation of different types of pads can be found in Cochrane reviews by Fader et al. (2009a, 2009b).

Penile sheaths

Penile sheaths (also referred to as 'condom catheters') (see Figure 9.11) consist of a soft, flexible sleeve that fits over the penis with an anti-reflux bulbous end leading to a short tube that attaches to any standard urinary drainage system (Kyle 2011b). They can provide a reliable form of containment for men with unresolvable urinary incontinence or as a temporary measure, but they should not be used for patients with urinary retention. NICE (2010b) suggests that penile sheaths should be offered to men, prior to considering in-dwelling catheterisation. They avoid the complications of long-term in-dwelling urethral catheters and, by diverting urine into a bag, prevent odour and contact of urine on skin (Pemberton et al. 2006). In the study by Saint et al. (2006), urinary sheaths reduced adverse outcomes, such as infection, and patients reported that they were comfortable and less painful than catheters. In many cases, patients can manage the system themselves or carers can be taught to do so but manual dexterity will be necessary.

ACTIVITY

Can you think of any patients for whom this method of dealing with urinary incontinence might be particularly unsuitable?

Patients with any skin soreness of the penis should not have a sheath applied. Patients with cognitive impairment may pull the device off, causing trauma (Williams and Moran 2006). Penile length is another important factor; there should be at least 1.5 inches (3.8 cm) of penile length available (Kyle 2011b). For men with significant retraction, a urinary sheath is unlikely to be successful as it will roll off the shaft of the penis. Kyle (2011b) advises that if the penile length is very short, an external device (the Clinimed Bioderm®) that fixes just to the glans of the penis can be used. The Bioderm is made of hydrocolloid, so it is hypoallergenic and latex-free, and it can be attached to any urinary drainage system.

If a patient is considered suitable for a penile sheath, selection of equipment should next occur with consideration to:

Material: A silicone sheath can be used if there is a history of latex allergy. A clear sheath as opposed to an opaque one allows observation of the penile skin.

Choice of one piece or two piece: The two-piece sheath requires application of an adhesive strip to the penis in a spiral manner, before rolling the sheath on, while the one-piece sheath has an integral adhesive coating.

Correct size: Dwivedi et al. (2012) report on a patient who developed a urethral diverticulum as a complication of wearing a sheath, and they stress the importance of avoiding over tight application and careful sizing. You should measure the circumference of the penis at its widest point and measure the length. If the sheath is too big there will be leakage as urine will seep under the sheath and loosen the adhesive, causing the sheath to slip off. Sheaths that are too small could cause sores and discomfort. Sheaths are available in a variety of widths (20–40 mm) and lengths (50–80 mm) and each manufacturer has a defined size range and provides their own measurement guide which must be used together (Williams and Moran 2006).

Box 9.18 outlines how to apply a penile sheath and subsequent care.

Support for people with continence problems

People with continence problems can benefit from support and advice, but they may often be unaware of what support is available, and where it can be accessed. Nurses should be aware of the resources available so that they can advise people with continence issues. There are many local self-help support groups that can be very beneficial to participants and these give people the opportunity to meet informally, and share ideas and experiences. The DH (2010) advises that best practice is for people with continence problems, and their carers, to be able to access other people and carers with similar problems in order to gain support. The Bladder and Bowel Foundation (www.bladderandbowelfoundation.org) provides information and support to people affected by bladder and bowel problems. Other organisations have also developed information leaflets for people who have continence problems, for example, the Alzheimer's Disease Society (www.alzheimers.org.uk).

Children: practice points – continence

In some situations, children who are usually toilet-trained may need to wear incontinence pads due to special needs or health conditions such as neuropathic bladder or congenital malformation. This can be upsetting for them so great sensitivity is needed. For changing an incontinence pad in a child, see

Himsworth, J. 2010. Caring for personal hygiene needs. In: Glasper. A, Aylott, M. and Battrick, C. (eds.) *Developing Practical Skills for Nursing Children and Young People.* London: Hodder Arnold, 188–202.

Children who are anxious or fearful may regress to day or night wetting. Bedwetting is a widespread and distressing condition that can have a deep impact on a child or young person's behaviour, emotional well-being and social life. It is also very stressful for the parents or carers (NICE 2010c). NICE (2010c) provides detailed guidelines for managing this distressing condition.

For further reading, see

Glasper, A., Aylott, M., and Battrick, C. (Eds). 2010. *Developing Practical Skills for Nursing Children and Young People.* London: Hodder Arnold, Chapter 14 Promoting children's continence, 220–41.

See also:

ERIC – Enuresis Website: http://www.eric.org.uk/

Pregnancy and birth: practice points – continence

There is an established association between urinary incontinence and pregnancy and childbirth (Herbruck 2008). The physiological changes occurring during pregnancy and the processes of childbirth have a detrimental effect on the structure and function of the muscles, nerves and connective tissue that make up the pelvic floor complex. Dysfunction of the pelvic floor complex can result in a wide range of symptoms including urinary or anal incontinence. Pelvic floor muscles and their associated structures are at risk of becoming weakened during pregnancy or of experiencing trauma and damage during delivery. Pelvic floor muscle training should be offered to women in their first pregnancy as a preventive strategy for urinary incontinence. There is evidence that pelvic floor muscle training used during a first pregnancy reduces the likelihood of postnatal urinary incontinence (NICE 2006).

Box 9.18 Application of penile sheath and subsequent care: key points

Preparation

- Carefully select the patient for suitability, explain the procedure and gain consent.
- Gather equipment (correctly sized sheath, urinary drainage system).
- Conduct hand hygiene and wear non-sterile gloves and apron.
- Ensure privacy during the procedure.

Procedure

- If provided, use the manufacturer's pubic hair guard over the penis to keep hair away from the adhesive. If necessary pubic hair can be trimmed but must not be shaved.
- Ensure the penis is clean and dry – avoid powder, cream or sprays.
- If using a two-piece sheath, apply the adhesive strip in a spiral fashion around the penis.
- Roll the sheath over the penis: leave a small space (1–2 cm) between the end of the penis and the outlet of the sheath. If the patient is uncircumcised, ensure that the foreskin remains over the glans and is not retracted.
- Gently squeeze the sheath to ensure adhesion.
- Attach the urine drainage bag and place it on a stand.
- Make the patient comfortable.
- Remove and dispose of gloves and apron and wash hands.

Subsequent care

- Ensure that the catheter tubing does not kink, to allow collection of urine and prevent pressure on the sheath, weakening the adhesive.
- Remove the sheath daily by gently rolling it off (preferably in the bath), and wash and dry the skin before reapplying.
- Observe the penile skin for any problems. Note that a patient with reduced or absent sensation will not be able to feel if the sheath is too tight or a sore is developing, so observe carefully for problems and teach the patient and/or carers to do so too.

Summary

- Nurses within almost any setting are likely to encounter people with continence issues, so an understanding of the underlying causes and the wide-ranging effects on people is important.
- Nurses should have knowledge about specialised services, such as the continence advisor and support organisations, so that they can advise and refer people accordingly.
- Promoting continence and managing incontinence requires careful assessment of each individual, and knowledge about appropriate strategies and products. Care for people with continence problems should be based on the best evidence available.

CHAPTER SUMMARY

This chapter has focused on assisting people with elimination, emphasising that quality care requires a sensitive and empathetic approach, effective communication skills and a sound, evidence-based knowledge. Implementing measures to prevent cross-infection, while assisting people with elimination, are also paramount. Urinalysis and specimen collection are very common investigations, but if not carried out with care they can lead to misleading results and inappropriate treatment. Constipation is a common problem and preventing and managing constipation was addressed. Urinary catheterisation is invasive and potentially harmful, but is nevertheless often necessary as a short- or long-term measure. An understanding of this procedure, and particularly how potential complications can be reduced, is also important. Nurses may encounter people with stomas in a range of acute and long-term settings and key aspects of stoma care were considered.

Continence is a huge topic and may require specialist involvement. Here, the practical skills in dealing with continence have been explored; students wishing to extend their knowledge should access the referenced material. To conclude, nurses need to value the care given in relation to patients/clients' elimination needs as, if effective, it can do much for comfort, well-being and self-esteem.

REFERENCES

Abd-el-Maeboud, K.H., el-Naggar, T., El-Hawi, E.M.M., et al. 1991. Rectal suppositories and mode of insertion. *The Lancet* 338: 798, 800.

Addison, R., Ness, W., Abulafi, M., et al. 2000. How to administer enemas and suppositories. *Nursing Times NT Plus: Continence* 96(6): 3–4.

Akpan, A., Gosney, M.A. and Barrett, J. 2006. Privacy for defecation and fecal incontinence in older adults. *Journal of Wound, Ostomy and Continence Nursing* 33(5): 536–40.

Alzheimer's Society. 2009. *Counting the Cost: Caring for People with Dementia on Acute Hospital Wards.* London: Alzheimer's Society.

Ananthapadmanabhan, K.P., Moore, D.J., Subramanyan, K., et al. 2004. Cleansing without compromise: The impact of cleansers on the skin barrier and the technology of mild cleansing. *Dermatological Therapy* 17(Suppl 1): 16–25.

Avery, J.C., Wilson, I. and Braunack-Mayer, A.J. 2006. Beliefs and barriers about seeking help for incontinence. *Australian and New Zealand Continence Journal* 12(1): 6.

Baatenburg de Jong, H. and Admiraal, H. 2004. Comparing cost per use of 3M Cavilon No Sting Barrier Film with zinc oxide oil in incontinent patients. *Journal of Wound Care* 13(9): 398–400.

Bale, S., Tebble, N., Jones, V., et al. 2004. The benefits of implementing a new skin care protocol in nursing homes. *Journal of Tissue Viability* 14(2): 44–50.

Bar, O. and Sowney, M. 2007. Inclusive nursing care for people with intellectual disabilities using urology services. *International Journal of Urological Nursing* 1(3): 138–45.

Bayer. 1997. *Urine Analysis: The Essential Information.* Newbury: Bayer.

Bayer. 1998. *A Practical Guide to Urine Analysis.* Newbury: Bayer.

Beeckman, D., Defloor, T., Verhaeghe, S., et al. 2010. What is the most effective method of preventing and treating incontinence associated dermatitis? *Nursing Times* 106(38): 22–5.

Beldon, P. 2012. Incontinence-associated dermatitis: Protecting the older person. *British Journal of Nursing* 21(7): 402–7.

Beynon, M. and Nicholls, C. 2004. Urological investigations. In: Fillingham, S. and Douglas, J. (eds.) *Urological Nursing,* 3rd edn. Edinburgh: Baillière Tindall, 25–42.

Billington, A. 2010. The management of stress urinary incontinence. *British Journal of Nursing* 19(Continence Care, Suppl 18): S20–5.

Black, P. 2011. Caring for the patient with a stoma and dementia. *Gastrointestinal Nursing* 9(7): 19–24.

Black, P. 2012. Choosing the correct stoma appliance. *Gastrointestinal Nursing* 10(7): 18–25.

Blake, D.R. and Doherty, L.F. 2006. Effect of perineal cleansing on contamination rate of mid-stream urine culture. *Journal of Pediatric and Adolescent Gynecology* 19(1): 31–4.

Bliss, D.Z., Zehrer, C., Savik, K., et al. 2006. Incontinence-associated skin damage in nursing home residents: A secondary analysis of a prospective, multicenter study. *Ostomy/Wound Management* 52(12): 46–55.

Bowers, B. 2006. Evaluating the evidence for administering phosphate enemas. *British Journal of Nursing* 15(7): 378–81.

Bradshaw, E., Collins, B. and Williams, J. 2009. Administering rectal suppositories: preparation, assessment and insertion. *Gastrointestinal Nursing* 7(9): 24–8.

British Geriatrics Society. 2007. *Behind Closed Doors: Delivering Dignity in Toilet Access and Use.* Available from: http://www.bgs.org.uk/campaigns/dignitypress.htm (Accessed on 1 January 2013).

British Infection Association and Health Protection Agency. 2011. *Diagnosis of UTI: Quick Reference Guide for Primary Care.* Available from: http://www.hpa.org.uk/webc/HPAwebFile/HPAweb_C/1194947404720 (Accessed on 6 January 2012).

Brown S.R., Wadhawan, H. and Nelson, R. 2013. Surgery for faecal incontinence in adults. *Cochrane Database of Systematic Reviews* 7. Art. No.: CD001757. DOI: 10.1002/14651858. CD001757.pub4.

Bucior, H. and Cochrane, J. 2010. Lifting the lid: A clinical audit on commode cleaning. *Journal of Infection Prevention* 11(3): 73–80.

Busuttil Leaver, R. and Leach, C. 2004. Psychological effects of urological problems. In: Fillingham, S. and Douglas, J. (eds.) *Urological Nursing.* Edinburgh: Baillière Tindall, 305–20.

Candy, B., Jones L., Goodman, M.L., et al. 2011. Laxatives or methylnaltrexone for the management of constipation in palliative care patients. *Cochrane Database of Systematic Reviews* 19(1) Art. No.: CD003448. DOI: 10.1002/14651858.CD003448.pub3.

Chelvanayagam, S. and Stern, J. 2007. Using therapeutic groups to support women with faecal incontinence. *British Journal of Nursing* 16(4): 214–18.

Chiarelli, P. and Weatherall, M. 2010. The link between chronic conditions and urinary incontinence. *Australian and New Zealand Continence Journal* 16(1): 7–14.

Chiarelli, P.E., Mackenzie, L.A. and Osmotherly, P.G. 2009. Urinary incontinence is associated with an increase in falls: A systematic review. *Australian Journal of Physiotherapy* 55: 89–95.

Clark, J. and Rugg, S. 2005. The importance of independence in toileting: The views of stroke survivors and their occupational therapists. *British Journal of Occupational Therapy* 68(4): 165–71.

Collett, K. 2002. Practical aspects of stoma management. *Nursing Standard* 17(8): 45–52, 54.

Coloplast. 2010. *High Impact Actions for Stoma Care. High Impact Action Steering Group.* Peterborough: Coloplast Ltd.

Colpman, D. and Welford, K. 2004. Urinary drainage systems. In: Fillingham, S. and Douglas, J. (eds.) *Urological Nursing*. Edinburgh: Baillière Tindall, 67–92.

Deering, C.G. and Cody, D.J. 2002. Communicating with children and adolescents: Children are all foreigners. *American Journal of Nursing* 102(3): 34–41.

de Hert, M., Dock, L., Bernagie, C., et al. 2011. Prevalence and severity of antipsychotic related constipation in patients with schizophrenia: A retrospective descriptive study. *BMC Gastroenterology* 11: 17.

Department of Health (DH). 2000. *Good Practice in Continence Services*. London: DH.

Department of Health (DH). 2003. *Winning Ways: Working Together to Reduce Healthcare Associated Infection in England and Wales*. London: DH.

Department of Health (DH). 2006. *Environment and Sustainability: Safe Management of Healthcare Waste*. Health Technical Memorandum 07-01. London: DH.

Department of Health (DH). 2009. *Health Action Planning and Health Facilitation for People with Learning Disabilities: Good Practice Guidance*. London: DH.

Department of Health (DH). 2010. *Essence of Care 2010: Benchmarks for Bladder, Bowel and Continence Care*. Gateway Reference 14641. London: The Stationery Office, DH.

Deutekom, M. and Dobben, A.C. 2012. Plugs for containing faecal incontinence. *Cochrane Database of Systematic Reviews* (4). Art. No.: CD005086. DOI: 10.1002/14651858.CD005086.pub3.

Dorey, G. 2007. Why men need to perform pelvic floor exercises. *Nursing Times* 103(26): 40–6.

Dwivedi, A.K., Singh, S. and Goel, A. 2012. Massive urethral diverticulum: A complication of condom catheter use. *British Journal of Nursing* 21(Urology, Suppl 9): S20–2.

Elstad, E.A., Taubenberger, A.S.P., Botelhoe, M., et al. 2010. Beyond incontinence: The stigma of other urinary symptoms. *Journal of Advanced Nursing* 66(11): 2460–70.

Ersser, S.J., Geliffe, K., Voegeli, D., et al. 2005. A critical review of the interrelationship between skin vulnerability and urinary incontinence and related nursing intervention. *International Journal of Nursing Studies* 42: 823–35.

Erwin-Toth, P. 2003. Ostomy pearls: A concise guide to stoma siting, pouching systems, patient education, and more. *Advances in Skin and Wound Care* 16(3): 146–52.

European Association of Urological Nurses (EAUN). 2012. *Catheterisation: Indwelling Catheters in Adults. Evidence-Based Guidelines for Best Practice in Urological Health Care*. EAUN Guidelines. Available from: http://www.uroweb.org/fileadmin/EAUN/guidelines/EAUN_Paris_Guideline_2012_LR_online_file.pdf (Accessed on 20 December 2012).

Eustice, S., Roe, B. and Paterson, J. 2009. Prompted voiding for the management of urinary incontinence in adults. *Cochrane Database of Systematic Reviews* (2). Art. No.: CD002113. DOI: 10.1002/14651858.CD002113.

Fader, M., Bain, D. and Cottenden, A. 2004. Effects of absorbent incontinence pads on pressure management mattresses. *Journal of Advanced Nursing* 48(6): 569–74.

Fader, M., Cottenden, A.M. and Getliffe, K. 2009a. Absorbent products for moderate-heavy urinary and/or faecal incontinence in women and men. *Cochrane Database of Systematic Reviews* (4). Art. No.: CD007408. DOI: 10.1002/14651858.CD007408.

Fader, M., Cottenden, A.M. and Getliffe, K. 2009b. Absorbent products for light urinary incontinence in women. *Cochrane Database of Systematic Reviews* (2). Art. No.: CD0014067408. DOI: 10.1002/14651858.CD001406.pub2.

Fillingham, S. and Fell, S. 2004. Urological stomas. In: Fillingham, S. and Douglas, J. (eds.) *Urological Nursing*. Edinburgh: Baillière Tindall, 207–26.

Floruta, C.V. 2001. Dietary choices of people with ostomies. *Journal of Wound, Ostomy and Continence Nursing* 28(1): 28–31.

Fraise, A.P. and Bradley, C. 2009. Decontamination of equipment, the environment and the skin. In: Fraise, A.P. and Bradley, C. (eds.) *Ayliffe's Control of Healthcare-Associated Infection,* 5th edn. London: Hodder Arnold, 107–49.

Gallagher, P.F., O'Mahony, D. and Quigley, E.M.M. 2008. Management of constipation in the elderly. *Drugs Aging* 25(10): 807–21.

Getliffe, K. 2002. Managing recurrent urinary catheter encrustation. *British Journal of Community Nursing* 7: 574–80.

Getliffe, K. and Dolman, M. (eds.) 2007. *Promoting Continence: A Clinical and Research Guide,* 3rd edn. Edinburgh: Baillière Tindall.

Getliffe, K. and Fader, M. 2007. Catheters and containment products. In: Getliffe, K. and Dolman, M. (eds.) *Promoting Continence: A Clinical and Research Guide,* 3rd edn. Edinburgh: Baillière Tindall, 259–308.

Gibney, L.E. 2010. Offering patients a choice of urinary catheter drainage system. *British Journal of Nursing* 19(15): 954–8.

Godfrey, H. and Fraczyk, L. 2005. Preventing and managing catheter-associated urinary tract infections. *British Journal of Community Nursing* 10(5): 205–12.

Gordon, M., Naidoo, K, Akobeng, A.K., et al. 2012. Osmotic and stimulant laxatives for the management of childhood constipation. *Cochrane Database of Systematic Reviews* (7). Art. No.: CD009118. DOI: 10.1002/14651858.CD009118.pub2.

Gould, D. 1994. Controlling infection spread from excreta. *Nursing Standard* 8(33): 29–31.

Greenstein, B. 2009. *Trounce's Clinical Pharmacology for Nurses,* 18th edn. Edinburgh: Churchill Livingstone.

Hägglund, D. 2010. A systematic literature review of incontinence care for persons with dementia: The research evidence. *Journal of Clinical Nursing* 19: 303–12.

Hansen, J.L., Bliss, D.Z. and Peden-McAlpine, C. 2006. Diet strategies used by women to manage fecal incontinence. *Journal of Wound, Ostomy and Continence Nursing* 33: 52–62.

Harari, D., Norton, C., Lockwood, L., et al. 2004. Treatment of constipation and fecal incontinence in stroke patients: Randomized controlled trials. *Stroke* 35(11): 2549–55.

Hay-Smith, E.J.C., Herderschee, R., Dumoulin, C., et al. 2011. Comparisons of approaches to pelvic floor muscle training for urinary incontinence in women. *Cochrane Database of Systematic Reviews* (12). Art. No.: CD009508. DOI: 10.1002/14651858.CD009508.

Health Protection Agency. 2012. UK standards for microbiology investigations: Investigation of urine. *Bacteriology B41* (7.1).

Heath, H. 2009. The nurse's role in helping older people to use the toilet. *Nursing Standard* 24(2): 43–7.

Herbison, G.P. and Dean, N. 2009. Weighted vaginal cones for urinary incontinence. *Cochrane Database of Systematic Reviews* (7). Art. No.: CD002114. DOI: 10.1002/14651858. CD002114.pub2.

Herbruck, L.E. 2008. Urinary incontinence in the child bearing woman. *Urologic Nursing* 28(3): 163–171.

Herderschee, R., Hay-Smith, E.J.C., Herbison, G.P., et al. 2011. Feedback or biofeedback to augment pelvic floor muscle training for urinary incontinence in women. *Cochrane Database of Systematic Reviews* (7). Art. No.: CD009252. DOI: 10.1002/14651858. CD009252.

Hodgkinson, B., Nay, R. and Wilson, J. 2007. A systematic review of topical skin care in aged care facilities. *Journal of Clinical Nursing* 16: 129–36.

Holland, K. and Hogg, C. 2010. *Cultural Awareness in Nursing and Health Care: An Introductory Text,* 2nd edn. London: Arnold.

Holman, C., Roberts, S. and Nichol, M. 2010. Preventing and treating constipation in later life. *Nursing Older People* 20(5): 22–4.

Jackson, S.L., Scholes, D., Boyko, E.J., et al. 2005. Urinary incontinence and diabetes in postmenopausal women. *Diabetes Care* 28(7): 1730–8.

Jahn, P., Preuss, M., Kernig, A., et al. 2007. Types of indwelling urinary catheters for long-term bladder drainage in adults. *Cochrane Database of Systematic Reviews* (3). Art. No.: CD004997. DOI: 10.1002/14651858.CD004997.pub2.

Jewell, D. and Young, G. 2009. Interventions for treating constipation in pregnancy. *Cochrane Database of Systematic Reviews* (2). Art. No.: CD001142. DOI: 10.1002/14651858.CD001142.

Karadag, A., Mentes, B. and Ayaz, S. 2005. Colostomy irrigation: Results of 25 cases with particular reference to quality of life. *Journal of Clinical Nursing* 14(4): 479–85.

Kristiansen, L. Björk, A., Kock, V.B., et al. 2011. Urinary incontinence and newly invented pad technique: Patients' close relatives' and nursing staff's experiences and beliefs. *International Journal of Urological Nursing* 5(1): 21–30.

Kyle, G. 2007a. Norgine risk assessment tool for constipation. *Nursing Times* 103(47): 48–9.

Kyle, G. 2007b. Bowel care. Part 5: A practical guide to digital rectal examination. *Nursing Times* 103(46): 28–9.

Kyle, G. 2009. Common bowel problems: Constipation risk assessment. *Nursing & Residential Care* 11(2): 76–9.

Kyle, G. 2010. The older person: Management of constipation. *British Journal of Community Nursing* 15(2): 58–64.

Kyle, G. 2011a. Constipation: Symptoms, assessment and treatment. *British Journal of Nursing* 20(22): 1432.

Kyle, G. 2011b. The use of urinary sheaths in male incontinence. *British Journal of Nursing* 20(6): 338.

Lewis, C.M., Schrader, R., Many, A., et al. 2005. Diabetes and urinary incontinence in 50–90 year old women: A cross-sectional population-based study. *American Journal of Obstetrics and Gynaecology* 193(6): 2154–8.

Macauley, M. 1997. Urinary drainage systems. In: Fillingham, S. and Douglas, J. (eds.) *Urological Nursing,* 2nd edn. London: Baillière Tindall, 90–130.

MacDonald, C. and Butler, L. 2007. Silent no more: Elderly women's stories of living with urinary incontinence in long-term care. *Journal of Gerontological Nursing* 33(1): 14–20.

Madersbacher, S., Schmidt, J., Eberle, J., et al. 2003. Long-term outcome of ileal conduit diversion. *Journal of Urology* 169(3): 985–90.

Maki, D.G. and Tambyah, P.A. 2001. Engineering out the risk for infection with urinary catheters. *Emerging Infectious Diseases* 7(2): 342–7.

Marsh, L., Capíes, M., Dalton, C., et al. 2010. Management of constipation. *Learning Disability Practice* 13(4): 26–8.

McNulty, C., Freeman, E., Smith, G., et al. 2003. Prevalence of urinary catheterisation in UK nursing homes. *Journal of Hospital Infection* 55(2): 119–23.

Mead, M. 1998. Stool culture. *Practice Nurse* 16(3): 170.

Medicines and Healthcare Products Regulatory Agency (MHRA). 2011. Urine dipsticks: Top tips. Crown. Available from: http://www.mhra.gov.uk/home/groups/dts-bi/documents/publication/con2023421.pdf (Accessed on 5 January 2013).

Mendoza, J., Legido, J., Rubio, S., et al. 2007. Systematic review: The adverse effects of sodium phosphate enema. *Alimentary Pharmacology and Therapy* 26(1): 9–20.

Midthun, S.J., Paur, R. and Lindseth, G. 2004. Urinary tract infections: Does the smell really tell? *Journal of Gerontological Nursing* 30(6): 4–9.

Milwain, E. 2010. The brain and person centred care. 4. Memory, belief, emotion and behaviour. *Journal of Dementia Care* 18(3): 25–9.

National Institute for Health and Clinical Excellence (NICE). 2006. *The Management of Urinary Incontinence in Women*. Clinical Guidelines 40. London: NICE.

National Institute for Health and Clinical Excellence (NICE). 2007a. *Urinary Tract Infection in Children: Diagnosis, Treatment and Long-Term Management*. Clinical Guidelines 54. London: NICE.

National Institute for Health and Clinical Excellence (NICE). 2007b. *Faecal Incontinence: The Management of Faecal Incontinence in Adults*. Clinical Guidelines 49. London: NICE.

National Institute for Health and Clinical Excellence (NICE). 2010a. *Constipation in Children and Young People: Diagnosis and Management of Idiopathic Childhood Constipation in Primary and Secondary Care*. Clinical Guidelines 99. London: NICE.

National Institute for Health and Clinical Excellence (NICE). 2010b. *Lower Urinary Tract Symptoms: The Management of Lower Urinary Tract Symptoms in Men*. Clinical Guidelines 97. London: NICE.

National Institute for Health and Clinical Excellence (NICE). 2010c. *Nocturnal Enuresis – The Management of Bedwetting in Children and Young People*. Clinical Guidelines 111. London: NICE.

National Institute for Health and Clinical Excellence (NICE). 2012a. *Prevention and Control of Healthcare-Associated Infection in Primary and Community Care*. Clinical Guidelines 139. London: NICE.

National Institute for Health and Clinical Excellence (NICE). 2012b. *Urinary Incontinence in Neurological Disease. Management of Lower Urinary Tract Dysfunction in Neurological Disease*. Clinical Guidelines 148. London: NICE.

National Patient Safety Agency (NPSA). 2007. *Using Bedrails Safely and Effectively*. London: NPSA.

Nazarko, L. 2009. Urinary tract infection: Diagnosis, treatment and prevention. *British Journal of Nursing* 18(19): 1170–4.

Nazarko, L. 2011. Understanding dementia: Diagnosis and development. *British Journal of Healthcare Assistants* 5(5): 216–20.

Newman, D.K. 2012. *Indwelling Urinary Catheters in Acute Care: A Step-by-Step Clinical Pathway for Nurses*. Available from: http://verathon.ca/portals/0/Uploads/ProductMaterials/_bsc/CAUTI/0900-2813-02-84.pdf (Accessed on 13 December 2012).

Nix, D. and Ermer-Seltun, J. 2004. A review of perineal skin care protocols and skin barrier product use. *Ostomy/Wound Management* 50(12): 59–67.

Norton, C. and Cody, J.D. 2012. Biofeedback and/or sphincter exercises for the treatment of faecal incontinence in adults. *Cochrane Database of Systematic Reviews* (7). Art. No.: CD002111. DOI: 10.1002/14651858.CD002111.pub3.

Ostaszkiewicz, J. 2006. The clinical effectiveness of systematic voiding programmes: Results of a metastudy. *Australian and New Zealand Continence Journal* 12(1): 5–6.

Ostaszkiewicz, J., Johnston, L. and Roe, B. 2010. Habit retraining for the management of urinary incontinence in adults. *Cochrane Database of Systematic Reviews* (2). Art. No.: CD002801. DOI: 10.1002/14651858.CD002801.pub2.

Ostaszkiewicz, J., Johnston, L. and Roe, B. 2011. Timed voiding for the management of urinary incontinence in adults. *Cochrane Database of Systematic Reviews*. (1). Art. No.: CD002802. DOI: 10.1002/14651858.CD002802.pub2.

Padmanabhan, A., Stern, M., Wishin, J., et al. 2007. Clinical evaluation of a flexible fecal incontinence management system. *American Journal of Critical Care* 16(4): 384–93.

Palmer, M.H. and Newman, D.K. 2006. Bladder control: Educational needs of older adults. *Journal of Gerontological Nursing* 32(1): 28–32.

Palmieri, B., Benuzzi, G. and Bellini, N. 2005. The anal bag: A modern approach to fecal incontinence management. *Ostomy/Wound Management* 51(12): 44–52.

Panagamuwa, C., Glasby, M.J. and Peckham, T.J. 2004. Dipstick screening for urinary tract infection before arthroscopy: A safe alternative to laboratory testing? *International Journal of Clinical Practice* 58(1): 19–21.

Parascandolo, M.E. and Doughty, D. 2001. Multiple ostomy complications in a patient with Crohn's disease: a case study. *Journal of Wound, Ostomy and Continence Nursing* 28(5): 236–43.

Pellatt, G. 2007. Clinical skills: Bowel elimination and management of complications. *British Journal of Nursing* 16(6): 351–5.

Pellatt, G.C. 2012. Non-containment management options of urinary continence. *Nursing & Residential Care* 14(2): 68–73.

Pemberton, P., Brooks, A., Erikson, C.M., et al. 2006. A comparative study of two types of urinary sheath. *Nursing Times* 102(7): 36–41.

Pratt, R.J., Pellowe, C., Wilson, J.A., et al. 2007. National evidence-based guidelines for preventing healthcare-associated infections in NHS England. *Journal of Hospital Infection* 65(Suppl 1): S1–64.

Rassin, M., Dubches, L., Libshitz, et al. 2007. Levels of comfort and ease among patients suffering from urinary incontinence. *International Journal of Urological Nursing* 1(2): 64–70.

Ratliff, C., Scarano, K.A., Donovan, A.M., et al. 2005. Descriptive study of peristomal complications. *Journal of Wound, Ostomy and Continence Nursing* 32(1): 33–7.

Resnick, B., Leilman, L.J., Calabrese, B., et al. 2006. Nursing staff beliefs and expectations about continence care in nursing homes. *Journal of Wound, Ostomy and Continence Nursing* 33(6): 610–18.

Richbourg, L., Thorpe, J.M. and Rapp, C.G. 2007. Difficulties experienced by the ostomate after hospital discharge. *Journal of Wound, Ostomy and Continence Nursing* 34(1): 70–9.

Richmond, J.P. and Wright, M.E. 2004. Review of the literature on constipation to enable development of a constipation risk assessment scale. *Clinical Effectiveness in Nursing* 8(1): 11–25.

Rigby, D. 2007. Medication for continence. In: Getliffe, K. and Dolman, M. (eds.) *Promoting Continence: A Clinical and Research Guide*, 3rd edn. Edinburgh: Baillière Tindall, 239–58.

Roe, B., Ostaszkiewicz, J., Milne, J., et al. 2006. Systematic reviews of bladder training and voiding programmes in adults: A synopsis of findings from data analysis and outcomes using metastudy techniques. *Journal of Advanced Nursing* 57(1): 15–31.

Royal College of Nursing (RCN). 2011. *Meeting the Health Needs of People with Learning Disabilities.* London: RCN.

Royal College of Nursing (RCN). 2012. *Management of Lower Bowel Dysfunction, Including DRE and DRF.* London: RCN.

Royal Marsden Hospital Manual of Clinical Nursing Procedures. 2011. 8th edn. Wiley Blackwell.

Saint, S., Kaufman, S.R., Rogers, M.A.M., et al. 2006. Condom versus indwelling urinary catheters: A randomized trial. *Journal of the American Geriatrics Society* 54(7): 1055–61.

Saye, D.E. 2007. Recurring and antimicrobial resistant infections: considering the potential role of biofilms in clinical practice. *Ostomy/Wound Management* 53(4): 46–52.

Schmelzer, M. and Wright, K.B. 1996. Enema administration techniques used by experienced registered nurses. *Gastroenterology Nursing* 19: 171–5.

Schumm, K. and Lam, T.B.L. 2010. Types of urethral catheters for management of short-term voiding problems in hospitalised adults. *Cochrane Database System Review* (2). Art. No.: CD004013. DOI: 10.1002/14651858.CD004013.pub3.

Scottish Intercollegiate Guidelines Network (SIGN). 2006. *Management of Patients with Dementia.* Available from: http://www.sign.ac.uk/pdf/sign86.pdf (Accessed on 1 September 2012).

Slater-Smith, S. 2010. Promoting children's continence. B) Childhood constipation. In: Glasper, A., Aylott, M. and Battrick, C. (eds.) *Developing Practical Skills for Nursing Children and Young People.* London: Hodder Arnold, 229–41.

Smith, B. 2010. Faecal incontinence in older people: Delivering effective, dignified care. *British Journal of Community Nursing* 15(8): 370–4.

Smith, P. and Smith, L. 2007. Continence training in intellectual disability. In: Getliffe, K. and Dolman. M. (eds.) *Promoting Continence: A Clinical and Research Resource,* 3rd edn. Edinburgh: Baillière Tindall, 173–202.

Steggall, M. and Cox, C. 2009. A step-by-step guide to performing a complete digital rectal examination. *Gastrointestinal Nursing* 7(2): 28–32.

Steggall, M.J. 2008. Digital rectal examination. *Nursing Standard* 22(47): 46–8.

Stewart, E. 2010. Treating urinary incontinence in older women. *British Journal of Community Nursing* 15(11): 526, 528, 530–2.

Stickler, D. 2008. Bacterial biofilms in patients with indwelling urinary catheters. *Nature Clinical Practice Urology* 5: 598–608.

Stoma Care. 2007. *An Educational Resource for Stoma Care Nursing,* DVD. Cambridgeshire: Burdett Institute of Gastrointestinal Nursing and Dansac Ltd.

Thompson, J. 2007. Falls and incontinence: Evaluation of a quality management project. *Australian and New Zealand Continence Journal* 13(1): 18, 20–1.

Tlaskalová-Hogenová, H., Štepánková, R., Hudcovic T., et al. 2004. Commensal bacteria (normal microflora) mucosal immunity and chronic inflammatory and autoimmune diseases. *Immunology Letters* 93: 97–108.

Vaillancourt, S., McGillivray, D., Zhang, X., et al. 2007. To clean or not to clean: Effect on contamination rates in midstream urine collections in toilet-trained children. *Pediatrics* 119: e1288–93.

Vickerman, J. 2003. The benefits of a lending library for female urinals. *Nursing Times* 99(44): 56–7.

Voegeli, D. 2008. Skin care and incontinence in the elderly. *Nursing and Residential Care* 10(10): 487–92.

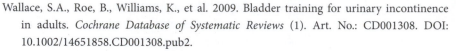

Wallace, S.A., Roe, B., Williams, K., et al. 2009. Bladder training for urinary incontinence in adults. *Cochrane Database of Systematic Reviews* (1). Art. No.: CD001308. DOI: 10.1002/14651858.CD001308.pub2.

Wareing, M. 2005. Lower urinary tract symptoms: A hermeneutic phenomenological study into men's lived experience. *Journal of Clinical Nursing* 14: 239–46.

Wells, M. and Wagg, A. 2007. Integrated continence services and the female Bangladeshi population. *British Journal of Nursing* 16: 516–9.

Williams, D. and Moran, S. 2006. Use of urinary sheaths in male incontinence. *Nursing Times* 102(47): 42–5.

Williams, J. 2012. Inserting suppositories and enemas into a colostomy. *Gastrointestinal Nursing* 10(1): 13–14.

Wilson, J. 2006. *Infection Control in Clinical Practice,* 3rd edn. Edinburgh: Baillière Tindall.

Wilson, M. 2011. Addressing the problems of long-term urethral catheterisation: Part 1. *British Journal of Nursing* 20(22): 1418–24.

Wilson, M. 2012. Addressing the problems of long-term urethral catheterisation: Part 2. *British Journal of Nursing* 21(1): 16–25.

Wolfman, A. 2010. Preventing incontinence-associated dermatitis and early-stage pressure injury. *World Council of Enterostomal Therapists Journal* 30(1): 19–24.

Woodford, H.J. and George, J. 2009. Diagnosis and management of urinary tract infection in hospitalized older people. *Journal of the American Geriatrics Society* 57: 107–114.

Woodward, S. 2012. Assessment and management of constipation in older people. *Nursing Older People* 24(5): 21–6.

Yates, A. 2012. Management of long-term urinary catheters. *Nursing and Residential Care* 14(4): 172–8.

10 Assessing and Meeting Fluid and Nutritional Needs

Sue Maddex

The European Nutritional Health Alliance (ENHA 2008) highlighted that air, water and nutrition are basic human needs. However, across Europe, malnutrition continues to compromise people's quality of life, health and well-being, delays the speed of recovery from disease and increases mortality rates. Malnutrition is frequently undetected and untreated, causing a wide range of adverse consequences (Carers UK 2012). It is estimated that 20%–50% of people are malnourished upon admission to hospital, which is of concern as malnutrition is associated with negative outcomes for patients (Barker 2008). Malnutrition inhibits cellular function and affects the function and recovery of every organ system (Lean and Wiseman 2008). The consequences of malnutrition include vulnerability to infection, delayed wound healing, impaired function of the heart and lungs, decreased muscle strength and depression (National Institute of Health and Clinical Excellence [NICE] 2006). Therefore, it is a fundamental part of a nurse's role to ensure that patients have adequate nutrition and hydration when receiving healthcare, but this role is sometimes overlooked while other care and treatment are prioritised.

The Nursing and Midwifery Council (NMC) (2010a) standards for preregistration nursing education includes an Essential Skills Cluster for 'Assessing and promoting adequate nutrition and hydration'; all aspects are addressed within this chapter, with activities to assist your learning. The Department of Health's (DH) (2010) Essence of Care Benchmarks include benchmarks for 'Food and drink', which are recommended as a resource.

This chapter includes the following topics:

- Nutrition in healthcare: Concerns and initiatives
- Recognising the contribution of nutrition to health
- Assessing and maintaining hydration
- Promoting healthy eating and addressing people's choices
- Nutritional screening
- Assisting people with eating and drinking
- Additional nutritional support strategies
- Enteral and parenteral feeding

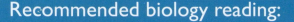
Recommended biology reading:

The following questions will help you to focus on the biology underpinning the skills in this chapter. Use your recommended textbook to find out:

- What are nutrients?
- Where do nutrients come from?
- What is a balanced diet?
- What advice would you give to patients regarding their '5-a-day' intake?
- How is food digested in the body?
- What process does the body adopt to use water in the body?
- Briefly explain these processes: mastication, consumption, absorption, defecation.
- How does fluid shift in the body?
- In a cell, what is the process of fluid shift across a membrane known as?
- What percent of your body weight is water?
- What should be the average fluid intake of a person each day?
- What is a calorie?
- How many calories should be ingested by a man each day?
- How many calories should be ingested by a woman each day?
- What is the difference between a macronutrient and a micronutrient?
- Why do we need these nutrients? What are their roles?
- How are macronutrients digested?
- Once digested, where do they go?
- What factors may affect the absorption of digested nutrients?
- How does nutrition affect health?
- What are the consequences of under-nutrition and over-nutrition?
- How do nutritional requirements alter across the lifespan?
- What features of different age groups (e.g. teenagers, young adults and older people) may impinge upon nutritional status?
- How does a 'health need' alter our nutritional demands (or supply)?

PRACTICE SCENARIOS

Nutrition is relevant for everybody. The following practice scenarios highlight situations where nutritional issues would be particularly important, and they will be referred to throughout this chapter.

Adult

Stroke

Cerebral damage caused either by decreased blood flow or haemorrhage. Effects vary, but a stroke often causes paralysis down one side of the body (hemiplegia), and speech and swallowing difficulty.

Miss Alice West is 84 years old and has been transferred from a medical ward to a rehabilitation unit following a **stroke** that has caused right-sided weakness. The medical ward staff who transferred her said that, although she initially had swallowing problems, she has since been assessed as being able to swallow. However, her appetite is very poor, and she often eats only a few small mouthfuls, refusing any more. The staff have been keeping a food chart and a fluid chart, which confirm her poor intake. She has dentures but they appear loose. Her niece is concerned that she is 'looking thin' and seems depressed. Miss West is often uncommunicative but on occasions expresses herself clearly. She is also registered partially sighted. Her weight on admission was 58 kg and is now 53 kg. Her height is 1.64 m.

Learning disability

Phillip Picton is a 31-year-old man with a learning disability who lives in a supported living scheme with three other people. Recently, he has become increasingly overweight. His obesity is beginning to interfere with his day-to-day activities. He has expressed concern about two issues: bending over to put his socks on and getting out of breath walking to the local shops. His carers took him to see his GP who referred him to the community team for people with learning disabilities. The community nurse for learning disabilities and the occupational therapist, who is Phillip's **health facilitator**, are going to visit him to carry out an assessment. Phillip does his own food shopping with support. His weight three years ago was 58 kg and is now 92 kg.

Mental health

Charles Cooper is an 88-year-old widower (his wife died 15 years ago). He lives alone in a bungalow in a small village. The village has very poor public transport services. The local shop has recently closed. Mr Cooper has a diagnosis of **dementia** for which he is prescribed medication. He is prompted to take this by a home carer who calls twice a day. Recently, community mental health nurse noticed that Mr Cooper had lost weight. When questioned about his dietary intake, Mr Cooper stated that he has a 'good appetite' and manages to prepare his own meals. On checking the kitchen, the nurse observed little evidence of recent food preparation or cooking. The refrigerator contained some dairy products, and these had all expired and were beginning to smell.

NUTRITION IN HEALTHCARE: CONCERNS AND INITIATIVES

The ENHA (2013) report that while malnutrition includes both over-nutrition (overweight and obesity) and under-nutrition, there has been a concentration on the problem of obesity, while the problem of under-nutrition has been largely neglected. In 70% of patients, **malnutrition** remains undiagnosed (Lean and Wiseman 2008).

Health facilitator

The role focuses on an individual's health outcomes and can be undertaken by a range of people including support workers, family carers, friends and advocates as well as health professionals, see *Health Action Planning and Health Facilitation for People with Learning Disabilities: Good Practice Guidance* (DH 2009).

Dementia

The term 'dementia' is used to describe the symptoms that occur when the brain is affected by specific diseases and conditions. Dementia is progressive; symptoms include loss of memory, confusion and problems with speech and understanding. See http://alzheimers.org.uk for more information.

Malnutrition

Malnutrition is a condition in which a deficiency, excess or imbalance of food intake, protein and other nutrients causes measurable adverse effects on tissue, body form (shape, size or composition), function, clinical outcome and quality of life.

> **LEARNING OUTCOMES**
>
> By the end of this section, you will be able to:
> 1 review reports which have highlighted concerns about malnutrition, particularly hospital patients;
> 2 discuss recommendations and initiatives to improve nutrition in healthcare.

Learning outcome 1: Review reports which have highlighted concerns about malnutrition, particularly hospital patients

This chapter's introduction highlighted the continuing problem of malnutrition in community and in hospitals.

ACTIVITY

Drawing on practice experiences, reflect on why people could be at risk of malnutrition, particularly in hospital?

Compare your thoughts with those from some of the reports:

Age Concern (2006, p. 6) raised the following as being problems in hospital:

- Appropriateness of the food on offer
- Availability of help with eating the food
- Monitoring of patients for signs of malnutrition
- Involvement of patients, relatives and carers
- Knowing how and who to raise concerns with

Age UK (2012) highlighted that these problems closely link to relationships between staff and patients and between different groups of staff, such as nurses and catering staff. Age Concern's (2006) original *Hungry to be Heard: The Scandal of Malnourished Older People in Hospital* included harrowing case studies of nutritional needs being neglected. The mental health charity MIND reported that 45% of respondents did not have access to snacks outside of mealtimes, and almost a third of people in inpatient units said they did not have enough access to hot and cold drinks (Baker 2001).

This problem is not just isolated to hospital settings. Carers UK (2012) revealed that the vital role of carers providing nutrition for their significant others is often overlooked; 60% reported worrying about the nutrition of the person they care for. In addition, 16% were caring for someone underweight and with a small appetite (indicators of malnutrition risk) and were worried, but they were receiving no support regarding nutrition. Referrals to healthcare professionals, including dieticians, were found to be suboptimal.

In the light of these reports, various recommendations and improvements have been initiated.

Learning outcome 2: Discuss recommendations and initiatives to improve nutrition in healthcare

ACTIVITY

What initiatives have you seen in practice to try to improve nutrition in healthcare settings?

You may have seen the following:

Protected mealtimes: These are periods on hospital wards when all non-urgent clinical activity stops so that patients can eat their meals uninterrupted, assisted by staff (DH 2007). Generally, visiting is stopped during protected mealtimes, but a family coming to assist a patient with eating should be welcomed.

Red trays/red jugs: The 'red tray' system is a simple way of alerting healthcare staff that a person needs help with eating. A red dot sticker on the person's menu sheet (or similar agreed system) signals to the catering department that the meal must be served on a red tray. Ward staff can then easily identify people who require help by looking out for a red tray and providing assistance quickly so that there is no compromise to the dignity of the patient or the quality of the meal (Royal College of Nursing [RCN] 2012). Red jugs may be used in a similar way, to alert staff to patients who need help drinking.

24-hour catering: Previously hot food was not always available outside mealtimes, but the traditional breakfast, lunch and supper at set times need to be challenged. 24-hour catering should ensure that hot food, snacks and drinks are available to patients at any time of day, to meet patients' needs. A DH (2010) best practice benchmark in *Essence of Care* is that 'People can access food and drink at any time according to their needs and preferences' (p. 130).

Familiar foods and snacks: Some wards with people with dementia have implemented tables with a variety of familiar snacks that patients can help themselves to. Some wards are implementing 'afternoon tea', where cakes are served mid-afternoon. These simple initiatives can improve calorific intake.

Sustainability and seasonality: This includes sourcing local food, which is likely to be fresher, using organic or fairly traded goods and reducing food waste.

Flexi-menu systems: These offer a fixed menu for lunch and evening meals, so that patients can choose food they like more than once.

Mealtime volunteers: Volunteers registered with the care setting who attend to patients assisting them to eat.

Nutrition champions: Staff members who have up-to-date knowledge about nutrition and strive to promote this to other staff.

Easy handling or assisted drinking devices: Devices such as the 'Hydrant bottle' to promote independence in drinking (see later discussion).

Take-aways and food from home: These can offer patients familiar choices in their diet.

Missed meals and replacements: Individualising mealtimes for patients and offering replacement meals, if a meal is missed.

Other innovations to address patients' nutritional needs include the Nutrition on Admission Card (DH 2007), where people can complete an overview of their appetite and dietary intake prior to admission to hospital. In the case of admission, the ambulance crew or significant other of the patient could give staff an overview of their nutritional needs on admission, if a patient is unable to do this for themselves. The Alzheimer's Society promotes the use of 'This is me', which is a simple tool to offer a snapshot view of people with dementia and their likes and dislikes, which includes preferences for food and drink.

The Council of Europe Alliance (2007) has identified ten key characteristics of good nutritional care in hospitals (see Box 10.1).

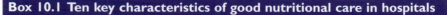
> **Box 10.1 Ten key characteristics of good nutritional care in hospitals**
>
> • All patients are screened on admission to identify the patients who are malnourished or at risk of becoming malnourished. All patients are re-screened weekly.
> • All patients have a care plan which identifies their nutritional care needs and how these are to be met.
> • The hospital includes specific guidance on food services and nutritional care in its Clinical Governance arrangements.
> • Patients are involved in the planning and monitoring arrangements for food service provision.
> • The ward implements Protected Mealtimes to provide an environment conducive to patients enjoying and being able to eat their food.
> • All staff have the appropriate skills and competencies needed to ensure that patients' nutritional needs are met. All staff receive regular training on nutritional care and management.
> • Hospital facilities are designed to be flexible and patient-centred with the aim of providing and delivering an excellent experience of food service and nutritional care 24 hours a day, every day.
> • The hospital has a policy for food service and nutritional care which is patient-centred and performance managed in line with home-country governance frameworks.
> • Food service and nutritional care are delivered to the patient safely.
> • The hospital supports a multidisciplinary approach to nutritional care and values the contribution of all staff groups working in partnership with patients and users.
>
> *Source*: Council of Europe Alliance (UK). 2007. Council of Europe resolution food and nutritional care in hospitals: 10 key characteristics of good nutritional care in hospitals. Available from: http://www.hospitalcaterers.org. With permission.

ACTIVITY

Consider the care environment you work in. Are all the characteristics in Box 10.1 being demonstrated? Discuss your findings with your practice mentor. If all ten factors are not addressed, what do you think might help to ensure they are?

In the United Kingdom (UK), government policies and action groups continue to ensure that nutrition stays at the forefront in the healthcare setting. For example, the British Dietetics Association (BDA 2012) report how their main objective of the 'Food Counts Group' is to improve the nutritional quality of food in hospitals and care settings. Various UK organisations have made recommendations for improving nutrition in healthcare settings; some of the initiatives outlined earlier relate to these recommendations. Age UK (2012) highlighted the following seven steps to address issues, which include that staff:

1. should listen to patients, relatives, significant others and carers about the person's diet;
2. should be food aware;

3. should follow their professional codes and be directed by their professional bodies;

4. should assess patients for signs of risks for malnutrition on admission and at regular intervals during their stay;

5. should follow guidance for protected mealtimes;

6. should implement systems for red tray meals;

7. should involve volunteers to help at mealtimes.

The Care Quality Commission (CQC) inspects all health and social care providers in nutrition. The CQC's 2012 inspections of nutrition in hospital revealed that more hospitals were meeting people's nutritional needs (CQC 2013). They found that many hospitals were now providing flexible catering, offering choices in meals, including portion size and when they could be ordered. In hospitals with good systems in place, staff completed nutritional risk assessments, recorded food and fluid intake accurately and recorded and monitored patients' weights as needed. Problems areas in a minority of hospitals were that patients were not helped to eat and drink, were not given food choices, or helped to wash their hands before eating.

Summary

- Patients' nutritional needs should be given high priority, but a number of reports have highlighted that patients' nutritional needs are not always met effectively, particularly in hospitals.
- Many initiatives are being implemented to address these concerns, and recommendations have been made.
- Nurses are well-placed to implement improvements, working with families and the multi disciplinary team, and other departments, for example, catering units.

RECOGNISING THE CONTRIBUTION OF NUTRITION TO HEALTH

An adequate supply of essential nutrients is required in the diet to maintain health. The term **diet** usually refers to the total food eaten, while **nutrients** refers to components of foodstuffs which have a role in body functioning. For example, bread is composed of the nutrients carbohydrate, protein, fat and some vitamins. It is important to understand the key components of a nutritious diet and to be able to identify factors that might prevent adequate nutrition.

LEARNING OUTCOMES

By the end of this section, you will be able to:

1 explain the major nutrients in the body;

2 discuss factors that might influence healthy people's nutritional needs;

3 reflect on situations in which an individual's nutritional status might be impaired.

Learning outcome 1: Explain the major nutrients in the body

Nutrients are derived from foods that we eat to promote normal growth, maintenance and repair. Most foods contain a variety of nutrients.

ACTIVITY

The major nutrients are listed below. For each of these, consider what are their main uses in the body? Refer to your biology book for details about:
. Carbohydrates and glucose
. Protein
. Fats (lipids)
. Vitamins
. Minerals
. Water

Some brief notes on each are given below:

Carbohydrates and glucose: These are used for body cells. Your brain and red blood cells rely on glucose to supply their energy: think of these as brain foods.

Protein: Essential to the body for growth and repair and maintenance.

Fats (lipids): Phospholipids are used to make up cell membranes; triglycerides are fuel for the body. Fats act as insulation for your body and help the body absorb vitamins.

Vitamins: A, B group, C, D, E and K are crucial in helping the body to use the other nutrients.

Minerals: Calcium, phosphorus, potassium, sulphur, sodium, chloride and magnesium are required for living organisms.

Water: An essential nutrient for hydration.

In the body, these nutrients become involved in a variety of biomechanical processes. Refer to your biology book to find out more about the important groups of nutrients and their role in maintaining health.

ACTIVITY

Consider your last meal and think about the nutrients in it:
• What nutrient(s) did you eat in large quantities?
• Were any nutrients missing?
• Now consider: On an average day, what quantity of water do you consume?
• Before moving on, think about what, if anything, you could change about your water and food intake.

We are all perhaps guilty of a missed meal, a reluctance to drink or not having time to drink enough. However, looking after ourselves is essential for us to care for others. Ganasegeran et al. (2012) reviewed factors which may affect university students' eating habits. They found that students skipped meals and did not include enough fruit and vegetables in their diet. They also found that students had a greater potential to snack while studying and commented that economic factors affected diet choices when shopping for food. They concluded that university students were at risk of having a poor diet and needed to eat healthy foods to prepare them for their future and avoid chronic diseases.

Whilst the media may bombard you with messages about what to eat, remember patients in your care may often look to you for advice about their diet, particularly if they are newly diagnosed with a disease or have experienced an illness or accident recently. Try to educate yourself about the components of a healthy diet and why this is essential. Gain an understanding of the role of nutrients in the body so that you may share your knowledge.

Learning outcome 2: Discuss factors that might influence healthy people's nutritional needs

The amounts of various nutrients required for health vary from individual to individual and throughout life.

ACTIVITY | What factors might influence a healthy person's nutritional needs?

You may have thought of the following:
- **Age**. In adulthood, the energy requirement decreases with age because older people have a lower metabolic rate than younger adults.
- **Gender**. Men require more energy because their relatively greater muscle mass results in a higher metabolic rate than that in women.
- **Height and build**. The bigger the body, the greater the amount of nutrients required to maintain cells.
- **Amount of physical activity**. As energy is used as fuel, the greater the physical activity, the higher the energy utilisation.
- **Pregnancy**. During the second and third trimesters of pregnancy, rapid growth of the foetus alters the woman's nutritional needs – see 'Pregnancy: practice points' box at the end of this section.
- **Lactation**. A breast feeding woman requires increased energy (as much as 500 calories/day or more), increased intake of calcium and vitamins A, C and D. She should drink enough fluids to satisfy her thirst.

Being aware of factors affecting nutritional demands in healthy people is important prior to considering factors that compromise nutritional status.

Learning outcome 3: Reflect on situations in which an individual's nutritional status might be impaired

There are many situations where people may be unable to meet their nutritional needs, leading to malnutrition, as a result of inadequate intake, inappropriate intake, increased nutritional demands or any combination of these factors.

What might predispose to an inadequate nutritional intake? The scenarios will give you some clues but also reflect on your experience in practice. Remember to think about psychological and socio-economic factors as well as physical factors.

There are many factors you could have identified and many of these interlink. Here are examples:

Loss of appetite. As you read, Miss West currently has a poor appetite. Appetite loss may be seen in older people and can be caused by pain, stress, anxiety, reduced physical activity and fatigue, which often accompany illness.

Stress. Digestion slows when adrenaline is produced; thus, people who are stressed may feel less able to eat.

Lack of knowledge and skills. People may not understand the importance of eating and could be unable to buy suitable food and prepare it. For example, although Phillip can eat independently and can shop with help, he might be unaware of the different nutrients he needs to stay healthy. Therefore, he may not be eating enough of the right food while eating too much of the food that might lead to obesity, such as a high-fat diet or excess sugar.

Dementia. Mr Cooper has dementia, which could affect his appetite and his ability to shop and prepare food, leading to an inadequate and inappropriate intake. People with dementia may not be able to eat independently, and in very severe cognitive impairment they may no longer recognise food (www.alzheimers. org.uk)

Paranoia. Some people may not eat because of fear of being poisoned; for example, people who have psychological problems may see food as poisonous.

Nausea and vomiting. These symptoms, which are caused by various illnesses and are side effects of some medicines, prevent people from eating even if they feel hungry (Holmes 2003).

Nil by mouth. Some people may be unable to eat for prolonged periods due to their condition (e.g. if they are unconscious) or treatment (e.g. following some types of surgery).

End of life. People nearing the end of their life may wish to withdraw from eating or drinking either due to physical lack of strength or loss of interest in food.

Physical factors. One example is dysphagia (difficulty in swallowing), which results from delayed or absent swallow reflex, for example, following a stroke (see www.rcslt.org). Initially, Miss West had this problem. Difficulty in chewing and pain caused by decayed teeth or ill-fitting dentures or mouth ulcers are other physical causes of inadequate intake. Limited dexterity causing difficulty in manipulating cutlery may make eating slow and difficult (e.g. people with cerebral palsy, stroke or rheumatoid arthritis). For example, Miss West's weak right arm

Emphysema

Lung disease characterised by over-inflation and destructive changes leading to lack of elasticity in the alveolar walls.

Basal metabolic rate

The amount of energy needed by the body for essential processes when at complete rest but awake.

Anorexia nervosa

Anorexia nervosa is an eating disorder in which people feel they need to have an unnatural control of what they are eating to avoid putting on weight. It is associated with irrational thoughts about becoming overweight. Extensive weight loss is often seen as people attempt to keep their weight under control.

Bulimia

Bulimia is an eating disorder that begins as a psychological issue, which in turn affects the person's ability to consume a balanced and nutritional diet. Bulimia is associated with eating too much in a short space of time, often referred to as a binge.

will cause difficulty manipulating eating utensils. The physical effort of eating may be too great for some people with chronic diseases such as heart failure or **emphysema**. Loss of taste (**dysgeusia**) may occur due to illness, for example, after a stroke (Stroke Association 2012). A loss of taste can make a big difference to the quality of life, and people find it to be a distressing and unexpected after-effect of a stroke.

Medication. Some medications hinder the taste of food, for example, ferrous sulphate or steroids, often giving patients a metallic taste in their mouth. Some medicines suppress the appetite (Holmes 2003).

Increased nutritional demands: Holmes (2003) describes how the body's reaction to injury, infection and surgery raises the **basal metabolic rate** and hence increases nutritional demands. Healing of wounds and fractures requires additional nutrients (see Chapter 7 for discussion of nutrition and wound healing). Some neurological conditions, such as some types of cerebral palsy, can cause excessive body movements, using up energy and thus increasing nutritional demands.

Dependency. People who are dependent on others and unable to express their needs are at risk of inadequate intake. Examples would be people unable to communicate as a result of intellectual or neurological impairment, or dementia.

Lack of finance. People who are living on a low income often have many demands on their limited funds, so nutrition may not be the top priority.

Food is sometimes found to be a source of comfort in periods of stress or anxiety. With Phillip, it would be important to consider whether these social and psychological factors are relevant. For example, are there sufficient activities for him to be involved in? Fad diets and erroneous health beliefs may lead people to follow diets that are too restricted to meet their needs. It is important that dietetic advice is sought.

Altered food intake due to mental health issues

Eating disorders, for example, **anorexia nervosa** or **bulimia**, obsessive compulsive disorder, addiction to drugs and alcohol, personality disorders, depression, bipolar disorder and schizophrenia could all affect a person's nutritional intake. Some people who experience mental health issues need to take medication as part of their treatment. Certain sedative medication may alter the person's desire for food either increasing or decreasing their appetite.

See NICE (2004) for details of management of people with eating disorders to assist you in understanding the issues which people face with an eating disorder. See also www.mind.org.uk for information about eating disorders. The Royal College of Psychiatrists (RCP 2012) (see http://www.rcpsych.ac.uk/) also provide guidance for healthcare professionals and the public, aiming to ensure that those caring for people with eating disorders address such issues as diet and exercise and electrolyte imbalance.

Children: practice points – nutrition

The UNICEF website provides useful information on infant feeding:

Formula feeding: http://www.unicef.org.uk/BabyFriendly/Resources/Resources-for-parents/A-guide-to-infant-formula-for-parents-who-are-bottle-feeding/

Breast-feeding: http://www.unicef.org.uk/UNICEFs-Work/What-we-do/Our-UK-work/Breastfeeding/

Bottle feeds must be prepared with scrupulous attention to hygiene.

In *Weaning: Starting Solid Food*, the DH (2008) recommends that solid foods are introduced from about 6 months and never before 4 months old.

For further reading, see:

Howe, R., Forbes, D. and Baker, C. 2010. Providing optimum nutrition and hydration. In: Glasper, A., Aylott, M. and Battrick, C. (eds.) *Developing Practical Skills for Nursing Children and Young People*. London: Hodder Arnold, 203–09.

Macqueen, S. Bruce, E.A. and Gibson, F. 2012. Nutrition and feeding. In: *The Great Ormond Street Hospital Manual of Children's Nursing Practices*. Chichester: Wiley-Blackwell. 473–511.

Pregnancy and birth: practice points – nutrition

A healthy, balanced diet is important for both the mother and her baby throughout pregnancy and after birth. Pregnant women have a number of additional dietary requirements. These include folic acid supplementation to prevent foetal neural tube defects/spina bifida and Vitamin D supplementation to increase the mother's own stores and reduce the risk of her baby developing rickets in childhood.

Obesity in women can significantly increase the risk of additional complications occurring in pregnancy and childbirth (raised blood pressure; pre-eclampsia; gestational diabetes; venousthromboembolism; difficulty with intubation during general anaesthetic). This means that all healthcare staff have a public health obligation in supporting pregnant women to eat healthily and exercise appropriately, to achieve the best possible birth outcome.

When caring for breastfeeding postnatal mothers in the general hospital setting, staff must ensure adequate hydration and a balanced diet with sufficient calories to maintain a good breast milk supply.

Further reading:

www.unicef.org.uk

www.eatwell.gov.uk

Summary

- An adequate intake of the correct balance of nutrients is essential to maintain health and prevent malnutrition.
- The nutritional needs of healthy people are affected by various factors, including their stage in the lifespan.

- Nurses care for many people who are unable to meet their nutritional needs due to a wide range of issues, and some will also have increased nutritional demands.
- Various mental and physical health conditions affect nutritional intake, with a potential adverse effect on health.

ASSESSING AND MAINTAINING HYDRATION

Whilst obtaining the necessary nutrients from food is important, water is also essential to life. The NMC (2010a) states that nurses must be able to assess fluid status of patients and act to ensure there is adequate intake, in partnership with patients. The body's fluid intake is mainly regulated by thirst. Dehydration refers to a fluid loss of 1% or greater of the total body mass (Campbell 2011). Medical conditions may inhibit or promote fluid intake; for example, when a person has dementia, the person may think they have just had a drink; at the onset of diabetes, the person cannot quench their thirst. Causes of inadequate fluid intake include dependency on healthcare workers, prolonged preoperative fasting, weakness, illness, reduced taste, loss of sensation due to ageing and restricted access to drink.

LEARNING OUTCOMES

By the end of this section, you will be able to:

1 identify the percentage of water in the body and the recommended fluid intake;
2 explain how to assess and monitor a patient's fluid status;
3 discuss ways of promoting adequate oral fluid intake for patients and initiatives in practice;
4 explain how supplementary fluids can be administered when the oral route is not available or sufficient.

Learning outcome 1: Identify the percentage of water in the body and the recommended fluid intake

Approximately 60% of the body is made up of water; for example, a 70 kg man is made up of about 42 L of total water. Scanlon and Sanders (2011) explain that about two-thirds of body fluid is found within body cells and is termed intracellular fluid (ICF). The other third is extracellular fluid (ECF) and is found in plasma, lymph, tissue fluid and specialised body fluids such as cerebrospinal fluid, ocular, pleural, peritoneal and synovial fluids.

The proportion of water in the body varies according to age. A new-born baby is composed of approximately 75% water whilst an older person is composed of approximately 50% water (Metheny 2012). The more muscular a person's body is, the more water it contains while, conversely, the more fat in the human body, the less the water content.

ACTIVITY

What do you think the recommended fluid intake is? Reflect on your own fluid intake yesterday: do you think you drank sufficient fluids?

There is currently no agreed recommended daily intake level for water in the UK, but estimates range from approximately 1.2 to 3.1 L per day (RCN 2007); how does that compare with your intake? Healthcare professionals are best placed to ensure that patients receive sufficient fluid whether it is oral or via other routes (see learning outcome 4). Simply administering fluids orally, when the patient's condition allows, can be life saving and life preserving. Occasionally, patients have medically restricted fluid intake, for example, in renal failure, but for all other patients, the recommended fluid intake should be the target.

Learning outcome 2: Explain how to assess and monitor a patient's fluid status

Nurses must be able to assess and monitor fluid balance (NMC 2010a). Fluid balance refers to the amount of fluid that is taken into the body (input) and the amount that is excreted (output). A negative fluid balance is where the output is greater than fluid ingested, and a positive fluid balance is where intake is greater than output (Shepherd 2011).

ACTIVITY

Review a fluid balance chart in your practice area.
- What do you note about the person's input and output?
- Are they in a negative or positive fluid balance?
- Why do you think this might be?

Now, review the possible causes of positive or negative fluid balance below and compare them with your answer:

Negative fluid balance: Could be due to dehydration resulting from excessive fluid loss from the body, through sweating, urination, vomiting, diarrhoea or haemorrhage, or may result from insufficient fluid intake.

Positive fluid balance: Due to fluid overload and electrolyte imbalance, in particular sodium. Could also be due to conditions that reduce the body's ability to eliminate fluid, for example, heart or renal failure.

A fluid balance chart to record input and output is readily available in many clinical care settings, and regular reviews of fluid balance charts is part of many ward routines. This tool assists you in identifying over a period of 24 hours if a patient is in a negative or positive fluid balance. There are often underlying health issues which lead to dehydration or fluid overload. Patients' biochemistry results are much more readily and quickly available, and results of these blood results can then be acted upon promptly. Consideration of vital signs, capillary refill time, elasticity of skin, body weight and urine output can all assist in fluid balance assessment.

ACTIVITY

What clinical signs would alert you that an adult is dehydrated?

Box 10.2 summarises signs of dehydration in adults, which you should be aware of.

Learning outcome 3: Discuss ways of promoting adequate oral fluid intake for patients and initiatives in practice

Fluid intake should be a consideration for all patients. Remember, if a patient is embarrassed about asking for the toilet or is worried about how they might manage

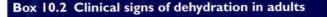

Box 10.2 Clinical signs of dehydration in adults

Mild to moderate dehydration:
- Thirst
- Dizziness or light-headedness
- Headache
- Tiredness
- Dry mouth, lips and eyes
- Concentrated urine (dark yellow)
- Passing only small amounts of urine infrequently (less than three or four times a day)

If mild or moderate dehydration is untreated, the person may become severely dehydrated.

Severe dehydration:
- Dry, wrinkled skin that sags slowly into position when pinched up
- An inability to urinate, or not passing urine for 8 hours
- Irritability
- Sunken eyes
- Hypotension
- A rapid, weak pulse
- Cool hands and feet
- Seizures
- Reduced consciousness, lethargy or confusion
- Blood in the stools or vomit

Source: NHS Choices. 2013. Signs of dehydration. http://www.nhs.uk/Conditions/dehydration/Pages/Introduction.aspx

in the hospital bathroom, even the most mobile of patients may refrain from drinking; thus, fluid intake should be considered for all people in care settings.

ACTIVITY

In your practice area, observe several mobile patients who are able to take oral fluids independently and reflect on whether they readily help themselves to drinks on a regular basis. If not, try to find a way to discuss this with them. Remember to offer them drinks when other less mobile patients are offered drinks too.

Do not assume that patients know they need to drink more while they are unwell nor assume that they know they are 'allowed' to drink outside mealtimes. Consider ways in which you can portray this message to patients in your practice area. Observe whether signage to drinks machines and water fountains are easily visible. If not, what could you do to rectify this? Is it ward or department policy that patients and visitors can help themselves to drinks?

Remember that drinking is a social event too. Events of happiness and sadness are often accompanied by drinking (alcoholic or non-alcoholic). If it is not policy for patients and family to drink together, then explore how to address this issue, which is especially important where people are in hospital for long periods. In long-stay settings, check if there are canteen facilities where patients and visitors can socialise and get beverages together and, if so, direct them to these facilities. Be proactive and see how you might bring about changes in your area.

In the community setting, consider ways in which you can assist patients to increase their fluid intake. Look at the placing of taps, kettles, cups, tea and coffee facilities when you visit their home. Consider ways in which you might assist them to easily make a cup of tea. Does the patient have a flask made up for them or is there someone who could assist them with drinks when you are not there? With the person's permission, are there items which can be placed nearer so that they can maintain their independence for accessing a drink? Again, be proactive, consider ways in which you may promote patients' hydration at home and with their permission set up their environment to promote their independence. Ask the patient to keep a log of when they take a drink and monitor this when you visit them. Offer information about why fluid intake is important and why omitting fluids for a long period of time is potentially harmful to them.

ACTIVITY — Have you observed any initiatives to promote hydration for patients?

There have been many initiatives within the NHS recently to try to ensure that patients receive enough hydration. Examples include the provision of a red jug to patients who require assistance to drink or need to drink more (Campbell 2011; Hollis 2011). The 'Hydrant' bottle is a water bottle devised for easy handling to assist people with limited mobility with their fluid intake (see http://www.hydrateforhealth.co.uk/the-hydrant.html). The Royal College of Nursing (RCN 2007), in conjunction with the National Patient Safety Agency (NPSA), published *Water for Health: Hydration Best Practice Toolkit.* as part of the Nutrition Now campaign. This toolkit aims to offer best practice guidance on hydration to all healthcare workers in England, Scotland and Wales and highlights that hydration is a patient safety issue. The toolkit highlights how ensuring patients receive adequate hydration has economic benefits and long-term health benefits for patients. In their extensive toolkit, they identify factors associated with poor hydration and offer tips on how to increase water content each day. The toolkit also stresses that carers play a vital role in ensuring patients receive adequate hydration.

McIntyre et al. (2012) proposed an 'intelligent fluid management bundle', aimed at getting the basics of hydration right. They recommended that all patients are assessed in terms of hydration needs, a plan is devised to ensure optimum hydration and fluid intake is continuously monitored. The aim is that dehydration is detected early and staff are educated regarding hydration (McIntyre et al. 2012).

Learning outcome 4: Explain how supplementary fluids can be administered when the oral route is not available or sufficient

Nurses must be able to safely administer fluids when patients cannot take them independently (NMC 2010a). In some instances, fluid intake by the oral route is not possible or insufficient to maintain hydration.

Reflect on experiences in practice and write down a list of routes for administering fluids, if the oral route is not suitable or sufficient.

You may have thought of the following:

- Intravenously (IV): into the vein.
- Subcutaneous (SC) (hypodermoclysis): into subcutaneous tissue. This route is a valuable alternative method of fluid delivery to the traditional intravenous route, particularly used for older people. It has many advantages over parenteral fluid administration, including ease of administration and fewer systemic side effects (Barton et al. 2004).
- Intra-osseous (IO): directly into the bone marrow of the antero-medial aspect of the tibia (most popular), femur, iliac crest or humerus.

In an emergency, the IV and IO routes are more likely to be used. The SC route is used for fluid administration when the intravenous route is not available, for hydration of an older person or at the end stages of life for rehydration.

Children: practice points – dehydration

Dehydration can develop very quickly in infants and young children as such a large proportion of body weight is water. There is a risk of dehydration if diarrhoea and vomiting occur or with other conditions, for example, acute respiratory conditions where the infant may not be feeding adequately. Nurses working with infants and young children should be alert and able to recognise signs of dehydration which may be:

Mild: loss of body weight (<5%), slightly dry mucous membranes, slightly decreased urine output, increased thirst, irritability.

Moderate: loss of body weight (5–10%), raised heart rate, poor tear production, decreased skin turgor, sunken eyes and fontanelles, decreased urine output, restless to lethargic.

Severe: loss of body weight (10–15%), low blood pressure, absent urine output, lethargic to comatose.

For mild to moderate dehydration, oral rehydration therapy is used. For moderate to severe dehydration, IV fluids are required.

For further reading, see:

Howe, R., Forbes, D. and Baker, C. 2010. Providing optimum nutrition and hydration. In: Glasper, A., Aylett, M. and Bat trick, C. (eds.) *Developing Practical Skills for Nursing Children and Young People.* London: Hodder Arnold, 203–9.

Macqueen, S., Bruce, E.A. and Gibson, F. 2012. Fluid balance. In: *The Great Ormond Street Hospital Manual of Children's Nursing Practices.* Chichester: Wiley-Blackwell. 143–65.

Summary

- Maintaining hydration is a fundamental part of care, along with other important care principles such as hand hygiene.
- Nurses must be proactive in ensuring that people in their care have an adequate fluid intake, whether in the hospital or community setting, in order to maintain hydration. Ease of access to fluids must be in place, 24 hours a day.
- Fluid intake must be assessed on admission to hospital and then monitored to ensure that adequate hydration is maintained during each person's care.
- Nurses must be alert to any signs of dehydration so that hydration status can be promptly addressed.
- When patients cannot take sufficient oral fluids to maintain hydration, other methods must be used that are suitable for the individual.

PROMOTING HEALTHY EATING AND ADDRESSING PEOPLE'S CHOICES

The British Dietetics Association (BDA) (2012) explains how food and fluid are a significant part of services provided to older people in residential care and are key to satisfaction with services. A best practice benchmark for 'Food and drink' is that 'people are encouraged to eat and drink in a way that promotes their health' (DH 2010, p. 9). Similarly, the Welsh Assembly Government (2011) states that people must be offered a choice of food and drink that meets their nutritional and personal requirements. A balanced diet consists of a particular selection of foods, in the correct proportions to meet the body cells' requirements and is essential for maintaining a healthy body that functions efficiently. We have already considered the nutrients necessary for a healthy diet and factors that affect nutritional status, but in care settings, achieving a healthy diet poses particular challenges. Considering people's food preferences is an important aspect of promoting healthy eating.

LEARNING OUTCOMES

By the end of this section, you will be able to:
1 discuss factors that should be considered to enable patients to make healthy food choices that are acceptable to them;
2 assist patients to select a healthy diet from a menu in a care setting.

Learning outcome 1: Discuss factors that should be considered to enable patients to make healthy food choices that are acceptable to them

The NMC (2010a) expects that nurses should assist patients to choose a diet that provides an adequate nutritional and fluid intake.

ACTIVITY

Thinking about the scenarios at the start of this chapter, reflect on factors that you would consider when helping patients to make healthy food choices.

Recognising and responding to patients' food preferences is paramount if people are to consume a balanced nutritional diet while in your care. Therefore, spending time with Miss West, Philip and Mr Cooper to find out what they like to eat and drink is key to promoting healthy eating for them. Family can also be involved, for example, Miss West's niece should be able to help with information about her usual diet. There is no replacement for asking the patient or significant other about personal preferences and making sure that you recognise the patient's individual choices. As mentioned earlier in this chapter, there should be written documentation of food preferences. For example, the Alzheimer's Society have developed 'This is me', which is a leaflet that, when completed, helps people with dementia to communicate their needs, preferences, likes and dislikes (see http://www.alzheimers.org.uk/thisisme).

Nurses must ensure that patients' cultural and religious beliefs are respected during food selection. Cultural differences in food preparation, serving and eating routines need to be considered to enable people to have choices in their diet. People's beliefs and values may lead them to require a vegetarian or vegan diet, for example. You should consider the person's religion as food preferences of some people are related to religious beliefs. It is important not to make assumptions about what people might eat according to their culture/religion, instead it is to be found out from the individual or the family concerned. For example, a person who follows Sikhism may refrain from eating beef, eggs or fish or may be a vegetarian (Holland and Hogg 2010). A person following Judaism is required to eat kosher food (food fit to be eaten in accordance with Jewish law), but there are many diverse practices concerning this (Collins 2002).

You should become familiar with any dietary restrictions that are advised for chronic diseases as some patients in your care may receive prescribed diets as part of their medical treatment, for example, low fat for a patient who has heart disease or high protein for a patient who has had extensive surgery. Dietary supplements may also be prescribed, and it is important that you work with the dietician to ensure that the patient receives these in a timely manner.

ACTIVITY

Arrange to meet with the dietician in your care environment and discuss with them what types of diet are recommended for patients in your care setting.

Learning outcome 2: Assist patients to select a healthy diet from a menu in a care setting

ACTIVITY

How might you assist a patient to choose a healthy diet from a menu?

When looking at the menu with a patient, you need to be prepared to explain the foods, as some items may be unfamiliar to people. You may need to read out menus and complete them for people; this would be necessary for Miss West, who is partially sighted. You can guide patients towards appropriate foods on the menu, ensuring there is a balance of the important food groups discussed earlier in this chapter, while taking preferences into account. Miss West requires food that is not only nourishing but also weight inducing, so you might encourage her to eat more carbohydrates and dairy products. Ford (2012) highlights how showing a person a picture of food on offer may support people in making informed choices. It can also assist them to try new foods that they have perhaps not considered. For some people, seeing pictures may help prompt them to make choices of their favourite foods.

Summary

- When promoting healthy eating, nurses should find out patients' food preferences, from the individual, their family or written information.
- Patients may need help with understanding and completing menus; pictures of food available will be helpful in some situations.
- Nurses should guide patients/clients regarding appropriate food choices, with respect for individual preferences, culture, religion, values and beliefs.
- Nurses should take account of any specific nutritional requirements, relating to patients' health conditions, liaising with the dietician accordingly.

NUTRITIONAL SCREENING

Nurses must be able to assess and monitor patients' nutritional status and formulate a plan of care in partnership with them (NMC 2010a). The *Essence of Care* benchmark for best practice is that 'People are screened on initial contact and those identified as at risk receive a full nutritional assessment' (DH 2010, p. 16). Learning how to use a nutritional screening tool is therefore an essential requirement. Nurses are in a unique position to identify people at risk of malnourishment and then take appropriate action. As recognised already in this chapter, there are many factors that can affect nutritional status. If nurses do not carry out nutritional screening carefully, patients can be put at unnecessary risk from the effects of malnourishment. A range of nutritional screening tools is available, but the Malnutrition Universal Screening Tool (MUST) is recommended (DH 2010).

LEARNING OUTCOMES

By the end of this section, you will be able to:
1 discuss how observations can contribute to nutritional assessment;
2 explain the purpose and use of nutritional screening tools;
3 carry out nutritional screening and recognise if people are at risk of malnutrition.

Learning outcome 1: Discuss how observations can contribute to nutritional assessment

Assessment should include a range of observations to gain insight into nutritional status and contribute to screening.

ACTIVITY

With reference to the scenarios, what observations could be carried out to assist nutritional assessment?

You may have identified many of the aspects listed below – most would be useful in assessing the patients/clients in the scenarios.

- Observe whether clothing, rings and dentures are fitting comfortably. If not, this could suggest an alteration in weight. These could be useful indicators as to whether Mr Cooper is losing weight. You will remember that Miss West's dentures are loose, and her niece might know whether her aunt's loose dentures are a new problem. Remember that patients may be deliberately trying to lose weight and so do not make assumptions.
- Look at the skin and check for excessive dryness, scaling and temperature.
- Check the eyes for brightness and whether they are sunken into their sockets, which could indicate dehydration. These would be important observations with both Mr Cooper (who may not be drinking enough) and Miss West, whose fluid intake we know is poor.
- Note the smell of the breath. Halitosis can indicate poor dental health or dehydration. This could lead you to review the state of the mouth, and to identify a problem, if any, with the teeth or gums. A sore mouth can indicate a poor diet. Chapter 8 considers oral hygiene in detail.
- Observe the level of mobility, for example, whether the person can move their arms adequately to eat independently, or can walk or manoeuvre to get access to food. This is particularly relevant to Miss West, but the community mental health nurse should also consider Mr Cooper's mobility in relation to obtaining and preparing food.
- Observe for drooling which could be a sign of poor swallowing, as well as poor lip seal. Although Miss West has been assessed as able to swallow now, these are signs that nurses should be aware of owing to her previous history.
- While the person is eating and drinking, observe their sequence of breathing and swallowing.
- Observe for non-verbal signals, gestures or signs that the person may use to communicate their wishes, such as pushing the dish away. It is important to respect people's wishes.
- In people's own homes, community nurses can observe what food is around and whether it is within the sell-by date. Out-of-date food could indicate that food is being bought but not actually eaten. These were important observations for Mr Cooper's community mental health nurse to make. Regarding Phillip, the community nurse for learning disability and occupational therapist could observe what food he is buying and storing.

- Observe food intake, which will indicate the amount of food that is actually being consumed. Such details recorded over several days allow for any day-to-day fluctuations. It was good practice that the staff on the medical ward from which Miss West was transferred were recording her food and fluid intake on a food chart. The nurses on the rehabilitation unit should check back over charts from previous days. Three days should be sufficient to assess a patient's eating habits, and then a decision can be made as to what additional support is needed. This may be by the nurse or may involve the dietician.

Learning outcome 2: Explain the purpose and use of nutritional screening tools

Nutritional screening is the process of identifying people at risk of malnourishment. The Malnutrition Advisory Group (MAG 2003), part of British Association for Parenteral and Enteral Nutrition (BAPEN), developed MUST for use with adults at risk of malnutrition (Todorovic et al. 2003). MUST is downloadable from www.bapen. org.uk along with detailed screening guidelines and is advocated as the tool that all healthcare settings should be using. Additional information for use with MUST is also available, in *The MUST Explanatory Booklet* (Todorovic et al. 2003). The components of the tool and its usage are presented next, but do refer to the website documents for further explanation and these documents may also be updated periodically.

Todorovic et al. (2003) explained that nutritional screening is the first step in identifying people who may be at nutritional risk or potentially at risk, and who may benefit from appropriate nutritional intervention. It is a rapid, simple and general procedure used by nursing, medical or other staff on first contact with patients so that clear guidelines for action can be implemented and appropriate nutritional advice provided. Todorovic et al. point out that repeated screening may be necessary when a person's condition and nutritional risk change, and that it is always better to prevent or detect problems early by screening than discover serious problems later. Box 10.3 presents the five steps in screening using MUST. These steps are explained next.

Step 1: Body mass index (BMI)

The BMI provides a 'rapid interpretation of chronic protein-energy status based on an individual's height and weight' (Todorovic et al. 2003, p. 5). Box 10.4 explains how to measure height and weight accurately. The formula to calculate BMI is:

$$\frac{\text{Weight in kilogrammes}}{(\text{Height in metres})^2}$$

The chart in Figure 10.1 displays BMI scores based on weight and height and the corresponding MUST score. In some care settings, entering the weight and height into an electronic patient record will automatically generate the BMI measurement. MAG (2003) suggests a variety of other indicators if weight and height measurements are not available.

Box 10.3 The five MUST steps

Step 1

Measure height and weight to get a BMI score using the chart provided. If unable to obtain height and weight, use alternative procedures, detailed in Malnutrition Universal Screening Tool (MAG 2003).

Step 2

Note percentage of unplanned weight loss and score using tables provided in Malnutrition Universal Screening Tool (MAG 2003)

Step 3

Establish acute disease effect and score.

Step 4

Add scores from Steps 1, 2 and 3 together to obtain overall risk of malnutrition.

Step 5

Use management guidelines and/or local policy to develop care plan.

Source: Reproduced with the kind permission of BAPEN. Available from: http://www.bapen.org.uk/pdfs/must/must-full.pdf

Box 10.4 Measuring height and weight

Height
- Use a height stick (stadiometer), if available. Ensure it is correctly positioned against the wall.
- Ask the person to remove their shoes and to stand upright, feet flat, heels against the height stick or wall (if height stick not used).
- Ask the person to look straight ahead. Lower the head plate until it gently touches the top of the head.
- Read and document height.
- Some people's height may need to be measured while lying in bed.

Weight
- Use clinical scales wherever possible and make sure they have been regularly checked for accuracy.
- Ensure that the scales read zero without the person standing on them.
- Weigh the person in light clothing and without shoes.
- Bed scales are available to weigh patients restricted to bed. Hoist scales are also available.

Source: Adapted from Todorovic, V., Russell, C., Stratton, R., et al. 2003. *The MUST Explanatory Booklet*. Redditch: BAPEN.

Height (feet and inches)

Weight (kg)	4'9½	4'10½	4'11	5'0	5'0½	5'1½	5'2	5'3	5'4	5'4½	5'5½	5'6	5'7	5'7½	5'8½	5'9½	5'10	5'11	5'11½	6'0½	6'1	6'2	6'3	6'3½	6'4½	Weight (stones and pounds)
100	47	46	44	43	42	41	40	39	38	37	36	35	35	34	33	32	32	31	30	30	29	28	28	27	27	15 10
99	46	45	44	43	42	41	40	39	38	37	36	35	34	33	33	32	31	31	30	29	29	28	27	27	26	15 8
98	46	45	44	42	41	40	39	38	37	36	36	35	34	33	32	32	31	30	30	29	28	28	27	27	26	15 6
97	46	44	43	42	41	40	39	38	37	36	35	34	34	33	32	31	31	30	29	29	28	27	27	26	26	15 4
96	45	44	43	42	40	39	38	38	37	36	35	34	33	32	32	31	30	30	29	28	28	27	27	26	26	15 2
95	45	43	42	41	40	39	38	37	36	35	34	34	33	32	31	31	30	29	29	28	27	27	26	26	25	14 13
94	44	43	42	41	40	39	38	37	36	35	34	33	33	32	31	30	30	29	28	28	27	27	26	25	25	14 11
93	44	42	41	40	39	38	37	36	35	35	34	33	32	31	31	30	29	29	28	27	27	26	26	25	25	14 9
92	43	42	41	40	39	38	37	36	35	34	33	33	32	31	30	30	29	28	28	27	27	26	25	25	24	14 7
91	43	42	40	39	38	37	36	36	35	34	33	32	31	31	30	29	29	28	27	27	26	26	25	25	24	14 5
90	42	41	40	39	38	37	36	35	34	33	33	32	31	30	30	29	28	28	27	27	26	25	25	24	24	14 2
89	42	41	40	39	38	37	36	35	34	33	32	32	31	30	29	29	28	27	27	26	26	25	25	24	24	14 0
88	41	40	39	38	37	36	35	34	34	33	32	31	30	30	29	28	28	27	27	26	25	25	24	24	23	13 12
87	41	40	39	38	37	36	35	34	33	32	32	31	30	29	29	28	27	27	26	26	25	25	24	24	23	13 10
86	40	39	38	37	36	35	34	34	33	32	31	30	30	29	28	28	27	27	26	25	25	24	24	23	23	13 8
85	40	39	38	37	36	35	34	33	32	32	31	30	29	29	28	27	27	26	26	25	25	24	24	23	23	13 5
84	39	38	37	36	35	35	34	33	32	31	30	30	29	28	28	27	27	26	25	25	24	24	23	23	22	13 3
83	39	38	37	36	35	34	33	32	32	31	30	29	29	28	27	27	26	26	25	25	24	23	23	23	22	13 1
82	38	37	36	35	35	34	33	32	31	30	30	29	28	28	27	26	26	25	25	24	24	23	23	22	22	12 13
81	38	37	36	35	34	33	32	32	31	30	29	29	28	27	27	26	26	25	24	24	23	23	22	22	22	12 11
80	38	37	36	35	34	33	32	31	30	30	29	28	28	27	26	26	25	25	24	24	23	23	22	22	21	12 8
79	37	36	35	34	33	32	32	31	30	29	29	28	27	27	26	26	25	24	24	23	23	22	22	21	21	12 6
78	37	36	35	34	33	32	31	30	30	29	28	28	27	26	26	25	25	24	24	23	23	22	22	21	21	12 4
77	36	35	34	33	32	32	31	30	29	29	28	27	27	26	25	25	24	24	23	23	22	22	21	21	20	12 2
76	36	35	34	33	32	31	30	30	29	28	28	27	26	26	25	25	24	23	23	22	22	22	21	21	20	12 0
75	35	34	33	32	32	31	30	29	29	28	27	27	26	25	25	24	24	23	23	22	22	21	21	20	20	11 11
74	35	34	33	32	31	30	30	29	28	28	27	26	26	25	24	24	23	23	22	22	21	21	20	20	20	11 9
73	34	33	32	32	31	30	29	29	28	27	26	26	25	25	24	24	23	23	22	22	21	21	20	20	19	11 7
72	34	33	32	31	30	30	29	28	27	27	26	26	25	24	24	23	23	22	22	21	21	20	20	20	19	11 5
71	33	32	32	31	30	29	28	28	27	26	26	25	25	24	23	23	22	22	21	21	21	20	20	19	19	11 3
70	33	32	31	30	30	29	28	27	27	26	25	25	24	24	23	23	22	22	21	21	20	20	19	19	19	11 0
69	32	32	31	30	29	28	28	27	26	26	25	24	24	23	23	22	22	21	21	20	20	20	19	19	18	10 12
68	32	31	30	29	29	28	27	27	26	25	25	24	24	23	22	22	21	21	21	20	20	19	19	18	18	10 10
67	31	31	30	29	28	28	27	26	26	25	24	24	23	23	22	22	21	21	20	20	19	19	19	18	18	10 8
66	31	30	29	29	28	27	26	26	25	25	24	23	23	22	22	21	21	20	20	19	19	19	18	18	18	10 6
65	30	30	29	28	27	27	26	25	25	24	24	23	22	22	21	21	21	20	20	19	19	18	18	18	17	10 3
64	30	29	28	28	27	26	26	25	24	24	23	23	22	22	21	21	20	20	19	19	18	18	18	17	17	10 1
63	30	29	28	27	27	26	25	25	24	23	23	22	22	21	21	20	20	19	19	19	18	18	17	17	17	9 13
62	29	28	28	27	26	25	25	24	24	23	22	22	21	21	20	20	20	19	19	18	18	18	17	17	16	9 11
61	29	28	27	26	26	25	24	24	23	23	22	22	21	21	20	20	19	19	18	18	18	17	17	17	16	9 8
60	28	27	27	26	25	25	24	23	23	22	22	21	21	20	20	19	19	19	18	18	17	17	17	16	16	9 6
59	28	27	26	26	25	24	24	23	22	22	21	21	20	20	19	19	19	18	18	17	17	17	16	16	16	9 4
58	27	26	26	25	24	24	23	23	22	22	21	21	20	20	19	19	18	18	18	17	17	16	16	16	15	9 2
57	27	26	25	25	24	23	23	22	22	21	21	20	20	19	19	18	18	18	17	17	16	16	16	15	15	9 0
56	26	26	25	24	24	23	22	22	21	21	20	20	19	19	18	18	18	17	17	17	16	16	16	15	15	8 11
55	26	25	24	24	23	23	22	21	21	20	20	19	19	19	18	18	17	17	17	16	16	16	15	15	15	8 9
54	25	25	24	23	23	22	22	21	21	20	20	19	19	18	18	17	17	17	16	16	16	15	15	15	14	8 7
53	25	24	24	23	22	22	21	21	20	20	19	19	18	18	18	17	17	16	16	16	15	15	15	14	14	8 5
52	24	24	23	23	22	21	21	20	20	19	19	18	18	18	17	17	16	16	16	15	15	15	14	14	14	8 3
51	24	23	23	22	22	21	20	20	19	19	19	18	18	17	17	16	16	16	15	15	15	14	14	14	14	8 0
50	23	23	22	22	21	21	20	20	19	19	18	18	17	17	17	16	16	15	15	15	14	14	14	14	13	7 12
49	23	22	22	21	21	20	20	19	19	18	18	17	17	17	16	16	15	15	15	14	14	14	14	13	13	7 10
48	23	22	21	21	20	20	19	19	18	18	17	17	17	16	16	15	15	15	14	14	14	14	13	13	13	7 8
47	22	21	21	20	20	19	19	18	18	17	17	17	16	16	16	15	15	15	14	14	14	13	13	13	12	7 6
46	22	21	20	20	19	19	18	18	18	17	17	16	16	16	15	15	15	14	14	14	13	13	13	12	12	7 3
45	21	21	20	19	19	18	18	18	17	17	16	16	16	15	15	15	14	14	14	13	13	13	12	12	12	7 1
44	21	20	20	19	19	18	18	17	17	16	16	16	15	15	15	14	14	14	13	13	13	12	12	12	12	6 13
43	20	20	19	19	18	18	17	17	16	16	16	15	15	15	14	14	14	13	13	13	12	12	12	12	11	6 11
42	20	19	19	18	18	17	17	16	16	16	15	15	15	14	14	14	13	13	13	12	12	12	12	11	11	6 9
41	19	19	18	18	17	17	16	16	16	15	15	15	14	14	14	13	13	13	12	12	12	12	11	11	11	6 6
40	19	18	18	17	17	16	16	16	15	15	15	14	14	14	13	13	13	12	12	12	12	11	11	11	11	6 4
39	18	18	17	17	16	16	16	15	15	15	14	14	13	13	13	13	12	12	12	12	11	11	11	11	10	6 2
38	18	17	17	16	16	16	15	15	14	14	14	13	13	13	13	12	12	12	11	11	11	11	11	10	10	6 0
37	17	17	16	16	16	15	15	14	14	14	13	13	13	13	12	12	12	11	11	11	11	10	10	10	10	5 12
36	17	16	16	16	15	15	14	14	14	13	13	13	12	12	12	12	11	11	11	11	10	10	10	10	10	5 9
35	16	16	16	15	15	14	14	14	13	13	13	12	12	12	12	11	11	11	11	10	10	10	10	9	9	5 7
34	16	16	15	15	14	14	14	13	13	13	12	12	12	11	11	11	11	10	10	10	10	10	9	9	9	5 5
33	15	15	15	14	14	14	13	13	13	12	12	12	11	11	11	11	10	10	10	10	10	9	9	9	9	5 3
32	15	15	14	14	13	13	13	13	12	12	12	11	11	11	11	10	10	10	10	9	9	9	9	9	9	5 1
31	15	14	14	13	13	13	12	12	12	12	11	11	11	10	10	10	10	10	9	9	9	9	9	8	8	4 12
30	14	14	13	13	13	12	12	12	11	11	11	11	10	10	10	10	9	9	9	9	9	8	8	8	8	4 10
Height (m)	1.46	1.48	1.50	1.52	1.54	1.56	1.58	1.60	1.62	1.64	1.66	1.68	1.70	1.72	1.74	1.76	1.78	1.80	1.82	1.84	1.86	1.88	1.90	1.92	1.94	

Score 0 (obese)
Score 0
Score 1
Score 2

Figure 10.1: Body mass index score. (Reproduced with kind permission of BAPEN. Available from: http://www.bapen.org.uk/pdfs/must/bmi-weight-loss-charts/must-table-up-to-100kg.pdf.)

ACTIVITY

Calculate:
- Phillip's BMI, if his weight is 92 kg and his height is 1.68 m;
- Mr Cooper's BMI, if his height is 1.9 m and his weight is 64 kg.
- Looking at Figure 10.1, what would their BMI scores be for the MUST screening?

Phillip's BMI is 33. The chart classifies this as 'obese', and his score for Step 1 of the MUST is 0. Mr Cooper's BMI is 18, giving his score for Step 1 of the MUST as 2.

Step 2

Todorovic et al. (2003) identify that unplanned weight loss over 3–6 months is 'a more acute risk factor for malnutrition than BMI' (p. 6). You can ask the person whether they have lost weight in the last 3–6 months and, if so, how much. You can also check their records. Then calculate how much weight has been lost using weight-loss tables (see MAG 2003) and identify the weight-loss score:

   <5% = 0

   5–10% = 1

   >10% = 2

Note: Take care when interpreting a patient's BMI or percentage weight loss in some circumstances, for example, fluid disturbances, pregnancy, lactation, critical illness and presence of plaster casts. Adjustments of body weight can be made for amputations (for details, see Todorovic et al. 2003).

Step 3

If the person has an acute illness and there has been no nutritional intake, or it is likely that there will be none for more than 5 days, they score 2.

Step 4: Overall risk of malnutrition

The scores from Steps 1, 2 and 3 are added to provide the overall risk of malnutrition:

Score 0 = low risk;   **Score 1 = medium risk;**   **Score 2 or more = high risk**.

Note: If neither BMI nor weight loss could be calculated, the score is assessed taking other criteria into account (see Box 10.5). The observations discussed earlier (in learning outcome 1) will contribute to this estimation.

Step 5: Management guidelines

Table 10.1 presents action required according to the MUST score. The MUST management guidelines advise that if the screening identifies a person is obese, this should be noted and that for those with underlying conditions, these are generally controlled before treating obesity.

Box 10.5 Other criteria

If height, weight or BMI cannot be obtained, the following criteria which relate to them can help form a clinical impression of an individual's overall nutritional risk. The factors listed below can either contribute to or influence the risk of malnutrition.

Note: Use of these criteria will not result in an actual score for nutritional risk but will help indicate whether or not a person is at increased risk of malnutrition.

BMI

- Clinical impression – thin, acceptable weight, overweight. Obvious wasting (very thin) and obesity (very overweight) can be noted.

Weight loss

- Clothes and/or jewellery have become loose fitting. History of decreased food intake, reduced appetite or dysphagia (swallowing problems) over 3–6 months and underlying disease or psychosocial/physical disabilities likely to cause weight loss.

Acute disease

- No nutritional intake or likelihood of no intake for more than 5 days.

Estimate a malnutrition risk score based on your evaluation.

Source: Todorovic, V., Russell, C., Stratton, R., et al. 2003. *The MUST Explanatory Booklet. Redditch:* BAPEN. Reproduced with kind permission of BAPEN.

Table 10.1: Management guidelines based on MUST score

0	1	2 or more
Low risk	**Medium risk**	**High risk**
Routine care	**Observe**	**Treat***
Repeat screening: • Hospital – weekly • Care Homes – monthly • Community – annually for special groups, for example, those >75 years	Document dietary intake for 3 days **If adequate** – little concern and repeat screening: • Hospital – weekly • Care Home – at least monthly • Community – at least every 2–3 months **If inadequate** – clinical concern – follow local policy, set goals, improve and increase overall nutritional intake, monitor and review care plan regularly	Refer to dietitian, nutritional support team or implement local policy Set goals, improve and increase overall nutritional intake Monitor and review care plan: • Hospital – weekly • Care Home – monthly • Community – monthly * Unless detrimental or no benefit is expected from nutritional support, for example, imminent death.

All risk categories:
- Treat underlying condition and provide help and advice on food choices, eating and drinking, when necessary.
- Record malnutrition risk category.
- Record need for special diets and follow local policy.

Source: Malnutrition Advisory Group (MAG). 2004. *Malnutrition Universal Screening Tool.* Available from: http://www.bapen.org.uk. Reproduced with kind permission of BAPEN.

Learning outcome 3: Carry out nutritional screening and recognise if people are at risk of malnutrition

Nutritional screening tools have been designed to enable nurses to make an accurate and quick assessment of patients/clients.

ACTIVITY

Using the information provided about Miss West in the scenario and MUST, work out her risk of malnutrition. Remember to use Figure 10.1 to calculate her BMI score. As discussed previously, you can use weight-loss tables to calculate her percentage weight loss – available from BAPEN (http://www.bapen.org.uk/pdfs/must/must-full.pdf).

Your assessment should have clearly identified Miss West as being at high risk. Compare your scoring with that given below:

- Step 1 – BMI. Figure 10.1 shows that Miss West's BMI is 20, so she scores 1.
- Step 2 – weight loss. Miss West has lost 5 kg since admission. The weight-loss table calculates that she has lost 5%–10% of her body weight, thus scoring 1. Miss West's loose dentures also suggest some weight loss.
- Step 3 – acute disease can affect risk of malnutrition. Miss West is eating small amounts, but this needs to be monitored, and she has had a stroke, so she scores 2 on this step.
- Step 4 – overall risk of malnutrition. Miss West scores 4, so she is at high risk; therefore, a plan of care needs to be initiated.
- Step 5 – management guidelines. According to MAG (2003), Miss West should be referred to the dietician. Goals to improve her nutritional intake must be set, and her weight should be monitored weekly. The next sections in this chapter detail likely interventions to improve her nutrition.

ACTIVITY

Practise using MUST with some other people:
- Find a willing colleague and assess their nutritional status by working through the screening tool; hopefully, their result falls into the low-risk category.
- Think back to a person you have been caring for recently and work through the tool. Are you surprised at the score you obtained?

You have now practised using the screening tool with several individuals. Once you have established that a person is at risk of malnutrition, you need to develop a plan of action. If the person is at high risk (like Miss West), she will need referral to a dietician for an in-depth nutritional assessment, and additional nutritional support may be needed. However, there are many ways in which nurses can help people to meet their nutritional needs, based on their individual assessment.

Children: practice points – nutritional assessment

Assessment on admission will include the method of feeding for infants (breast, formula or combination) and likes and dislikes for children. Weight is an important measurement; infants should be weighed without clothes or nappy on. Weights must be recorded with total accuracy; medication doses are calculated on weight. Infants' growth is recorded on standard percentile charts.

For further reading see:

Howe, R., Forbes, D. and Baker, C. 2010. Providing optimum nutrition and hydration. In: Glasper, A., Aylott, M. and Battrick, C. (eds.) *Developing Practical Skills for Nursing Children and Young People.* London: Hodder Arnold, 203–9.

Macqueen, S., Bruce, E.A. and Gibson, F. 2012. Assessment. In: *The Great Ormond Street Hospital Manual of Children's Nursing Practices.* Chichester: Wiley-Blackwell, 16–17.

Summary

- Observations can usefully contribute to assessment of nutritional status.
- Nutritional screening allows rapid identification of patients at risk of malnutrition, and MUST is recommended for adults in all settings.
- After screening is completed, an appropriate action plan must be developed and implemented.

ASSISTING PEOPLE WITH EATING AND DRINKING

The *Essence of Care* benchmark for best practice is that 'People receive the care and assistance they require with eating and drinking' (DH 2010, p. 20). Most people eat independently. However, physical or mental impairment, debilitating illness or generalised weakness may make people physically unable to eat and drink without assistance. NICE (2012a) guidelines specify that patients should be provided with an adequate quality and quantity of food and fluid in an environment conducive to eating, with encouragement and help given as needed. Some people will be able to eat independently, as long as they are well prepared and supported (e.g. by positioning, appropriate equipment). These aspects are discussed in detail in this section. Other patients will need complete assistance with eating, and then nurses must do everything possible to make this a pleasant experience and to ensure that their nutritional intake is adequate. When handling food in care settings, good food hygiene is essential and this is also discussed.

To gain the most from this section, you need the opportunity to assist someone with eating, so you might like to work through the section with a colleague, or another willing volunteer. You will also need a variety of foods: hot, cold, chewy and soft.

Learning outcome 1: Identify how food hygiene can be promoted

The NMC (2010a) requires that nurses must assist in creating an environment that is conducive to eating and drinking. One aspect of this is food hygiene. Chapter 3 focused on preventing cross-infection, and when involved with food, nurses must adhere to the principles discussed. This is important for people of all age groups but particularly people who are vulnerable to cross-infection, such as people who are immune-compromised and older people, such as Miss West and Mr Cooper. Hand hygiene is a key skill in relation to food hygiene.

ACTIVITY

When next in the practice setting, actively observe what precautions nurses and other staff take when handling food. Also, find out if there is a local policy on food hygiene and, if so, access this to read.

You should have observed staff performing hand hygiene before serving meals, wearing a clean apron (perhaps a different colour to that worn for other care activities), and keeping food covered and utensils clean, with one serving utensil per menu item.

Good food hygiene must be practised in all areas; this is a government requirement under the Food Safety Act (1990), the Food Safety (General food hygiene) Regulations (1995) and Food Hygiene (Eng) Regulations (2006). All aspects are covered in the legislation and regulations, including how food is stored and handled. Food poisoning outbreaks in healthcare settings are not uncommon; stringent steps to prevent occurrences are essential. See the Food Standards Agency for further information (http://www.food.gov.uk/).

Learning outcome 2: Assist people with eating and drinking

It is important to consider the environment in which patients are eating.

ACTIVITY

What do you think nurses can do to make the environment in a care setting conducive for eating in?

You might have considered removing any unpleasant odours and sights and making sure that the table is cleaned. Some care settings have a separate dining area, so if possible assist people to leave the bedside and sit at a dining table to eat. The table should be set properly. Ward cleaning and bed-making must never be carried out during mealtimes, and patients should not be disturbed by other healthcare professionals carrying out ward rounds. As discussed in an earlier section, 'protected mealtimes' are recommended so that people can eat undisturbed and with sufficient staff available to assist.

ACTIVITY

How might nurses help patients to eat and drink? Consider how Miss West can be helped to eat independently, and the correct technique for assisting her.

The following aspects are all important points to consider.

Oral hygiene

Ensure that your patient's mouth is clean and that dentures have been washed. Many people leave dentures in soak overnight, so prior to serving breakfast ensure that they have been cleaned, rinsed and reinserted.

Comfort and hygiene

Offer use of the toilet before eating and offer a handwash prior to meals.

Environment

Try to create a pleasant and calm environment at mealtimes. Remove obstructions from the patient's eating area (e.g. Zimmer frames, commodes, urine bottles). If appropriate, help Miss West to move to the area she wishes to eat in – patients should have the freedom to choose where, and with whom, they sit.

Positioning

Miss West should be helped into a safe and comfortable position for eating. Patients should always eat and drink in an upright position, as close to 90 degrees as possible and in the midline. This lessens the risk of food passing into the respiratory tract, causing choking. Sitting out of bed in a comfortable chair is preferable to sitting up in bed. Ideally, the person should sit upright with their feet on the ground, their body well supported and their head tipped slightly forward. There may be circumstances when it is not possible for people to be positioned upright, and then a side-lying position can be substituted. For useful information about how to support people who have had a stroke with eating and drinking, including positioning, see Stroke4Carers (http://www.stroke4carers.org/).

Clothing protection

Offer the patient a serviette or protection for their clothing if they would like it. Avoid using plastic bibs or paper towels because this will reduce self-esteem and dignity.

Giving food choices

Tell the patient what the choices of food are. Ideally, show the patient the food as the smell can induce appetite, and appearance also influences food choice. Help your patient choose their meal – ensure you understand what is on the menu, particularly when describing casseroles, for example, whether it is lamb or beef, and so on. Explain clearly anything they do not understand. Encourage them to eat food that is appropriate for their needs, such as soft diet, low in sugar and low in fat.

Individual dietary needs

Ensure that patients have expressed their individual dietary requirements to the staff. Do not presume about ethnic meal requirements.

Food presentation

Try to ensure that food is well presented, at the right consistency and temperature to encourage the patient. The food should be prepared on a tray that is clean with an appropriate drink, a napkin and cutlery. Try to set the meal out so that it tempts the appetite and is enticing to eat.

Condiments

Provide a range of condiments – individual sachets of salt, pepper, mustard, vinegar, mint sauce, horseradish – and allow the patient time to choose.

Portion size

Serve food in sensible portions to suit the patient's needs. For a person with a poor appetite (like Miss West), presentation and portion size might influence whether the food will be eaten. A large meal could be overwhelming, so a small portion is better. Second helpings can then be offered, if wished.

Correct consistency

Ensure specific advice from the multidisciplinary team (MDT) is followed regarding diet as appropriate; for example, puree diet/thickened fluids as recommended by the speech and language therapist (SLT). Many people with eating difficulties (like Miss West) need texture-modified food and fluids, for example, pureed/liquidised or thickened. Where food needs to be liquidised, each item should be liquidised separately to preserve distinctive flavours. The SLT may recommend thickened fluids to help to prevent the choking that can occur with liquid.

Positioning of food

Ensure that the food is within Miss West's reach and inform her that the food is in front of her. This is particularly important as she is partially sighted.

The clock method

As Miss West has a visual impairment, make her aware of the position of the food on the plate using the clock method to explain (see Figure 10.2). Ensure that the plate is not the same colour as the table, as this helps people who have a visual impairment to identify the plate.

Providing the correct equipment

Ensure the patient has access to specialist equipment, if required, for eating and drinking (e.g. adaptive cutlery, plate guard, wide-spouted beaker). You may need to liaise with the occupational therapist on this. Non-slip mats prevent the plate from moving around and are useful for people (like Miss West) who can use only one hand. Lipped plates are high-rimmed plates and bowls that prevent the food from being pushed off or over the side. This allows people with erratic hand and arm movements to manage with a degree of independence. Plate guards work in a similar way. Two handle cups and sports bottles may be used to assist a patient to drink.

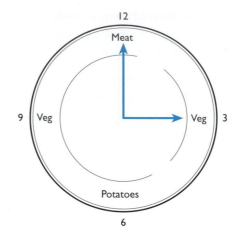

Figure 10.2: The clock method. This is a means of helping people with visual impairment to find their food. Place the food on the plate roughly at the quarter hours. Explain to the person that the meat is at the 12 o'clock position on the plate and that the vegetables are at quarter past and quarter to the hour, and the potatoes are at the half-past position. Ensure that you keep the foods separate.

Insulated beakers can be useful for people who are slow to eat or drink as this keeps the liquid hot for longer.

Knowing people's likes and dislikes
Find out about people's dietary likes and dislikes; if they are unable to communicate these, or to recall what meals or fluids they prefer, then talk to their family or look for other information, for example, accompanying notes from a care home, an Age UK Nutrition card, an Alzheimer's Society (2012) 'This is me' leaflet (discussed earlier).

Cultural and dietary needs
Know what may offend your patient; a vegetarian receiving meat or a Muslim who is fasting receiving food will indicate a lack of understanding of your patient. Be aware of allergies and foods which are restricted in the person's diet and avoid offering them these.

Assisting people to eat
You need to assess exactly how much help Miss West needs. This might range from cutting up food and giving verbal encouragement and reinforcement, to total assistance if she is unable to feed herself at all. The technique for this is discussed in detail next. With some people, it is a matter of giving time and not hurrying. Do open cartons, remove lids, cut up food and spread butter on bread, because for some people this is all they need to eat independently. Someone who has cerebral palsy might take up to three times as long to eat. They would also need some assistance to ensure that they can safely regulate the flow of liquid. You should observe for signs of fatigue and offer to help when necessary.

Assisting people who cannot eat unaided
When assisting with eating, nurses must demonstrate a caring attitude, appreciating that people who cannot eat independently may experience feelings of helplessness and loss of self-esteem and dignity. Try to encourage social contact at mealtimes.

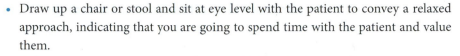

- Draw up a chair or stool and sit at eye level with the patient to convey a relaxed approach, indicating that you are going to spend time with the patient and value them.
- Ask the person in what order they would like the food and drink. They may communicate this through non-verbal rather than verbal communication, and it is important to observe reactions closely. Food should be cut into bite-sized proportions. If a soft diet is being given, adjust the portion according to the size of the mouth.
- Use normal cutlery/crockery appropriate to the food, as in a fork for the main course, a spoon for the pudding.
- Help your patient eat in a socially acceptable manner. If necessary, help the person to wipe away excess food from the mouth, clothes or hands after eating.
- Offer drinks that the patient may enjoy during and after mealtime. Establish when they want it (during or after) and what they would like.
- Allow patients to eat at their own pace. Allow time for the person to chew and swallow the food and drink, before offering the next mouthful. Do not hurry the person.
- Observe for any signs of choking, for example, coughing or poor colour, and stop if you suspect this. Be especially vigilant if you know that the person has a history of swallowing problems, which may accompany neurological impairment.
- Ensure specific safe swallowing strategies as recommended by the MDT are followed as appropriate (e.g. encourage clearing swallows, use of teaspoons).
- Offer second helpings, if possible.
- When the person indicates that they have finished, remove the equipment and offer further drink and the opportunity to clean their mouth and teeth. Particles of food left in the mouth may cause dental decay, or sores can develop around the gums.
- Complete documentation (discussed later), evaluate the care provided with the patient, and check whether they have any other care needs.

ACTIVITY

With a willing colleague, practise giving each other a variety of food and drink – cold, hot, soft and chewy. Then try some of the following positions for eating:
- sitting in a scrunched up position;
- sitting on your hands with a blindfold covering your eyes;
- lying fairly flat on your side and pretending that you cannot move.
  (As discussed above, this is not a recommended position for eating and should be used only for a person who, for medical reasons, has to lie flat.)

Now ask your colleague about your technique: What did they feel you did well? What do they feel you could do better in? Then reflect on the experience:
- How did this activity feel?
- What would have made the experience better?
- What have you learned from this activity?

Reporting/evaluating/documenting

After assisting a person with eating and drinking, you should complete any relevant documentation, such as filling in the food chart and/or fluid balance chart. Remember to report any unusual occurrence to the nurse in charge. Review the plan of care and evaluate. Is it still appropriate? Does it need to be changed?

Other approaches

For people who are in non-acute hospital settings, other approaches may be employed. For example, in some mental health units, nurses eat with clients so that they can encourage and prompt them to eat. For people with paranoia, it may dispel fear of poisoning if the nurse is eating the same meal from the same source. In some settings, facilities to make snacks, for example, sandwiches, are available, and for a person with paranoia it may be less frightening to make their own food from raw materials than to eat pre-cooked food, which they may fear has been poisoned. Alternatively, they may accept food brought in by their own family.

Alzheimer's Society (2009) identified that nurses and carers reported concerns related to eating and drinking for people with dementia. In response, Alzheimer's Society developed some 'Top tips'. Box 10.6 includes some of these additional points. Other members of the multidisciplinary team will be a valuable resource (see next section).

Box 10.6 Eating and drinking for people with dementia: Top tips for nurses

- Offer regular prompts and encouragement to eat and drink. Place the cutlery in the person's hands and guide their movements to start with. Similarly, place a cup in the person's hands and guide it to their mouth.
- If using cutlery is difficult, offer finger foods to maintain independence at mealtimes.
- Allow sufficient time for eating as coordination difficulties can make eating slow; prevent the person from feeling pressurised.
- Mealtimes should be relaxed and unhurried; a noisy busy ward can be distracting for people with dementia at mealtimes, resulting in food left uneaten.
- Be flexible as to when food is offered; a person with dementia may develop patterns of eating that fall outside of fixed mealtimes. Ensure there are nutritious snacks available throughout the day and night.
- A person with dementia may struggle to make a menu choice from words alone; pictures of food may help.

Source: Summarised from Alzheimer's Society. 2013. Top tips for nurses: Eating and drinking. Available from: http://www.alzheimers.org.uk/site/scripts/documents_info.php?documentID=1211&pageNumber=3

Summary

- Good food hygiene is essential in care settings.
- When assisting with oral intake of food and drink, the nurse should prepare the person, the environment and the food carefully, and try to promote mealtimes as enjoyable and relaxed events.
- The nurse's approach should ensure that the person feels valued and does not feel rushed.
- Good hygiene should be maintained, including handwashing and oral care for the patient.
- Monitoring and recording food intake is important, especially when a person has been assessed as at high risk of malnutrition.
- Reviewing the plan of care is vital after every meal.

ADDITIONAL NUTRITIONAL SUPPORT STRATEGIES

Nurses have a responsibility to assist and support patients in meeting nutritional needs. This section considers how the MDT can be involved to support nutrition and how the nutritional value of a person's oral intake can be improved.

LEARNING OUTCOMES

At the end of this section, you will be able to:

1 identify other healthcare professionals who may be involved in nutritional care and explain their roles;
2 discuss how the nutritional value of a person's oral intake can be enhanced.

Learning outcome 1: Identify other healthcare professionals who may be involved in nutritional care and explain their roles

ACTIVITY

List healthcare professionals who might be able to help people with meeting their nutritional needs; some have already been mentioned in this chapter. Think back to the scenarios and identify healthcare professionals who might support nutrition.

You might have identified that there are a wide range of professionals who contribute to nutritional care. Their roles are explained next.

Dieticians

Dieticians are experts in nutrition, capable of performing comprehensive assessments of people's nutritional status and needs. They are capable of offering general healthy eating advice, guidance for the use of dietary supplements and specific advice for dietary management in relation to medical disorders. Some dieticians specialise in certain age groups, for example, older people. As Miss West's screening identified she was at high risk of malnutrition, she must be referred to the dietician. If Mr Cooper is found to be high risk when nutritional screening is carried out, referral to a dietician would be appropriate for him too. A dietician can educate Phillip about eating healthily and his carers too, so that they can support Phillip in making healthy food choices, and also educate Phillip and his carers about the implications of not making dietary changes.

Speech and language therapists

SLTs are capable of assisting people of all ages and abilities with chewing and swallowing problems; these can occur in people with dementia or people like Miss West, who had dysphagia following a stroke. It could be worthwhile asking an SLT to reassess Miss West's swallowing as she is still having problems eating. SLTs will advise on whether it is possible for people to take food orally and, if so, whether special precautions are necessary, such as using thickening agents.

Physicians

Dietary supplements may need to be prescribed by a doctor. For some people, there may be an underlying medical problem affecting their nutrition, which needs to be treated. In some instances, weight gain, as experienced by Phillip, can be caused by an underlying medical condition, for example, an underactive thyroid gland (hypothyroidism).

Pharmacists

Pharmacists may advise other health professionals in medication-related issues and may be involved in aspects of enteral and parenteral nutrition.

Dentists

Dentists may assist people with dental or denture problems. If Miss West's dentures fitted properly, it could help considerably with her eating. The community mental health nurse should check whether referral to a dentist would be appropriate for Mr Cooper too.

Community support

Some health centres have health advisors for older people, and this could be relevant to Miss West when she is discharged and for providing additional support for Mr Cooper.

Psychologists

A referral to a psychologist would be appropriate if a person has an eating disorder but could also be relevant to Miss West in relation to her possible depression.

Physiotherapists

Physiotherapists can assist people with motor problems, for example, following a stroke, and help with their positioning. This is likely to be helpful for Miss West.

Occupational therapists

An occupational therapist may be able to identify suitable aids to assist with eating and drinking and positioning, thus promoting independence. Miss West would be likely to benefit from this help. They may also be able to suggest equipment to assist people with dementia. The occupational therapist could assist Phillip in improving his skills in food preparation.

Social workers

A social worker would be involved in arranging home care packages, including home-carers to serve meals and shop. This may well be essential to enable Miss West to maintain her nutrition after discharge from hospital. The community mental health nurse visiting Mr Cooper will be part of a multidisciplinary team that will include social workers. The different members of the team will appear on his Care Programme Approach plan, with their input identified. His plan may well need reviewing and additional support planned.

Another source of help for Phillip could be attending a 'Healthy lifestyles' course, aimed at his age group, covering a range of issues such as nutrition and exercise, which will be run by a group of professionals, including the dietician, occupational therapist and community nurse for learning disabilities.

Learning outcome 2: Discuss how the nutritional value of a person's oral intake can be enhanced

Sometimes, if appetite is poor or a person is very unwell, food intake may be insufficient to meet nutritional needs. Oral supplements may need to be prescribed by the dietician to assist in supplementing oral intake.

ACTIVITY

What supplements have you seen in practice to increase the nutritional value of a person's oral intake?

A wide range of dietary supplements are available, some of which are designed to be added to the normal diet (e.g. powdered glucose polymers such as Maxijul and Polycal), or to be taken as a drink between normal meals (e.g. Fresubin, Fortisip and Enlive). The purpose of these is to increase the nutritional value of oral intake; some provide just calories while others provide proteins, vitamins and minerals in addition. A dietician can advise which is most appropriate for an individual person following a comprehensive nutritional assessment. There are a wide variety of flavours available, some probably acceptable to both Miss West and Mr Cooper. These supplements can be a very good way of increasing nutritional intake. However, it should be remembered that these supplements should be prescribed, monitored and their usefulness assessed on a regular basis. These substances fall into the British National Formulary, Borderline substances category, and as such need close monitoring (Aneurin Bevan Health Board 2013).

Even with the use of supplements, it may not be possible for some people to fully meet their nutritional needs with oral intake. Other people may not be able to take food and drink orally at all owing to an inability to swallow. This may be for a temporary period (e.g. if a person is unconscious for a few days), but for some people it can be permanent. In these situations, you might have seen people fed by tube (enteral feeding) or through an intravenous infusion (parenteral feeding). The next sections explore these methods.

Summary
- A multidisciplinary approach to promoting nutrition will optimise specialist skills and knowledge, giving people the best chance of having their individual nutritional needs met in full.
- If nutritional needs cannot be met through a person's usual oral diet, other alternatives must be found. These could be oral supplements, enteral feeding or parenteral feeding. The dietician's input and advice are essential in these situations.

ENTERAL AND PARENTERAL FEEDING

The NMC (2010a) requires that nurses must ensure that people who cannot take food by mouth receive adequate fluid and nutrition and can safely administer fluids when they cannot be taken independently. Enteral feeding may be achieved via a **nasogastric tube** (a tube passed via the nose down the oesophagus and into the stomach), or via a **gastrostomy tube**, which is an opening in the abdominal wall through which a tube is passed to allow feeds to enter the stomach directly. Both these procedures are invasive, and consent must be gained from the patient – written consent for gastrostomy, which is a surgical procedure. A gastrostomy provides more secure nutritional provision than nasogastric tube feeding.

Enteral feeding may be used to supplement or completely replace oral intake. Enteral feeding might be done to maintain adequate nutrition for a person with severe neurological impairment as a result of cerebral palsy or stroke where swallowing is extremely difficult or hazardous, or for people whose nutritional needs exceed their oral intake, owing to a health problem. Both these methods have benefits and hazards associated with them. Medicines may be prescribed via the enteral tube route, and this procedure is also included in this section. In some circumstances, the enteral route cannot be used, and this section also identifies the role of parenteral nutrition and intravenous fluid administration. The use of enteral feeding has gained popularity over recent years, and many people now receive home parenteral and enteral nutrition. Wanten (2011) explains how home parenteral nutrition is the treatment of choice for patients with long-term intestinal failure. NICE (2006) provides detailed, evidence-based guidelines relating to enteral and parenteral feeding; these are recommended further reading. See also the NICE's (2012b) *Quality Standard for Nutritional Support in Adults*.

LEARNING OUTCOMES

By the end of this section, you will be able to:
1 discuss nasogastric tube insertion and the associated care;
2 explain the specific care needed following gastrostomy;
3 identify key principles for administering enteral feeds;
4 discuss the process of administering medicines by the enteral route;
5 identify the role of parenteral nutrition and intravenous fluid administration in maintaining patient nutrition.

Learning outcome 1: Discuss nasogastric tube insertion and the associated care

Note: This section focuses mainly on nasogastric tubes (NGTs) for feeding, but the insertion of NGTs for gastric drainage will also be discussed in a subsection.

It is essential that you follow your organisation's policy about who can pass an NGT for feeding and the preparation and competency assessment required.

Prior to NGT insertion, key issues to consider are:

- whether the need for the tube is clinically indicated, appropriate and documented;
- whether the use of an NGT is for drainage or feeding;
- how to ensure the position of the tube is checked after insertion;
- what the on going management of the tube will entail.

Inserting an NGT for feeding

The decision to pass an NGT for feeding must be made by two competent health professionals, to include the person's senior doctor, and the decision must be balanced carefully against the risks with the rationale documented in the person's notes (NPSA 2011a). NGTs must only be inserted by healthcare professionals who have been assessed as competent to do so and should not be inserted out of hours except in urgent situations as there should be radiology staff available to check tube placement, if required (NPSA 2011a).

ACTIVITY

Find out what NGTs are used in your care setting. You may also be able to look at these tubes in the skills laboratory. What are their key features?

NGTs used for feeding people vary according to care setting but should be fine-bore feeding tubes. A decision must be made whether or not to insert a tube within 24 hours of identifying the need and appropriateness of enteral feeding. Consent must be gained from the patient, and any potential contraindications to passing the NGT should be identified, such as:

- previous surgery/trauma;
- oesophageal varices, stricture or other upper gastrointestinal pathology;
- complex head and neck problems (e.g. tumour, altered anatomy);
- trauma from poisoning (e.g. oral consumption of bleach);
- poor level of consciousness.

Any of the above should be discussed with the clinical team as the doctor or gastroenterology team may be required to insert the NGT under radiological guidance.

Table 10.2 presents the procedure for passing a nasogastric feeding tube, with the rationale explained; be sure to follow local guidelines. Figure 10.3 shows how to measure the length of tube required, and Figure 10.4 illustrates some of the steps in NGT insertion. Checking of the NGT position is an essential element which is discussed in more detail in the next section.

Table 10.2: Insertion of a nasogastric feeding tube

Note: Ensure that you follow local guidelines for this procedure.

Wash hands and then prepare equipment:

Clinically clean tray/trolley, fine-bore nasogastric tube (NGT) with guide wire, sterile receiver, cotton buds and tissues, non-sterile gloves and apron, sterile water, 50 mL syringe, 20 mL syringe, hypoallergenic tape, adhesive patch from NGT packet, glass of water, pH paper/indicator strips

Action	Rationale
Prepare the patient. Arrange a signal by which the patient can communicate, if they want the nurse to stop the procedure (e.g. by raising their hand)	Reduces fear by giving the patient some control over the procedure
Assist the patient into an upright position in the bed or chair with head supported by pillows; or if unconscious, on their side, supported by pillows	Ensures patient comfort and allows for easy passage of the tube
The head should not be tilted backwards or forwards	Enables easy swallowing and ensures that the epiglottis is not obstructing the oesophagus
Ask the patient to blow their nose, if possible	Ensures nostrils are clear, aiding insertion
Clean the mucus/encrustations around the nostrils with cotton buds, moistened with warm water	Helps with ease of insertion and ensures patient comfort
Perform hand hygiene and put on non-sterile gloves and apron	Minimises the risk of cross-infection. Standard principles must be observed when dealing with body fluids
Estimate the length of the tube to be passed by selecting the appropriate distance mark on the tube by measuring the distance on the tube from the tip of the nose to the earlobe and then to the xiphisternum (see Figure 10.3)	Gives the estimated length of tube required to enable the tip of the tube to rest in the stomach
Assess if the patient has a gag/swallow reflex by consulting medical notes	Absence of a gag/swallow reflex highlights the increased risk of misplacement of the tube which may lead to aspiration
Lubricate the tube, as per manufacturer's instructions/local policy	Lubrication reduces friction between mucous membranes and tube during insertion
At all times during the procedure, talk to and reassure the patient	Instills confidence in the patient and allays fears
Insert the proximal end of the tube (with the guide wire introducer in position) into the clearest nostril, passing along the floor of the nasopharynx to the oropharynx (see Figure 10.4a). If any obstruction is felt, withdraw the tube and try again in a slightly different direction, or try the other nostril	Facilitates the passage of the tube into the oesophagus
As the tube passes down into the oropharynx, ask the patient to swallow. To assist the passage of the tube, ask the patient to take sips of water (if not contraindicated). If the patient is unconscious then stroking the throat can stimulate the swallow reflex	Swallowing closes the epiglottis and reduces the risk of inadvertent endotracheal placement, enabling the tube to pass into the oesophagus
Advance the tube through the oropharynx, down the oesophagus into the stomach until the estimate mark on the tube reaches the external nares	Sufficient length of tube has been passed for it to enter the stomach
If at any time the patient shows signs of distress, for example, coughing, gasping, cyanosis, remove the tube immediately	The tube may have entered the trachea, not the oesophagus

(Continued)

Table 10.2: (Continued)

Action	Rationale
Confirm the position of the tube by attaching the 50 mL syringe to the guide wire introducer (Figure 10.4b). Gently aspirate a small amount of fluid (0.5–1 mL) to test with pH indicator strips (Figure 10.4c). The pH should be 1–5.5. The NPSA (2011a) recommends that a second competent person checks any readings that fall within the pH range of 5–6, as it may be difficult to differentiate readings in this range.	A pH reading of 1–5.5, can reliably exclude pulmonary placement of the NGT (NPSA 2011a). *Note:* a pH of 1–5.5 does not necessarily confirm gastric placement of the NGT; there is a small possibility that the tube is in the oesophagus, which carries a higher risk of aspiration (NPSA 2011a). See text for further discussion.
If there is any doubt about the position of the tube, and if repeated attempts to obtain aspirate are unsuccessful, a chest x-ray will be required to verify the position of the tube (NPSA 2011a)	To ensure the tube is in the correct position prior to administering anything down it
Remove the guide wire only after the correct position of the tube has been confirmed	While present, it makes the tube more radio-opaque, enabling repositioning of the tube, if necessary
To remove the guide wire, attach a 20 mL syringe and inject 5 mL of fresh tap water down the tube (or as per manufacturers' instructions)	Injecting water activates the lubricant on the guide wire, enabling easy removal
Hold the tube end firmly at the tip of the nose and gently and carefully withdraw the guide wire, disposing of it appropriately	Ensures that the tube stays in position as the guide wire is removed
Secure the tube in place by taping around it and across the nose (a fixing device should be in the pack) (see Figure 10.4d)	Secures the tube easily and comfortably: less likely to cause nasal pressure ulcers
Using an indelible marker, mark the tube at the point where it leaves the nose	To have a visual reference point and allow easy detection of dislodgement of the tube
Document in the patient's records, including the method of testing position (NPSA 2011a)	To ensure that there is documented evidence of insertion and confirmation of position of the tube

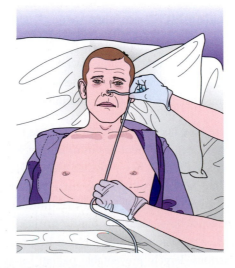

Figure 10.3: Measuring nasogastric tube length.

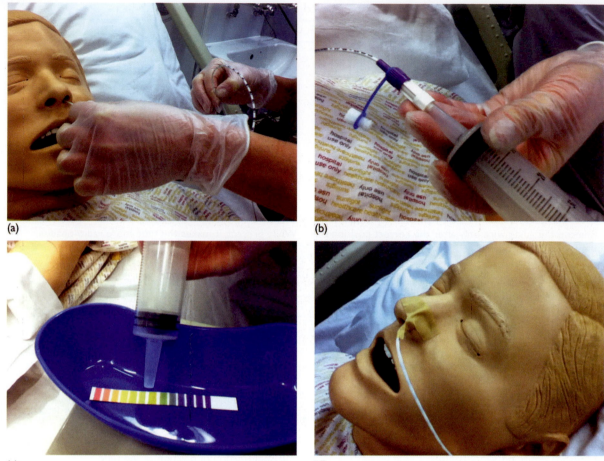

(a)   (b)

(c)   (d)

Figure 10.4: Insertion of a nasogastric tube. (a) Inserting the nasogastric tube; (b) Attaching the syringe for aspiration; (c) Testing aspirate with the pH strip; (d) Securing of the nasogastric tube to the nostril.

Checking NGT position

Potential position complications include:

- passage of the tube into the trachea;
- coiling of the tube into the posterior pharynx;
- trauma/haemorrhage or perforation of any of the surrounding tissues.

There have been a number of incidents where incorrect positioning of NGTs for feeding has led to patient deaths or illness (NPSA 2005, 2011a, 2012). Consequently the NPSA (2011a) has provided detailed guidelines, and also a 'decision tree', regarding how to confirm the correct position of nasogastric feeding tubes; do access these documents for further information and detailed guidance including the evidence base. Also, look out for further guidance being released. Feeding into a lung via a misplaced NGT is a Never Event in England (NPSA 2009). Never Events are 'serious, largely preventable patient safety incidents that should not occur if the available preventative measures have been implemented' (NPSA 2010, p. 2).

NGTs must not be flushed, nor any liquid or feed introduced through the tube following initial placement, until the tube tip is confirmed by pH testing or x-ray, to be in the stomach (NPSA 2011a, 2012).

If there are problems obtaining aspirate for pH testing, the NPSA (2011b) recommends trying each of the following techniques:

- if possible, turn the person, onto their left side;
- inject 10–20 mL air into the tube using a 50 mL syringe;
- wait for 15–30 minutes before aspirating again;
- advance or withdraw the tube by 10–20 cm;
- give mouth care to patients who are nil by mouth as this stimulates gastric secretion of acid.

If aspirate is obtained it can then be tested but otherwise, an x-ray must be performed to check the position of the NGT.

The NPSA (2011a) advises that further placement checks should be made daily (see BAPEN guidance at www.bapen.org.uk/res_drugs.html) before administering each feed and before giving medicines. It is also advisable to check the tube's position following vomiting, retching or coughing (as this could dislodge the tube) or if the tube appears to be displaced (e.g. tape undone, tube appears to have moved).

Documentation

It is the responsibility of the professional who inserted or reinserted the NGT to document:

- date and time inserted and by who;
- type, size and batch number of tube;
- length to which the tube was inserted (e.g. '60 cm at right nostril'); at the time of its initial placement, the tube must be marked with an indelible pen at the point it enters the nostril;
- patency of the tube and details of pH testing (NPSA 2011a):
  - whether aspirate was obtained;
  - what the aspirate pH was;
  - who checked the aspirate pH;
  - when it was confirmed to be safe to administer feed and/or medication (i.e. gastric pH between 1 and 5.5).
- any additional comments (difficulties in insertion, etc.)
- expected date for review or removal.

The NGT packaging may include a sticky label with space for these details, for insertion in the patient's notes.

After initial insertion, a record of subsequent tube position checks should be maintained, along with the tube length, and any tube-related issues, until it is removed (NPSA 2011a). The NPSA (2011a) provides examples of charts for documentation. If there is any indication that the tube length has changed, appropriate action should be taken to assess tube tip position prior to using the NGT (NPSA 2011a).

ACTIVITY

Take the opportunity to practise NGT insertion, if available. You may have the opportunity to practise on a manikin in the skills laboratory. When in practice, if a patient is to have a NGT inserted, ask if you can observe the procedure, with the patient's consent. Discuss with your mentor the reasons why the patient requires a NGT.

Management of NGTs and feed administration

The tape used to secure the tube should be checked daily to highlight any inflammation, irritation or signs of the beginnings of a nasal pressure ulcer. The tape should be changed if it is not secure or irritation has occurred. During feeding, the patient should be lying at a 45-degree angle (semi-upright position) at all times. The type of feed prescribed and administered should be as recommended by the dietician. Always ensure that the feed has not expired and is in a sealed, sterile bottle. The length of time the tube is *in situ* prior to removal or reinsertion must comply with manufacturer's guidelines. Box 10.7 provides guidelines for removal of NGTs.

NGT insertion for drainage

The NGTs routinely used for drainage are larger than feeding tubes and produced in various sizes. The clinical need will determine the size of tube that is appropriate, but the smallest (i.e. narrowest) tube appropriate for the patient's management should be used. Prior to inserting an NGT for drainage, first identify whether the tube is being inserted for free drainage, aspiration or intermittent drainage. For free drainage, you will require a bile bag for attachment. Also, identify the purpose of the NGT, for example, is the tube for conservative measures, that is, bowel

Box 10.7 Removal of nasogastric tube

Ensure that the tube is clinically no longer required or there is a clear documented reason for removal.
- Prepare equipment – waste bag, gloves, tissues, spigot (optional).
- Prepare the patient for the removal of the tube. Explain and discuss each step.
- Ensure that the patient is seated upright, if they are able to.
- Wash hands and put gloves on.
- Ensure the feed has been stopped and detached from the feeding line, and the tube contents have been drained.
- Remove tape.
- The patient may find taking a deep breath during the removal helpful.
- Remove the tube in one swift action and dispose of in the waste bag.
- Wipe the patient's nose.
- Remove gloves, wash hands and dispose of waste appropriately.
- Document removal in the patient's medical and nursing notes.

obstruction or following surgery to prevent aspiration or to relieve vomiting due to gut stasis/ileus?

As with any procedure, you should explain and obtain verbal consent from the patient. Check for potential contraindications: previous head, face or gut surgery or trauma including basal skull fracture, a depressed level of consciousness, oesophageal varices, cancer/tumour or complex head and neck problems, upper gastrointestinal pathology (i.e. strictures) or coagulation problems should all be taken into account. If contraindications are present, the patient may need a surgeon or gastroenterology team to insert the tube under radiological guidance.

The key principles of passing an NGT for drainage are the same as for insertion of NGTs for feeding (see Table 10.2, and Figures 10.3 and 10.4), including measuring the length of the tube to be passed, checking of tube position and record keeping. However, the tube should preferably have been stored in a fridge for at least half an hour before the procedure is to begin, to ensure a rigid tube that can be passed easily. Also, have a vomit bowl available or – if there is likely to be a large gastric residual volume – ensure that appropriate suction equipment is available. Prior to passing the tube, check the patient's nostrils are patent by asking them to sniff with one nostril closed and repeat with the other nostril. The tube can be passed by oral route if necessary. About 15–20 cm of the tube should be lubricated with a thin coat of lubricating jelly placed on a swab, thus reducing friction between the mucous membrane and the tube.

Learning outcome 2: Explain the specific care needed following gastrostomy

Gastrostomy is indicated in patients where dysphagia has been present or is likely to be present for 28 days or more. Usually, it is not required in patients who have oesophageal obstruction since other methods of treatment are available. Neurological causes of dysphagia (stroke and other chronic diseases such as motor neurone disease) are the most common reasons for referral.

There are two methods of placing gastrostomy; **percutaneous endoscopic gastrostomy** (PEG) is the most frequently used. **Percutaneous radiological gastrostomy** (PRG) is the other method, and it is particularly indicated for patients with a high risk of pulmonary aspiration following gastro-oesophageal reflux. Both techniques can be complicated by abdominal wall sepsis (including necrotising fasciitis) and peritonitis. The type of tube placed and the date of placement are recorded in the medical notes.

In general, gastrostomy is contraindicated where death is likely in a very short time, even if feeding were started. Survival of patients after gastrostomy is determined mainly by selection criteria. The majority of patients who receive gastrostomy feeding have had a stroke. The immediate procedure-related mortality for PEG is about 2%, and the 30-day mortality is about 30% (Sanders et al. 2000, 2002). Gastrostomy placement is not a trivial decision, and complications of gastrostomy can lead to death.

Necrotising fasciitis

Rare bacterial infection of the deeper layers of skin and subcutaneous tissue.

Peritonitis

Inflammation of the peritoneum, which lines the inside of the abdomen and covers the internal organs, usually due to bacterial infection.

ACTIVITY

If you are caring for anyone with a gastrostomy currently, discuss the rationale for its insertion with your mentor. Also, find out about local guidelines for immediate and long-term care following insertion.

Learning outcome 3: Identify key principles for administering enteral feeds

Most enteral feeds come prepared from the manufacturers. Feeds may be given continuously, overnight or by bolus at regular intervals, and dieticians will decide on the most appropriate feed regimen. The feeds are administered by an enteral feed pump, so that the rate can be set accurately. It is increasingly common for people to administer their own enteral feeds at home, with training and support from community nurses.

ACTIVITY

If a person is unable to take food or fluids orally and is being fed enterally, what special care do you think they would need?

You might have included the following:
- Observe fluid intake and output.
- Ensure that the prescribed feeding regimen is adhered to. Store feeds according to manufacturer's instructions.
- Observe for and report any untoward effects (like vomiting, diarrhoea or constipation).
- Maintain mouth care (see Chapter 8).
- Ensure that the position of the tube is maintained (e.g. that a nasogastric tube is secured adequately) (see earlier section regarding placement checks).
- Take measures to prevent cross-infection (e.g. hand hygiene, aseptic technique when connecting the feed administration set and the feeding tube).
- Ensure that the tube remains patent. Flush with water before and after feeds and medicine are administered.
- Be aware of, and try to minimise, the psychosocial effects of enteral feeding; for example, effects on body image (see Chapter 2) and the loss associated with inability to enjoy eating and join in with the associated social aspects.

Patients with enteral tubes may be administered medication via this route, which is discussed next.

Learning outcome 4: Discuss the process of administering medicines by the enteral route

Patients who are unable to take medicines orally and have a NGT or a gastrostomy tube may have some medication administered via a syringe attached to the tube's connector. Other routes (e.g. topical) should be used where possible. Community patients can learn how to self-administer their medicines via the enteral tube route.

ACTIVITY What difficulties or risks might there be of administering medicine via the enteral tube route? Consider how these might be addressed.

You could have thought of these points:

- The NGT route can be hazardous as the tube could dislodge from its position in the stomach. Therefore, the tube's position must be checked prior to medicine administration, as discussed earlier.
- Absorption and preparation of medicines for the enteral tube route may differ from oral medication. Therefore, nurses must work with the pharmacist who can advise about medicines being prescribed and dispensed in a suitable format, with consideration of any drug interactions. Some liquid preparations are suspensions of small granules and are therefore not suitable and others contain sorbitol, which is a laxative (BAPEN 2004a). The medicines will usually be prescribed as liquids or soluble tablets.

Note: Tablets must not be crushed nor capsules opened as this could alter the medicine's therapeutic action, making it ineffective and thus invalidating the product's licence (NMC 2010b).

- Enteral tubes can become blocked. Common causes are inadequate flushing and using the wrong formulation of medicine (BAPEN 2004b). BAPEN (2004a) suggests that if blockage occurs, aspiration to remove particles can be tried followed by a warm water flush, but excessive pressure must not be applied due to risk of tube fracture.
- A syringe is used to prepare the medicine, and there have been reports of enteral medicines being given intravenously by accident with serious consequences (NPSA 2007); this is identified as a Never Event (DH 2012). Therefore, syringes used to draw up and administer medication via enteral tubes must comply with NPSA (2007) guidance, to prevent administration errors. The syringes used must not be able to be connected to intravenous (IV) cannula, should be labelled and may be of a different colour to distinguish them from IV syringes (NPSA 2007).

ACTIVITY Look at an enteral medication syringe – in practice or in the skills laboratory. Note how it differs from other syringes.

All safety aspects of medicine administration (see Chapter 5) must be adhered to when administering medicines by enteral tube. You must maintain infection control precautions: wash hands and put on non-sterile gloves. You should prepare the correct dose as prescribed in an enteral syringe. The pharmacist's specific instructions regarding the medicine and its preparation and administration must be followed. Liquids should be shaken well and thick liquids diluted with an equal amount of water; soluble tablets should be dissolved in 10–15 mL of water (BAPEN 2004b).

ACTIVITY What specific aspects will be necessary when administering a medicine via the enteral tube route? *Consider:* the patient may have a feed in progress, or the tube may be closed off with a spigot.

Remember, as discussed previously, for NGTs, if there is no feed in progress, you must first check if the tube's position is in the stomach (see earlier discussion). BAPEN (2004b) advises the following method for administration:

- If the patient has a feed in progress, switch this off. Sometimes, there will need to be a break from feeding before and/or after medicine administration – the pharmacist will advise.
- Use a non-touch technique to attach the syringe to the tube's connector. Flush the tube with at least 30 mL of water (or as directed).
- Administer the medicine, flushing with 10 mL of water in between each medicine given.
- Give a final flush of at least 30 mL of water and restart the feed (unless a break is advised).

Learning outcome 5: Identify the role of parenteral nutrition and intravenous fluid administration in maintaining patient nutrition

In some instances, it may not be possible to provide nutrition enterally. Parenteral feeding (often referred to as total parenteral nutrition – TPN) may be used when a person is unable to use the gastrointestinal tract for nutrition, either temporarily or in the long term. An example would be a person who has had major surgery to the gastrointestinal tract. In parenteral nutrition, nutrients and micronutrients are administered directly into the circulation intravenously via a device in the vein and therefore only qualified nurses can administer TPN.

The aim of IV therapy is to maintain or restore normal fluid and electrolyte balance. IV therapy should always be approached with caution if fluid overload, fluid deficit, fluid shifts and unwanted alterations in electrolyte concentrations are to be avoided. It is essential that all fluid replacement regimes are tailored to the individual's requirements.

Assessment of the need for IV fluids and electrolytes should include:

- vital signs;
- fluid intake and output measurements;
- daily weight;
- skin turgor – this can be assessed by pinching a fold of skin. In a well-hydrated person, the skin will immediately fall back to its normal position when released. It is best practice to pinch the skin over the sternum or the inner thigh (Davies 2010);
- capillary refill time (see Chapter 11);
- central venous pressure (CVP) measurements (see Chapter 11);
- serum electrolyte levels;
- arterial blood gas results (See Chapter 11);
- urinary specific gravity.

See Metheny (2012) for further reading of fluid and electrolyte balance. IV fluid does not provide nutrition for patients, and it merely provides hydration which is crucial for life. Chapter 5 includes a section on IV fluid administration, focusing on the medicine administration aspects.

> ### 🛏 Children: practice points – nasogastric tube insertion
>
> Nasogastric tube insertion is invasive and traumatic for children and parents. As with adults, it is essential to check that the nasogastric tube position is correct prior to administering medication or feeds; see NPSA (2011a) and also the NPSA's (2011c) decision tree for NGT placement checks in children and infants.
>
> For details on nasogastric tube insertion and feeding see:
>
> Howe, R., Forbes, D. and Baker, C. 2010. Providing optimum nutrition and hydration. In: Glasper, A., Aylott, M. and Battrick, C. (eds.) *Developing Practical Skills for Nursing Children and Young People*. London: Hodder Arnold, 203–9.
>
> Macqueen, S., Bruce, E.A. and Gibson, F. 2012. Nutrition and feeding. In: *The Great Ormond Street Hospital Manual of Children's Nursing Practices*. Chichester: Wiley-Blackwell, 488–91.

Summary

- Enteral feeding is required when nutritional needs cannot be sufficiently met through the oral route.
- NGT insertion and gastrostomy insertion are invasive procedures with potential complications. There must be good rationale for their instigation.
- NGT insertion must be carried out carefully and skilfully, and practitioners must follow national guidance about confirming gastric tube position prior to any fluid administration, and checks thereafter. Insertion can be a difficult procedure for people to tolerate, and they need psychological support.
- Medicine administration via the enteral route must be carried out safely and in liaison with the pharmacist.
- If enteral feeding is not possible, parenteral feeding can provide nutrition. Intravenous fluid administration can maintain hydration and electrolyte balance.

CHAPTER SUMMARY

This chapter has highlighted throughout the importance of nutrition and hydration for the maintenance of health. Nurses are in an excellent position to screen people for nutritional risk as part of their assessment and should work collaboratively with other healthcare professionals to identify and implement strategies to meet the differing nutritional needs of individuals.

This chapter has included general principles that apply across a range of ages and settings. However, nutrition is a vast subject; you are encouraged to undertake further reading if you wish to enquire into specialist areas in more depth.

ACKNOWLEDGEMENT

The author acknowledges the contribution of Lesley Marsh to this chapter in the third edition of this book.

REFERENCES

Age Concern. 2006. *Hungry to Be Heard: The Scandal of Malnourished Older People in Hospital.* England: Age Concern.

Age UK. 2012. *Still Hungry to Be Heard: The Scandal of People in Later Life Becoming Malnourished in Hospital.* London: Age UK.

Alzheimer's Society. 2009. *Counting the Cost: Caring for People with Dementia on Acute Hospital Wards.* London: Alzheimer's Society.

Alzheimer's Society. 2012. 'This is me' leaflet. Available from: http://www.alzheimers.org.uk/site/scripts/documents_info.php?documentID = 1290 (Accessed on 30 January 2013).

Aneurin Bevan Health Board. 2013. *Guidelines for the Treatment of Under Nutrition in the Community Including Advice on Oral Nutritional Supplement (SIP Feed) Prescribing.* Available from: http://www.wales.nhs.uk/sites3/Documents/814/TreatmentOfMalnutrition%5BCommunity%5D-ABHBguidelinesJune2013.pdf (Accessed on 30 January 2012).

Baker, S. 2001. *Environmentally Friendly: Patients' Views of Conditions on Psychiatric Wards.* London: MIND.

Barker, H. 2008. *Nutrition and Dietics for Health Care,* 10th edn. London: Elsevier Health Sciences.

Barton, A., Fuller, R. and Dudley, N. 2004. Using subcutaneous fluids to rehydrate older people: Current practices and future challenges. *Quality Journal of Medicine* 97(11): 765–8.

British Association for Parenteral and Enteral Nutrition (BAPEN). 2004a. *Drug Administration via Enteral Feeding Tubes: A Guide for General Practitioners and Community Pharmacists.* BAPEN. Available from: http://www.baben.org.uk (Accessed on 2 February 2013).

British Association for Parenteral and Enteral Nutrition (BAPEN). 2004b. *Administering Drugs via Enteral Feeding Tubes: A Practical Guide.* BAPEN. Available from: http://www.bapen.org.uk (Accessed on 2 February 2013).

British Dieticians Association (BDA). 2012. *Nutrition and Hydration Digest: Improving Outcomes through Food and Beverage Services.* Available from: http://www.bda.uk.com/publications/NutritionHydrationDigest.pdf (Accessed on 30 January 2013).

Campbell, N. 2011. Dehydration why is it still a problem? *Nursing Times* 107(22): 12–15.

Care Quality Commission (CQC). 2013. *Time to Listen in NHS Hospitals: Dignity and Nutrition Inspection Programme 2012.* Available from: http://www.cqc.org.uk/sites/default/files/media/documents/time_to_listen_-_nhs_hospitals_main_report_tag.pdf (Accessed on 24 September 2013)

Carers UK. 2012. *Nutrition.* Available from: http://www.carersuk.org/help-and-advice/care-with-nutrition (Accessed on 8 February 2013).

Collins, A. 2002. Nursing with dignity. Part 1: Judaism. *Nursing Times* 98(9): 34–5.

Council of Europe Alliance (UK). 2007. Council of Europe Resolution food and nutritional care in hospitals: 10 key characteristics of good nutritional care in hospitals. Available from: http://www.hospitalcaterers.org (Accessed on 2 February 2013).

Davies, A. 2010. How to perform fluid assessments in patients with renal disease. *Journal of Renal Nursing* 2(2): 76–80.

Department of Health (DH). 2007. *Improving Nutritional Care: A Joint Action Plan from the Department of Health and Nutrition Summit Stakeholders.* Gateway Reference 8813. London: DH.

Department of Health (DH). 2008. *Weaning: Starting Solid Food.* London: DH.

Department of Health (DH). 2009. *Health Action Planning and Health Facilitation for People with Learning Disabilities: Good Practice Guidance.* London: DH.

Department of Health (DH). 2010. *Essence of Care 2010.* Gateway Reference 14641. London: DH.

Department of Health (DH). 2012. *The Never Events Policy Framework: An Update to the Never Events Policy.* Gateway Reference 17891. London: DH.

European Nutrition for Health Alliance (ENHA). 2005. *Malnutrition within an Ageing Population: A Call to Action.* London: ENHA.

European Nutritional Health Alliance (ENHA). 2008. Nutrition is a basic need: Let's treat it like one. Available from: http://www.european-nutrition.org/images/uploads/Nutrition_is_a_basic_need_flyer.pdf (Accessed on 24 September 2013).

European Nutritional Health Alliance. 2013. Oral nutritional supplements to tackle malnutrition – A summary of the evidence base. Available from: http://www.european-nutrition.org/index.php/news/news_post/oral_nutritional_supplements_to_tackle_malnutrition_a_summary_of_the_eviden (Accessed on 2 September 2013).

Ford, S. 2012. East Kent trust pioneers new nursing tool. *Nursing Times* 108: 34–5.

Ganasegeran, K., Al-Dubai, S.A.R., Qureshi, A.M., Al-abed A.A., Rizal A.M. and Aljunid, S.M. 2012. Social and psychological factors affecting eating habits among university students in a Malaysian medical school: A cross-sectional study. *Nutritional Journal* 11(14). Doi:10.1186/1475-2891-11-48.

Holland, K. and Hogg, C. 2010. *Cultural Awareness in Nursing and Healthcare: An Introductory Text,* 2nd edn. London: Hodder Arnold.

Hollis, S. 2011. Using red jugs to improve hydration. *Nursing Times* 107(28): 21.

Holmes, S. 2003. Undernutrition in hospital patients. *Nursing Standard* 17(19): 45–52.

Lean, M. and Wiseman, M. 2008. Malnutrition in hospitals. *British Medical Journal* 336: 290.

Malnutrition Advisory Group (MAG). 2003. *Malnutrition Universal Screening Tool.* Available from: http://www.bapen.org.uk/pdfs/must/must_full.pdf (Accessed on 24 September 2013).

McIntyre, L., Munir, F. and Walker, S. 2012. Intelligent fluid management bundle to support practitioners to ensure patient get adequate hydration. *Nursing Times* 108(28): 18–20.

Metheny, N.M. 2012. *Fluid and Electrolyte Balance: Nursing Considerations,* 5th edn. Philadelphia, PA: Lippincott.

National Institute for Health and Clinical Excellence (NICE). 2004. *Eating Disorders – Core Investigations in Treatment and Management of Anorexia Nervosa, Bulimia Nervosa and Related Eating Disorders.* Clinical Guidelines 9. London: NICE.

National Institute for Health and Clinical Excellence (NICE). 2006. *Nutrition Support in Adults Oral Nutrition Support, Enteral Tube Feeding and Parenteral Nutrition.* Clinical Guidelines 32. London: NICE.

National Institute for Health and Clinical Excellence (NICE). 2012a. *Patient Experience in Adult NHS Services: Improving the Experience of Care for People Using Adult NHS Services.* Clinical Guidelines 138. London: NHS.

National Institute for Health and Clinical Excellence (NICE). 2012b. *Quality Standard for Nutritional Support in Adults.* London: NICE.

National Patient Safety Agency (NPSA). 2005. Patient safety alert: Reducing the harm caused by misplaced nasogastric feeding tubes. Available from: http://www.nrls.npsa.nhs.uk/resources/?EntryId45=59794 (Accessed on 24 September 2013).

National Patient Safety Agency (NPSA) 2007. Promoting safer measurement and administration of liquid medicines via oral and other enteral routes. Available from: http://www.nrls.npsa.nhs.uk/resources/?entryid45 = 59808 (Accessed on 30 January 2013).

National Patient Safety Agency (NPSA). 2009. Misplaced naso or orogastric tube not detected prior to use. Available from: http://www.nrls.npsa.nhs.uk/resources/collections/never-events/core-list/misplaced-naso-or-orogastric-tube-not-detected-prior-to-use/ (Accessed on 2 February 2013).

National Patient Safety Agency (NPSA). 2010. *Never Events – Framework: Update for 2010–11.* Gateway Reference 13969. London: NPSA.

National Patient Safety Agency (NPSA). 2011a. Patient Safety Alert NPSA/2011/PSA002: Reducing the harm caused by misplaced nasogastric feeding tubes in adults, children and infants: supporting information. Available from: http://www.nrls.npsa.nhs.uk/resources/?entryid45=129640&q=0%c2%acnasogastric+tube%c2%ac (Accessed on 30 January 2013).

National Patient Safety Agency (NPSA). 2011b. Nasogastric feeding tubes – decision tree Adults. Available from: http://www.nrls.npsa.nhs.uk/resources/?entryid45=129640&q=0%c2%acnasogastric+tube%c2%ac (Accessed on 30 January 2013).

National Patient Safety Agency (NPSA). 2011c. Nasogastric feeding tubes – Decision tree children and infants. Available from: http://www.nrls.npsa.nhs.uk/resources/?entryid45=129640&q=0%c2%acnasogastric+tube%c2%ac (Accessed on 30 January 2013).

National Patient Safety Agency (NPSA). 2012. Rapid Response Report. NPSA/2012/RRR001. Harm from flushing of nasogastric tubes before confirmation of placement. Available from: http://www.nrls.npsa.nhs.uk/resources/?EntryId45=133441 (Accessed on 2 February 2013).

NHS Choices. 2013. Signs of dehydration. Available from: http://www.nhs.uk/Conditions/dehydration/Pages/Introduction.aspx (Accessed on 8 February 2013).

Nursing and Midwifery Council (NMC). 2010a. *Standards for Pre-Registration. Nursing Education.* London: NMC.

Nursing and Midwifery Council (NMC). 2010b. *Standards for Medicines Management.* Revised edition (First published 2007). London: NMC.

Royal College of Nursing (RCN). 2007. *Water for Health: Hydration Best Practice Toolkit for Hospitals and Healthcare.* London: RCN.

Royal College of Nursing (RCN). 2012. *Supporting and Assisting People.* Available from: http://www.rcn.org.uk/development/practice/cpd_online_learning/supporting_peoples_nutritional_needs/supporting_and_assisting_people (Accessed on 8 February 2013).

Royal College of Psychiatrists (RCP). 2012. *Eating Disorder Guidelines.* Available from: www.rcpsych.ac.uk (Accessed on 2 February 2013).

Sanders, D.S., Carter, M.J., D'Silva, J., et al. 2000. Survival analysis in percutaneous endoscopic gastrostomy: A worse outcome in patients with dementia. *American Journal of Gastroenterology* 95: 1472–5.

Sanders, D.S., Carter, M.J., D'Silva, J., et al. 2002. Percutaneous endoscopic gastrostomy: A prospective audit of the impact of guidelines in two district general hospitals in the United Kingdom. *American Journal of Gastroenterology* 97: 2239–45.

Scanlon, V.C. and Sanders, T. 2011. *Essentials of Anatomy and Physiology*. 6th Ed. Philadelphia: F.A. Davis Co.

Shepherd, A. 2011. Measuring and managing fluid balance. *Nursing Times* 107(27): 12–16.

Stroke Association. 2012. Taste changes after stroke, Factsheet 39. Available from: http://www. stroke.org.uk (Accessed on 2 February 2013).

Todorovic, V., Russell, C., Stratton, R., et al. 2003. *The MUST Explanatory Booklet*. Redditch: BAPEN.

Wanten, G. 2011. Managing adult patients who need home parenteral nutrition. *British Medical Journal* 34: d1447.

Welsh Assembly Government. 2011. *Fundamentals of Care. Guidance for Health and Social Care Staff: Improving the Quality of Fundamental Aspects of Health and Social Care for Adults*. Available from: http://wales.gov.uk/topics/health/publications/health/guidance/care/?lang=en (Accessed on 30 January 2012).

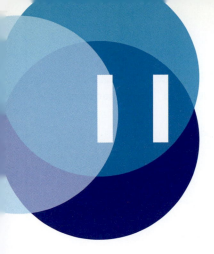

Assessing Physical Health and Responding to Sudden Deterioration

Sue Maddex and Tracey Valler-Jones

Recognising, monitoring, interpreting and responding to changes in a patient's health status are core nursing skills. In 1999, the Audit Commission highlighted that hospitals should review services for acutely ill patients, recommending the training of ward staff to deal with deterioration in patients' conditions and the availability of outreach services. In 2000, the Department of Health (DH) advised that outreach teams should be an integral part of critical care services. Outreach teams that respond to deteriorating patients have been established, but the National Patient Safety Agency (NPSA 2007) reported that the deterioration of some patients is still not recognised or acted upon. Patient Safety First (2008) made recommendations towards improving the identification and management of deteriorating patients, which included the introduction of a communication tool to convey information.

Since the publication of these reports, many hospitals have strived to address care deficits and improve the care of people who are acutely ill. In 2011, the NPSA identified some improvements but challenges remained. The National Confidential Enquiry into Patient Outcome and Death (NCEPOD 2012) provided a detailed review of the situation, finding a succession of system and performance failures that compromised patient safety and well-being throughout the care pathway. The report revealed that systems sometimes leave junior staff to assess patients and that early warning systems sometimes failed to track the deterioration of vital signs effectively and trigger an emergency response. Clearly, there are still improvements needed and hence the importance of this chapter's topic.

This chapter addresses the immediate care management of acutely ill adult patients, explaining a systematic approach to recognising and responding to sudden deterioration. The chapter explores skills relevant to managing airway obstruction, breathlessness, circulatory problems and unconsciousness. Some relevant skills are discussed in the other chapters of this book, so you can refer to them as appropriate. In particular, Chapter 4 includes monitoring vital signs (temperature, pulse, respiration, oxygen saturation and blood pressure) and neurological assessment.

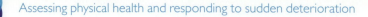

This chapter includes the following topics:

- Recognising and responding to people who are deteriorating: An overview
- Airway management problems and related skills
- Breathing problems and related skills
- Circulatory problems and related skills
- Unconsciousness and related skills

Recommended biology reading:

At the beginning of Chapter 4, there were questions related to biology underpinning measurement of vital signs. Check those again to ensure that you understand the principles. The following questions will help you to focus on the biology underpinning this chapter's skills. Use your recommended textbook to find out:

- What is homeostasis?
- Why is glucose important to the body?
- What is the role of insulin in the body?

Airways and breathing

- What is the structure of the airways?
- How is oxygen transported in the body?
- What role do cilia play?
- How does the respiratory system respond to respiratory tract infection?
- What other situations could cause respiratory distress or dysfunction?
- Where is bronchial smooth muscle located?
- What is the consequence of bronchoconstriction?
- Where are the pleural membranes? What functions do they have?
- What is surfactant? How does it prevent lung collapse?
- How can lung function be assessed? What factors could affect lung function?
- What do you understand by the term acid–base balance?

Circulation

- How is blood pressure controlled within the body, and how might this be affected if a patient is in shock?
- What are baroreceptors and where are they found in the body?
- What is the basic structure of the heart? Name its layers.
- What is the electroconduction system of the heart?
- What is the function of the sino-atrial node?

Nervous system

- What is the role of the medulla oblongata in the body?
- Describe the structure of the brain.

Parkinson's disease

There is a loss of dopamine-producing neurons within the brain, causing a chronic, progressive degenerative neurological disease with symptoms such as tremor, rigidity and bradykinesia (slow movement). It affects many activities, including eating, with a risk of food aspiration.

Asthma

A respiratory disorder characterised by recurrent episodes of difficulty in breathing, wheezing on expiration, coughing and viscous mucoid bronchial secretions.

PRACTICE SCENARIOS

The following scenarios illustrate situations where sudden deterioration in a person's condition might occur in different settings. These scenarios will be referred back to throughout the chapter.

Adult community setting: Airway obstruction

Mrs Mary Wyatt, aged 89 years, is resident in a care home. She has a history of **Parkinson's disease** and sometimes has difficulty eating. Today, during lunch, she started to choke on a piece of meat. Staff initially encouraged her to cough but Mary was becoming tired and her colour was deteriorating. The staff attempted first aid to clear her airway obstruction, which was not successful, and they called an emergency ambulance. The ambulance crew have used suction and given oxygen therapy. Mary has now arrived in the accident and emergency department, where a team of staff are awaiting.

Mental health setting: Breathing problem

Tina Lunn is 58 years old and has a long history of mental illness. She has been admitted to an acute mental health unit owing to her deteriorating mental state. She is known to have **asthma**, has becotide (a **corticosteroid**) and salbutamol (a **bronchodilator**) inhalers and takes oral prednisolone (also a corticosteroid). The staff are encouraging her to manage her asthma, to monitor her peak flow and take her inhalers as prescribed. However, one morning after a restless night, her respiration is so laboured that she has difficulty completing sentences and she is very distressed and wheezy. Her peak flow is about half her normal measurement. A salbutamol nebuliser (prescribed on an as-required basis) is administered via oxygen with some effect. The doctor diagnoses a chest infection and asks for a sputum specimen to be collected.

Adult hospital setting: Circulatory problem

Sira Patel, a 67-year-old woman, has just returned from the operating theatre after undergoing a left total hip replacement. She is known to have **atrial fibrillation** which is managed with 62.5 micrograms of **digoxin** daily. The anaesthetist has requested that she has cardiac monitoring for the first 24 hours postoperatively and has a 12-lead electrocardiogram (ECG) performed the following morning. She has **patient-controlled analgesia** in progress, and oxygen is being delivered at 5 litres per minute via a face mask. She also has an intravenous infusion in progress. While conducting her postoperative observations, you find that her blood pressure has decreased, her heart rate is increasing and is irregular and her respiratory rate is also rising. Furthermore, she has excessive drainage from her wound.

Learning disability setting: Impaired conscious level

Enid Campbell is a 52-year-old woman with a severe learning disability and very limited verbal communication. She lives in a group home. She is overweight and was diagnosed with **type 2 diabetes** six years ago. It was initially treated with oral hypoglycaemic

Corticosteroid
Inhaled corticosteroids such as becotide are used for asthma as a preventative treatment. They reduce bronchial mucosal inflammation, thus decreasing oedema and secretion of mucus in the airway. Corticosteroids can be administered via most other routes. Prednisolone is an oral preparation.

Bronchodilator
A drug that relaxes the smooth muscle of the bronchioles to improve ventilation to the lungs. Commonly used examples are salbutamol and terbutaline.

Atrial fibrillation
A common arrhythmia where, rather than the impulse originating from the sino-atrial node, there is disorganised electrical activity in the atria, leading to irregular and often fast ventricular contraction.

Digoxin
A cardiac glycoside that increases the force of myocardial contraction and reduces conductivity within the atrioventricular node. It is commonly used to control atrial fibrillation.

Patient-controlled analgesia
Patient-controlled analgesia (PCA) is a pain management system in which the patient controls the dose and frequency of analgesic delivered up to a predetermined limit. PCA usually refers to an intravenous system that delivers opioids when the patient presses a demand button. See Chapter 12 for more information.

agents; but owing to her blood glucose level being persistently high, she was started on insulin injections, which are administered by her carers. This morning the community nurse for learning disability is visiting to advise on her hydration and nutrition. When the nurse arrived, Enid's carers reported that a short while ago Enid slumped forward in her wheelchair and seemed unable to hold herself up. Some twitching of her right arm and leg was noticed. Enid has no history of epilepsy. When a staff member spoke to her, she was initially unable to respond but is now responsive though 'not her usual self'. The carers checked her blood glucose and it was within Enid's usual range. Her general practitioner (GP) has been contacted and is on her way to Enid's home.

EQUIPMENT REQUIRED FOR THIS CHAPTER

Find out what equipment is available within your skills laboratory or your practice area for monitoring acutely ill patients. In particular, look for:

- Resuscitation Council (UK) guideline posters (you can also look at these on www.resus.org.uk or via a smartphone application);
- cardiac monitoring equipment 3-lead or 5-lead;
- 12- or 15-lead ECG machine;
- National Early Warning Score (NEWS) chart or Early Warning Score (EWS) chart;
- peak flow meter;
- blood glucose monitoring equipment.

RECOGNISING AND RESPONDING TO PEOPLE WHO ARE DETERIORATING: AN OVERVIEW

The NCEPOD's (2012) report found that survival to discharge after in-hospital cardiac arrest was 14.6%. Cardiac arrest often follows a period of slow and progressive physiological derangement that may be poorly recognised and treated (Kause et al. 2004). This deterioration is usually preceded by changes in the physiological parameters that represent failing respiratory, cardiovascular and neurological systems. Recognition of these changes and dealing with them appropriately can help prevent further decline or even death. Traditionally, the identification of critically ill and deteriorating patients relied on clinical intuition (Bright et al. 2004). The introduction of physiological 'track-and-trigger' systems such as the EWS has enabled staff to identify patients at risk, assisting in the early detection of critical illness (Smith et al. 2006). As healthcare practitioners, you will be responsible for caring for people who become acutely ill, and so learning about the use of track-and-trigger assessment tools is essential.

Note: The assessment and management of patients who are critically ill is constantly under review so you must keep abreast of new documents and guidelines which may influence your practice.

Decisions about resuscitation

People who, due to their condition, will not benefit from resuscitation will have a 'Do not attempt resuscitation' order signed. Decisions must be made on the basis of an individual assessment of each patient and effective communication about this decision is essential.

Where no explicit decision has been made in advance, there should be an initial presumption in favour of resuscitation; see www.resus.org.uk for further guidance.

> ### LEARNING OUTCOMES
>
> By the end of this section, you will be able to:
>
> 1 explain the components of an Early Warning Score chart, understand how scores are calculated and decide the action to be taken;
> 2 discuss how to use a communication tool in the acute/emergency setting;
> 3 appreciate the key aspects of an ABCDE approach for assessing and managing an acutely unwell person;
> 4 locate and recognise emergency equipment.

Learning outcome 1: Explain the components of an Early Warning Score chart, understand how scores are calculated and decide the action to be taken

AVPU score

A = Alert
V = (responds to) Voice
P = (responds to) Pain
U = Unresponsive

The early warning score (EWS) is a tool for patient evaluation based on five physiological parameters: systolic blood pressure, pulse rate, respiratory rate, temperature and **AVPU score** (Oakey and Slade 2006; Royal College of Physicians [RCP] 2012). The EWS allocates points to measurements outside the 'normal' parameters, alerting staff to the patient's deteriorating condition. These tools are used in primary care, for ambulance service assessments and in hospital (Mann and Bowler 2008; RCP 2012). They can be used for any patient where there are concerns about their health, such as post operatively, following severe trauma or if the patient has a serious acute medical condition.

The use of physiological track-and-trigger systems is effective in reducing mortality and morbidity of acutely ill patients as well as preventing admissions to the intensive therapy unit (ITU) (Buist et al. 2002). If detected early enough, simple interventions such as fluid or oxygen administration can help prevent further deterioration. The National Institute for Health and Clinical Excellence (NICE 2007) recommended their use to monitor all adult patients in acute hospital settings. Odell et al. (2009) highlighted how intuition contributes to nurses' detection of deterioration but the EWS is sometimes used to validate this intuition. Odell (2010) acknowledged that the use of the EWS has helped early detection and management but she warned that their limitations need to be considered too. As with any tool in clinical practice, the value and constraints of the EWS should be appraised. Ensure that you refer to Trust guidelines and become familiar with Trust-validated tools, which you can use to validate your feelings or hunches, and report any concerns immediately.

A nationally recognised aggregate-weighted track-and-trigger system has been advocated (Prytherch et al. 2010) and the Royal College of Physicians (RCP 2012) has now presented the National Early Warning Score (NEWS) (see Figure 11.1). The RCP (2012) is encouraging the widespread use of the NEWS to generate a robust, evidence-based assessment system.

Chronic obstructive pulmonary disease

A chronic respiratory disease, which includes conditions such as emphysema, chronic bronchitis and chronic asthma. It causes debilitating breathlessness which affects day-to-day living.

Note: For patients with **chronic obstructive pulmonary disease** (COPD), their chronically altered pathophysiology may make the NEWS tool hypersensitive. Therefore, ask your practice mentor for guidance when assessing a patient with COPD.

Observation chart for the National Early Warning Score (NEWS)

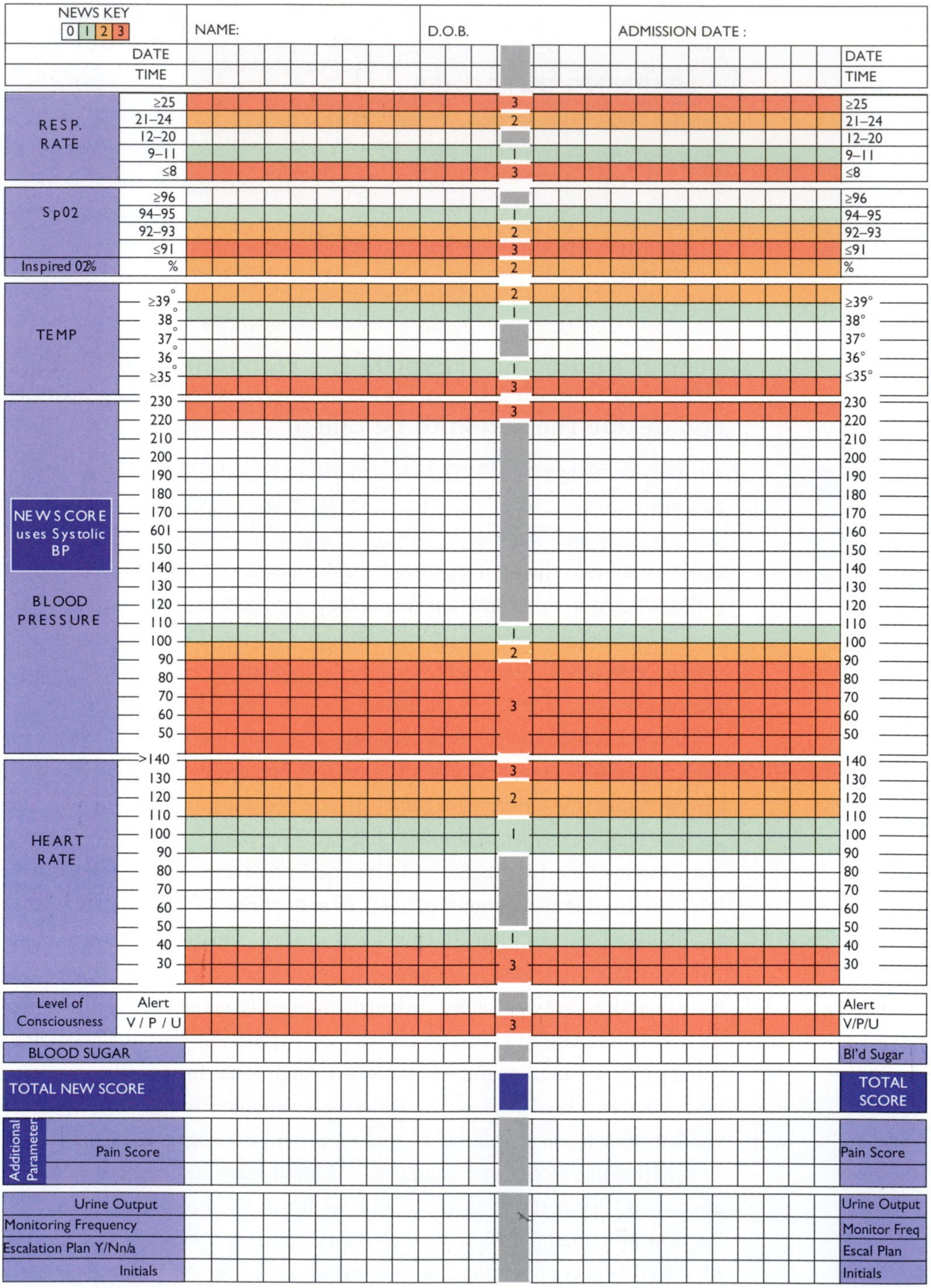

Figure 11.1: The National Early Warning Score (NEWS). (From Royal College of Physicians. 2012. *National Early Warning Scores: Standardising the Assessment of Acute Illness Sensitivity in the NHS*. Available from: http://www.rcplondon. ac.uk.)

ACTIVITY

Within your clinical area, find out what EWS/NEWS chart is used and what protocol should be followed to ensure that the appropriate staff are called to assist. Try calculating the EWS/NEWS for patients who are not acutely unwell and observe the differences that the scores reveal.

Although the level of response is dependent on the facilities available, the RCP (2012) outlines the following actions when using the NEWS:

- A **low score** (NEW score of 1–4) should prompt assessment by a competent registered nurse who should decide whether to change the frequency of clinical monitoring or initiate an escalation of clinical care.
- A **medium score** (NEW score of 5–6) should prompt an urgent review by a clinician competent in the assessment of acute illness – usually a ward-based doctor or acute team nurse, who should consider whether escalation of care to a team with critical care skills is required (i.e. critical care outreach team).
- A **high score** (NEW score of 7 or more) should prompt emergency assessment by a clinical team/critical care outreach team with critical care competencies and usually transfer of the patient to a higher dependency care area.

The RCP (2012) advises that the NEWS tool should NOT be used in children under the age of 16, or women who are pregnant, because the physiological response to acute illness can be modified in children and by pregnancy. However, modified tools may be used; see 'Practice points' boxes at the end of this section.

Using technology to assist you with assessment

Increasingly, healthcare practitioners can use technology to assist them in assessing acutely ill or deteriorating patients. Smartphone applications, web devices and hand-held bedside computers, for example, VitalPAC, are available to assist in recording and analysing data from patients' observations. Ensure that you discuss these applications and devices with your practice mentor and use only accredited and trusted sources for these purposes. Many systems that are designed specifically for practice areas work well with Trust protocols and analysers to enable informed decisions to be made about their patient care. These also incorporate EWS systems to prompt healthcare professionals that a patient may be at risk. There can however be no replacement for observing and assessing patients visually yourself and learning key skills that you will use throughout your career.

ACTIVITY

In your practice area, identify which electronic devices are used to record patient data and ensure that you receive adequate training to use them.

Learning outcome 2: Discuss how to use a communication tool in the acute/emergency setting

Gaining assistance early is essential to help manage a clinical emergency. Effective communication is the cornerstone of good healthcare but is difficult to master (Pritchard 2010); poor communication can have serious consequences and put lives at risk (Greenberg et al. 2007). The Royal College of Nursing (RCN) (2013) recommends the use of communication tools to help improve patient safety.

ACTIVITY

When you are next in clinical practice, find out what communication tools are being used as there are a variety of tools available.

Examples of communication tools are SBAR (Situation–Background–Assessment–Recommendation) and RSVP (Reason–Story–Vital Signs–Plan) (Featherstone et al. 2008). A communication tool helps practitioners to focus conversations in often difficult circumstances and helps to convey a message to summon help quickly. Box 11.1 displays the SBAR tool with examples of information for each component. National Health Service Trusts have developed their own versions of the tool, but the principles of using this communication tool remain.

ACTIVITY

Reread Mrs Patel's scenario, presented at the start of this chapter, and identify the vital signs you will assess to complete her NEWS (see Figure 11.1). Then consider how a nurse might use SBAR (Box 11.1) when contacting the doctor to seek help with Mrs Patel.

The **situation** you would want to report would be Mrs Patel's NEWS and her excessive wound drainage. In explaining the **background,** you would include her recent surgery and current treatment (e.g. oxygen, PCA, cardiac monitoring), her history of atrial fibrillation and its treatment. Your **assessment** might include your concern that she is developing shock due to excessive bleeding. Your **recommendation** is likely to be that you request an immediate visit.

Ensure that you understand these tools so that you can use them to assist you in everyday situations when asking for help. Using them regularly will help if you need to use them effectively in an emergency situation.

Box 11.1 The SBAR communication tool

Situation – explain the reason for calling your location, the patient you are calling about and their diagnosis, the issue of concern, for example, EWS/NEWS, pain, wound drainage, urine output

Background – supporting background information – further information: reason for admission and treatment, patient's mental status, skin (e.g. pale, clammy), oxygen therapy

Assessment – state what your assessment is, for example, 'I think the problem is …' or state that you do not know what the problem is but the patient is deteriorating

Recommendation – state your recommendation for intervention, treatment, for example, 'I would like you to see her now'. Clarify whether any further tests should be carried out or treatment changed

Source: Summarised from Patient Safety First. 2008. *The 'How to Guide' for Reducing Harm from Deterioration.* Available from: http://www.patientsafetyfirst.nhs.uk (Accessed on 1 February 2013).

Learning outcome 3: Appreciate the key aspects of an ABCDE approach to assessing and managing an acutely unwell person

When a patient is acutely ill or at risk of deterioration, it is vitally important that they have an initial assessment and are frequently reassessed to evaluate interventions used and to ensure there is no further deterioration. Immediate assessment involves the ABCDE approach:

- Airway (consider **cervical spine protection**)
- Breathing
- Circulation
- Disability (involves assessment of neurological status)
- Exposure (enables a full examination to be undertaken)

This order of assessment and interventions is used because airway obstructions kill faster than disordered breathing, which in turn kills faster than haemorrhage or cardiac dysfunction (Smith 2003). Thim et al. (2012) advocate the use of ABCDE approaches in any clinical emergency for immediate assessment and treatment. They add that high-quality ABCDE skills amongst all team members can save valuable time and improve team performance which should in turn influence patient outcomes. Remember that you can use the ABCDE system in any location: in the street, in the patient's home or within the hospital situation.

Each step will now be considered in more detail.

Airway: Does the patient have a patent airway? (with cervical spine protection)

A patent airway is essential to ensure that there is adequate oxygen circulating in the body. If airway compromise – or a potential for compromise – is present, you must protect and maintain it, otherwise hypoxic brain damage will occur. When a person becomes unconscious, there is a reduction in their muscle tone, so the tongue can fall back and occlude the airway. Blood, secretions and vomit may also be present. There are various airway adjuncts available which are discussed later. If someone needs help to maintain a patent airway, they must be constantly observed to ensure the airway does not become occluded.

Breathing: Is the patient breathing? If so, is it sufficient?

Once the airway is established and secured, you must evaluate breathing. You should perform a rapid assessment of respiratory rate and rhythm, any presence of hypo- or hyperventilation and oxygen saturation level. If breathing is compromised, then supplementary oxygen by nasal cannulae, non-rebreather oxygen mask, **bag–valve–mask (BVM)** ventilation or mechanical ventilation should be applied. Oxygen administration is considered later in this chapter.

Cervical spine protection

In the event of suspected trauma, the patient's cervical spine should be immobilised as per Trust trauma guidelines, usually through the use of a rigid cervical collar with head restraint.

Bag–valve–mask

A hand-held device used to provide ventilation to a patient who is not breathing or breathing inadequately.

Circulation: What do you note about the patient's circulation? Is it sufficient?

Circulatory assessment must be performed rapidly in someone who is acutely ill. If perfusion is compromised, then hypoxia and tissue damage occur quickly. Restoring adequate circulating blood volume is essential if oxygen deficit and inadequate tissue perfusion are present. Three of the most common indicators of inadequate circulatory function are hypotension (low blood pressure), tachycardia (increased heart rate) and oliguria (decreasing urinary output). The pulse rate may rise for various reasons and is not necessarily specific to hypovolaemia (low blood volume). Various pre-existing medical conditions or medications may cause tachycardia, for example, patients like Mrs Patel who has a cardiac conduction disturbance.

Note: A person with a high spinal cord injury may have bradycardia, not tachycardia. A simple assessment of the circulation can be obtained by the capillary refill time (see later in the chapter).

Blood pressure data can be misleading or unreliable. However, typical compensatory mechanisms used to maintain perfusion to the heart and brain may produce a normal systolic pressure. Loss of up to 15% of the circulating volume (700–750 mL for a 70 kg patient) may produce few obvious symptoms, while loss of up to 30% of the circulating volume (1.5 L) may result in mild tachycardia, tachypnoea and anxiety (Garrioch 2004). Hypotension, marked tachycardia (pulse rate 110–120 bpm) and confusion may not be evident until more than 30% of the blood volume has been lost, while loss of 40% of circulating volume (2 L) is immediately life threatening (Garrioch 2004; Harbrecht et al. 2004). If hypotension is present, it requires immediate attention and treatment. Systolic blood pressure measurement and analysis is now advocated in the NEWS scale (RCP 2012) to indicate altered pathophysiology.

Disability: Is the patient conscious? Assess the patient's level of consciousness

A rapid neurological evaluation is conducted once the airway is secured, breathing is adequate and circulatory issues have been dealt with. To do this, the patient's level of consciousness can be assessed using the Glasgow Coma Score (GCS), as described in Chapter 4. However, a more rapid assessment is the AVPU system (defined earlier in this chapter).

You should also check the pupil reaction to light (see Chapter 4). Pupillary responses can give important information about the causes of neurological problems. If the pupils are both dilated, it can denote stress, fear and so on, and it can also indicate that sympathetic stimulants have been taken (e.g. tricyclic antidepressants, adrenaline). If the pupils are both constricted, it can indicate that opiates have been taken (e.g. morphine) or that the brain stem has been affected (Smith 2003). However, a dilated pupil on one side can indicate a unilateral space-occupying lesion such as haematoma, tumour or abscess which is a medical emergency.

A decreased level of consciousness may indicate cerebral injury. However, factors such as hypoxia, hypovolaemia, alcohol and/or drugs may alter the level of consciousness. If the GCS is less than 8, the patient's level of consciousness is severely compromised and they will require help to maintain their airway. It is also important to undertake a blood glucose recording (discussed later in this chapter).

Exposure: Look for other information which will assist you

The patient should be completely undressed to be thoroughly examined. In acute deterioration or traumatic injury, it may be necessary to cut off the clothes. Patients' dignity must be protected and they should not be exposed unnecessarily. The patient must be warmed with blankets or other warming devices to prevent the rapid onset or continued state of hypothermia. When combined with rapid infusions of cold fluids or blood products and exposure, hypothermia can have potentially fatal results, if left untreated. Hypothermia is associated with arrhythmias, coagulopathies and higher mortality (Spahn et al. 2007). Generally, patients with a temperature of less than 32°C should be rapidly warmed.

Remember: Always reassess ABCDE regularly and do not progress from one stage to another until you have dealt with the first.

Learning outcome 4: Locate and recognise emergency equipment

In any new placement area, always familiarise yourself with emergency equipment and its location. Emergency equipment must be checked regularly to ensure it remains in working order, and it should be rechecked after each usage. The necessary equipment might be on a resuscitation (cardiac-arrest) trolley, or the items – including oxygen, suction and defibrillator (see Box 11.2) may be available in separate locations. The Resuscitation Council (UK) (2008) advises on appropriate equipment for cardiac-arrest trolleys (see: www.resus.org.uk).

ACTIVITY

When in your next or current practice placement, locate the emergency equipment and ask your mentor to check the equipment with you.

Box 11.2 The defibrillator

A defibrillator is a device that delivers electrical current across the myocardium. It is used when the heart is suffering from disorganised electrical activity (e.g. ventricular fibrillation). By passing electricity through the heart in a controlled dose, the heart can be stopped briefly with the intention of restoring organised spontaneous electrical activity (see www.resus.org.uk).

The shock is administered by charging up the defibrillator to the appropriate dosage, placing the paddles or attaching pads on the patient's chest and pressing the discharge button. People using defibrillators require specialist training as it is a complex and potentially dangerous skill. There are automatic external defibrillators (AEDs) available that can automatically recognise rhythms and give instructions for defibrillation. These are becoming increasingly available both inside and outside the hospital setting.

Children: practice points – assessment in emergencies

If faced with a sick child, remember to use an ABCDE approach and act upon your findings until skilled help arrives. If you are required to care for children, you must become familiar with the EWS chart in use and seek advice from your practice mentor to develop confidence in assessing children using an ABCDE approach. In practice areas which care for children, there will be a separate paediatric resuscitation trolley.

Useful resources:

The Department of Health's website (www.spottingthesickchild.com) aims to support healthcare professionals in the assessment of acutely ill children.

For resuscitation advice visit: www.resus.org.uk

See also:

Heath, J. 2010. Undertaking emergency life support. In: Glasper, A., et al. (eds.) *Developing Practical Skills for Nursing Children and Young People*. London: Hodder Arnold, 167–87.

Macqueen, S. Bruce, E.A. and Gibson, F. 2012. Resuscitation practices. In: *The Great Ormond Street Hospital Manual of Children's Nursing Practices*. Chichester: Wiley-Blackwell, 663–91.

Pregnancy and birth: practice points – assessment in emergencies

Pregnancy and birth is, for the majority of women, a normal, physiological process (King's Fund 2008). However, a few may develop unexpected complications when specialist care is required (DH 2007). Severely ill pregnant women may be cared for in a variety of non-midwifery settings; theatre; theatre recovery; general high-dependency unit (HDU); intensive care unit (ITU). Care must be managed by the multidisciplinary team, including specialist medical staff, anaesthetists, obstetricians and midwives. Detecting signs of deterioration in the physical health of pregnant women can be difficult due to an altered physiology, and healthcare professionals can fail to identify warning signs of impending collapse (Confidential Enquiry into Maternal and Child Health 2007). Modified early obstetric warning scoring (MEOWS) systems improve the detection of life-threatening illness.

In an emergency, the mother and unborn child must receive appropriate, timely and specialised care immediately. Remember to stay calm; the initial assessment and management priorities for caring for a deteriorating pregnant woman and her resuscitation follow an ABCDE approach, with some adaptations and additional skills needed. An unconscious woman in her third trimester of pregnancy should be positioned on her left side to avoid compression of the inferior vena cava. For further information, visit www.resus.org.uk

Summary

- Patients should be assessed, monitored and cared for using current guidelines to ensure that they receive the most appropriate and effective care.
- Patients' deterioration can be recognised through recording vital signs and calculating the EWS/NEWS. Scores must then be responded to by promptly and appropriately using Trust protocols.
- The use of a communication tool in an acute/emergency setting will assist you to convey your message and seek help urgently.
- An ABCDE approach to assessing an unwell person is systematic and ensures that priorities of care are addressed.
- It is essential to be familiar with emergency equipment and its location in any care setting you are working in – hospital or community.

AIRWAY MANAGEMENT PROBLEMS AND RELATED SKILLS

There are many reasons why a person's airway becomes compromised, including infection, smoke inhalation, allergic reaction, foreign body obstruction or trauma. Foreign bodies may cause either a mild or a severe airway obstruction and are usually inhaled bits of food such as meat, boiled sweets and fruit, or vomit or blood. Acute allergic reactions (e.g. a bee sting, peanuts, penicillin) can cause the trachea or throat to swell until it is closed.

Resuscitation Council (UK)

The Council's evidence-based guidelines are reviewed approximately every five years. Current guidance for 2010 is available from: Resuscitation Council (UK). 2010. *Resuscitation Guidelines.* http://www.resus.org.uk/ pages/guide.htm. (Accessed on 2 February 2013).

LEARNING OUTCOMES

By the end of this section, you will be able to:

1 recognise the signs of an obstructed airway and take appropriate action;
2 identify and discuss the different types of airway adjuncts available;
3 explain reasons for oxygen administration and discuss how it can be delivered safely through different delivery devices;
4 discuss how suction equipment is used in practice.

Learning outcome 1: Recognise the signs of an obstructed airway and take appropriate action

An airway can obstruct very suddenly, so it is important to be able to recognise the signs and act on them. Your mandatory basic life-support training will address this topic. Visit www.resus.org.uk for up-to-date guidelines on airway management.

ACTIVITY

Looking at Mary Wyatt's scenario, how do you think care home staff knew she had an obstructed airway? What first aid should the staff have attempted?

Mary was eating at the time and she may have clutched her neck. The **Resuscitation Council (UK)** (www.resus.org) suggests that in mild airway obstruction, the person is able to speak, breathe and cough, and can verbally respond to the question: 'Are you choking? However, with a severe obstruction (as in Mary's case), she would not have been able to speak but might have nodded and her attempts at coughing would have been silent.

To recognise an airway obstruction, the recommended method is 'look, listen and feel' (www.resus.org.uk)

- **Look to see whether there are any chest and abdominal movements**. In normal respiration, the chest and abdomen move outwards during inspiration and inwards during expiration, but with respiratory compromise there is a seesaw pattern of movements. Other signs include using accessory muscles: neck and shoulders and a pulling in of the trachea.
- **Look at the person's colour**. As hypoxia develops, the peripheries gain a grey/blue tinge (cyanosis). Peripheral cyanosis is seen in areas like hands and toes. Central cyanosis (blueness in the tongue and lips) is a late sign of airway obstruction.
- **Listen for sound of breathing**. Normal breathing should be quiet – noise indicates a partially obstructed airway. Respiratory sounds can indicate the position of the obstruction:
  - *Stridor*, a high-pitched sound usually heard during inspiration, is due to partial blockage of the trachea, larynx or pharynx.
  - *Gurgling* can indicate fluids such as blood or vomit in the upper airways.
  - *Snoring* indicates partial blockage of the pharynx usually by the tongue or soft palate.
  - *Expiratory wheeze* can be heard when the airways collapse during expiration (e.g. asthma).

  However, a silent chest is a bad sign too as it indicates a totally occluded airway.
- **Feel**. Feel for breath by placing your cheek or your hand close to the person's mouth. You should be able to feel the air movement at the mouth.

Airway opening

You will learn airway opening in your mandatory basic life-support sessions. The steps to follow are:

- If it is possible, turn the patient onto their back.
- To perform a **head tilt and chin lift**, rest one hand on the patient's forehead and place the fingertips of your other hand on to the chin, taking care not to press on the soft tissue under the chin which can obstruct the airway. Gently push down on the forehead and lift up the chin to open the airway.
- A **jaw thrust** should be used if there is suspected neck injury. To perform this manoeuvre, kneel (or stand if the patient is on a bed) near the top of the patient's head. Grasp the angles of the patient's lower jaw on both sides with your fingers and lift. This displaces the mandible (jawbone) forward while tilting the head backward.

Dealing with someone who has an airway obstruction can be alarming. If the person is showing signs of a mild airway obstruction, they should be encouraged to cough to help clear their airway. You should observe them closely in case they deteriorate and require intervention.

If (as in Mary Wyatt's case) the airway obstruction is severe or their cough becomes ineffective, you should help them to clear the airway. It is important to remain calm, talk to the person and explain what you are doing, as struggling to breathe can be a very frightening experience. The Resuscitation Council (UK) explains the steps to take.

- Give up to *five* sharp blows between the shoulder blades using the heel of your hand. Stand behind the person and lean them forward, so when the object is dislodged it will come out of the mouth and not back down the airway.
- If these back blows are unsuccessful, give up to *five* abdominal thrusts. Stand behind the person and put both arms around their upper abdomen. Make a fist with one hand and place it in-between the navel and the bottom end of the sternum. Clasp the other hand around it and pull sharply inwards and upwards. Ensure that you do not have your face directly behind their head as the movement can cause their head to move upwards, causing you an injury. If the person is seated or small you, may need to kneel behind them.
- If after five abdominal thrusts the object has still not been expelled, then give further back blows and abdominal thrusts until the object is expelled.
- If the person loses consciousness, support them to the floor and begin basic life support (see the guidelines at www.resus.org.uk).

What you are attempting to do is to increase the intrathoracic pressure, thus forcing the object out – similar to the effect of coughing. As there is risk of internal damage, the person should always be medically assessed following abdominal thrusts.

Learning outcome 2: Identify and discuss the different types of airway adjuncts available

ACTIVITY

In the skills laboratory, look at different types of airway adjuncts. Which ones have you seen in practice? How do you think they would be used?

You may have identified any of the airway adjuncts summarised in Table 11.1. The paramedics attending Mary Wyatt may have inserted one of these. You might have seen these devices used in emergency situations or in the operating theatre. There are other methods to help secure an airway, including endotracheal tubes and tracheostomies. All airway adjuncts must be inserted by trained professionals who will have learned how to select the correct size for each patient and how to insert them safely. In a situation where a patient's airway is compromised, it is imperative that their airway is cleared as rapidly as possible and that their oxygen levels are monitored and maintained.

ACTIVITY

When next in your clinical area, find out what airway adjuncts are available and their location. Ensure that you can recognise these pieces of equipment. Ask your mentor for guidance, if necessary.

Table 11.1: Airway adjuncts

Basic oropharyngeal airway

- A rigid curved plastic tube used for unconscious patients
- The patient's mouth is checked to ensure that nothing could be pushed back during insertion
- Inserted upside down until it has passed the teeth to prevent the tongue being pushed back, then rotated into the correct position
- If any signs of gagging or straining occur, it must be removed immediately

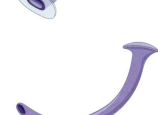

Nasopharyngeal airway (NPA)

- Can be used when an oropharyngeal airway cannot be tolerated, or inserted (e.g. patients with facial injuries or clenched jaws)
- Should not be used if there is a suspected basal skull fracture, owing to risk of penetrating the brain tissue (Ellis et al. 2006)
- The NPA, once in place, can be used for suctioning
- However, the vagus nerve can be stimulated, producing bradycardia (Pryor and Prasad 2008) – in which case, suctioning should stop and senior staff should be alerted

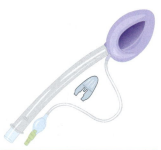

Laryngeal mask airway (LMA)

- Has an inflatable cuff that is inserted into the pharynx
- When the tube is inserted, the cuff is inflated, creating an airtight seal
- Bag-valve apparatus and oxygen can be attached to ventilate the patient, which has been shown to reduce risk of gastric regurgitation (Resuscitation Council (UK))

Learning outcome 3: Explain reasons for oxygen administration and discuss how it can be delivered safely through different delivery devices

Breathing normally involves a process of inspiration and expiration. This is achieved by expansion of the thoracic cavity and air being forced down into the lungs. The oxygen we need is gained from the atmospheric air around us. Oxygen constitutes approximately 21% of air at sea level. Oxygen therapy is the administration of extra oxygen to enable a higher inspiration of oxygen than that achieved during normal breathing. Oxygen delivery equipment is essential in emergency situations and is available in all acute settings and many community care environments too. Oxygen delivery relies on a patent airway.

Oxygen therapy may be a short-term measure in acute illness or long-term therapy for chronic respiratory disease. For all patients, other than in an emergency situation, oxygen concentration is prescribed (see www.bnf.org) to achieve specified target oxygen saturation measurements (O'Driscoll et al. 2008).

Hypercapnic respiratory failure

Inadequate gas exchange by the respiratory system where there is a build-up of carbon dioxide.

For most acutely ill adults, the target oxygen saturation is 94–98%, but it is 88–92% for people at risk of **hypercapnic respiratory failure** (O'Driscoll et al. 2008). Correct procedures and local guidelines must be followed for oxygen delivery. Refer to British Thoracic Society (BTS) guidelines (O'Driscoll et al. 2008) for use of oxygen therapy.

ACTIVITY

Reflect upon a situation when you have seen oxygen therapy being used within the hospital or community? When might people benefit from oxygen therapy?

Hypoxaemia

Low O_2 tension or partial pressure of O_2 (PaO_2) in the blood.

O'Driscoll et al. (2008) advise that oxygen is a treatment for **hypoxaemia**, not breathlessness, so oxygen saturation measurements should guide whether oxygen is administered. You may have thought of the following situations where hypoxaemia might occur:

- After a general anaesthetic;
- In emergency situations such as cardiac or respiratory arrest, shock and airway obstruction (as with Mary Wyatt);
- In chest injuries following trauma;
- In acute respiratory disease (e.g. asthma, as with Tina);
- In chronic respiratory conditions such as COPD and cystic fibrosis where long-term oxygen therapy may be needed, usually for a minimum of 15 hours per day;
- in heart disease where cardiac output is reduced (e.g. **myocardial infarction**)

Myocardial infarction

A myocardial infarction (MI) occurs when there is interrupted blood supply to the myocardium, causing death of tissue and usually resulting in severe chest pain which may radiate to the arms, jaw and/or neck, often accompanied by sweating. 'Heart attack' is the lay term for this condition.

Oxygen supplies

In hospital, oxygen is obtained either from a cylinder (black with white shoulders) or a wall-mounted piped oxygen supply. If cylinders are used, the dial showing the remaining oxygen must be inspected regularly as they can run out quite quickly. It is also imperative that equipment is checked to ensure good working order. Between 2004 and 2009, there were 103 incidents of risk or harm caused to patients by faulty oxygen equipment in acute hospitals, a further four from community hospitals and two from mental health or learning disability care settings (NPSA 2009). In the home, in England and Wales, oxygen is supplied by the NHS on a regional tendering service (review due 2014). These companies supply the equipment and oxygen as part of an integrated service. In Scotland and Northern Ireland, supply is by local contractors. Home oxygen is usually administered from an oxygen concentrator (McLauchlan 2002), which takes in room air and removes nitrogen through filtration but without depleting the surrounding air. The concentrator runs off electricity (an emergency cylinder is supplied in case of power failure), can deliver up to 4 L per minute and is supplied with up to 15 m of tubing, allowing movement around the home (Baird 2001).

Delivery devices

Different concentrations of oxygen are administered according to clinical need, which affects oxygen administration devices used. For example, for someone like Tina, who is very breathless and mouth breathing, a mask must be used. Nurses must record details of oxygen concentration, delivery device and commencement and termination of therapy, and sign for oxygen administration on the drug chart at each drug round (O'Driscoll et al. 2008).

ACTIVITY

Either in your clinical setting or in the skills laboratory, look at oxygen delivery devices. How do you think different concentrations are achieved?

Choice of oxygen delivery system

Oxygen therapy can be delivered at varying concentrations, often measured in percentages (e.g. 24%, 28%, 35%, and 40%); please refer to O'Driscoll et al. (2008) for further information. The oxygen flow is measured in litres per minute using a flow meter. Devices include simple oxygen masks, Venturi masks, nasal cannulae and non-rebreathing masks (Figure 11.2). These are disposable and packaged separately and each individual has their own equipment. Masks should be cleaned regularly, especially if the patient has a productive cough (please refer to manufacturer's guidelines for cleaning instructions and recommended length of use). If a mask or nasal cannulae is worn for an extended period of time, there is a risk of pressure ulcer development, particularly on the bridge of the nose or behind the ears. Therefore, masks and cannulae must be correctly applied, a good fit, and replaced regularly.

O'Driscoll et al. (2008) suggest the following options for stepping up or down oxygen doses:

- Venturi 24% mask at 2–4 L/min or nasal cannulae at 1 L/min
- Venturi 28% mask at 4–6 L/min or nasal cannulae at 2 L/min
- Venturi 35% mask at 8–10 L/min or nasal cannulae at 4–6 L/min
- Venturi 40% at 10–12 L/min or simple face mask at 5–6 L/min
- Venturi 60% at 12–15 L/min or simple face mask at 7–10 L/min
- Non-rebreather mask at 15 L/min

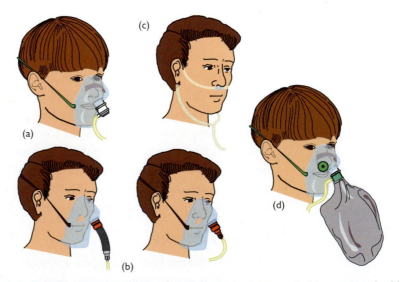

Figure 11.2: Devices for administering oxygen: (a) simple oxygen mask; (b) venturi masks; (c) nasal cannulae and (d) non-rebreathing mask.

Each device will now be considered in more detail.

Nasal cannulae

These may be used for people with acute or chronic respiratory disease where low levels of oxygen are required. They are well tolerated and administer oxygen directly into the nostrils. Oxygen flow is adjusted using the oxygen flow meter. Estimated oxygen concentration in the range of 25% to 40% can be obtained using a flow rate of 2–6 L per minute. However, flow rates of more than 4 L per minute are not recommended due to the drying effect on the nasal mucosa (Vines et al. 2000). Administration may not be very accurate, as actual oxygen intake varies according to how much the patients breathe through their mouth (Khaw et al. 2008). To make the nasal cannulae fit closely, move the ends of the tubes through the horizontal piece of tubing across the nose and also the adaptor on the tubing below the chin. With nasal cannulae, people can eat, drink and talk more easily than with masks. Procedures such as mouth care can be carried out without disrupting oxygen administration. Zevola and Maier (2001) found that nasal cannulae were considered comfortable and were better tolerated than masks; some patients find an oxygen mask claustrophobic. New materials like Softech® make the cannulae easy to tolerate and comfortable to wear (see www.teleflex.com).

Simple face mask

Sira Patel is currently receiving oxygen via a simple face mask. These are referred to as Hudson, medium concentration (MC) or semi-rigid. To make the mask fit comfortably, the strap should be adjusted to fit behind the ears. The oxygen amount delivered is adjusted by using the flow meter and the exact amount delivered depends on the rate and depth of breathing. If a patient is breathing rapidly, large amounts of room air are drawn into the mask. This mixes with the oxygen therefore diluting the concentration (Pruitt and Jacobs 2003). Oxygen can be delivered at 4–15 L per minute, achieving concentrations of 35–70% (see manufacturer's guidelines for the mask you are using). Rates of below 4 L per minute should not be used as, with a low flow rate, rebreathing of carbon dioxide may occur due to exhaled carbon dioxide accumulating within the mask (Khaw et al. 2008).

Venturi mask system

In the Venturi system, the oxygen concentration is not significantly affected by the rate and depth of breathing and a set concentration can thus be achieved (Higgins 2005).The mask is supplied with different coloured fittings, each clearly marked with an oxygen percentage and the required flow rate. The device ensures that oxygen flow is accurately diluted with entrained air. You can thus administer the exact percentage prescribed by fitting the correct device and setting the correct flow rate.

Non-rebreathing masks

These have a large reservoir for oxygen with valves to allow the patient to inhale only oxygen and prevent it from mixing with expired gases. Oxygen concentration is determined by the flow meter. They can provide up to 85% oxygen (Gwinnutt 2006), particularly for short periods of time, for example, postoperatively or in an emergency such as Mary's. The valve must be pressed to enable the chamber to fill with oxygen.

Other oxygen delivery devices

Some patients need additional technology in order to delivery oxygen to them and assist their breathing; Box 11.3 summarises the use of these devices.

Hazards of oxygen therapy

ACTIVITY

Can you think of any hazards that might arise from oxygen therapy?

The two main hazards are fire and the delivery of oxygen to people with chronic pulmonary disease who retain carbon dioxide.

Fire hazard

You have probably attended fire lectures or completed an e-learning activity where the fire triangle was outlined. Can you remember the three factors necessary for fire? Oxygen, fuel and heat are needed; if one of these is missing the fire cannot start or will quickly go out. Oxygen supports combustion and thus enhances the inflammable properties of other materials, such as cigarettes, grease and oil (Sheppard and Davis 2000). Administration of oxygen could therefore be a fire hazard.

Box 11.3 Other devices to deliver oxygen

Continuous positive airway pressure (CPAP)
Used in cases of respiratory failure. During the delivery of oxygen via a tight-fitting mask, the device delivers positive- and negative-pressure ventilation to the patient.

Non-invasive positive pressure ventilation (NIPPV)
This process involves positive-pressure ventilation being administered to the patient through a tight-fitting mask or similar device.

Ventilation
A mechanical ventilator machine can support or replace a patient's breathing when a patient is experiencing extreme respiratory dysfunction or is unable to breathe due to injury or disease. The patient is intubated via the nose or mouth and attached to the ventilator machine. Mechanical ventilation is used after a full respiratory assessment indicates no other alternatives to assist breathing. Patients receiving this type of treatment will be cared for in a high-dependency acute area or in theatre.

Source: Summarised from O'Driscoll, B.R., Howard, L.S. and Davison, A.G. 2008. BTS guideline for emergency oxygen use in adult patients. *Thorax* 43(Suppl vi): vi1–vi68; see http://www.brit-thoracic.org.uk/guidelines.aspx.

What precautions will be needed to reduce the risk of fire during oxygen therapy?

You could have thought of:

- No smoking signs.
- Devices that can spark.
- Educating patients and relatives about the risk of smoking during oxygen administration and alcohol-based sprays (e.g. in perfume).
- Knowledge of fire procedure and equipment.
- Oxygen cylinders in the home should be kept away from gas fires, naked flames and hot radiators (NHS 2011).

People who retain carbon dioxide

Normally, rising levels of CO_2 stimulate respiration. However, some patients with chronic respiratory disease may continuously have a high level of CO_2 in their blood and therefore their chemoreceptors are no longer stimulated by this. For these patients, who retain CO_2, the less important hypoxic drive predominates, which means that breathing is only stimulated by lack of oxygen. However, oxygen therapy can improve the patient's outcomes. Croxton and Bailey (2006) reported improved survival rates in people with COPD who have long-term oxygen therapy. People with chronic respiratory disease are, therefore, normally prescribed less than 28% oxygen (via a Venturi mask) or 2 L per minute (via nasal cannulae) initially and would only be prescribed a higher amount if indicated by arterial blood gas analysis or pulse oximetry (NICE 2010; O'Driscoll et al. 2008). These patients should carry an oxygen alert card (O'Driscoll et al. 2008).

ACTIVITY If an adult with hypoxia and confusion is not tolerating oxygen therapy, what could you do?

Patients who understand how and why they need oxygen are more likely to tolerate it (Baird 2001), so clear explanations are necessary. An adult who is confused due to hypoxia may resist oxygen therapy. Repositioning to improve ventilation, for example, sitting upright in a chair or in bed, will be helpful. Nasal cannulae rather than a mask may be better tolerated. Support and explanations from a familiar relative may help. If a person with learning disabilities needs oxygen therapy, you must consider level of understanding and learning ability. Demonstration of the mask/cannulae in position on a carer or nurse, and an explanation of the associated sensations and sounds, may be reassuring.

Humidification of oxygen devices

Oxygen can dry the mucous membranes of the upper airway (Pilkington 2004). The National Heart, Lung and Blood Institute (2012) reports how oxygen therapy can cause dryness, bloody nose, skin irritation and mucus dryness. Dryness of nostrils and mouth can be prevented through good oral hygiene, application of E45 cream and adequate fluid intake. However, never use petroleum jelly near oxygen, because of its potentially flammable nature (NHS 2011). Oxygen administered for more than a short period can be humidified, particularly if the concentration administered is high, for example, over 35%, or at a rate of 4 L per minute or above (O'Driscoll et al. 2008).

ACTIVITY

Locate humidification equipment either in the skills laboratory or in the clinical setting. What sort of water is to be used and why? What hazards might be associated with humidification equipment?

Humidification provides a moist environment and so may encourage bacterial growth. Therefore, sterile water must be used to minimise bacterial contamination (Porter-Jones 2002) and the water should be changed daily. The bottles themselves should be changed according to the manufacturer's instructions.

Learning Outcome 4: Discuss how suction equipment is used in practice

If the airways become obstructed by secretions, blood or vomit, a suction device should be used. However, suctioning is a traumatic procedure and can have serious side effects (Moore 2003). It is important to assess the patient during and after the suctioning and ensure that any oxygen device is repositioned immediately. Suctioning should only be done if clinically indicated.

ACTIVITY

While in the clinical setting, locate a suction device. With your mentor, check whether it is working efficiently. What attachments are there and which might you use for Mary?

Suctioning devices can be wall mounted or portable and have a negative-pressure regulator so that the degree of suction can be altered accordingly. The amount of suction required depends on the viscosity of the secretions but the recommended amount is between 100 and 150 mmHg (Cuthbertson and Kelly 2007; Pryor and Prasad 2008).

To collect the debris, it will also have a reservoir, which must be kept clean and clear. A correct sized tubing should be connected, with enough length to reach the patient and a suitable suction tip. This can be a wide bore rigid tip, for example, a Yankauer sucker, which can be used to clear vomit or secretions from the mouth, or a soft flexible catheter that can be used in conjunction with an airway adjunct. In Mary's case, a Yankauer sucker could have been used in an attempt to remove the piece of meat initially. When she had an airway inserted, *it would then* be possible to insert a flexible suction catheter down the airway as well as use the Yankauer sucker to clear her mouth. Box 11.4 outlines the procedure for suctioning the mouth.

Box 11.4 Procedure for suctioning the mouth

- Check whether the suctioning equipment is functioning correctly and collect other equipment.
- Maintain standard infection control precautions throughout.
- Explain the procedure to the patient/carer.
- Connect one end of the suction connecting tubing to the machine's suction post and the other end to a clean catheter or Yankauer sucker.
- Set the suction machine pressure at the recommended amount.
- Prepare the patient for the procedure and if possible ask their to open the mouth, so that you are able to see where the secretions are.
- Insert the catheter or sucker into the mouth but do not apply suction.
- Gently withdraw the catheter whilst applying suction.
- Clean the catheter by sucking through some clear water.
- Repeat the procedure, if necessary.
- Dispose of the used equipment appropriately.
- Rinse the suction tubing using sterile water.
- Make sure the patient is comfortable after suctioning.
- Assess the patient to ensure that they have suffered no adverse effects from the suctioning.
- Empty and clean the suction jar as necessary.

Source: Adapted from Moore, T. 2003. Suctioning techniques for the removal of respiratory secretions. *Nursing Standard* 18(9): 47–54.

All suctioning equipment should be checked daily along with emergency equipment, before and after use to ensure its proper working. A suction device should only be used by staff who have had appropriate training.

Children: practice points – airway management

Choking is common in small children and often characterised by respiratory distress associated with coughing, gagging and/or stridor. Choking in children mainly occurs during feeding or playing. For guidance on choking management, see: www.resus.org.uk

In areas where children are cared for, there will be airway adjuncts, oxygen and suction equipment in smaller sizes to cover all ages.

For airway management in children, see: Heath, J. 2010. Undertaking emergency life support. In: Glasper, A., et al. (eds.) *Developing Practical Skills for Nursing Children and Young People.* London: Hodder Arnold, 167–87.

For oxygen therapy in children, see: Aylott, M. 2010. Non-invasive respiratory therapy: Oxygen therapy. In: Glasper, A., et al. (eds.) *Developing Practical Skills for Nursing Children and Young People.* London: Hodder Arnold, 357.

Further reading:

Macqueen, S., Bruce, E.A. and Gibson, F. 2012. Resuscitation practices. In: *The Great Ormond Street Hospital Manual of Children's Nursing Practices.* Chichester: Wiley-Blackwell, 681–84.

Pregnancy and birth: practice points – choking

For women in the third trimester who are choking, if back blows are unsuccessful, **do not** use abdominal thrusts but alternate backslaps with chest thrusts: see www.resus.org.uk

Summary

- When dealing with a patient who is deteriorating, it is vital to seek help immediately.
- Recognising an airway obstruction and dealing with it quickly and effectively can prevent further deterioration.
- Oxygen therapy is given to treat hypoxaemia and must be given in accordance with recommended guidelines using an appropriate delivery device.
- Suction should be used to clear secretions from the airway but should only be performed by an appropriately trained person.

BREATHING PROBLEMS AND RELATED SKILLS

Breathing problems resulting in tachypnoea (rapid breathing) and dyspnoea (difficulty in breathing) can indicate significant disease. Jevon (2010) notes how the patient's respiratory rate is the first parameter to rise when a patient is deteriorating. The Royal College of Nursing (RCN 2011) identified that respiratory disease is the main cause of death in people with learning disabilities – who are at risk of respiratory tract infections caused by aspiration or reflux if they have swallowing difficulties. There are many causes of breathing problems; some originate from the respiratory system (e.g. asthma, COPD) but other causes are due to problems with other body systems, for example, heart or renal failure. Francis (2006) offers an overview of respiratory diseases in detail.

All people who experience acute breathing problems should be evaluated by a healthcare professional immediately. There are a range of skills needed to assess and care for people with breathing problems. Many are included elsewhere in this book and in other sections of this chapter; you will be referred to these during this section.

LEARNING OUTCOMES

By the end of this section, you will be able to:

1 discuss the signs and symptoms of a person who is having difficulty breathing;
2 outline assessment skills, investigations and interventions for a person with an acute breathing problem;
3 measure and record a person's peak expiratory flow rate;
4 describe how sputum expectoration can be encouraged and sputum specimens collected.

Learning outcome 1: Discuss the signs and symptoms of a person who is having difficulty breathing

ACTIVITY

What are the signs and symptoms of a person who is having difficulty breathing? Consider a person, like Tina, who is acutely breathless – her scenario will give some clues.

You may have considered the following:
- Tachypnoea (rapid breathing)
- Tachycardia (rapid pulse)
- Noisy breathing, for example, wheezing
- Cyanosis
- Delayed capillary refill time (see explanation later in this chapter)
- Inability to speak in full sentences
- Use of accessory muscles for breathing
- Coughing
- Pursed lips
- Flared nostrils
- The person may lean forward and hold their chest
- Confusion or disorientation due to hypoxia.

In extreme situations, patients who have breathing difficulties will continue to deteriorate despite healthcare interventions. Their respiratory muscles become fatigued as they fail to sustain respiratory function. Oxygen therapy or mechanical support (artificial ventilation) may not maintain adequate gaseous exchange. Healthcare professionals should explain the seriousness of the situation to the patient, family and significant others, giving time, support and understanding to make decisions about their own or their family member's care. Patients in this situation may deteriorate very quickly. If the respiratory system suddenly ceases, then apnoea occurs and respiratory arrest follows. Resuscitation Council (UK) guidelines should then be followed (see www.resus.org.uk). Immediate causes of respiratory failure will be considered and treated accordingly.

Learning outcome 2: Outline assessment skills, investigations and interventions for a person with an acute breathing problem

Patients with acute breathing difficulties (like Tina Lunn) can use up considerable energy in trying to breathe and are often extremely anxious and frightened. Prompt and careful assessment and management of their breathlessness must occur. You should adopt a calm and confident approach with your patients to alleviate their fears. Chapter 2 addresses communication in detail.

ACTIVITY

What assessment skills, investigations and interventions will be carried out to assess and care for a patient with an acute breathing problem? Tina Lunn's scenario will give some clues.

As discussed earlier, using an ABCDE framework will promote a systematic approach. You might have included the following:

Assessment:

- airway patency (see earlier section);
- observation of effort, depth, rhythm and sound of breathing (see Chapter 4);
- pulse oximetry for measuring oxygen saturation (see Chapter 4);
- blood pressure and pulse measurement (see Chapter 4);
- capillary refill assessment (discussed later in this chapter);
- peak flow measurement (discussed later in this section);
- observation of sputum and sputum specimen collection (discussed later in this section);
- cardiac monitoring and electrocardiogram recording (discussed later in this chapter);
- temperature measurement (see Chapter 4) – as infection may be an underlying cause.

Investigations:

- chest x-ray;
- blood tests – specifically arterial blood gas analysis (see Box 11.5).

Interventions:

- oxygen therapy (see previous section);
- administration of inhalers and nebulisers (see Chapter 5);
- positioning in an upright position to aid lung expansion.

Observation of respiration and other vital signs are relevant to all the patients in this chapter's scenarios. Mrs Patel may have a chest x-ray performed if there is concern about her developing a chest infection or heart failure. If Tina's condition does not improve with the nebulisers and oxygen prescribed, she might need to have a chest x-ray, which could require her being transferred to the emergency department at a different hospital. Mrs Patel, Mary and Tina may have blood gas analyses performed and all will require oxygen therapy. Tina will have her peak flow rate recorded, and a sputum specimen needs to be collected.

Learning outcome 3: Measure and record a person's peak expiratory flow rate

Peak expiratory flow rate (PEFR) is a simple test of lung function. The peak flow meter measures an individual's ability to exhale. PEFR is recorded in litres per minute and is the maximum flow rate achieved on forced expiration, when starting at full inspiration. As previously identified, Tina is an asthmatic, so the measurement of her PEFR is particularly helpful. Asthma leads to a reduction of lung volume and variable obstruction of the airways. Asthma UK (a charity which supports people with asthma – see www.asthma.org.uk) recommends that people with asthma monitor their PEFR regularly. It is particularly useful for people who have difficulty recognising that their asthma control is worsening (McGrath et al. 2001).

Box 11.5 Arterial blood gas analysis

- Arterial blood gas (ABG) is a blood test performed on arterial blood.
- Its purpose is to measure oxygen, carbon dioxide, bicarbonate levels and hydrogen concentration (pH) levels in the blood, thus providing an overview of the person's gaseous exchange, respiratory status and acid–base balance.
- The body's ability to regulate acid–base balance is crucial for survival; enzymes essential for biochemical reactions in cells function best within certain ranges of pH. Thus, impairment of body functions results from abnormal acid–base balance.
- The results of blood gas analysis affect treatment, such as administration of medicines to adjust acidosis, and oxygen therapy.

For normal values and a discussion of ABG interpretation, see Woodrow (2004).

Procedure

- Taking an arterial sample of blood is an advanced skill that is carried out by a healthcare professional who has received appropriate training – doctors or registered nurses with additional education.
- Radial and femoral arteries are commonly used.
- The test can be painful and patients undergoing the test need support.
- Local anaesthesia should be used, except in emergencies or if the patient is unconscious or anaesthetised (O'Driscoll et al. 2008).
- After the needle has been withdrawn, pressure needs to be applied for about 5 minutes to prevent bleeding.
- The sample is analysed, and its components can offer vital evidence of the patient's well-being.
- Patients requiring regular blood gas analysis (e.g. those who are being mechanically ventilated) will have an arterial line setup, from which blood can be extracted when necessary.

See Coggan (2008a, 2008b) for further reading.

Equipment for PEFR measurement

A peak flow meter is needed with a disposable mouthpiece for each person. Peak flow meters are increasingly used by people with asthma to monitor and manage their condition and are often available on prescription. There are several types of peak flow meters available; the same peak flow meter should be used for a particular individual to ensure consistency. Figure 11.3 shows a peak flow meter which adheres to EU standard EN 13826 (see www.peakflow.com for details). Electronic peak flow meters are now available, and many patients have their own devices. The standard meter measures up to 1000 L per minute but low reading or paediatric meters are also available. These should be used for children and for adults with widespread airways disease.

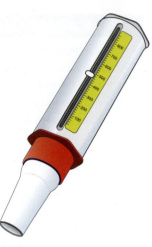

Figure 11.3: A peak flow meter which adheres to EU standard EN 13826.

ACTIVITY

Access a peak flow meter and mouthpiece. Using the instructions and diagrams in Box 11.6, measure your PEFR, noting the measurements. Now work through the instructions/questions below:
1 Try measuring your PEFR while in a semi-upright position. How does it compare with your original reading? What does that tell you about positioning of patients prior to PEFR measurements?
2 What would you do if a measurement seemed low?
3 How could PEFR measurements be recorded?
4 How often might PEFR be measured?

Points which you may have considered:
1. PEFR measurements can be misleading if the person is not positioned upright and does not use the correct technique.
2. If a low reading is obtained, you should confirm that the person's position and technique are correct. Then, as with any other observation, you would report the abnormal measurement to a qualified nurse. Little can usually be deduced from a single PEFR measurement as a series is required to produce a comprehensive picture. However, a single low reading may need a quick response. Obviously, the person's general condition and other observations will be considered too.
3. In hospital, PEFR is often recorded simply as a figure at the bottom of the observation chart. There are special charts available, particularly for ongoing monitoring; these are often used for home PEFR monitoring.
4. Generally, twice-daily (morning and early evening) measurements are sufficient, except during acute episodes. PEFR measurements are often necessary to monitor medication effects, for example, inhaled bronchodilators. The PEFR is then measured before and 30 minutes after medication (when the medication is having the maximum effect).

> **Box 11.6 Measuring peak expiratory flow rate**
>
> - With the mouthpiece attached, hold the peak flow meter with the scale uppermost and the pointer at zero.
> - Stand upright. Take a deep breath, close your lips around the peak flow meter and blow as hard as possible as if blowing birthday candles out.
> - Take note of the reading and return the pointer to zero.
> - Repeat the test twice more, taking note of each reading. Record the highest result.

What are normal PEFRs?

Patients are normally advised about their baseline PEFR, according to age, height and gender. European standards, EN 13826, for measuring PEFR (see www.peakflow.com), offer a chart for average PEFR readings. Generally, an adult should achieve 400–600 L per minute, but males achieve a higher figure than females, and greater height increases the measurement. Even in individuals without asthma, there are variations in the measurement, with the morning figure being lower, and the highest being achieved in early evening. This tendency is likely to be exaggerated in people with asthma, such as Tina. Currie et al. (2005) recommend that all patients who have asthma should be aware of their own personal PEFR values and judge their deterioration or improvement on their own values rather than relying on predicted values. They also recommend these values should form part of the person's asthma action plan, which is their personal plan for managing their asthma, developed with the health care team. Tina may have her own asthma action plan and her PEFR should be compared to her 'normal' value and her immediate care should be based upon this plan.

ACTIVITY

Why might teaching people who have asthma to measure their PEFR be useful in managing their condition?

You may have considered:

- To find out how well their asthma is controlled.
- Regular measurements may reveal a gradual (and possibly asymptomatic) deterioration, which requires action (e.g. change of medication) to prevent an acute episode. If the reading falls below 80% of an individual's best level, then preventive medicine (usually an inhaled steroid) should be increased (see www.asthma.org.uk).
- Without PEFR monitoring, people can be unaware of worsening symptoms; the measurement may fall by up to 50% before symptoms are noticed.
- Circumstances affecting measurements may be identified (e.g. contact with a cat), thus enabling asthma triggers to be recognised.
- The measurement may indicate the severity of the asthma at that particular time. The lower the measurement, the narrower the airways. A measurement of below 50% of the baseline requires immediate medical attention.
- To monitor how any change in medication is affecting respiratory status.

British Thoracic Society/Scottish Intercollegiate Guidelines Network (BTS/SIGN 2008) emphasised that teaching people to use inhalers and volumatic spacer devices and monitoring their PEFR should be only part of a comprehensive asthma management programme. This should also include instruction about avoiding asthma triggers, correct use of medication, identification of warning signs of worsening asthma and what action to take. On going education and monitoring can be achieved through attending asthma clinics where the correct technique in PEFR measurement can be checked. Manual dexterity and coordination for using peak flow meters need to be assessed. Asthma UK recommends that patients keep a peak flow diary to identify significant issues or readings. The diary also offers the patient and the healthcare team an overview of what is happening in their lungs, how effective are medications in treating breathlessness and average PEFR readings over a given period of time.

Despite the potential benefits of PEFR monitoring, long-term levels of use can be low, even in motivated patients who have taken part in an educational programme. However, the introduction of electronic devices in 2004 coupled with asthma health education programmes at asthma clinics are just some of the steps which have been taken to improve this situation. Booker (2007) identifies how in some instances, for example, non-acute settings, PEFR monitoring has been superseded by **spirometry.** The spirometer can be used for diagnosing and monitoring people with conditions such as COPD. This assessment can take place in the community setting to ensure that patients are fully aware of their diagnosis and can monitor the effects of their treatment. Spirometry offers further objective feedback to the patient with asthma.

> ### Spirometry
>
> A test which can help diagnose lung function and identify how respiratory disease affects the lungs. Uses a spirometer, a device consisting of a mouth piece attached to a machine which measures the amount of air exhaled.

Learning outcome 4: Describe how sputum expectoration can be encouraged and sputum specimens collected

Adults normally produce about 100 mL of mucus in the respiratory tract daily, but it goes unnoticed as it is usually swallowed (Law 2000). However, in some diseases, excess mucus is produced, and smoking also stimulates excessive mucus production. The mucus expectorated from the lungs is termed sputum. Sputum consists of lower respiratory tract secretions, nasopharyngeal and oropharyngeal material (including saliva), microorganisms and cells (Rubin 2002). Clearance of secretions is very important to maintain a clear airway and reduce the risk of infection (Rubin 2002). However, Law (2000) notes that patients may deny the existence of sputum due to social stigma or lack of awareness. Some, particularly women, feel embarrassed to expectorate, and they are more likely to swallow their sputum.

ACTIVITY How can you encourage Tina to expectorate her sputum?

First, Tina needs to understand why it is important to clear her secretions. She will be able to cough more easily if in a well-supported, upright position, and a sputum pot and tissues should be provided. If she is well hydrated, her sputum will

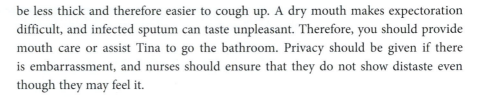

be less thick and therefore easier to cough up. A dry mouth makes expectoration difficult, and infected sputum can taste unpleasant. Therefore, you should provide mouth care or assist Tina to go the bathroom. Privacy should be given if there is embarrassment, and nurses should ensure that they do not show distaste even though they may feel it.

ACTIVITY

How would you describe normal sputum? What do you think might cause sputum to look abnormal?

Sputum (or mucus) is odourless, clear and thin, but people who have respiratory disease may expectorate sputum which is altered in colour and consistency. When assessing, it is important to identify what the individual's sputum is like normally. Signs of respiratory infection are sputum which is green, yellow or rust coloured, and it may be odorous. Purulent green sputum in patients with an acute exacerbation of their COPD is highly associated with infection (Stockley et al. 2000). A *pseudomonas* infection produces thick green sputum with a characteristic odour.

A stringy mucoid specimen often occurs with bronchial asthma (Law 2000). If blood is present, the sputum will be rust coloured or red and is termed **haemoptysis**. It may be a sign of infection but can also occur in cancer, heart failure and pulmonary embolus. Haemoptysis can be distressing to patients. It is important to check whether it has actually come from the lungs and has not been vomited (**haemetemesis**) or come from the nose (**epistaxis**). Haemoptysis is worsened by vigorous coughing, chest trauma, chest physiotherapy, anticoagulant therapy and activity. When assessing the amount being produced, it is best to ask in terms of teaspoons, tablespoons or cups. Patients may comment on the sputum's taste which may be unpleasant if infected or salty with cystic fibrosis.

When sputum is being produced, especially in suspected respiratory disease, a specimen is often required for laboratory examination. You will remember that Tina has been asked to produce a sputum specimen as she may have a chest infection. The goal of sputum collection is to gain a fresh, uncontaminated specimen of secretions from the tracheobronchial tree (Warrell et al. 2012). The lower respiratory tract can be colonised by many different bacteria; collection of a sputum specimen can help identify which bacteria are causing an infection.

ACTIVITY

Why might a sputum specimen need to be sent to the laboratory?

A sputum specimen may be sent for microbiological examination if infection, including tuberculosis (TB), is suspected. It may also be sent for cytology – examination for abnormal (e.g. cancerous) cells. Box 11.7 outlines the equipment needed, and the procedure and additional points are discussed below.

Box 11.7 Key points in collecting a sputum specimen

Equipment needed
- A sterile specimen container with a leak-proof lid or cap, and tissues.

Key points
- An early-morning specimen is best, as bacteria counts are probably highest then.
- Careful explanation is needed.
- The mouth should be rinsed with water and teeth brushed to prevent contamination with oral microbes.
- The sputum should be expectorated directly into the labelled container and the lid reapplied immediately.

When a sputum specimen is collected, it must come from the lower airways rather than being cleared from the throat or saliva. This needs to be explained carefully to the person, taking into account level of understanding. You can explain that the specimen must come from the 'windpipe'. Sputum is usually more viscous and purulent than saliva; if the specimen appears to be saliva, it should be discarded. A physiotherapist can assist people who have difficulty expectorating.

When sputum is being sent for testing for TB, the specimen should be at least 10 mL. Three early-morning specimens taken on different days are required as *Mycobacterium tuberculosis*, which causes TB, may only be present in small

Children: practice points – breathing problems

Asssessment and management of airway and breathing in infants and children is significantly different in comparison to adults due to the anatomical and physical features. Children are more likely to suffer a respiratory arrest, whereas adults are more likely to suffer a cardiac arrest.

For respiratory assessment, see:

Macqueen, S. Bruce, E.A. and Gibson, F. 2012. Resuscitation practices. In: *The Great Ormond Street Hospital Manual of Children's Nursing Practices*. Chichester: Wiley-Blackwell, 663–91.

Royal College of Nursing (RCN). 2011. Standards for assessing, measuring and monitoring vital signs in infants, children and young people. Available from: http://www.rcn.org.uk/__data/assets/pdf_file/0004/114484/003196.pdf

Resuscitation Council (UK): http://www.resus.org.uk/SiteIndx.htm

Gormley-Fleming, E. 2010. Assessment and vital signs: A comprehensive overview. In: Glasper et al. (eds.) *Developing Practical Skills for Nursing Children and Young People*. London: Hodder Arnold, 109–47.

For PEFR measurements in children, see:

Aylott, M. 2010. Non-invasive respiratory therapy: A) Aerosol therapy. In: Glasper, A., et al. (eds.) *Developing Practical Skills for Nursing Children and Young People*. London: Hodder Arnold, 342–56.

numbers, particularly in the disease's early stages (Wilson 2006). As *Mycobacterium tuberculosis* has very resistant cell walls, it is stained using a special dye which cannot be removed by acid or alcohol. This method is termed the 'acid-fast bacilli' or AFB test (Wilson 2006). Most bacteria grow within 24–48 hours, but the *Mycobacterium tuberculosis* can take up to 6 weeks to grow (Wilkins et al. 2010). Nevertheless, microscopic examination of the sputum can lead to an initial tentative diagnosis.

Summary

- There are many reasons for acute breathing problems. These situations can be frightening for patients and so a calm, confident approach is necessary.
- You need to understand the assessment skills, investigations and interventions that may be needed and develop your skills to assist people with acute breathing problems.
- Peak flow measurements are important indicators of respiratory function, particularly in people who have asthma. They must be recorded accurately and consistently, as they may influence treatment.
- Nursing measures can encourage expectoration of sputum, which can then be observed for colour, consistency, amount and odour.
- Careful explanations can help to ensure that an uncontaminated sputum specimen is obtained.

CIRCULATORY PROBLEMS AND RELATED SKILLS

An effective circulation requires a functioning cardiovascular system and adequate blood volume. A range of symptoms result when abnormalities occur, so effective assessment skills and interventions are needed to support patients with circulatory problems.

LEARNING OUTCOMES

By the end of this section, you will be able to:

1 identify common causes of acute circulatory problems and key aspects of assessment;
2 describe the term 'capillary refill time' and be able to perform the skill;
3 attach a patient to a cardiac monitor and recognise sinus rhythm;
4 outline how a 12-lead electrocardiograph is recorded.

Learning outcome 1: Identify common causes of acute circulatory problems and key aspects of assessment

There are many causes of circulatory problems.

ACTIVITY

Re read Mrs Patel's scenario. Can you identify possible causes of a circulatory problem?

You read that Mrs Patel has an abnormality in her heart's conduction system (atrial fibrillation) which will affect her circulation. You also know that she would have lost blood from her circulation during surgery and is continuing to do so. A reduction in blood volume (due to fluid loss or haemorrhage) can lead to hypovolaemia and then shock. Shock is a complex condition leading to a cascade of physiological reactions in the body. It is caused by an underlying medical condition or trauma; if left unmanaged, it can be life-threatening. Your biology book will give a detailed explanation – see Box 11.8 for a few key points.

In shock, a reduction in the person's cardiac output is seen and significant changes occur in their vital signs. It is important to find the cause of shock and treat it quickly. Mrs Patel has a lot of drainage from her wound and changes in her vital signs. Thus, her rate of intravenous fluid administration may be increased to boost the circulating fluid volume, or a blood transfusion may be commenced (see Chapter 5).

Anaphylactic shock is caused by an allergic reaction, when a person is exposed, and reacts, to a trigger suddenly, bringing about airway compromise, breathing difficulties and circulatory compromise, associated with urticaria (raised itchy rash). The incidence of allergic reaction within the United Kingdom (UK) is increasing and related fatalities have been reported. The Resuscitation Council (UK) (see www.resus.org.uk) produces guidelines to help practitioners recognise and respond to allergic reactions immediately. Please refer to these guidelines for up-to-date information on actions and drugs of choice in dealing with this emergency situation.

Box 11.8 Shock: key points

- Shock is a potentially recoverable but significant reduction in circulating blood volume that leads to inadequate tissue perfusion.
- The inability to deliver oxygen and nutrients to body tissues leads to metabolic and functional impairment and hypoxia.

Types of shock

- Hypovolaemia – low blood volume.
- Cardiogenic shock – due to the heart's inability to pump blood around the body efficiently (e.g. following myocardial infarction).
- Anaphylactic shock – a severe allergic reaction (see 'Preventing and managing anaphylaxis' in Chapter 5).
- Septic shock – occurs in severe infection. The systemic inflammatory response causes vasodilatation of peripheral blood vessels, increased capillary permeability and thus extravascular fluid loss.
- Neurogenic shock – rapid loss of vasomotor tone leads to vasodilation and a severe decrease in blood pressure.
- Emotional shock – emotion triggers parasympathetic stimulation leading to vasovagal syncope (unconsciousness). Spontaneous recovery usually occurs within a few minutes.

How will you know a person is in shock?

There are four stages of shock: initial, compensatory, progressive and refractory (Garretson and Malberti 2007; Hand 2001):

- *Initial* – the body shows signs of reduced cardiac output.
- *Compensatory* – the body attempts to restore homeostasis and improve tissue perfusion.
- *Progressive* – the body loses its ability to compensate, bringing about acidosis and electrolyte imbalance.
- *Refractory* – irreversible cell damage occurs and the body organs are affected.

As the patient's condition deteriorates, their vital signs change. The body first tries to compensate by moving fluids around from within cells to the circulation, attempting to maintain blood pressure in a normal range. However, there may be a slight rise in the heart rate. As the body loses the ability to compensate, respiratory rate rises as the body tries to apply as much oxygen as possible on to the remaining red blood cells and deliver them to the cells. As this body mechanism fails, the body becomes overwhelmed. Acidosis and electrolyte imbalance follow, with the patient becoming cold, clammy, less responsive and confused.

ACTIVITY

Look back at Mrs Patel's scenario. Are there any indications that she is developing shock?

Mrs Patel has lost a lot of blood, so she will start to show signs of shock at an early stage. You read that her heart rate and respiratory rates are rising and her blood pressure falling. However, the body has an ability to compensate for a short time during shock responses, and each patient responds to shock differently.

Assessment and management of a patient who is in shock should take a systematic ABCDE approach, as discussed earlier in this chapter. Measuring vital signs – including capillary refill time, conscious level, heart rate, blood pressure and urine output – are all important for patients in shock. Thus, the patient in shock may have a urinary catheter inserted, with hourly urine measurements being recorded (see Chapter 9 for urinary catheterisation procedure). To further assist with monitoring, critically ill patients might have a central venous pressure line inserted and/or an arterial line.

Central venous pressure line

A central venous catheter might be inserted, so that central venous pressure (CVP) monitoring can commence. Typically, a CVP line is inserted into the jugular, subclavian or brachial veins; the catheter tip will lie in the superior vena cava. CVP monitoring assists in assessment of a patient's circulating blood volume and identification of circulatory failure. CVP measurements must be interpreted in conjunction with other vital signs, with the trend assessed rather than a single measurement. If Mrs Patel continued to deteriorate, CVP monitoring might be commenced as it would help to carefully manage fluid replacement while preventing overloading her – a particular danger with her cardiac condition. CVP monitoring is an advanced skill; Cole (2007) explains this procedure in detail. Complications can include infection, embolus or haemorrhage.

ACTIVITY

When in the practice setting, identify whether any patients are having CVP measured. Ask your mentor to explain why the patient is having CVP monitoring and how this procedure is carried out. Discuss what the patient's CVP measurements indicate about their condition.

Arterial line

An arterial line is inserted into an artery. As with central lines, this is an invasive procedure with potential complications, many of which are similar to those associated with central lines. The main reason for inserting an arterial line is to allow continuous arterial blood pressure monitoring and arterial blood sampling, with arterial BP recordings having greater accuracy than the non-invasive methods for BP recording (Woodrow 2004) as arterial lines allow direct measurement via the cannula placed in the artery. A variety of arterial sites may be used to achieve this recording (e.g. radial, brachial and femoral). This is an advanced skill carried out by qualified practitioners; however, you may be required to assist with this procedure.

ACTIVITY

In your practice area, identify if any patients have arterial lines in situ. Ask your mentor to explain how these patients' lines are managed according to Trust policy.

Learning outcome 2: Describe the term 'capillary refill time' and be able to perform the skill

To assess capillary refill time, cutaneous pressure is exerted on the person's fingertip for 5 seconds and released. The finger should be held at heart level or just above and the pressure should be enough to cause blanching (Resuscitation Council (UK)). The test indicates capillary perfusion. Normally, capillary refill time is less than 2 seconds. Situations where capillary refill time is increased include shock, dehydration, aortic aneurysm, aortic occlusion, cardiac tamponade, hypothermia and **Raynaud's syndrome**.

> **Raynaud's syndrome**
>
> A condition causing constriction of small blood vessels, usually in the hands and feet.

ACTIVITY

Depress the tip of your finger for 5 seconds, then release the pressure and watch the blood return to your capillaries. Now, repeat the test and time the return of the blood to your finger. This should be less than 2 seconds, usually the time it takes you to say 'capillary refill'.

Learning outcome 3: Attach a patient to a cardiac monitor and recognise sinus rhythm

You read that Mrs Patel had a cardiac monitor attached postoperatively. The paramedics probably attached cardiac monitoring to Mary, which will be continued on her arrival at the hospital. Cardiac monitoring is carried out for many acutely ill patients and where heart rhythm is, or may become, abnormal (e.g. cardiac conditions, electrolyte imbalance, poisoning, hypothermia). You may have seen this equipment on placement or in the skills laboratory.

ACTIVITY

When you are next in your practice area, see what types of cardiac monitoring equipment are available. How many leads are attached to the patient and where?

You may have observed 3 or 5 leads being attached for monitoring. With 3-lead monitoring, there are three standard bipolar leads, I, II and III: red, yellow and green (or black) (see Figure 11.4). With 5-lead monitoring, lead colours can vary so check the equipment coding and seek your mentor's guidance. The monitor leads are connected to adhesive electrode pads placed on the patient's chest. The cardiac monitor detects voltage differences within the body surface and amplifies and displays these as a signal (Jones 2005). The device can offer useful information to healthcare professionals, such as indicating myocardial ischaemia and cardiac arrhythmias.

Box 11.9 outlines key points for cardiac monitoring. The ECG produces a graphic recording of the heart's electrical impulses producing a **PQRST complex** (Jowett and Thompson 2007). Figure 11.5 shows the PQRST complex and briefly

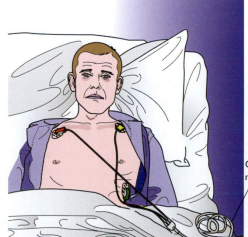

Connected to monitor

Figure 11.4: Placement of cardiac monitoring leads for 3- or 5-lead monitoring.

Box 11.9 Cardiac monitoring: key points

- First establish the patient's identity and rationale for cardiac monitoring.
- Inform the patient about the procedure and gain their cooperation and verbal consent.
- Check that the patient does not have a cardiac pacemaker *in situ*. If they do, seek advice before connecting any monitoring equipment, as some devices can interfere with cardiac pacemakers.
- Assemble all equipment: cardiac monitor and ECG leads, skin-pad electrodes, alcohol wipe and razor.
- Ensure that the patient's skin is clean and free from grease as the electrodes will not adhere to the chest fully otherwise. With consent, shave or trim any chest hair to ensure that the electrodes will stick.
- Place electrodes on the chest (see Figure 11.4).
- Turn on the monitor and adjust the setting to lead I, II or III as directed. Lead II is usually chosen as it shows a positive R wave and a clear P wave.
- Check whether the patient is comfortable and that the cardiac monitor is recording. Take note of the rate and rhythm of the patient's heart and report if there is an abnormality. If unsure, ask a senior colleague to review your patient with you.
- Record that you have commenced cardiac monitoring in the patient's notes.

identifies what each part of the complex denotes (see Hampton 2008 for more detail).

Once connected to a monitor, you may observe that the patient has a 'normal' heart rhythm (**sinus rhythm**), portraying that electrical impulses are travelling from the sino-atrial node to the atrioventricular node, down the septum of the heart, into the Bundle of His and then the left and right bundle branches and the Purkinje fibres. If you need to remind yourself about this physiology, re read the heart's conduction system in your biology book. However, Mrs Patel's heart rhythm is known to be atrial fibrillation.

ACTIVITY

Look at the two rhythm strips in Figure 11.6 that show sinus rhythm and atrial fibrillation. What differences can you see? Look at the following for each strip:

- the rate – frequency of the complex;
- the regularity of each complex occurring;
- whether P waves are present and precede each QRS.

Now, think about what you would feel if taking Mrs Patel's pulse. How might it differ from the pulse of a person with sinus rhythm?

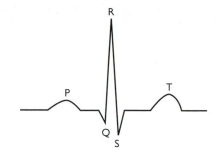

P wave: represents atrial depolarisation prior to atrial contraction.
QRS: represents depolarisation of the ventricles prior to ventricular contraction:
– **Q:** the first downward deflection
– **R:** the first upward deflection
– **S:** the first downward deflection following the R wave
T wave: the next positive wave which shows ventricular repolarisation.

Figure 11.5: The PQRST complex.

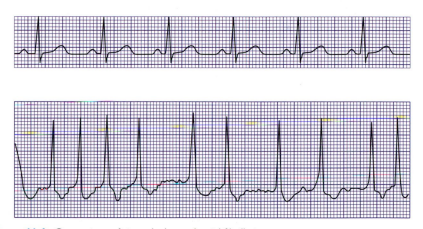

Figure 11.6: Comparison of sinus rhythm and atrial fibrillation.

You will have noticed that, unlike in sinus rhythm, in atrial fibrillation, 'P' waves cannot be identified. This is because the atria are 'fibrillating' rather than contracting, and the impulses are conducted through the atrioventricular node irregularly, so the QRS complexes appear irregularly. You will see that the QRS complexes occur more frequently as often uncontrolled atrial fibrillation leads to a more rapid heart rate. If you were feeling Mrs Patel's pulse, it would feel irregularly irregular. This observation is an important indicator of atrial fibrillation and it should be reported. In this section, you have learned how to attach a cardiac monitor, how to observe a rhythm strip and how to recognise one common arrhythmia, atrial fibrillation.

ACTIVITY

You may be able to practise attaching a cardiac monitor to a colleague in the skills laboratory. If so, ask them to move around and then to simulate cleaning teeth. Note how this muscle movement affects the cardiac monitor's rhythm display.

There are many textbooks and websites that look in detail at interpreting arrhythmias, so access them for further reading about arrhythmias.

Remember: Observing a cardiac monitor is no substitute for observing your patient. The observations previously discussed – vital signs and capillary refill – must also be carried out during your assessment.

Learning outcome 4: Outline how a 12-lead electrocardiograph is recorded

The 12-lead ECG is a useful diagnostic tool and can comprehensively portray the patient's heart rhythm and rate.

ACTIVITY

> Mrs Patel is to have an ECG recorded as she is known to have atrial fibrillation. In what other situations might an ECG be recorded? Think back to when you have seen an ECG recorded in practice.

ECGs are often recorded as a routine investigation before anaesthesia, particularly in older people, to identify myocardial ischaemia, in people with electrolyte imbalances and when the heart may be affected by drugs. The ECG is also recorded in emergency situations, for example, patients who have collapsed, and people with a history of a fall. Therefore, Enid might have an ECG recorded, either in the community, when her GP visits, at the health centre by the practice nurse or if she is referred to a hospital.

Electrical impulses precede cardiac muscle (myocardium) contraction, so this electrical impulse is captured and recorded in an ECG. Waveforms vary in different leads placed on the person's body, and the ECG records the conduction of electrical impulses through the heart from different points. Think of taking a picture with a camera and obtaining a 360° view of the patient's heart from various positions around their bed. For more detail about the physiology underpinning ECGs and their interpretation, refer to your physiology textbook and specialist cardiology books (e.g. Jowett and Thompson 2007). This section focuses on the practice of recording an ECG; Box 11.10 provides key practice points for recording ECGs.

Placement of the 4 ECG leads on the limbs

The 12-lead ECG uses 10 electrodes (sometimes referred to as 'leads') to obtain the reading: six are placed on the person's chest and one on each of the four limbs. All ECG machines use the same principle of recording electrical impulses from the heart but more wireless machines are now available. The placement of these electrodes offers 12 views of electrical activity in different areas of the heart – hence, the name 12-lead ECG.

The four limb leads (which are labelled) are placed as follows:

- RA on right arm;
- LA on left arm;

Box 11.10 Recording ECGs: key points

- Assemble the equipment: ECG machine, alcohol wipes, tissues, razor (to trim chest hair, if necessary), disposable pre-gelled electrodes.
- Identify the patient, explain the procedure and gain their verbal consent.
- Ensure the patient's privacy and dignity is maintained during the procedure.
- Position the patient in a semi-recumbent position if their clinical condition allows; otherwise, record the ECG in the position they are comfortable in.
- Plug in the ECG machine to the DC power supply, or ensure that the machine's battery is fully charged.
- Perform hand hygiene.
- Clean the patient's skin, where the electrodes are to be applied, with an alcohol wipe and remove excess chest hair if the electrodes will not adhere to the skin.
- Apply the electrodes to the limbs and chest: for chest lead positions, see Figure 11.7.
- Connect the ECG leads to these electrodes, placing the lead box on the patient's abdomen.
- Switch on the ECG machine, check calibration of the machine and ECG size.
- Set the paper speed at 25 mm/s unless otherwise instructed.
- Enter the patient's name, date of birth, date and time of procedure if the ECG machine has these facilities.
- Inform the patient you are going to now record the ECG and advise them not to move, speak or cough but to breathe normally. Print the ECG. Remember that movement will affect the reading and be seen as an artefact on the ECG, and then the test will have to be repeated.
- Advise the patient that you have completed the test. Attempt to reassure the patient as this may be an anxious time.
- Advise that the ECG will now be reviewed by a nurse or doctor trained in this procedure. Do not make any attempt to offer a diagnosis to the patient at this stage, and avoid suggesting the test was 'all right' as a patient may misinterpret this as an indication of their ECG showing no signs of disease or problem.
- Labelling – If this has not been entered before the procedure, note the patient's details now on the ECG printout. Do not allow anyone to remove the ECG from the machine before you label it. Record if the patient has chest pain or not at this stage. If this is a serial ECG, also write the number on it. If it was a 15-lead ECG, note this too.
- Disconnect the ECG leads from the patient, make the patient comfortable and assist them to redress, if necessary.
- Document that you have recorded an ECG.
- Clean the ECG machine before returning it to its storage place and reconnecting it to the DC power supply.
- Show the ECG to a competent practitioner and assist in any treatment that the patient now requires.

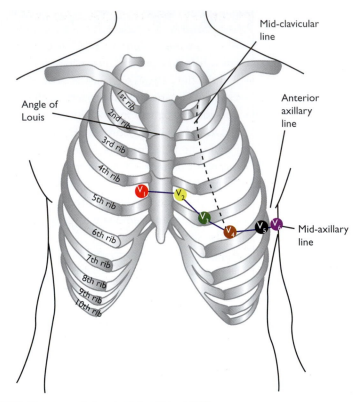

Figure 11.7: Placement of chest leads for 12-lead ECG.

- LL on left leg;
- RL on right leg – this plays no part in the actual reading other than providing an earth.

If the patient is an amputee, place the electrode on the stump.

The placement of these leads forms six standard leads: three bipolar leads (I, II, III) and three augmented vector leads (aVR, aVL, aVF). These limb leads record electrical activity in the following areas (see Hampton 2008):

- I, II and aVL – the lateral aspect of the heart;
- III and aVF – the inferior aspect of the heart;
- aVR – the right atrium.

Placement of the 4 limb leads on the torso

In some clinical situations, the limb leads may be placed on the torso when the limbs cannot be used. There will be a difference in the depth and height of the waves recorded if leads are placed on the torso rather than the limbs which will affect the reading of the ECG. Ask your mentor to show you the differences in what you see. You may have observed a shift in the cardiac axis to the right, a smaller R wave in lead 1 and smaller Q waves in the inferior leads.

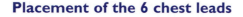

Placement of the 6 chest leads

The six chest leads provide the other six views and are colour-coded and labelled: red (V1), yellow (V2), green (V3), brown (V4), black (V5) and purple (V6). These leads are placed on the torso (see Figure 11.6):

- V1 – at the fourth intercostal space, approximately 1–2 cm right of the sternum;
- V2 – at the fourth intercostal space, approximately 1–2 cm left of the sternum;
- V4 – at the left side of the chest at the fifth intercostal space on the mid-clavicular line;
- V3 – midway between V2 and V4;
- V5 – at the fifth intercostal space at level of V4 (anterior axilla, halfway between V4 and V6);
- V6 – at the same level as V4 and V5, at the mid-axilla line.

These chest leads record electrical activity in the following areas (see Hampton 2008):

- V1 and V2 – right ventricle;
- V3 and V4 – septum and anterior wall of the left ventricle;
- V5 and V6 – anterior and lateral walls of left ventricle.

ACTIVITY

Look at Figure 11.7 and try feeling for the 4th and 5th intercostal spaces on your own chest in front of the mirror.

Additional electrodes for ECG recording

The ECG lead placement can be extended to improve the views of the heart. In some instances, in practice, you may see 15-lead ECGs being recorded using extra leads. Additional leads sometimes used in ECG recordings are:

- Posterior leads: V7, V8, V9: these are positioned in order following V6, along the 5th intercostal space.
- Right-sided leads: Leads can be placed on the right side of the chest in order to enable better views of the right ventricle. These are placed in a 'mirror image' of the left chest leads and will be labelled accordingly: V2R, V3R, V4R, V5R, V6R. Not all of these will necessarily be used – V4R is most often used in practice.

You must ensure that the ECG is labelled to indicate the additional leads used. Where additional leads are placed may vary so follow local policy and guidance.

ACTIVITY

If possible, while in your healthcare setting, observe an ECG being recorded and then record one under supervision. An ECG technician, or a nurse, might be able to assist you with this activity. Look at the ECG recorded and observe the differences in how the PQRST complex appears in the 12 different views. In some practice areas, you may see a 15-lead ECG being recorded as many 12-lead ECG machines can be reconfigured to record 15-lead views. It is important that you ascertain which machine you are likely to use in practice and discuss its capabilities of 15-lead ECG recording with your mentor.

Children: practice points – circulatory problems

For management of circulatory problems in children, see the following sources:

Macqueen, S. Bruce, E.A. and Gibson, F. 2012. Resuscitation practices. *The Great Ormond Street Hospital Manual of Children's Nursing Practices*. Chichester: Wiley-Blackwell, 663–91.

Royal College of Nursing (RCN). 2011. Standards for assessing, measuring and monitoring vital signs in infants, children and young people. Available from: http://www.rcn.org.uk/__data/assets/pdf_file/0004/114484/003196.pdf

Resuscitation Council (UK): http://www.resus.org.uk/SiteIndx.htm

For ECGs in children, see:

Gormley-Fleming, E. 2010. Assessment and vital signs: a comprehensive review. In: Glasper, A., et al. (eds.) *Developing Practical Skills for Nursing Children and Young People*. London: Hodder Arnold, 167–87.

Summary

- Assessment of a patient's circulatory volume and measurement of vital signs are important aspects of the ABCDE assessment.
- Recognising and responding to signs of shock in patients is essential in nursing practice.
- Clinical skills such as measuring capillary refill are simple to learn and greatly assist in your patient's assessment. Practise these skills and take time in refining them.
- Cardiac monitoring and the recording of a 12-/15-lead ECG are more complex skills that will require direct supervision at first, and then as you gain knowledge and experience in a variety of settings, you will become competent in these skills and understand their significance.

UNCONSCIOUSNESS AND RELATED SKILLS

Our awake state is known as consciousness, whilst unconsciousness is defined as when an individual's awareness no longer exists. Normal reflexes protecting conscious patients are lost and so healthcare professionals must maintain their safety and provide all care needed. For initial assessment of an unconscious person, look back to Chapter 4 for an overview of how to carry out a neurological assessment – AVPU and the GCS – and ensure that you can conduct these assessments before continuing with this section as they are necessary for anyone with altered conscious level. There are many causes of unconsciousness including abnormal temperature, oxygen or blood glucose levels, infection (e.g. encephalitis, meningitis), drug intoxication, seizures, focal head injury (trauma), hypoxia, hypercarbia (high levels of carbon dioxide in the circulating blood) or vascular events (shock, stroke). Investigations will be conducted to determine the underlying cause. In this section, general care of an unconscious person is considered, followed by a review of blood glucose monitoring, which will be carried out for a person with altered consciousness and management of seizures.

By the end of this section, you will be able to:

1 appreciate the general care required for people who are unconscious;
2 discuss the principles of blood glucose monitoring;
3 explain how to deal with seizures.

Learning outcome 1: Appreciate the general care required for people who are unconscious

ACTIVITY

Reflect on how unconsciousness will affect a person's ability to self-care. What general care might an unconscious person require?

You should have identified that an unconscious person's airway must be maintained, and oxygen and suction could be necessary (see earlier sections). The person will also need care to prevent complications of immobility (Chapter 6), personal hygiene care, including mouth and eye care (Chapter 8), care of their elimination (Chapter 9) and maintenance of their fluid and nutrition (Chapter 10). It is also important to consider whether they are experiencing pain, and ensure their comfort (see Chapter 12 for more information).

Communication is vital when dealing with unconscious patients. When people lose consciousness, they may still be aware of their surroundings and sensitive to touch and speech. Thus, Enid's carers should have talked to her calmly while she appeared unresponsive. It is very important to talk to unconscious patients and explain what you are going to do. Social conversation is also helpful so that the person is aware of your presence. Family members and significant others should be encouraged to talk to the unconscious person. They might need your help and support in doing this initially.

Learning outcome 2: Discuss the principles of blood glucose monitoring

Hypoglycaemia or hyperglycaemia can cause unconsciousness. Glucose is generated in the body from the foods we eat and is circulated in the blood. Insulin is necessary to enable glucose to enter the cells to provide energy for cellular metabolism. Check your biology textbook or the Internet for a detailed explanation about this process. If glucose levels rise or fall outside the normal range (4–7 mmol/L; 3.6–5.8 mmol/L fasting), then the person's conscious level is affected and they can become extremely unwell. Blood glucose monitoring is therefore often carried out by or for people known to have diabetes. However, other underlying medical conditions and traumatic incidents can affect a person's blood glucose levels without them having diabetes. So, most unconscious patients or medically unwell people will have their blood glucose levels assessed to identify if these are within the normal range.

Organisations have varying policies about who can carry out blood glucose monitoring, so you must go by local policy as to whether you can carry it out in practice. You must be trained how to use your organisation's particular blood glucose monitoring equipment.

ACTIVITY

Find out about blood glucose monitoring in your own practice setting. Investigate:

• what equipment is used;
• what training is given to use this equipment;
• whether there are training updates;
• who can carry out blood glucose monitoring.

The Diabetes UK website (www.diabetes.org.uk) is regularly updated and very informative about managing diabetes; ensure that you review this regularly as management interventions change rapidly. In particular, do look up recognition and management of hypoglycaemia on this website. Also, there are NICE guidelines about managing diabetes and National Service Frameworks and guidelines for all four UK countries, which you can access via their websites.

Blood glucose monitoring is part of the daily routine of many people with diabetes, who know their normal blood glucose levels and are aware of how to control their blood glucose. In Enid's instance, her carers know her usual blood glucose level. When a person becomes unwell due to infection, disease, trauma or a mental health problem, they may be unable to control their diabetes. Blood glucose levels are measured by carrying out a finger prick and gaining a blood sample which is then analysed using a glucose meter. There are different types of glucose meters available. Alternatively, a blood sample can be taken to the biochemistry laboratory for analysing glucose levels. This test usually takes a little time to perform and is therefore not useful in an emergency situation. Treatment will need to be administered according to the blood glucose level. Box 11.11 lists key points in blood glucose measurement.

ACTIVITY

Read Box 11.11 carefully and identify possible reasons for blood glucose tests being inaccurate. Now categorise these causes under the following headings: 'Problems with technique' and 'Problems with equipment'. What could be the consequences of obtaining an inaccurate blood glucose result – either too high or too low?

Box 11.11 Blood glucose monitoring: Key points

Equipment

• Finger-pricking device, gauze/cotton wool for cleaning finger with water and drying, glucose meter, reagent strips

Technique

• Remember infection control: perform hand hygiene before the procedure and apply non-sterile gloves.
• The glucometer must be maintained and checked as per manufacturer's instructions and the strips should be correctly stored (airtight container) and in-date. The user must be trained to use the specific meter and strips.
• Fingers used should be third, fourth or fifth on either side of the end of the finger – but not the top, as this is more painful. This gives 12 possible sites

(Continued)

> **Box 11.11 (Continued)**
>
> and the site should be rotated to avoid causing neurological damage over time with repeated finger pricks. The thumb and second finger are not used as these are most important for touch.
> - If the hand is very cold, ensure that the patient is warm first.
> - The finger site must be washed and dried with water as contamination by food, etc., can affect the accuracy of the test.
> - The finger should not be squeezed/milked from the base.
> - After the finger has been pricked, apply blood to the reagent strip and then insert the strip into the meter for reading, as per the manufacturer's instructions.
> - Ensure safe sharps disposal, dispose of gloves and perform hand hygiene.
> - Record the result in the person's notes.
> - Show the results to a competent practitioner and assist in any treatments that are necessary.

You must pay attention to both technique and the equipment used to gain accurate results. Examples of technique error include failing to wash the finger (consider how the result might be affected if the person has just been eating grapes or chocolate), squeezing the finger leading to interstitial blood entering the blood sample and insufficient blood being obtained. Equipment problems can include reagent strips that have been exposed to air or are out of date, and a machine that has not been quality checked as per manufacturer's instructions.

Gaining inaccurate results of any test is potentially very dangerous. Blood glucose monitoring directly affects treatment. For example, a sliding-scale insulin pump is adjusted according to the blood glucose result. If the result obtained was higher than it really is, the person might be administered more insulin than they really need, with the risk of developing hypoglycaemia. If the result is lower than it really is, the person might not be administered enough insulin and could become increasingly hyperglycaemic. Recording and reporting results from the test is important because, like other information obtained in assessment, it directly impacts on care. If a blood glucose result was very high or very low, immediate action might be necessary.

ACTIVITY

Arrange to observe blood glucose being measured and, if allowed within your organisation's policy, and if you have been trained on the meter used, carry out blood glucose monitoring under supervision. Ensure that you document the result and discuss its implications with your mentor.

Learning outcome 3: Explain how to deal with seizures

A seizure is caused by a sudden burst of excess electrical activity in the brain, causing a temporary disruption in the normal message passing between brain cells, resulting in the brain's messages becoming halted or mixed up (see www.epilepsy.org.uk for more information). Some people experience a seizure on a one-off basis, where no diagnosis is given, and seizures can be caused by medical conditions in some instances. However, some people experience seizures on a regular basis and are then said to have epilepsy. People should be referred to as having epilepsy rather than being 'an epileptic' which is a label (www. epilepsy society.org.uk). They may wear jewellery alerting that they have epilepsy or carry a card indicating the medication they are prescribed.

All healthcare practitioners should be able to recognise and respond appropriately to a person experiencing a seizure. There are thought to be around 40 different types of seizures which vary in severity. Epilepsy has been estimated to affect between 362,000 and 415,000 people in England (NICE 2012). While epilepsy affects about 1% of the population, a third of people with learning disabilities have epilepsy; nearly half the people with severe learning disabilities have epilepsy (RCN 2011).

NICE (2012) guidelines address the importance of healthcare practitioners remaining up to date in the management of epilepsy. Their updated guideline specifies the different drug options that doctors should prescribe their patients, both according to their type of seizure (i.e. when a diagnosis has not yet been confirmed) and according to the epilepsy syndrome.

People who experience an epileptic seizure can progress through several stages. There are many classifications available but the International League Against Epilepsy (2006) offers the following international classification for seizures, which is based on work by Dreifuss (1989):

- *partial seizures*, either local or focal in origin;
- *generalised seizures* (convulsive or non-convulsive), involving the whole brain;
- *unclassified epileptic seizures*, including all seizures that have incomplete data to aid classification.

When a person with epilepsy has a seizure, it should always be treated as an emergency situation and prompt action should be taken in a systematic manner. Some people who experience epileptic seizures have prolonged episodes; these are known as **status epilepticus**.

Convulsive stages and interventions

Immediate care

A person should be assessed using an ABCDE approach (see earlier section) and interventions as per Resuscitation Council (UK) guidelines should be followed as required. Drug therapy may be needed; for example, buccal diazepam may be given or midazolam may be administered rectally by an appropriately trained person (see Chapter 9).

During the seizure, **do**:

- protect the person from further harm and provide privacy;
- maintain their airway (see earlier section);
- stay with the person and reassure them by speaking calmly.

During the seizure, **do not**:

- restrain the person in any way;
- put any object in the person's mouth;
- attempt to rouse the person.

Status epilepticus

A seizure that lasts 30 minutes or longer, or a series of seizures without consciousness being regained in between (see http://www.epilepsy.org.uk/info/treatment/status-epilepticus).

Subsequent care

Monitoring using the ABCDE approach must continue, with recording of vital signs and consideration of possible causes of the seizure. After convulsions have ceased, move the patient into the recovery position to protect their airway (see www.resus.org.uk for further details of this position). Sometimes, incontinence occurs during a seizure, so be sensitive and promote dignity.

Hospitalisation usually follows if the person does not recover spontaneously. At this stage, maintenance of vital signs (as discussed in Chapter 4) should continue. Assessment of arterial blood gases, monitoring of blood glucose levels, cardiac monitoring and recording of a 12-lead ECG, as discussed earlier in this chapter, will be carried out as indicated.

See NICE (2012) Clinical Guideline for full details about the management of people with epilepsy (www.nice.co.uk).

Children: practice points – neurological problems

The NICE (2012) guideline 137 covers epilepsy in children as well as adults.

Febrile seizures (or convulsion due to fever) is relatively common in children up to 7 years of age (3%–8%: Sadleir and Scheffer, 2007). Febrile seizures are commonly associated with an acute infection.

For blood glucose monitoring in children, see:

Gormley-Fleming, E. 2010. Assessment and vital signs: A comprehensive overview. In: Glasper, A., Aylott, M., Battrick, C.(eds.) *Developing Practical Skills for Nursing Children and Young People*. London: Hodder Arnold, 109–47.

For neurological care in children, see: Macqueen, S. Bruce, E.A. and Gibson, F. 2012. Neurological care. In: Glasper, A., et al. (eds.) *The Great Ormond Street Hospital Manual of Children's Nursing Practices*. Chichester: Wiley-Blackwell, 437–64.

Pregnancy and birth: practice points – neurological problems

- An unconscious woman in her third trimester of pregnancy should be positioned on her left side to avoid compression of the inferior vena cava. For further information, visit www.resus.org.uk
- The NICE (2012) guideline 137 covers in detail the care of women with epilepsy during pregnancy.
- Rarely, pre-eclampsia in pregnancy can lead to eclampsia, which is a type of seizure that is life threatening to the mother and baby.

Summary

- People who are unconscious need support and monitoring of their airway, breathing and circulation as well as pressure area care, support for hygiene, elimination and nutrition, and comfort and communication.
- Blood glucose monitoring can assist in identifying the cause for a patient's deterioration. This skill should be observed in your practice setting, and

appropriate training on using specific equipment should be obtained before practising this skill. Local policies must be adhered to.

- Dealing with seizures and recognising the stages of convulsion and responding appropriately are important skills for all nurses.

CHAPTER SUMMARY

This chapter has reviewed how to identify, assess and manage an acutely ill adult patient. The systematic ABCDE assessment approach was discussed. Appropriate emergency skills and care interventions have been highlighted. Since ABCDE assessments are performed rapidly in acute settings, you may not have an opportunity to talk to your colleagues about what is happening at the time. Try to find an opportunity to review emergency assessments with your colleagues after the event when you will be able to learn more about the situation and the patient's assessment and management. ABCDE assessment forms part of many track-and-trigger systems and you should familiarise yourself with your local organisation's charts, methods of record keeping and protocols. It can take considerable time to become confident in these acute skills. The recognition, assessment and management of the person who is acutely ill remains a challenge for all healthcare practitioners. It is important that you work with your mentor to develop these skills in practice settings. Practise your skills of assessment regularly, learn how to observe for signs of deterioration, measure vital signs accurately and communicate your findings immediately using a communication tool. Keep up to date with changes in protocols and procedures of caring for the person who is acutely ill.

REFERENCES

Audit Commission. 1999. *Critical to Success: The Place of Efficient and Effective Critical Care Services within the Acute Hospital.* London: Audit Commission.

Baird, A. 2001. Concordance with long-term oxygen therapy. *Practice Nursing* 12: 457–9.

Booker, R. 2007. Understanding why we use spirometry: Part 1. *Nursing Times* 103(45): 46–8.

Bright, D., Walker, W. and Bion, J. 2004. Outreach: A strategy for improving the care of the acutely ill hospitalized patient. *Critical Care* 8: 33–40.

British Thoracic Society/Scottish Intercollegiate Guidelines Network (BTS/SIGN). 2008. *Guidelines on the Management of Asthma.* Available from: http://www.brit-thoracic.org.uk/Portals/0/Guidelines/AsthmaGuidelines/sign101%20revised%20June%2009.pdf (Accessed on 5 September 2013).

Buist D., Moore, G., Bernard, S., et al. 2002. Effects of a medical emergency team on the reduction of incidence of and mortality from unexpected cardiac arrests in hospital: Preliminary review. *British Medical Journal* 324: 387–90.

Coggan, J.M. 2008a. Arterial blood gas analysis 1. Understanding ABG reports. *Nursing Times* 104(18): 28–9.

Coggan, J.M. 2008b. Arterial blood gas analysis 2. Compensatory mechanisms. *Nursing Times* 104(19): 24–5.

Cole, E. 2007. Measuring central venous pressure. *Nursing Standard* 22(7): 40–2.

Confidential Enquiry into Maternal and Child Health. 2007. *Saving Mothers' Lives to Make Motherhood Safe*. Available from: http://www.hqip.org.uk/assets/NCAPOP-Library/CMACE-Reports/21.-December-2007-Saving-Mothers-Lives-reviewing-maternal-deaths-to-make-motherhood-safer-2003-2005.pdf *(Accessed on 24 September 2012)*.

Croxton, T.L. and Bailey, W.C. 2006. Long-term oxygen treatment in chronic obstructive pulmonary disease: Recommendation for future research. *American Journal of Respiratory and Critical Care Medicine* 174: 373–8.

Currie, G., Deveraux, G., Lee, D. and Ayres, J. 2005. Recent developments in asthma management. *British Medical Journal* 330: 585–9.

Cuthbertson, S. and Kelly, M. 2007. Support of respiratory function. In: Elliott, D., Allen, L. and Chaboyer, W. (eds.) *ACCCNs Critical Care Nursing*. Marrickville: Elsievier, 263–306.

Department of Health (DH). 2000. *Comprehensive Critical Care: A Review of Adult Critical Care Services*. London: DH.

Department of Health (DH). 2007. *Maternity Matters: Choice, Access and Continuity of Care in a Safe Service*. London: DH.

Dreifuss, F.E. 1989. Classification of epileptic seizures and the epilepsies. *Pediatric Clinics of North America* 36: 265–79.

Ellis, D.Y., Lambert, C. and Shirley, P. 2006. Intracranial placement of nasopharyngeal airways: Is it all that rare? *Emergency Medicine Journal* 23: 661.

Featherstone, P., Chalmers, T. and Smith, G.B. 2008. RSVP: A system for communication of deterioration in hospital patients. *British Journal of Nursing* 17(13): 860–4.

Francis, C. 2006. *Respiratory Care: Essential Clinical Skills for Nurses*. Oxford: Blackwell.

Garretson, S. and Malberti, S. 2007. Understanding hypovolaemic, cardiogenic and septic shock. *Nursing Standard* 50(21): 46–55.

Garrioch, M.A. 2004. The body's response to blood loss. *Vox Sanguinis* 87(Suppl 1): S74–6.

Greenberg, C.C., Scott, E., Regenbogen, S.E., et al. 2007. Patterns of communication breakdowns resulting in injury to surgical patients. *Journal of the American College of Surgeons* 204(4): 533–40.

Gwinnutt, C. 2006. *Clinical Anaesthesia*. Oxford: Blackwell Publishing.

Hampton, J. 2008. *ECG Made Easy,* 7th edn. London: Churchill Livingstone.

Hand, H. 2001. Shock. *Nursing Standard* 15(48): 45–52.

Harbrecht, B.G., Alarcon, L.H. and Peitzman, A.B. 2004. Management of shock. In: Moore, E.E., et al. (eds.) *Trauma*, 5th edn. New York: McGraw-Hill, 201–25.

Higgins, D. 2005. Oxygen therapy. *Nursing Times* 101(4): 30–2.

International League Against Epilepsy. 2006. Classification of seizures. Available from: http://www.ilae.org (Accessed on 8 February 2013).

Jevon, P. 2010. How to ensure patient observations lead to prompt identification of tachynoea. *Nursing Times* 106(2): 12–14.

Jones, I. 2005. *Cardiac Care: An Introductory Text*. London: Whurr.

Jowett, N. and Thompson, D. 2007. *Comprehensive Cardiac Care,* 4th edn. London: Baillière Tindall.

Kause, J., Smith, G., Prytherch, D., et al. (2004). A comparison of antecedents to cardiac arrests, deaths and emergency intensive care admissions in Australia and New Zealand, and the United Kingdom – The ACADEMIA study. *Resuscitation* 62: 275–82.

Khaw, K.S., Ngan Kee, W.D., Tam, Y.H., et al. 2008. Survey and evaluation of modified oxygen delivery devices used for suspected severe acute respiratory syndrome and other high-risk patients in Hong Kong. *Hong Kong Medical Journal* 14(Suppl 5): 27–31.

King's Fund. 2008. *Safe Births: Everybody's Business. An Independent Enquiry into the Safety of Maternity Services in England.* London: King's Fund.

Law, C. 2000. A guide to assessing sputum. *Nursing Times Plus* 96(24): 7–10.

Mann, S. and Bowler, M. 2008. Using an early warning score tool in community nursing. *Nursing Times* 104(20): 30–1.

McGrath, A.M., Gardner, D.M. and McCormack, J. 2001. Is home peak expiratory flow monitoring effective in controlling asthma symptoms? *Journal of Clinical Pharmacy and Therapeutics* 26(5): 311–17.

McLauchlan, L. 2002. Supplementary oxygen therapy in the community. *Nursing Times Plus* 98(40): 50–2.

Moore, T. 2003. Suctioning techniques for the removal of respiratory secretions. *Nursing Standard* 18(9): 47–54.

National Confidential Enquiry into Patient Outcome and Death (NCEPOD). 2012. Time to intervene. Available from: http://www.ncepod.org.uk/2012report1/downloads/CAP_fullreport.pdf (Accessed on 5 September 2013).

National Health Service (NHS). 2011. Using oxygen at home: A patient and carer's guide. Available from: http://www.nhs.uk/Conditions/home-oxygen/Documents/Oxygen%20leaflet%20printer%20friendly.pdf (Accessed on 5 September 2013).

National Heart, Lung and Blood Institute. 2012. Explore oxygen administration. Available from: http://www.nhlbi.nih.gov/ (Accessed on 8 February).

National Institute for Health and Clinical Excellence (NICE). 2007. *Acutely Ill Patients in Hospital: Quick Reference Guide*, Clinical Guideline 50. London: NICE.

National Institute for Health and Clinical Excellence (NICE). 2010. *Chronic Obstructive Pulmonary Disease: Management of Chronic Obstructive Pulmonary Disease in Adults in Hospital.* Available from: http:// publications.nice.org.uk/chronic-obstructive-pulmonary-disease-cg101 (Accessed on 5 September 2013).

National Institute for Health and Clinical Excellence (NICE). 2012. *The Epilepsies: The Diagnosis and Management of the Epilepsies in Adults and Children in Primary and Secondary Care.* Clinical Guidelines 137. London: NICE.

National Patient Safety Agency (NPSA). 2007. *Safer Care for the Acutely Ill Patient: Learning from Serious Incidents*, 5th report. London: NPSA.

National Patient Safety Agency (NPSA). 2009. Rapid Response Report NPSA/2009/RRR006: Oxygen safety in hospitals. London: NPSA.

Oakey, R. and Slade, V. 2006. Physiological observation track and trigger system. *Nursing Standard* 20(27): 48–54.

Odell, M. 2010. Are early warning scores the only way to rapidly detect and manage deterioration? *Nursing Times* 106(8): 24–6.

Odell, M., Victor, C. and Oliver, D. 2009. Nurses' role in detecting deterioration in ward patients: systematic literature review. *Journal of Advanced Nursing* 65(10): 1992–2006.

O'Driscoll, B.R., Howard, L.S. and Davison, A.G. 2008. BTS guideline for emergency oxygen use in adult patients. *Thorax* 43(Suppl vi): vi1–vi68.

Patient Safety First. 2008. *The 'How to Guide' for Reducing Harm from Deterioration.* Available from: http://www.patientsafetyfirst.nhs.uk (Accessed on 1 February 2013).

Pilkington, F. 2004. Humidification for oxygen therapy in non-ventilated patients. *British Journal of Nursing* 13(2): 111–15.

Porter-Jones, G. 2002. Short-term oxygen therapy. *Nursing Times Plus* 98(40): 53–6.

Pritchard, M.J. 2010. How effective communication skills can reduce anxiety in elective surgical patients. *Nursing Times* 107: 3.

Pruitt, W.C. and Jacobs, M. 2003. Breathing lessons: basics of oxygen therapy. *Nursing.* 33(10): 43–5.

Pryor, J.A. and Prasad, S. A. 2008. *Physiotherapy for Respiratory and Cardiac Problems in Adults and Paediatrics,* 4th edn. Edinburgh: Churchill Livingstone.

Prytherch, D., Smith, G., Schmidt, P., et al. 2010. ViEWS towards a national early warning score for detecting adult inpatient deterioration. *Resuscitation* 81(8): 932–7.

Resuscitation Council (UK). 2008. Cardiopulmonary resuscitation: Standards for clinical practice and training. Available from: http://www.resus.org.uk/pages/standard.pdf (Accessed on 24 September 2013).

Resuscitation Council (UK). 2010. Resuscitation guidelines. Available from: http://www.resus.org.uk/pages/guide.htm. (Accessed on 2 February 2013).

Royal College of Nursing (RCN). 2011. *Meeting the Health Needs of People with Learning Disabilities.* London: RCN.

Royal College of Nursing (RCN). 2013. Tools, techniques and taking action. Available from: www.rcn.org.uk/development/practice/cpd_online_learning/making_sense_of_patient_safety/tools_and_techniques_for_you_to_improve_patient_safety (Accessed on 5 September 2013)

Royal College of Physicians (RCP). 2012. *National Early Warning Scores: Standardising the Assessment of Acute Illness Sensitivity in the NHS.* Available from: http://www.rcplondon.ac.uk (Accessed on 2 February 2013).

Rubin, B.K. 2002. Physiology of airway mucus clearance. *Respiratory Care* 47: 761–8.

Sadleir, L.G. and Scheffer, I.E. 2007. Febrile seizures. *British Medical Journal* 334: 307.

Sheppard, M. and Davis, S. 2000. Oxygen therapy – 1. *Nursing Times* 96(29): 43–4.

Smith, G. 2003. *ALERT: A Multiprofessional Course in Care of the Acutely Ill Patient*, 2nd edn. Portsmouth: University of Portsmouth.

Smith, G.B., Prytherch, D.R., Schmidt, P., et al. 2006. Hospital-wide physiological surveillance: A new approach to the early identification and management of the sick patient. *Resuscitation* 71(1): 19–28.

Spahn, D.R., Cerny, V., Caoats, T.J., et al. 2007. Management of bleeding following major trauma: A European guideline. *Critical Care* 11: R17.

Stockley, R.A., O'Brien, C., Pye, A., et al. 2000. Relationship of sputum colour to nature and outpatient management of acute exacerbations of COPD. *Chest* 117: 1638–45.

Thim, T., Krarup, N.H., Grove, E.L., et al. 2012. Initial assessment and treatment with the airway, breathing, circulation, disability, exposure (ABCDE) approach. *International Journal of General Medicine* 5: 117–21.

Vines, D.L., Shelledy, D.C. and Peters, J. 2000. Current respiratory care. Part 1: oxygen therapy, oximetry, bronchial hygiene. *Journal of Critical Illness* 15: 507–10, 513–15.

Warrell, D., Cox, T. and Firth, J. 2012. *Oxford Textbook of Medicine,* 5th edn. Oxford: Oxford University Press.

Wilkins, R.L., Dexter, J.R. and Heuer, A.J. 2010. *Clinical Assessment in Respiratory Care,* 6th edn. St. Louis, MO: Elsevier Mosby.

Wilson, J. 2006. *Infection Control in Clinical Practice,* 3rd edn. London: Baillière Tindall.

Woodrow, P. 2004. Arterial blood gas analysis. *Nursing Standard* 18(21): 45–52.

Zevola, D.R. and Maier, C.B. 2001. Use of nasal cannula versus face mask after extubation in patients after cardiothoracic surgery. *Critical Care Nurse* 21(3): 47–53.

USEFUL WEBSITES

- Asthma UK: www.asthma.org.uk
- British Lung Foundation: http://www.blf.org.uk
- British National Formulary: www.bnf.org/bnf
- British Thoracic Society: www.brit-thoracic.org.uk
- Diabetes UK: www.diabetes.org.uk
- Epilepsy Action: www.epilepsy.org.uk
- Resuscitation Council (UK): www.resus.org.uk
- Peak flow information: www.peakflow.com

12 Managing Pain and Promoting Comfort and Sleep

Dee Burrows, Lesley Baillie and Stephanie Forge

Clients and patients in all healthcare settings experience pain and discomfort, whether it is physical, emotional or spiritual. Studies suggest that over 50% of patients have severe pain after surgery (in hospital and following discharge) and that more than 30% of patients in medical wards report their pain as being severe (Macintyre et al. 2010). Furthermore, 7.8 million people – or one in seven of the United Kingdom (UK) population – have chronic pain (Donaldson 2009). Managing pain and promoting comfort are therefore essential skills in nursing practice.

Pain and discomfort impact many aspects of individuals' lives including sleep. Around 20%–30% of the UK population suffer from problems related to falling asleep, staying asleep, waking early and feeling un-refreshed when they do wake up (Patient.co.uk 2011). Pain and discomfort are among the factors that disturb sleep. Understanding the consequences of poor sleep and how to improve sleep are further key components of nursing.

This chapter aims to help you understand how nursing skills may be used to reduce pain and promote comfort and sleep.

The chapter includes the following topics:

- Managing pain in a variety of settings – the nature of pain, pain assessment, pain management using medication, and non-pharmacological approaches to managing pain
- Promoting comfort – the nature of comfort care, using presence and developing relationships, touch, verbal interactions, physical actions and integrating comfort care skills in practice
- Promoting sleep – normal sleep physiology across the age range, restorative versus non-restorative sleep, hints and tips for sleep at home and discussion of how these can be applied in hospital and residential settings.

Recommended biology reading-pain

Crohn's disease

Chronic inflammation of the intestines, especially the colon and ileum.

The following questions will help you to focus on the biology underpinning the skills used in pain management. Use your recommended textbook to find out:

- How is pain defined?
- What is Melzack's 'body-self neuromatrix'?
- Is pain useful? Why?
- What are the three distinct parts of the nociceptive pathway?
- What are the differences between C-fibres and Aδ-fibres?
- To which part of the nociceptive pathway does the 'gate-control theory of pain' relate?
- Name three parts of the brain which are involved in the perception of pain.
- What affects pain perception and how does this relate to the concept of the neuromatrix?
- What physiological signs may indicate that a person is in acute pain?
- How does chronic pain differ from acute pain?

Enhanced recovery programme

Often referred to as rapid recovery, this is a new, evidence-based model of care that creates fitter patients who recover faster from major surgery. See: http://www.improvement. nhs.uk/enhancedrecovery/ (Accessed 18th July 2012).

Recommended biology reading-sleep

Laparotomy

A surgical procedure involving a large incision through the abdominal wall to gain access into the abdominal cavity.

The questions below will help you to focus on the biology underpinning the skills used in sleep management. Use your recommended textbook and web resources to find out:

- What is sleep?
- How much sleep do children, teenagers, adults and older people need?
- What are the different types and stages of sleep?
- How long does each stage last in a young adult and what is its purpose?
- What is a sleep cycle?
- How quickly do we become sleep deprived?
- What happens in sleep deprivation?

Ileostomy

A surgical operation in which a piece of the ileum is diverted to an artificial opening in the abdominal wall.

PRACTICE SCENARIOS

The following scenarios illustrate when managing pain, promoting comfort and sleep may be needed. They will be referred to throughout this chapter.

Adult

Epidural

An injection of local anaesthetic or other pain-relieving medicines into the epidural space surrounding the spinal cord, temporarily numbing the nerves.

Thomas is 34 years old, married, with young children. He is a self-employed graphic designer who contracts out for work. Some time ago, Thomas was diagnosed with **Crohn's disease**, the impact of which has been affecting his home, work and leisure activities. He was admitted via the **enhanced recovery programme** for a **laparotomy** and formation of **ileostomy**. Post operatively he was transferred to the high dependency unit (HDU) overnight. He initially had an **epidural** for pain relief, was converted to oral analgesics after 2 days and was discharged home at six days with pain and stoma advice.

Learning Disability

Maria is a 58-year-old woman with a moderate learning disability who has been living in a group home for the last five years. She has long-standing **diabetes mellitus** treated with insulin and has recently developed **painful diabetic neuropathy**. She has pain in both legs below the knees, which she finds particularly distressing when she is walking and during the night; her sleep is disturbed. She is in the care of both her GP and the Diabetic Team at her local hospital. Maria's mother, who is 85 years old and recently widowed, visits on a weekly basis and is concerned about Maria's distress. Her Community Learning Disability Nurse would like to understand more about how he can support Maria, her mother and the group home staff on how to manage Maria's pain and increase her comfort.

Mental Health

Violet Davies, aged 76 years, has moderate **Alzheimer's disease**. She has been admitted to a care home for respite as her husband is physically and emotionally exhausted and needs a break. He has refused help in the past as he has been determined to look after his wife, but he has now agreed to take a holiday visiting friends. Violet is physically well, but she is also known to have **osteoarthritis** in her right hip and knee. She looks permanently worried and is agitated; she keeps repeating the same phrase over and over. Mr Davies looks shaky and tearful at the thought of leaving his wife for a week.

MANAGING PAIN IN A VARIETY OF SETTINGS

LEARNING OUTCOMES

By the end of this section, you will be able to:
1 discuss the nature of pain;
2 consider the biopsychosocial complexity of pain;
3 identify appropriate pain assessment tools for different client groups;
4 demonstrate understanding of pharmacological approaches to managing pain;
5 explore non-pharmacological approaches to managing pain.

Learning outcome 1: Discuss the nature of pain

ACTIVITY

Reflect back on your practice experiences. Write down a few examples of people you have met with pain and the setting in which you met them.

Pain is all around us. It is something we cannot see and others cannot see in us. People have to deal with pain at home, in work and during leisure activities. Some 27%–40% of children and young adults, rising to 59% of those aged 75 and over experience pain (Breivik et al. 2006; Bridges 2012). People with chronic pain consult their GP around five times more frequently than those without (see http://www.rcgp.org.uk). Around 70%–90% of older people in residential care report pain (Patients Association 2007; Zanocchi et al. 2008). The amount of pain in hospitals has been mentioned earlier in the chapter. Managing pain is, therefore, a key element of day-to-day nursing practice in all healthcare settings.

Defining pain

> Think back to a time when you have experienced pain, and write down the experience. Looking at your notes, how would you define pain?

Pain is a complex, personal experience that has been defined in various ways. For example, the International Association for the Study of Pain (IASP) defines pain as:

> An unpleasant sensory and emotional experience associated with actual or potential tissue damage, or described in terms of such damage. (IASP Subcommittee on Taxonomy 1979, p. 250)

This definition clearly recognises that pain comprises both physical and psychological components. It continues 'Pain is always subjective. Each individual learns the application of the word through experiences related to injury in early life'. This idea of the subjectivity of pain was used by Margo McCaffery in 1968:

> Pain is whatever the experiencing person says it is, existing when the experiencing person says it does. (McCaffery 1968, cited in Sofaer 1998, p. 95)

McCaffery's definition is an operational definition as it aims to guide real practice, and nurses following it believe the person and try to manage their pain. This may appear an obvious statement, as compassion includes alleviating suffering and pain (Hudacek 2008) but patients' pain is not always believed. Perhaps you can recall an occasion when you have found it difficult to believe what a patient is telling you about their pain. However, hard you may find it, it is worth remembering that Moskow (1987) points out:

> Pain occurring in unicorns, griffins, and jabberwockies is always imaginary pain, since these are imaginary animals: patients on the other hand are real, and so they always have real pain. (Moskow 1987, p. 68)

In order to make sense of the concept that all pain is real, we need to explore the different ways in which pain is perceived.

Experiencing pain

> With reference to your biology reading and the scenarios, what factors may affect the perception and experience of pain?

Go back and review the body-self matrix which Melzack (2005) proposes and look at the explanatory diagram in Figure 12.1. Which of the factors you identified belong to each of the cognitive, sensory or emotional inputs?

Sensory signalling systems

When there is tissue damage in the periphery, there is a response from the cells that initiates an inflammatory response. Various chemicals (sometimes called the 'sensitising soup') are released reducing the firing threshold of the nociceptors (or pain fibres). When these fibres are activated, the action potential travels to the dorsal

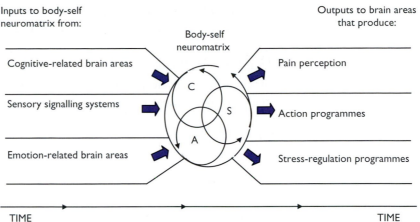

Inputs to body-self
neuromatrix from:

Outputs to brain areas
that produce:

Body-self
neuromatrix

Cognitive-related brain areas

Pain perception

Sensory signalling systems

Action programmes

Emotion-related brain areas

Stress-regulation programmes

C

S

A

TIME

TIME

Figure 12.1: Factors that contribute to the patterns of activity generated by the body-self neuromatrix. (C = cognitive, A = affective/emotional, S = sensory) (Adapted from Melzack, R. 2005. Evolution of the neuromatrix theory of pain. *Pain Practice* 5(2): 85–94.)

Box 12.1 Sensory signalling – definitions and information

Action potential

The process by which neurons (cells within a nerve) alter their electrical charge so that impulses are carried down the nerve

A-fibres

The $A\beta$-fibres are large myelinated fibres; they transmit touch, mild pressure, joint position sense and vibration. When pain occurs, the gate is 'opened' by the signals travelling up the $A\delta$- or C-fibres and 'closed' by the $A\beta$-fibres, thus blocking pain signals.

Central sensitisation and wind-up

For more information, visit http://www.wellcome.ac./en/pain/microsite/science4.html (Accessed 14th September 2012)

---

horn in the spinal cord. There are two main groups of nociceptors $A\beta$- or C-fibres. The $A\beta$-fibres are larger and myelinated and transmit impulses more quickly than the C-fibres. The $A\beta$-fibres conduct 'fast pain', often described as sharp pain, and the C-fibres conduct aching pain. These pains are called nociceptive (see Box 12.1).

The impulses from the periphery arrive at the dorsal horn of the spinal cord where they can be modified before continuing their journey to the brain. Melzack and Wall (1996) described the gate control theory of pain in 1965, which proposed that input from other neurones could change the messages being sent to the brain. The message could be enhanced – causing central sensitisation and 'wind-up' – or it could be decreased by the descending messages from the brain or from the $A\beta$-fibres in the periphery. Hence, the idea of a 'gate' which can be opened to let more messages through or closed to stop messages going on in the system. Box 12.1 provides a link to further information on central sensitisation and wind-up.

Finally, the impulse travels to the brainstem and higher centres in the brain. The various parts involved are referred to as 'the pain matrix', and information from the sensory signalling system is linked with those from the emotion-related brain areas (the limbic system) and the cognitive-related brain areas. When all this comes together, the person will perceive pain. These emotional and cognitive-related areas can activate impulses back down the system to change things at the 'gate'.

Pain can also be caused by damage to the nerves themselves, either in the periphery or centrally, which is called neuropathic pain. Sometimes, people may have both nociceptive and neuropathic pain. For example, people with multiple sclerosis may experience neuropathic pain because of demyelination of the axon and subsequent scar formation of the nerves and nociceptive pain due to mechanical stimulation arising from altered muscle balance and muscle spasms (Multiple Sclerosis Trust 2007).

With reference to the scenarios at the start of the chapter:

- Thomas will have pain as a consequence of the surgical incision and the resultant tissue damage, activating the sensory signalling system. His pain is clearly related to his injury and is expected to heal and eventually subside. This is acute pain. If he has had a lot of pain preoperatively, he may feel relieved that the surgery has been done and that he can start getting better (emotional and cognitive input). This will affect his perception of his pain, and he may report less pain than you expect as his descending mechanisms are brought into use by the stress-regulating programmes.

- Maria's leg pain is due to damage to the nerves by the progression of her diabetes. The damaged nerves continuously send messages, which are perceived as painful. She may struggle to understand why she has pain; therefore, using cognitive skills to modify or reduce the pain perception can be challenging for her carers. The underlying problem causing Maria's pain is unlikely to heal, and this long-term pain is known as chronic or persistent pain.

- Violet's situation is complex, with pain caused by the mechanical stimulation of osteoarthritis and changes to her brain arising from her Alzheimer's disease that appear to alter her emotional and cognitive processing. Her agitation activates the **reticular activating system**, a part of the brain involved in the pain pathways. These combined influences may make it difficult for her to change the pain perception (and the changes in her brain may also make it difficult for her to communicate – we will look at pain assessment for Violet later in the chapter).

- Violet's husband may be suffering from social isolation in addition to his mental and physical exhaustion. He may need comforting and active support if he is going to be able to look after his wife at home again in the future.

Reticular activating system

A network of brain cells concerned with arousal and awareness.

ACTIVITY

- How often have you or friends commented that someone has a 'high (or low) pain threshold'? Think for a minute what you meant by this. Jot down your feelings about people with a low threshold and those with a high threshold.
- Now consider what you understand by the word 'tolerance'.

In pain management, 'threshold' refers to the level at which the population at large perceives a stimulus as painful, rather than uncomfortable. In theory, we all feel pain at about the same level. Therefore, pain threshold is essentially a physiological measurement. Beacroft and Dodd (2010) comment that practitioners erroneously believe that people with learning difficulties have higher pain thresholds than the rest of the population. In fact, Maria's pain threshold will be much the same as that of Thomas.

What makes us feel pain differently is pain 'tolerance'. This refers to the amount of pain an individual can tolerate, or put up with, at any given time. It is not affected by age, gender or culture, but rather by the thoughts and feelings we are experiencing at that point in time, and it is thus an outcome of the combination of sensory, cognitive and emotional input and processing. In struggling to communicate her pain, Maria may have a lower tolerance than Thomas whose surgery should see an improvement in his condition.

To illustrate pain tolerance, imagine you are experiencing a really bad headache while attending a lecture. What would you do? Perhaps you would take painkillers or go home. You still have a headache but need to get ready for a party or meal out. What would you do? It is possible that you would go to the social event and within a short space of time forget your headache!

ACTIVITY

Using the idea of cognitive and emotional input, try to map your different responses to both situations above. How might these affect your perception of the pain and the action you take?

Pain tolerance varies from one individual to the next and within an individual from one minute to the next. Some factors that increase or decrease pain perception are listed in Box 12.2.

ACTIVITY

Look at the scenario of Violet and list the factors that may be influencing her pain perception. Note down an explanation for each factor.

- Mr Davies's emotional and physical exhaustion, his desire to support Violet at home and his tearfulness may be transmitted to Violet and increase her worry.
- The strange and potentially frightening environment may reduce Violet's sense of personal control and enhance her feelings of social isolation.
- The prolonged nature of Violet's osteoarthritis may have reduced her pain coping strategies.
- Violet's agitation will prevent her from relaxing and increase her tension.
- The lack of information about the immediate future may reduce Mr and Mrs Davies's abilities to maintain any sense of cognitive control.
- The pathophysiology of Alzheimer's disease may alter Violet's pain experience (covered further in learning outcome 3).

Knowing and understanding the factors that reduce pain perception can help guide your approach to pain management. A further concept you need to consider is pain behaviour.

> **Box 12.2 Examples of factors that increase or decrease our perception of pain**
>
> Increasing
> - Anxiety, fear, worry, tension
> - Lack of control
> - Tiredness
> - Prolonged or recurrent pain
> - Previous poor experiences with pain
>
> Decreasing
> - Information
> - Relaxation, distraction
> - Control
>
> Analgesics
> - Touch, social interaction, reassurance
> - Known positive outcome
> - Previous positive experience with pain

ACTIVITY

Again, thinking about headaches:
- How do you behave when you have a headache?
- How does your best friend behave?
- How do other people you know behave?

Perhaps one of the people you thought of wants attention, while others prefer to be on their own. Maybe some frown, grimace and become irritable, while others try to relax their facial expression and carry on as normal. As with non-verbal and social responses, verbal and vocal responses (e.g. shouting, moaning) also vary. These are all different pain behaviours or pain expressions.

Pain expression and pain behaviour are learned through our families and culture; see Box 12.3 for an example.

Cultural beliefs are a strong determinant of pain expression and behaviour.

ACTIVITY

- Think of the different pain behaviours you have seen. List the ones you think Thomas, Maria and Violet might be adopting.
- Scenarios often push you into stereotyping (as do handovers). Consider the behaviours you have listed for each scenario and ask yourself why you identified those particular ones.
- Access Lovering's (2006) article online and make some notes about the different cultural perspectives of those involved in her study.

During this activity, keep in mind that what the person says about their pain is invariably true and is a much better indicator of pain than behaviour and physiological signs, although sometimes one has to rely on the latter, such as in Violet's case.

> **Box 12.3 An example of how pain expression and behaviour is learned through families and culture**
>
> My own experience and research in the South Asian communities within Leicester and Milton Keynes has shown vast differences. South Asian people attending the pain clinics in Leicester have similar pain beliefs to the white population, perhaps because the South Asian community has been established in Leicester for many years. This is in contrast with my own clinical practice in Milton Keynes, where the South Asian population is very new in comparison to Leicester. They have very different beliefs, attitudes and ways of presenting their pain. For many of these people, the concept of self-management is alien. Hobbies and interests other than the family and politics seem to be unknown. If pain can't be cured they may think the doctor is useless, but accept that it is God's will that they should live with the pain, so one of my challenges is how to engage these people in self-management.
>
> (Dr Sue Peacock, Health Psychologist, Milton Keynes NHS Trust, personal communication, September 2012)

In summary, an appreciation of the differences between pain threshold, pain tolerance and pain behaviour will help you to understand how people's pain and their reactions to it vary.

You may want to re-read this section to ensure that you understand the knowledge underpinning some of the practical skills that will be discussed later.

Learning outcome 2: Consider the biopsychosocial complexity of pain

We have already suggested above that pain is a complex mix of physical sensation, emotions and cognitions that influence pain perception and behaviour. Both acute and chronic pain have these components.

ACTIVITY

Many of you will be familiar with the biopsychosocial model. If you are not, you will need to look up the model before completing this activity. Thinking of a patient you have recently nursed:
- What was the cause of your patient's pain sensation?
- What were the patient's worries and fears?
- What were the patient's home, leisure and, if appropriate, work circumstances?
- How did all of this impact on your patient's pain?

Thomas's biopsychosocial experience might look something like that shown in Figure 12.2.

As a self-employed graphic designer, Thomas is likely to both want and need to get back to work sooner than healthcare practitioners might advise. This is a good example of where using a biopsychosocial model differs from the bio-medical model.

Maria's more complex chronic pain experience is shown in Figure 12.3.

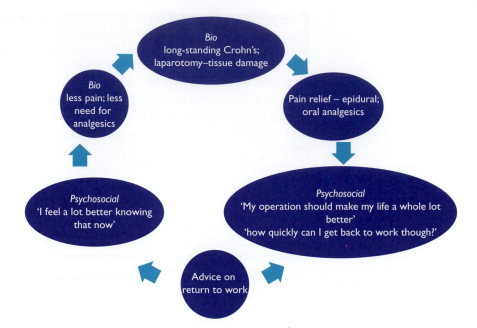

Figure 12.2: Thomas's biopsychosocial experience.

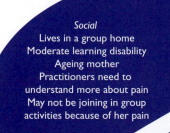

Figure 12.3: Maria's biopsychosocial experience.

Have a go at drawing your own diagram for Violet. Once you have done so:

- Give some thought to the knowledge and skills that you would need to improve Violet's pain management and reduce her pain perception
- Find an article that discusses biopsychosocial pain. Depending on your learning needs and stage of course, this could be an opinion article, a research paper or a video such as those available on the Pain Community Centre website (http://www.paincommunitycentre.org)

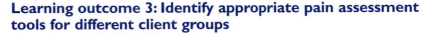

Learning outcome 3: Identify appropriate pain assessment tools for different client groups

Pain is assessed in a variety of ways in different clinical settings. It is a key aspect of pain management and research has consistently demonstrated that accurate pain assessment is a prerequisite of effective pain management (Wood 2008). All patients and clients should have their pain assessed and recorded at the beginning of each episode of care and at suitable intervals thereafter.

Unidimensional pain assessment

Earlier in the chapter, we learned that sensory signalling and emotional and cognitive inputs are involved in the perception of pain. It makes sense then, that in order to assess someone's pain we need to consider those different domains. In some settings, we prioritise the domain that we assess. For instance, in Thomas's situation on a busy HDU, it may be appropriate to simply ask:

- 'Have you any pain or discomfort?' or 'Are you sore? (Not everyone will call pain 'pain')'
- 'Where is the pain/where is it sore?'
- 'How bad is it when you are still? What about when you move?'

These questions help identify the whereabouts (location) and intensity of the person's pain.

To help patients respond to the last two questions, some nurses and doctors ask: 'On a scale of zero to ten, with zero being no pain and ten being the worst pain you can imagine, what is your pain?' Imagining a 0–10 scale when you are anxious, experiencing intense pain and possibly feeling very ill can be difficult. It may be more effective to show patients a scale and to ask them to point to the level that their pain is at. Figure 12.4 is an example of this type of numerical rating scale.

Other types of scales are the visual analogue scale (see Figure 12.5), the verbal rating scale (Figure 12.6) and combined verbal and numerical scale (Figure 12.7). Many acute hospitals use a numerical rating score of 0–3 which links closely to the verbal descriptors none, mild, moderate and severe (Figure 12.8). In turn, these levels

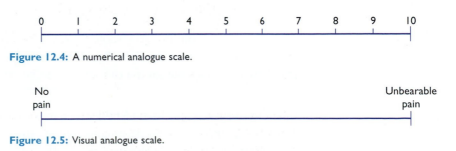

Figure 12.4: A numerical analogue scale.

Figure 12.5: Visual analogue scale.

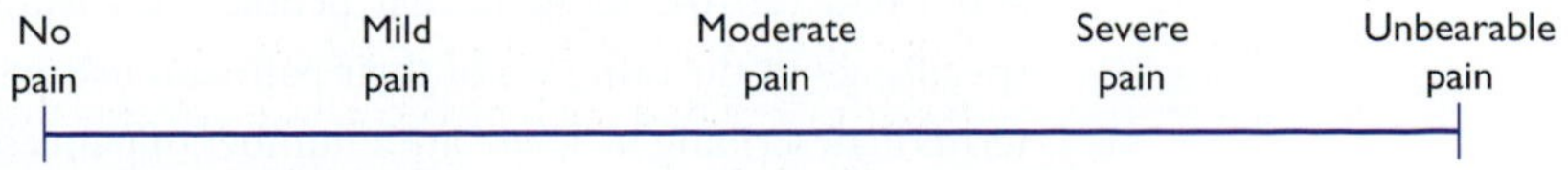

Figure 12.6: Verbal rating scale.

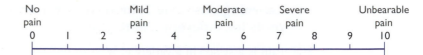

Figure 12.7: Combined verbal and numerical scale.

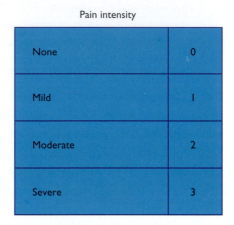

Figure 12.8: Categorical pain assessment scale.

of pain intensity may be linked to pharmacological strategies (see the next section). This combined approach tends to be the easiest to use, with some 96% of cognitively sound adults able to describe pain intensity in this way (Closs et al. 2003; Closs 2007); they are also useful for people with cognitive impairments such as Violet.

Kovach et al. (1999) developed an index of the behaviours associated with discomfort and pain in people with Alzheimer's disease. The most frequently occurring signs were tense body language, sad facial expression, fidgeting, repetitive verbalisations and verbal outbursts. Agitation, which is one of Violet's symptoms, was also listed. These behaviours have been drawn together in developing pain assessment tools for people with communication difficulties. The Abbey Pain Scale is an example of a tool for assessing pain in older people with severe cognitive impairment (Abbey et al. 2004). A copy of this scale is available on the British Pain Society website (www.britishpainsociety.org/book_pain_older_people.pdf). Using this scale together with discussion with Mr Davies would facilitate accurate assessment of whether or not Violet has pain.

ACTIVITY

Make some notes on how you would approach Violet to assess her pain, taking into account ways of communicating with people who have Alzheimer's disease and how you could explain the chosen scale to her and her husband.

Pain assessment has also been identified as a major issue with people with learning disabilities as they can struggle to communicate their pain effectively. A study by Stone-Pearn (2002), which continues to be cited by various authors, including Beacroft and Dodd (2010), suggests that people with learning difficulties tend to be non-specific about the duration of their pain and use external body locations and unusual terms in describing it. There are a number of pain assessment tools available including the FLACC Scale, which was developed for pain assessment with children, and which

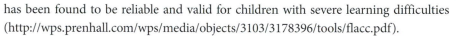

has been found to be reliable and valid for children with severe learning difficulties (http://wps.prenhall.com/wps/media/objects/3103/3178396/tools/flacc.pdf).

A fascinating service development by Kingston and Bailey (2009) describes the development of a protocol for assessing and managing pain with adults with learning difficulties. The protocol includes a 'pain story' template that enables individuals and their family to talk about their pain in a systematic and reflective manner. A visual pain diary and pictorial body chart were also trialled, amended and implemented. Maria's Community Learning Disability Nurse might be encouraged to contact the Portsmouth team who undertook this work to discuss their ideas and request a copy of the protocol.

Learning disability nurses and those working with adults with cognitive difficulties, such as those Violet experiences, should be aware of and be able to detect subtle behavioural changes which might indicate the presence of pain and distress. They need to be cautious about attributing behavioural change to cognitive impairments (McKay and Clarke 2012). In Maria's case, the focus on family involvement and liaison across the multidisciplinary team will help practitioners determine the underlying causes of behavioural change.

Body charts or verbal questions about pain location can also be useful in acute pain assessment, particularly when used with a categorical or numerical scale to provide insight into the areas that are the most painful. It is important to be aware that just because someone is complaining of pain in one area does not mean that they do not have pain elsewhere. In postoperative settings, it is not unusual for nurses to give opioids in response to a patient's complaint of pain, when the problem is a post-intubation sore throat or long-standing back pain, rather than incisional pain. Thomas may also have discomfort or pain resulting from his cannula and/or catheter. Many people with chronic pain also have multiple pain foci.

Multidimensional pain assessment

Tools for multidimensional pain assessment are useful for people with complex needs and those experiencing chronic pain. One of the best known tools is the short-form McGill Pain Questionnaire (SF-MPQ) (Melzack 1987). Through the use of descriptor words, it enables practitioners to identify the nature and quality of pain.

Another example of a multidimensional tool is the Disability Distress Assessment Tool or DisDAT (©2005 Northgate & Prudhoe NHS Trust and St Oswald's Hospice), which ends with the poignant words 'Distress may be hidden, but it is never silent'. This tool measures distress, rather than pain specifically, but it might be a useful tool for the community learning disability nurse to complete with Maria and her mother to gain an in-depth understanding of the way in which Maria is currently, or might in the future, express her distress. The findings can then be used to inform analgesic and non-pharmacological management. Violet's team might want to consider the Discomfort Scale for Dementia of the Alzheimer's Type (DS-DAT) available at http://prc.coh.org/PainNOA/DS-DAT_Tool.pdf. However, Liu et al. (2010) found that the Abbey Pain Scale was more reliable and valid in assessing osteoarthritis pain in older people, of varying cognitive abilities, when they were engaged in an exercise programme.

Psychological and coping strategies assessment

There are many tools available to assess the psychological components of pain and the ways in which people cope with their pain. These measurements are generally administered by pain experts and tend to be used with people with chronic pain. They include anxiety and depression scales, such as the PHQ-9 (http://www.patient.co.uk/doctor/patient-health-questionnaire-phq-9), coping strategy questionnaires, impact of pain on function and physical activity profiles. One that tries to capture the wide impact that pain can have is the Brief Pain Inventory.

Figure 12.9 shows the Pain Strategies Questionnaire. The tool was developed from the strategies recorded by 200 adults attending surgical outpatient clinics for the first time. The tool was then used in a randomised controlled trial to test whether identifying and supporting patients' own strategies in the hospital setting would reduce patients' postoperative anxiety, pain and distress, as well as other outcomes (Burrows 2010). The study findings are discussed later under learning outcome 6.

ACTIVITY

Complete column A of the Pain Strategies Questionnaire in Figure 12.9.

Depending on your past experience of pain, you may or may not have been aware of some of the strategies you use when in pain. We will consider how you might support patients' own strategies later in the chapter.

In summary, there are a variety of approaches to pain assessment. Each has its place with different client groups and different dimensions of pain. Whatever the approach, the response should be recorded so that it can be compared with the pain experience following an intervention. In acute pain settings, recordings should be made at rest and upon movement. As deep breathing, leg movements and mobilisation are important to postoperative recovery and the prevention of complications; it is imperative that pain does not prevent movement and rehabilitation. In chronic and palliative pain, post-intervention comparisons are likely to be more wide ranging.

ACTIVITY

Investigate what pain assessment tools are used in your locality for different client groups.

Analgesic

A drug for relieving pain ('painkiller').

Learning outcome 4: Demonstrate understanding of pharmacological approaches to managing pain

Knowledge of pharmacology and **analgesic** management may help to enhance **analgesia**, which in turn can decrease anxiety, increase functional activity, improve mood and promote comfort and sleep.

Key principles in promoting analgesia include:
- assessing pain at the beginning of each episode of care and at appropriate intervals thereafter;
- giving analgesics before or as soon as acute pain begins;

Analgesia

Another word for pain relief.

Pain Strategies Questionnaire

Many people use strategies at home to help relieve pain. We have found that if you continue to use them in hospital it can help to reduce the amount of pain you experience. Please help us to find out what you use by filling in the table below and handing this sheet to your nurse:

Please place a ✓ in column A, against all of the strategies that you use when in pain.

In column B, please place a ✓ against any of the strategies you would like to use in hospital

Strategy	Column A	Column B
None/not sure		
Painkillers (state which if known)		
Distraction, e.g. TV, reading		
Relaxation		
Breathing exercises		
Imagery (using your senses to imagine a place or experience)		
Music		
Massage		
Warmth		
Cold		
Resting alone: e.g. lying down, trying to sleep, peace and quiet PLEASE STATE WHICH		
Grin and bear, mind over matter, positive thinking		
Mobilising: e.g. walking, moving about, exercise PLEASE STATE WHICH		
Positioning: e.g. changing position, support painful area PLEASE STATE WHICH		
Treatment: e.g. seeking medical attention to treat the cause or pain, advice or information PLEASE STATE WHICH		
Reassurance: e.g. talking about the pain, physical contact with someone else, confidence in someone else PLEASE STATE WHICH		
General help with activities		
Other: PLEASE STATE WHAT		

Thank you for completing this questionnaire

Figure 12.9: Pain Strategies Questionnaire. (Reproduced from Burrows, D. 2000. *Engaging Patients in Their Own Pain Management: An Action Research Study.* Unpublished PhD thesis. Brunel University.)

- giving sufficient and regular analgesics to ensure patient comfort;
- considering drugs other than the true analgesics for chronic and neuropathic pain;
- assessing pain relief and side effects;
- balancing medication approaches with non-pharmacological strategies;
- never letting pain get out of control;
- remembering that pain is the fifth vital sign (Chronic Pain Policy Coalition 2007).

ACTIVITY **Why should you never let pain get out of control?**

You may have come up with a number of ideas, such as that it is inhumane, places patients at risk of physical and emotional complications and increases the likelihood of hospital admissions for those living in the community or residential homes.

Pharmacological management of pain is a team effort, involving the person with pain, their family, the doctor, pharmacist, nurse, physiotherapist and others. Nurses should:

- listen to patients and their relatives, demonstrating compassion;
- record patients' pain assessments, believing what they say about their pain;
- manage and evaluate pain competently and confidently;
- work with relevant members of the multidisciplinary team towards effective pain control;
- ensure that their knowledge is sufficient to achieve patient comfort;
- work to educate patients/clients and their families.

Patients should be encouraged to request pain relief and take sufficient regular and as required (p.r.n.) medication to enable them to carry out appropriate activities, readjusting dosages, if necessary. It is important to involve the family in determining medication management of pain whether in acute, chronic or palliative care settings.

ACTIVITY **Make a list of medicines used in your locality for pain relief.**

The true analgesics

The World Health Organization (WHO 1996) suggested that analgesic administration should be based on a pain ladder, where simple analgesics are used for mild pain, weak opioids for moderate pain and strong opioids for severe pain. First developed for use in cancer and palliative care, the principles have been extrapolated to acute and chronic pain management. The ladder allows for drugs from different levels of the ladder to be coprescribed and administered as patients move from one level to another. Table 12.1 gives an example of analgesics from each level of the ladder. You may also come across drugs such as co-codamol, co-dydramol and Tramacet. These drugs combine paracetamol with a weak **opioid**. While paracetamol is a relatively safe drug, opioids can have significant side effects such as respiratory depression when used postoperatively and serious effects on the immune and endocrine systems in long-term use (British Pain Society 2010).

Good practice principles advocate administration through oral and transdermal (across the skin) routes as the mode of choice for most pain medications. Transdermal patches provide continuous drug delivery over a set number of days before the patch has to be changed. Fentanyl patches are used in palliative pain management and buprenorphine patches in chronic pain management. The dose of the latter determines whether it sits as a weak or strong opioid on the ladder.

Opioids

Drugs that bind with opioid receptors in the central and peripheral nervous systems to reduce the intensity of pain signals.

Table 12.1: Examples of commonly used analgesics and their position on the ladder

Drug	Location on ladder	Administration	Side effects
Paracetamol	Simple analgesic; helpful for mild pain, but effect often underestimated; potentiates (enhances) the effect of weak and strong opioids	Adult: One/two 500 mg tablets every 4 hours; maximum 8 per day, unless otherwise directed	Rare; potentially fatal liver damage following overdose
Codeine	Weak opioid; helpful for moderate pain	Adult: 30–60 mg every 4 hours; maximum 240 mg per day	Constipation; initial drowsiness or dizziness not unusual; at least 8% of the population are unable to metabolise codeine
Tramadol	Weak opioid; helpful for moderate pain	Adult: 50–100 mg every 4–6 hours; maximum 400 mg per day	Constipation; initial drowsiness or dizziness not unusual
Morphine Oxycodone Fentanyl Tapentadol	Strong opioid	Adult: varies; discuss dose examples with qualified MDT	Most commonly nausea, vomiting; may also experience light-headedness, confusion, pruritus, constipation, respiratory depression

Studies suggest that around 20% of doctors and nurses fear that patients will become addicted to opioids (Mann and Carr 2006). In fact, hospital-prompted addiction occurs in less than 0.5% of admissions (Ferrell et al. 1992). Addiction is caused by cravings, and this is another reason why we should ensure that patients receive sufficient analgesics to be comfortable. People with long-term pain, being managed by integrated care teams, may have opioid contracts; an agreement between the patient and health professionals to ensure safe and effective use of opioids by patients.

Drugs for neuropathic pain

Transdermal Lidocaine medicated plasters and Capsaicin creams and patches are used for focal neuropathic pain including post-shingles pain and painful diabetic neuropathy. Lidocaine works by blocking sodium at the periphery and thus preventing the electrical nerve impulse from building up. Capsaicin, which is the active ingredient in chilli peppers, works as a counter irritant interfering at peripheral nerve endings with substance P, a neurotransmitter involved in pain processing. As well as being indicated for neuropathic pain, Capsaicin is also used for hand and knee osteoarthritis pain. Both Lidocaine and Capsaicin should be used for 2–4 weeks before determining whether there is any benefit. Although relatively side-effect free, concordance can be an issue as some people do not respond well to the cooling sensation of Lidocaine or the burning of Capsaicin, although others, of course, find these effects pain relieving.

The analgesic properties of certain antidepressants and antiepileptic drugs have also been found to be useful for neuropathic pain. Box 12.4 shows some

> **Box 12.4 Examples of drugs used in neuropathic pain management**
>
> - Antidepressants – Amitriptyline, Nortriptyline, Duloxetine, Venlafaxine
> - Anticonvulsants – Gabapentin, Pregabalin, Carbamazepine
> - Local anaesthetic – Lidocaine plasters
> - Rubefacients – Capsaicin

of the common antidepressants and anticonvulsants used in pain management. Amitriptyline and Nortriptyline are tricyclic antidepressants, while Duloxetine and Venlafaxine are serotonin and noradrenalin reuptake inhibitors (SNRIs) acting on central nervous system pain processing. The antiepileptic drugs Gabapentin and Pregabalin are predominantly used in chronic pain management; however, a recent meta-analysis (Clarke et al. 2012) supports their use perioperatively to reduce the incidence of long-term postsurgical pain, which is a significant issue for 10%–30% of patients (Bruce and Quinlan 2011). Carbapamazine is used for trigeminal neuralgia, a type of facial neuropathic pain.

ACTIVITY

Visit the NICE website and look at guideline 96: 'Neuropathic pain: The pharmacological management of neuropathic pain in adults in non-specialist settings, 2010, http://www.nice.org.uk/guidance/CG96
How would you manage Maria's painful diabetic neuropathy pharmacologically?

Drugs for inflammatory pain

Non-steroidal anti-inflammatory drugs (NSAIDs) reduce inflammation and are effective for mild to moderate pain. They are available in oral, transdermal and topical preparations. They are commonly used postoperatively in combination with analgesics and are also the drug of choice in conditions such as arthritis and some other chronic pain conditions. Ibuprofen 400 mg and Diclofenac 50 mg have been shown to be as effective as 10 mg intramuscular morphine in the treatment of acute pain (McQuay and Moore 1998). Side effects include gastric irritation, bleeding and renal failure. More recently, evidence of the cardiovascular risks of Diclofenac 100–150 mg has been identified, while Naproxen was associated with a lower risk (McGettigan and Henry 2013). Nurses need to be conscious that a past history of asthma, gastritis, ulcers, kidney problems, myocardial infarction and stroke may exclude an individual from using NSAIDs and be observant for side effects.

Violet has osteoarthritis in her right hip and knee; this can cause pain on movement and gradually worsen towards the end of the day. NSAIDs, such as Naproxen, could be effective in combatting her pain, allowing her to mobilise more easily and perhaps decrease her agitation.

ACTIVITY

Make a list of the different medications you think might help Maria and Violet. Look up these drugs and understand their effects, side effects, doses and how long they should be given prior to review. You might find the article by Huizinga and Peltier (2007) useful when thinking of Maria.

Other routes for administering analgesia

There are a variety of other routes for administering pain relief over and above oral and transdermal routes. Some of these are explained below.

Patient-Controlled Analgesia (PCA) is an approach to pain management in which the patient controls the dose and frequency of analgesic up to a predetermined limit. When practitioners refer to PCA, they generally mean the intravenous system that delivers opioids, such as morphine or Fentanyl when the patient presses a demand button. These systems are most commonly used in surgical settings and their management is covered by local protocols that include the administration of oxygen to minimise respiratory depression.

Epidurals are another route for administration, involving the infusion of a local anaesthetic, with or without an opioid, through a fine catheter into the **epidural space** (Middleton 2006). Reviews indicate that epidural analgesia tends to provide better pain relief than PCA or oral opioids in the immediate postoperative period (Nishimori et al. 2007; Werawatganon and Charuluxanun 2007).

> **Epidural space**
>
> The space between the spinal canal and dura mater.

> **ACTIVITY**
>
> Look up your local protocols for PCA and epidural. List the recordings that must be made by nurses and state why. Think about how the epidural protocol applies to Thomas.

Entonox is a 50:50 mixture of nitrous oxide and oxygen delivered through a hand-held mask or mouthpiece. If the patient becomes drowsy, as a consequence of the drug, their hand and therefore the delivery set will fall away. As such, entonox is another form of PCA. It should not be used by people with Vitamin B12 deficiency and caution should be applied to those at risk of deficiency (MacIntyre et al. 2010). It is effective for mild to moderate, short-lasting pain and is used by paramedics, in emergency care, for procedural pain and during labour. MacIntyre et al. (2010) recommend that entonox is avoided during early pregnancy, 'although this will depend on the relative harm of alternative methods' (p. 83).

Syringe drivers should be considered when oral or transdermal routes are no longer feasible for those approaching end of life. Syringe drivers involve a fine needle being inserted just under the skin of the abdomen or arm, attached to tubing, which in turn is attached to the pump. Analgesics, such as diamorphine, are made up to a 24-hour dose and delivered via the syringe driver so that the individual receives a continuous dose. Other medications such as anti-emetics can also be added.

> **ACTIVITY**
>
> Access the National End of Life Care Programme at http://www.endoflifecare.nhs.uk/. Have a look at the resource packs
> - 'Care Towards the End of Life for People with Dementia'.
> - 'The Route to Success in End of Life Care – Achieving Quality for People with Learning Disabilities'.
>
> Write some notes on the ideas you have for managing pain with people who have dementia or learning disabilities and are coming to the end of their lives. How might you involve their families?

Both documents emphasise that identifying and managing pain and distress (both physical and mental) are crucial. They also recommend the use of the Abbey Pain Scale and the DisDAT referred to earlier.

Resources

Many resources are available to help nurses develop their pharmacological knowledge. These include standard pharmacological and pain management texts, specialist texts such as those by MacIntyre et al. (2010), websites such as the British National Formulary (BNF) site (www.bnf.com), pharmaceutical literature, journal articles and nursing, medical and pharmacist colleagues. Understanding the way a drug works can be a rewarding addition to a nurse's knowledge base and practice.

Learning outcome 5: Explore non-pharmacological approaches to managing pain

While pain-relieving medications can modify the pain processing systems so as to reduce pain intensity and distress, they should not be the only approach in managing the biopsychosocial complexity of pain.

Heat and cold are useful non-pharmacological pain-relieving strategies. Heat can be comforting, improving blood flow and relaxing muscles. It should not be used for acute pain as it can increase swelling. In these instances, ice might be used, although neither should be applied directly over wounds as they can interfere with healing. There are also cautions expressed over the use of heat for cancer pain as tumour growth is a possibility and in body areas where sensation is altered, such as with painful diabetic neuropathy.

In a small randomised controlled trial, Yilidrim et al. (2010) found that 20 minutes of heat application every second day improved pain stiffness and physical function in people with osteoarthritis of the knee. Given that usual recommendations are 15–20 minutes 3–4 times daily, these results suggest that heat may be an under-used resource in pain management. Demir and Khorshid (2010) found that cold packs helped to reduce pain during and after chest drain removal and recommend its use for procedural pain.

Heat can be applied using covered hot water bottles, wheat bags, heat pads, disposable single use wraps and creams and via warm baths and showers. Cold tends to be applied for 5–10 minutes 3–4 times daily using ice packs, cold packs and cold gels. With both approaches, care should always be taken to ensure the skin is protected against burns.

Information and education are important to increase understanding and reduce anxiety. Studies indicate that it can also reduce postoperative and cancer pain, with the most recent meta-analysis suggesting that educational interventions in the management of cancer pain may be more effective than medication management (Bennett et al. 2009).

In chronic pain, management resources such as the Pain Toolkit (http://www.paintoolkit.org/) are available to aid self-management. A recent survey found that of the 12 strategies, patients found the most useful to be activity pacing, acceptance of the long-term nature of the pain condition, being patient with oneself, stretching and exercising and learning to prioritise and plan (Sanderson and Cole 2011).

ACTIVITY

- Go to the Pain Toolkit website at http://www.paintoolkit.org/ and read about the different self-management strategies.
  - Could Maria and Violet benefit from any of these approaches and, if so, how might they be put into practice in residential and group settings?
  - *Consider:* Could Violet's husband be able to make use of any of the approaches with Violet at home?
  - How do these strategies help to counteract the biopsychosocial experience of pain?

- Next, have a look at the following link to the NHS Institution for Innovation and Improvement. Available from: http://www.institute.nhs.uk/quality_and_service_improvement_tools/quality_and_service_improvement_tools/enhanced_recovery_programme.html (Accessed on 21 February 2013). quality_and_service_improvement_tools/quality_and_service_improvement_tools/enhanced_recovery_programme.html
  - What information might Thomas benefit from preoperatively?
  - How might this help him manage any pain and distress postoperatively?
  - How does this fit with his biopsychosocial experience of pain outlined earlier in this chapter?

Self-generated strategies (i.e. those developed by the individual, rather than being taught) can be useful in reducing postoperative pain, distress, anxiety and opioid consumption (Burrows 2000; Burrows and Taylor 2009). The caring role of the nurse in the context of people using self-generated strategies is to support people in using their strategies effectively when the experience of illness and a strange environment may disrupt their expertise. This may mean being compassionate to the person's needs by simply giving them permission to use the technique, being confident in offering ideas on how to adapt the strategy to a clinical setting, being committed to reminding the person to use their strategy and/or being competent to work with patients to rehearse and use their techniques. Table 12.2 outlines some of the approaches that Burrows and coworkers (2000, 2009) found; Thomas might make use of strategies such as distraction, relaxation and positioning but may need support and reassurance in doing so postoperatively.

TENS (transcutaneous electrical nerve stimulation) is a form of electrotherapy that is used in both acute and chronic pain management. A small battery-powered device delivers an electric current via adhesively attached electrodes, with the aim of blocking the pain messages to the brain and, in low-frequency TENS, of producing the body's natural painkillers: endorphins. The latter can produce analgesia for 5 minutes to 18 hours post-stimulation. Breaks between treatments are advised to reduce **habituation** in long-term use (Wright 2012). TENS is not recommended as a

Habituation

This is where the nervous system becomes accustomed to the stimulation resulting in reduced pain relief.

Table 12.2: Examples of supporting patients in using their own pain-relieving strategies

Identify the strategies the person uses	Understand how the strategy works	Work with the person to enable them to use their strategy in the clinical setting
Distraction	Focusing on something other than pain Useful for brief periods Can increase perception of self-control and reduce pain intensity	May include watching TV, reading, listening to music, visits from family and friends. For example: if a patient says they watch television help them to the day room
Relaxation	Directs attention away from pain Useful for mild to moderate pain Can reduce muscle tension, distress, anxiety and fatigue	Find out the person's technique and support them with it if asked Ensure periods of relative peace and quiet to enable them to use the strategy. Teach short and long techniques
Imagery	Using imagination to create mental pictures: directs attention away from pain by imaging sights, sounds, odours, taste and touch (e.g. a garden on a warm summer's day). Can alter pain experience	Find out the person's preferred image and talk them through it if asked. Ensure periods of relative peace and quiet to enable them to use the strategy
Warmth	Promotes relaxation and comfort, reduces muscle tension	Hot water bottles cannot be used in hospital settings for safety reasons Wheat packs, heat pads and wraps, warm water, baths and showers are alternatives
Cold	May help reduce inflammatory pain Should not be used over wounds, as cold will decrease healing rate	Provide cold flannels, water, ice or cold packs and gels. Even better, in the clinical area, show the patient/family where to access them
Positioning	Eases stiffness and enhances comfort	Help the person to adopt the most comfortable position, using own special pillows or cushions Encourage changes of position

sole treatment but should rather be used in combination with other pharmacological and non-pharmacological strategies.

A systematic review by Walsh et al. (2009) found that only one of six studies examined showed TENS to be significantly superior to placebo, but it can have adjunct benefits as identified in a meta-analysis by Bjordal et al. (2003) who concluded that use of TENS reduced the need for analgesics postoperatively. In chronic pain management, research outcomes on the use of TENS are more equivocal, although Bennett et al. (2011) point out that many of the primary studies are methodologically poor. Nevertheless, Dubinsky and Miyasaki (2010) found some evidence for the use of TENS to treat painful diabetic neuropathy; hence, it could be considered for Maria with careful explanation.

There are a number of contraindications and cautions to the use of TENS, which are succinctly outlined by Wright (2012).

Relaxation is a form of pain management that aims to reduce the physical and mental tension that enhances pain and pain perception. It is not 'relaxing in front of the TV', rather it must be purposeful. There are a variety of techniques such as breathing, imagery and meditation, among others. A systematic review by Kwekkeboom and Gretarsdottir (2006) found evidence of effect for progressive muscle relaxation for arthritis pain and a systematic relaxation intervention for postoperative pain. Morone and Greco (2007) also found support for progressive muscle relaxation for osteoarthritis pain, as well as for guided imagery. In both reviews, many of the primary studies were methodologically weak. Relaxation is often thought to be quite personal, with some individuals preferring one method over another; it maybe that this also influences the studies.

ACTIVITY

Visit NHS Choices at
http://www.nhs.uk/Conditions/stress-anxiety-depression/Pages/ways-relieve-stress.aspx
(Accessed on 14 September 2012). Although this page is about stress, anxiety and depression, the relaxation techniques described can also be used for pain.

There are many other non-pharmacological approaches, some of which you are likely to come across during your nursing studies. Not all strategies are appropriate for all people, in all situations. Those with neuropathic pain may actively avoid massage and touch because of altered sensation. Touch is considered further in the next section on comfort. In summary:

ACTIVITY

Look again at the list of factors that may be influencing Violet's pain perception. What strategies might be used to counter these?

You might have thought of:
- supporting Mr Davies in his role of being a carer, for example, by referring him to the resources of the Carers Trust, www.carers.org. You might want to go onto the site yourself and type 'pain' into the search box to see what you come up with;
- ensuring that Violet has familiar objects around her;
- using a mix of pharmacological and non-pharmacological pain and comfort measures to help her relax, reducing muscle tension, agitation and pain;
- increasing cognitive control by providing information about the techniques you are using in an understandable format, perhaps using pictures as well as verbal explanations.

For most patients, the most effective approach to pain management is to listen to what the person and their families say about his/her pain and its effect on their home, leisure and work activities; to work with the multidisciplinary team, individual and his/her family to combine pharmacological and non-pharmacological strategies; and to monitor the effectiveness of pain relief with all involved.

Children: practice points – pain management

Effective pain assessment and management are essential for infants and children. There are pain assessment charts specifically developed for use with children so, if working with children, ensure that you seek out guidance about using your organisation's pain assessment tool for children. Many of the pain management techniques discussed in this section are used for children too, including distraction, relaxation and guided imagery as well as analgesics, but all will need to be administered appropriately depending on the child's age and development stage, with analgesics prescribed according to weight.

For further information see:

Dickin, L. and Green, H. 2010. Pain assessment and management. In: Glasper, A., Aylott, M., Battrick, C. (Eds) *Developing Practical Skills for Nursing Children and Young People*. London: Hodder Arnold, 277–294

The Royal College of Nursing's resource for recognizing and assessing acute pain in children:

http://www.rcn.org.uk/development/practice/pain

Pregnancy and birth: practice points – pain management

- No medications for pain are guaranteed to be safe in pregnancy.
- Paracetamol is believed to be safe.
- Morphine may be beneficial to the mother but will affect the baby – foetal opioid dependency.
- For neuropathic pain, the only drug which has no evidence of causing damage to the foetus is amitriptyline. However, lack of evidence does not mean it is safe.
- Pregnant women may rely on non-pharmacological pain relief such as keeping active, warm baths, relaxation techniques, deep breathing and back massages, to assuage their discomfort.
- Always seek expert advice.

Women experiencing miscarriage or undergoing termination of pregnancy for foetal abnormality are often cared for in gynaecology or general wards. Without doubt, most will experience discomfort or pain adding significantly to their emotional distress. A compassionate approach is essential, and nurses should do everything they can to relieve pain and promote comfort.

If a recently delivered ill mother and/or baby are admitted to the general healthcare setting, then rest and adequate sleep are vital for their recovery. Staff should consider caesarean section or perineal wounds when assessing these mothers' pain scores. Pharmaceutical or medical advice should be sought regarding safety of medications in breastfeeding mothers.

Summary

- Pain is a subjective, multidimensional experience, unique to each individual.
- Nurses need to differentiate between the terms 'pain threshold', 'pain tolerance' and 'pain behaviour'.
- Effective pain assessment is the key to successful pain management, and pain assessment tools can facilitate communication about pain.
- Pain management comprises both pharmacological and non-pharmacological approaches.

PROMOTING COMFORT

People can usually promote their own comfort, but when they are unwell, physically or mentally, particularly when outside their own environment, their usual ways of seeking comfort may not be possible. Promoting comfort is closely aligned with compassion as it requires nurses to recognise and respond to a person's distress by taking action to alleviate discomfort and promote comfort.

LEARNING OUTCOMES

By the end of this section, you will be able to:

1 discuss the nature of comfort care;
2 reflect on how presence and developing relationships can provide comfort;
3 consider how touch can be used in comfort care;
4 explore how verbal interactions can be used to promote comfort;
5 select physical actions that can be used to promote comfort;
6 integrate comfort care skills in different circumstances.

Learning outcome 1: Discuss the nature of comfort care

There are many situations where comfort care is necessary.

ACTIVITY

Review the scenarios at the start of this chapter. What discomfort might these people experience and why?

- Violet appears to be suffering discomfort which might be emotional due to her change of environment and her mental condition. However, she might also have physical discomfort as she could be in pain due to her osteoarthritis or she may need to pass urine but be unable to express this verbally. She could be too hot or too cold, or hungry or thirsty. It is important not to make assumptions about the reasons underlying discomfort.
- Thomas has had major surgery for a serious health condition. Postoperatively, he could experience physical discomfort not only associated with pain and his wound but also due to the various tubes attached to his body which could restrict his movement, and the strangeness of the ileostomy bag. Having such major surgery would have been a big decision for Thomas and he may experience emotional discomfort relating to the significant change to his body and bowel function.

- Maria obviously has discomfort due to the pain caused by her peripheral neuropathy. She is likely to have emotional discomfort due to this new complication, and associated anxiety.

Discomfort is often associated with hospitalisation, as well as the procedures related to diagnosis or treatment (Williams et al. 2009), and people with health issues within the community often experience discomfort too, as illustrated in Violet's and Maria's scenarios. Williams et al. (2008) found that physical discomfort led to patients not feeling valued, which could affect their dignity. Williams and Irurita (2006) found that emotional discomfort exacerbated physical discomfort and involved feelings such as fear, frustration, sadness, worry, anger, stress, anxiety and embarrassment. Emotional comfort was defined by patients as positive feelings including optimism, happiness and being high in spirit; a central feature was found to be personal control, the ability to influence situations or the environment, which enhanced feelings of worth and self-esteem (Williams and Irurita 2006).

Promoting comfort is a fundamental skill all nurses need to develop; Hudacek (2008) found that providing comfort is one of the seven dimensions of professional nursing practice. Comfort care involves actions to promote comfort; for some people, total comfort may not be possible, due to the effects of illness or surgery, so the aim is then to promote comfort as far as possible using different approaches. Kolkaba (1995, 2003) has developed theories of comfort and applied these to care in different settings. She asserts that when comfort care is successful, patients feel well cared for and comforted because the care was efficient, individualised, targeted to the whole person and creative. Wilby (2005) found that when patients felt comforted, they were more relaxed and better able to accept their situation. She also identified actions that were discomforting, which included treating patients as though they were unimportant, ordering patients to do things, forgetting to do things for patients and giving inaccurate information.

ACTIVITY

Reflect on a situation where you comforted someone in distress: what personal qualities did you use?

The qualities of staff that promote comfort include kindness, gentleness and friendliness (Tutton and Seers 2004) and concern and compassion (Wilby 2005). Williams and Irurita (2004) found that competent staff, who portrayed ability and confidence, promoted emotional comfort by helping patients to feel secure.

An individualised and holistic approach is necessary for promoting comfort. For example, Roche-Fahy and Dowling (2009) found that a holistic approach with attention to emotional, spiritual, psychosocial and family needs, along with physical needs, helped to provide comfort for palliative care patients. In a care home, Bland (2007) identified that what constituted comfort and how it could be attained was different for each individual resident.

ACTIVITY

Reflect on a practice situation where a person needed comfort. What did you do to:
1 find out what would provide comfort for the person as an individual?
2 help the person to feel that you were interested in them as an individual?

Using effective communication skills, particularly listening and questioning skills, is key to understanding what will be comforting to an individual person and to help people to feel that you are interested in them; Chapter 2 addresses these skills in detail.

ACTIVITY

Maria's scenario mentions that she experiences distressing pain during the night. What could the staff do to promote Maria's comfort?

The staff could try to be with Maria as much as possible – 'being there' or 'presence' is well recognised as a comfort strategy. The unit staff will have an established relationship with Maria, which she should derive comfort from; they will also know how best to comfort Maria, for example, they may know that she finds touch comforting. The staff could talk to Maria and explain why her legs are painful; the community healthcare team will therefore need to educate the care home staff about peripheral neuropathy and how they can best explain this to Maria. The staff should administer prescribed analgesics and use other non-pharmacological pain-relieving strategies, as discussed earlier in this chapter, and monitor the effect of these. The staff should promote Maria's general physical comfort, ensuring that she is in a comfortable position, and check whether she has any other needs, such as a drink. Thus, in promoting comfort for Maria, staff would use:

- presence and their relationship with her;
- touch;
- verbal interactions;
- physical actions.

The next sections look at each of these ways of promoting comfort in more detail.

Learning outcome 2: Reflect on how presence and developing relationships can provide comfort

Presence is about 'being there' with someone who is in distress and needs comfort. Zerwekh's (1997) description of presence suggests planned, professional nursing action – 'presencing' is defined as a fundamental nursing intervention involving 'deliberate focused attention, receptivity to the other person, and persistent awareness of the other's shared humanity' (p. 261) Mottram (2009) found that trust in the health professional promoted comfort for day surgery patients and she described 'befriending', conveyed through empathic understanding and practical support, from which patients received emotional comfort and reassurance. Conversely, Bundgaard and Nielsen (2011) found that for patients undergoing endoscopy, a lack of nursing presence was associated with feelings of insecurity and discomfort.

Studies in various care settings have confirmed that the presence of nurses is a source of comfort (Cantrell and Matula 2009; Mottram 2009; Fridh et al. 2009).

Williams et al. (2008) found that patients felt more secure when they perceived that assistance was available to them when it was needed. While nurses are present with a patient, they can monitor their condition, observing and checking the person's mental and/or physical condition, asking about symptoms and assessing pain, as described earlier in this chapter. Williams and Irurita (2004) found that staff promoted emotional comfort through spending time with patients, getting to know them as people and making frequent contact. In a day surgery based study, Mottram (2009) highlighted that presence needs to be not just physical but actual engagement with the patient – listening and showing an interest. While some patients preferred a constant presence of the nurse, others were content with a nurse being close by. The patients identified that the presence of nurses was a therapeutic, comforting experience and some appreciated continuity of the nurse during their day surgery stay (Mottram 2009).

Rasin and Kautz (2007) emphasised the importance of staff getting to know residents with dementia, as person-centred knowledge led to staff being able to anticipate needs and know when something was 'not right'. The care home staff will need to get to know Violet as a person so that they can promote her comfort during her stay. Alzheimer's Society (2013) has developed a leaflet 'This is me', which when completed by the person with dementia and their family, provides a useful communication tool for staff to quickly find out about a person with dementia and their preferences. The care home staff could invite Mr Davies to complete 'This is me' with Violet.

ACTIVITY

Think about when you have sat with someone who was distressed, either in the healthcare setting or in everyday life. Were you comfortable doing this or was it difficult in any way?

It is not always easy to be with someone who is in distress, particularly if you are unable to fully relieve their discomfort. If someone has received bad news, perhaps about a serious diagnosis or death of a loved one, nothing you can say or do can take that away. The group home staff may find it quite distressing to sit with Maria during the night if she is in pain. Nurses often feel more comfortable when they can 'put things right': relieve mental distress, pain, vomiting or breathlessness. If they are unable to do this, being present with a person who, despite medication and other measures, continues to express feelings of hopelessness and is in pain, vomiting or acutely breathless, can engender feelings of helplessness. Nevertheless, nurses should be aware that their presence will be comforting for the person, even though it may be an uncomfortable situation for the nurse. The presence of a relative or friend (rather than a nurse) can be the best source of comfort for patients. When relatives or friends are providing comfort by being present, nurses should then support them to be with their loved one, remembering that they may find it difficult to be there.

Learning outcome 3: Consider the use of touch in comfort care

The use of touch to comfort is well supported by research (Fridh et al. 2009; Mottram 2009; Picco et al. 2010; Bundgaard and Nielsen 2011). There are two main types of touch used in nursing care: instrumental (or procedural) touch and comforting touch:

Instrumental touch is used while carrying out nursing actions such as repositioning someone or recording their pulse manually. This type of touch is diminishing as care increasingly uses technology, for example, electronic blood pressure measurement equipment. Bundgaard and Nielsen (2011) found that patients undergoing endoscopy-associated technical skills with the nurses' touch as if the skills were performed safely and properly, patients quickly developed trust in the nurse.

Comforting touch is used intentionally to comfort a person through putting an arm around a patient's shoulder or holding their hand. In Bundgaard and Nielsen's (2011) study, patients found that comforting touch helped in developing trust and confidence in the nurse and helped patients to feel secure, one patient saying: 'I need to know that someone is watching over me, I may need a hand to hold, so that I feel their presence and know that they will take care of me' (p. 37). Box 1.1 gives an example of how both instrumental touch (used to assist with washing and dressing) and comforting touch (touching the shoulder) were used to comfort one of this chapter's authors following her surgery.

Comforting touch can be combined with other comfort measures such as presence; for example, Bundgaard and Nielsen (2011) found that for patients undergoing endoscopy, touch conveyed presence. Touch can also be combined with assessment and monitoring of a patient's condition; for example, if Thomas was in distress, the nurses looking after him could observe his breathing while holding his hand, to comfort him. In Bundgaard and Nielsen's (2011) study, nurses described how, while holding patients' hands, they monitored patients' responses. For example, they could feel anxiety or calmness.

ACTIVITY

- Think back to a recent experience when you were comforting someone: did you use touch? If so, how did you use it? Reflect on how comfortable you feel about using touch to comfort.
- Now, ask three close family members or friends: how would they feel about nurses using touch to comfort them. Compare their responses.

People vary in how comfortable they feel about using and receiving touch; some people are much more 'touchy' than others. Some nurses use touch a great deal and feel comfortable to use touch in a variety of ways, while others shy away from using touch. Indeed, in the study by Picco et al. (2010), some nurses reported that they rarely used touch to comfort. In an article in *The Observer*, Colin Ludlow (2008) recalled how, when feeling 'fretful, feverish and frightened' in the intensive care unit, he asked for his wife to sit with him for comfort but that, as the message never reached her, he remained alone. He described how he asked the nurses if they would hold his hand for a few moments to 'calm and settle him'. Although the nurses were 'tremendously caring' and carried out physical actions like putting a cold compress on his forehead, the request appeared to embarrass the nurses as rather than holding his hand, they replied 'When I've finished this' or 'When I've done that' but he could not recall any of them holding his hand as he had asked. It seemed that Ludlow yearned for a comforting touch but he perceived that the nurses felt uncomfortable about using touch, while being attentive to physical comfort care actions. In contrast, in Arman and Rehnsfeldt's (2007) study, a patient described how a particular nurse was a comfort: 'She would sit and hold my hand when I was sad and in tears. It makes such a difference' (p. 378).

While many people respond well to touch as a means to comfort them, nurses should be sensitive to any non-verbal cues that indicate patients do not want to be touched. In some care situations, use of touch could be misconstrued, and some people might view touch as an invasion of privacy and personal space. Touch has cultural significance and also has different meanings and rules according to the gender of those involved. In Gleeson and Higgins's (2009) study, mental health nurses emphasised the importance of respecting clients' personal space, therefore taking care in using touch with people who the nurses did not know, clients who were experiencing psychosis and those from different cultural backgrounds. Gleeson and Higgins (2009) suggest that mental health nurses need to be careful in the use of touch; for example, being sensitive to how male nurses touching female clients might be perceived. Maria's carers will know how she responds to touch as a means of comfort. Violet's husband can explain to care home staff how best to comfort Violet and whether she responds well to touch.

As with any care, you should evaluate the effect, so observe for responses to touch. For example, if a nurse attempts to use comforting touch with Violet, does she become calmer or more agitated? Does she grasp the nurse's hand tightly or snatch her hand away? In some situations, it is appropriate to ask: 'Would you like to hold my hand during this (procedure)?'

Learning outcome 4: Explore how verbal interactions can promote comfort

Tutton and Seers (2004) found that nurses' interpersonal approach to patients was central in promoting comfort and, as discussed in Chapter 2, interpersonal skills comprise verbal and non-verbal communication.

ACTIVITY — Reflect on a situation in practice where you comforted a patient or family member. What verbal interactions did you use?

Consider your responses, as you continue to read this section: what type of interactions did you use?

Hawley (2000) identified four types of comforting talk which emergency unit patients described nurses using:

- *Reassuring talk* – phrases like 'Don't worry, we'll take care of you';
- *Coaching talk* – helps patients to stay in control and cope with pain and anxiety;
- *Explanatory talk* – giving information about what is happening and answering questions;
- *Empathetic talk* – conveys understanding and caring, for example, 'I understand this is really hard for you – I am so sorry'.

A pattern of talk – 'comfort talk' – has been identified (Morse and Proctor 1998), which nurses use to help patients get through difficult situations or painful procedures. This appears to be what Hawley (2000) referred to as 'coaching'. Comfort talk is slow and rhythmic, with short simple sentences and uses phrases such as 'We're almost there', 'You're doing well' along with other emotionally supportive statements (Proctor et al. 1996). Morse and Proctor (1998) suggested that comfort talk helps patients to endure the situation, allows an information exchange and communicates a sense of caring. They emphasised that nurses' comfort talk is accompanied by being face-to-face with the patient, holding the patient's hand and focusing on their eyes.

The comforting effect of appropriate verbal interactions is supported by a number of studies. Palliative care nurses expressed that to promote mental comfort, they would sit with the patient, talking to them and addressing any anxieties through explanations (Roche-Fahy and Dowling 2009). Williams and Irurita (2004) found that explaining openly and honestly about what to expect and being encouraging provided emotional comfort for patients, as did 'chit-chat' and social conversation. Wilby (2005) highlighted that the way explanations are given can be as important as the content, so you should be aware of the tone used during your verbal communication. Techniques to promote relaxation, such as guided imagery and distraction, also use verbal interactions; these strategies were discussed in relation to pain relief earlier in this chapter.

Learning outcome 5: Select and apply physical actions for promoting comfort

Appropriate physical actions play an important role in comfort as highlighted in several research studies. Wilby (2005) found that, to achieve physical comfort, the relief of physical symptoms (especially pain) is necessary. Roche-Fahy and Dowling (2009) identified that in palliative care, physical comfort was important, and it was promoted through actions such as repositioning, personal hygiene and pain control. The way in which physical comfort measures are carried out will affect how they are perceived, and physical actions can be combined with other aspects of comfort care: presence, touch and verbal interactions.

ACTIVITY

What physical actions have you used in practice, or seen used, to promote comfort?

There are a wide range of physical actions that can help promote people's comfort.

- *Administering medicines.* Obvious examples include analgesics (see earlier in this chapter), anti-emetics (to prevent nausea and vomiting), antipyretics (to reduce high temperature) and bronchodilators (via nebulisers or inhalers) to reduce dyspnoea. However, many other prescribed medicines also reduce discomfort from unpleasant symptoms. Examples include drugs to regulate the heart rate and rhythm, thus stopping palpitations, and antibiotics which relieve fever-related symptoms such as headache, aching and malaise by treating infection.
- *Repositioning.* Assisting a breathless person into a sitting position well supported by pillows or in a chair, turning people to provide relief from pressure and positioning limbs to prevent contractures are all examples of using repositioning to promote comfort. Positioning for both Thomas and Maria will be important in relieving physical discomfort.

- *Providing a comfortable bed.* For a person who is in bed for all or part of the day, a comfortable bed and appropriate bedding are fundamental. A comfortable, pressure-relieving mattress should be provided (see Chapter 6). Clean, unwrinkled bed-linen, covers that are not too hot, too heavy or too cold, and sufficient supportive pillows are all essential.
- *Assisting with hygiene.* Wilby (2005) found that people were comforted by being helped with hygiene care. Chapter 8 covers all aspects of this in detail, and attention should be paid to mouth care, hair care and shaving, as well as the skin. Hygiene is an important comfort measure for people who are vomiting. Teeth cleaning, mouthwashes, hand and face washes, and changing of clothes can help patients feel more comfortable.
- *Assisting with elimination.* Incontinence causes both physical and psychological discomfort. Chapter 9 looks in detail at assisting people with elimination, and promoting continence and managing incontinence in ways that promote comfort.
- *Providing food and drink.* Hunger and thirst cause discomfort, as you will almost certainly have experienced yourself. Chapter 10 looks in detail at how to assist people with eating and drinking. Wilby (2005) found that people were comforted by being helped with eating. For people who are 'nil by mouth' (like Thomas was postoperatively), it is important to explain why they cannot eat and drink and to offer mouthwashes to reduce the discomfort of a dry mouth.
- *Modifying the environment.* You need to observe whether the environment is too hot or too cold for the people you are caring for, and modify the temperature where possible. Remember, patients who lack mobility can quickly become cold and may need a blanket around them while sitting. Nurses should reduce excessive or unpleasant noise, for example, avoid banging waste bin lids. Music can be comforting (Lee et al. 2005; Leow et al. 2010), as can a pleasant décor, plants and pictures. For Violet, having some familiar items from home, such as framed photos, could be comforting. The psychological environment in which care takes place is also important for comfort; a calm, confident and relaxed atmosphere where there is good teamwork can all engender comfort for patients.

In many instances, people may not request the physical actions listed above owing to communication difficulties or because they feel unable to ask, so nurses must be proactive in assessing people's needs for these comfort measures.

Learning outcome 6: Integrate comfort care skills in different circumstances

The previous sections discussed different skills to promote comfort, but integrating skills is often more effective in comfort care. Competent physical actions are fundamental aspects of a nurse's role, but to provide comfort these need to be integrated with presence, touch and verbal interactions. These latter measures are the ones that nurses often feel they do not have time for, but the art of comfort care is about smoothly integrating comfort during other nursing actions.

One way in which comfort care can be integrated is through 'intentional rounding'.

Intentional rounds ('care rounds', 'comfort rounds')

'Intentional rounding', also known as 'care rounds' or 'comfort rounds', is a way of promoting comfort, as well as possibly patient safety (Kings College London 2012). Intentional rounds involve a nurse going to each patient every 1 or 2 hours to check on four key elements – the four Ps: **positioning** – making sure the patient is comfortable and assessing pressure ulcer risk; addressing any **personal needs**, such as taking the patient to the toilet; **pain assessment**; and **placement** – making sure the patient can reach everything they need (Kings College London 2012). Other elements of intentional rounds are that: the nurse starts with an introduction that puts the patient at ease; assesses the care environment, for example, the temperature, any fall hazards; asks the patient 'Is there anything else I can do for you before I go?'; informs the patient when the next round is. The nurse must document the round: what time it took place, and any actions taken. In some settings, depending on local protocols, a student nurse or nursing assistant may carry out these rounds, and they must report any necessary follow-up actions, such as the need for analgesics, to a registered nurse.

ACTIVITY

From the description above, reflect on your practice experience: have you seen intentional rounding being used? If so, what were patients' responses to intentional rounding? What benefits might there be, both for patient comfort and care quality?

From the evidence available, Kings College London (2012) identified possible benefits as: better pain management, decreased falls, reduction in pressure ulcers and increased patient satisfaction. In relation to comfort, the regular presence of a nurse, the interactions and the potential to build up a relationship will promote comfort as well as the actions to promote physical comfort. The practice of proactively checking on patients on a regular basis, rather than responding to needs reactively, is not new, but what is more recent is the supporting evidence and standardised ways of conducting intentional rounds.

ACTIVITY

While Thomas is in the HDU, there will be nurses close by nearly all the time. When he is transferred to the surgical ward, how might intentional rounding make him more comfortable?

Patients who have been in a high dependency area with a constant nurse presence can feel anxious when they transfer to a busy ward where the staff:patient ratio is lower. If the admitting nurse explains to Thomas when a nurse will be coming round to check if he is comfortable, has any personal needs and can reach everything he needs, he is likely to feel reassured that although there will not be a nurse there all the time, a nurse will attend to him regularly.

Children: practice points – comfort

Parents (or usual carers) are the most important presence for children and know how best to comfort their child. They are encouraged to stay with their child in hospital; care should be family-centred with nurses supporting the whole family and providing comfort during what is likely to be an anxious, stressful time. Cantrell and Matula (2009) found that children and young people with cancer were comforted by being treated as individuals with interests, not only people with cancer; simply being asked how they were doing was comforting.

Summary

- Promoting comfort is a key role of nurses in many different settings and is fundamental to a caring approach.
- Promoting comfort requires a holistic approach and the integration of presence and building a relationship, touch, verbal interactions and physical actions, encompassing a range of skills and knowledge, as applicable for each individual.

PROMOTING SLEEP

Sleep is a state of rest during which our eyes close, muscles and nerves relax and our mind becomes unconscious. It is something that we all need, no matter what our age, colour or creed. It can also be something we crave.

LEARNING OUTCOMES

By the end of this section, you will be able to:

1 reflect on the importance of sleep for health;
2 examine factors that may affect sleep for people with acute and long-term health conditions;
3 apply a range of strategies to promote sleep for people with health needs.

Learning outcome 1: Reflect on the importance of sleep for health

ACTIVITY

On a scale of 0–10, how happy are you with your sleep?

0 _____ 10

Totally happy
with my sleep

Totally unhappy
with my sleep

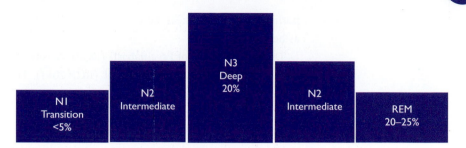

Figure 12.10: Sleep cycle showing the different stages.

Through your biology reading, you will have learned that there are different types and stages of sleep. For us to be satisfied with our sleep, each type and stage needs to be experienced in full during a sleep cycle. Sleep cycles last 90–120 minutes, and we will have several of them during each period of normal sleep. Figure 12.10 shows how the stages of sleep follow each other during a single sleep cycle.

You may have found in your reading that the stages were talked of as 1, 2, 3 and 4, with stage 2 being called light sleep; however, these were reclassified as in Figure 12.10 in 2007 (Iber et al. 2007). The two N2 stages equate to 40%–50% of sleep in total.

Sleep can be either restorative when the person wakes feeling rested and refreshed, or non-restorative. Although the usual definition of non-restorative sleep refers to light, restless, poor quality sleep, in the chronic pain syndrome fibromyalgia, there is evidence that individuals can appear to sleep well, having fallen asleep within a reasonable time and maintained their sleep for many hours. However, they wake unrested and unrefreshed (Doghramji and Deane 2010).

It is not unusual to wake for a few moments at the end of each sleep cycle. We are often not aware of doing so, unless there is something disturbing us – such as the noise of clinical equipment that might disturb Thomas in the HDU, the pain and associated distress that Maria is experiencing, the worry and anxiety that is affecting Mr Davies and the concerns that you might be experiencing regarding your next course assignment. Waking is of itself not an issue; the speed of falling back asleep and the degree of restoration are more important.

It is often said that the average adult needs 7½–8 hours sleep. However, optimum sleep is related to the circadian rythum and needs to occur at the 'right' time. Sleep needs also vary greatly at different ages and between different individuals.

ACTIVITY

Ask your family and friends across different ages (child, teenage, young adult, mature adult, older person) how much sleep they think they get and how much they think they need. It might also be worth asking whether they feel rested and refreshed on waking.

You may find that, as an example, a 40-year-old family member says that he is in bed from 23.00 to 06.30, wakes frequently and wishes he could sleep like he did as a teenager. Yet when you ask him if his sleep refreshes him, he says, 'yes'. A 40 year old gets half the deep sleep of a 20 year old and is more likely to have family worries,

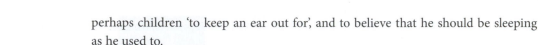

perhaps children 'to keep an ear out for', and to believe that he should be sleeping as he used to.

The Royal College of Psychiatrists (RCP) website offers a number of useful leaflets including one on sleep 'Sleeping well' (RCP 2011). They suggest that:

- Babies sleep around 17 hours each day.
- Older children sleep for 9 or 10 hours each night.
- Adults sleep around 8 hours each night.
- Older people often have only one period of deep sleep during the night, usually in the first 3 or 4 hours. After that, they wake more easily.

Adults' individual sleep requirements in fact vary from perhaps 3 or 4 hours up to 11 hours. However, the amount we sleep can affect how long we live, with 6–7 hours per night proving optimal and much more than this being linked to increased mortality (Patel et al. 2004, 2006). In 2007, a longitudinal survey involving 10,308 civil servants showed that those who had reduced their sleep from 7 hours in 1985–88 to 5 hours by 1992–93 had a 1.7-fold increase in mortality overall and twice the risk of dying from cardiovascular disease as those who had not reduced their sleep (Ferrie et al. 2007). Sleep disturbance is also linked to increased cardiovascular disease in adolescents (Narang et al. 2012).

Losing one hour of sleep per night for one week can leave you feeling sleepy and irritable the following day; reactions are slower, concentration is poor, heart rate increases and you feel cold. Everything is an effort and by the time you go to bed you

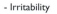

- Irritability
- Cognitive impairment
- Memory lapses or loss
- Impaired moral judgement
- Severe yawning
- Hallucinations
- Symptoms similar to ADHD
- Depression
- Anxiety

- Impaired immune system

- Risk of diabetes Type 2

- Increased heart rate variability
- Risk of heart disease

- Decreased reaction time and accuracy
- Tremors
- Aches

Other
- Growth suppression
- Risk of obesity
- Decreased temperature

Figure 12.11: Effects of sleep deprivation.

either fall asleep immediately or lie awake worrying whether you will get to sleep. Figure 12.11 summarises some of the effects of sleep deprivation on the body and mind.

Speigel et al. (2005) found significant alterations in glucose metabolism, with decreased glucose tolerance and insulin sensitivity, in a group of healthy young adults. The study supports increasing evidence that short sleep duration is associated with diabetes and obesity. It is possible that Maria had a history of poor sleep pre-dating the onset of her diabetes. Daytime napping (Berr et al. 2012) and sleeping for less than 5 hours or more than 9 hours per night (Devore et al. 2012) have been found to be associated with an increased cognitive decline and risk of dementia. Again, it is possible that Violet has a history of less night time sleep and daytime napping preceeding the onset of her Alzheimer's disease.

In acute settings, there have been various studies examining sleep disturbance in intensive care units (ICU) and HDUs. Thomas had an overnight stay in HDU following his surgery. Sleep disruption is common in these environments with sleep fragmentation, frequent arousals and loss of deep and rapid eye movement (REM) sleep. Van Rompaey et al. (2012) cite a number of studies that suggest that one consequence is an increase in delirium, by as much as 60%.

Sleep is important for patient health, our own health and the health of the population at large. A salutory report on explanatory factors in work-related accidents found that fatigue was almost twice as likely as alcohol to be listed as a causative factor (Department for Transport 2005), yet it is drink driving that takes precedent in public campaigns.

Learning outcome 2: Examine factors that may affect sleep for people with acute and long-term health conditions

ACTIVITY

What factors do you think might be affecting:
- Thomas's sleep in the HDU?
- Maria's sleep?
- Violet and her husband's sleep?

The sleep of those with acute pain is frequently disturbed by the intensity of their pain and anxiety. In the case of Thomas, his sleep in HDU may also be disturbed by environmental noise. Xie et al. (2009) list staff conversations and alarms as the most disturbing noises in ICU. The WHO recommends that noise levels in hospital wards are kept below 30dBA (Berglund et al. 1999), while the Environmental Protection Agency suggests 35dBA during sleeping hours and 45dBA in waking hours. Levels in ICU have been found to be at 50–103dBA (Al-Samsam and Cullen 2005). It is not surprising that environmental sound is thus disturbing many of our patients' sleep in intensive care and HDUs. It should be noted that noise above 85dBA for 8 hours is considered to be a risk factor for hearing loss.

At the age of 58, Maria may be menopausal, which is likely to disturb her sleep. As she has diabetes mellitus, alterations in blood sugar may also rouse her. Her painful diabetic neuropathy is likely to interfere with sleep quantity and quality. Brevik et al.

(2006) found that 50% of people with chronic pain feel tired all of the time. Finally, as a consequence of the natural ageing process, Maria will be having less deep sleep than she did when she was younger; the factors listed above are therefore even more likely to interfere with her sleep.

Violet's husband is exhausted. The USA National Sleep Foundation (2011) website page on Dementia and Sleep starts:

> Alzheimer's disease and senile dementia are characterised by frequent sleep disturbance, both for those diagnosed and their caregivers. In fact, many caregivers cite sleep disturbances, including night wandering and confusion, as the reason for institutionalising the elderly.

Sleep patterns can alter for people with dementia; they tend to wake more often and stay awake for longer at night, while being drowsy during the day. Some 20% also experience late afternoon/early evening restlessness and agitation, which has been termed 'sundowning'. The Alzheimer's and Dementia Caregiver Centre (http://www.alz.org/care/alzheimers-dementia-sleep-issues-sundowning.asp) has eight hints and tips on coping with sundowning. Some of these will be discussed later under learning outcome 3.

Insomnia is a significant issue for the population with 25–35% prevalence (Bartlett and Ambrogetti 2006). In today's society, many individuals operate a voluntary sleep restriction programme going to bed late and getting up early. This may be for school, work, family or social reasons; it frequently becomes a difficult habit to break. Bedrooms have become living room extensions with televisions, sound systems, computers and telephones all designed to stimulate the individual. Doghramji and Choufani (2011) list the following dietary and lifestyle issues as potential factors affecting sleep:

- Caffeine and alcohol consumption before bedtime
- Nicotine (both smoking and cessation)
- Large meals or excessive fluid intake within 3 hours of bedtime
- Exercising within 3 hours of bedtime
- Utilising the bed for non-sleep activities (work, telephone, Internet)
- Staying in bed while awake for extended periods
- Activating behaviours up to the point of bedtime
- Excessive worrying at bedtime
- Clock-watching before sleep onset or during nocturnal awakenings
- Exposure to bright light before bedtime or during awakenings
- Keeping the bedroom too hot or too cold
- Noise
- Behaviour of a bed partner (e.g. snoring, leg movements)

While many of these may not be directly appropriate to the hospital setting, patients may be admitted to hospital having developed these habits. Many of them will be applicable in primary and community care settings. The next section moves onto consider strategies for promoting sleep.

Learning outcome 3: Apply a range of strategies to promote sleep for people with health needs

Establishing a bedtime routine and good habits creates the right associations for sleep. We invest time helping young children establish a pattern that fits with the family way of life. As we get older, changes in lifestyle and circumstances alter these patterns. Unfortunately, bad habits and poor routines can develop. Recognising unhelpful patterns and creating helpful associations is the first step in identifying what needs to be changed to improve sleep; see Box 12.5 for questions about sleep.

ACTIVITY

Review Box 12.5. Can you think of any other relevant questions to add to this list? Complete the list of questions, first for yourself and then with a friend or family member. Compare the responses and reflect on the differences.

Box 12.5 Questions about sleep

Sleep pattern
1 What time do you usually go to bed?
2 Do you go off to sleep straight away? If not, why not?
3 Do you wake during the night? If so, how often and why?
4 What time do you usually wake up in the morning?
5 How do you feel when you wake in the morning?

Sleep hygiene
6 What time do you eat your evening meal?
7 How do you spend your time most evenings?
8 What is your routine prior to going to bed?

Sleep environment
9 How old is your mattress? What is it made of?
10 Is it soft, medium or hard?
11 How many pillows do you use and what are they made of?
12 What position do you sleep in?
13 Do you find your bedroom a relaxing and pleasant place to go? If not, why not?
14 Is your room noisy or quiet?
15 Do you watch television in bed?
16 Is your room at a comfortable temperature for you?

Sleep anxieties
17 Do you look forward to bedtime?
18 Do you spend time thinking about the things you have to do the following day or worrying about things at night?
19 Do you 'try' to sleep?

Sleep Pattern

Much of sleep is a habit; we should go to bed when we are tired, but we frequently stay up, for example, to watch the 22.00 news, which may then stimulate us and delay sleep onset. There are some parameters that are essential when thinking of sleep pattern; see Table 12.3. Sleep specialist centres will also measure non-REM and REM sleep stage percentages and the time taken to the first period of REM when analysing individuals' sleep profiles (Castronovo 2006). A further parameter is how restorative sleep is perceived to be by the individual.

There are a number of sleep assessment tools available; however, they tend to be used by sleep specialists. Asking Maria about her sleep and perhaps maintaining a sleep diary may provide additional insight into how her pain is interferring with her sleep pattern.

Sleep hygiene

Sleep is the opposite of arousal. Unfortunately in today's 24/7 society, there is much to maintain arousal at a time of day when our circadian rhythm is synchronised to sleep. Light is the strongest environmental stimulus to the sleep/wake cycle in humans (Ambrogetti 2006). During daylight hours, melatonin production is suppressed and cortisol, which promotes wakefulness, is released. As darkness falls, melatonin is released to cause a fall in body temperature and a slightly hypnotic state (Bartlett and Ambrogetti 2006). Turning lights down in the evening and reducing light stimulation from electronic devices will aid sleep.

Napping after 15.00 will reduce sleep debt and interfere with nighttime sleep. Large meals should be eaten several hours before bedtime, although a carbohydrate snack or malted milk drink, half an hour before bedtime, may promote the release of tryptophan, which is a precursor to increasing melatonin levels. Exercise needs to cease, to allow the body to cool down, 5 hours before bedtime, if it is vigourous, and 1–2 hours for gentle exercise, such as walking (Bartlett and Ambrogetti 2006). Warm baths should be taken at least an hour before bedtime for the same reason. Nicotine, caffeine and alcohol all affect sleep and should be avoided before bedtime as should other stimulants.

Table 12.3: Parameter of sleep

Parameter	Accepted abbreviation	Definition
Sleep latency	SL	Amount of time required to fall asleep
Wakefulness after sleep onset	WASO	Amount of time awake after initial sleep onset
Time in bed	TIB	Time spent in bed
Total sleep time	TST	Actual time spent in bed
Sleep efficiency	SE	Ratio between TIB and TST

Source: Castronovo, V. 2006. Basic concepts of polysomnography. In: Ambrogetti, A., Hensley, M.J. and Olson, L.G. (eds.) *Sleep Disorders: A Clinical Textbook*. Chapter 7. London: Quay Books, 211–76.

Another important factor is a signal or cue that it is time for sleeping. We often associate two things together, such as tea and biscuits, bread and cheese, sun and sand. Creating an association between time and sleepiness and with bed and sleep can be very helpful.

Sleep environment

Bedrooms should be dark and cool, with the bed being cosy. All electronic devices should be turned off to reduce noise and light and to decrease the frequency and length of time awake after initial sleep onset. People who do not draw their curtains, who have the television or radio on in their bedrooms and who complain of poor sleep can improve sleep by attention to these environmental factors.

Mattresses should be supportive of body curves, neither too hard nor too soft; mattress toppers may be useful to promote comfort, particularly for people with pain and insomnia. Pillows should be sufficient to fill the area between the edge of the shoulder and neck so as to maintain cervical posture in side lying. A bolster pillow under the top arm and firm pillow between the knees and ankles can help to maintain spinal alignment.

Tidy, relaxing bedroom environments will help to decrease brain stimulation.

Sleep anxieties

People who are anxious about their sleep are more likely to have disturbed sleep. Bartlett and Ambrogetti (2006) comment:

> Watching the clock at night tends to increase anxiety about sleep. Good sleepers see 2.00 am on the clock when they wake and think 'Wonderful, four more hours in bed'. Poor sleepers see the same and think 'Disaster – I am never going to get back to sleep'. (p. 244)

There is no evidence that the poor sleepers will not get back to sleep, unless perhaps having had the same thought the night before resulting in no further sleep. Catastrophic thinking – trying to get to sleep and worrying about sleep – disrupts sleep, which requires mental and physical relaxation.

People who spend the night planning or worrying about the following day should consider 'brain dumping' 2–4 hours before bedtime; make your list of work priorities at work, do the shopping list when cooking supper, plan your weekend over the meal, dump your worries in a journal for attention the following day; after all, there is little one can do about them during the night hours.

The Sleep Hygiene Hints & Tips Check List (Table 12.4) was developed by one of the author's (Dee Burrows) in her work with people with chronic pain and is used by her and colleagues on a regular basis.

ACTIVITY

- Complete the checklist for yourself and then complete it with someone you know (e.g. relative, friend) who has difficulty sleeping.
- Pick two of the strategies this person will try for the next 2–4 weeks and look up the evidence base.

- Next make a list of which strategies you might try with Maria whose sleep is disturbed by painful diabetic neuropathy.
- Finally, think about which, if any, of the strategies could be applied in a hospital setting. Is there any difference between what could be offered in a mental health unit, an acute hospital ward, and an intensive care unit (ICU) or high dependency unit (HDU).

For Maria, you might have thought of a pictorial busy brain journal for her to dump her worries in and a relaxation technique (see below). You may also need to undertake a bedroom environment assessment.

In ITUs and HDUs, a crucial sleep enhancing strategy is to reduce noise and light stimulation. Thomas is in a strange environment and a strange bed, with a surgical wound, new ileostomy, attached to an epidural and intravenous infusion

Table 12.4: Sleep Hygiene Hints & Tips Check List ©Dee Burrows

Sleep hygiene hints and tips that I could use	Tried but no longer doing ✓	I always do this ✓	I will try this for 2–4 weeks ✓
Aim to wake at the same time each day – set your alarm!			
Make sure you are exposed to bright light during the day.			
Exercise daily physically and mentally – but not late at night.			
Limit day time napping – unless you are Meditteranean!			
Limit caffeine, nicotine and alcohol – unless you are having the same amount now that you were before you developed sleep problems.			
Consider a busy brain journal – to dump your worries and over-active brain into.			
Proteins for lunch, carbohydrates for supper (4 hours before bedtime) and a milky Horlicks or Ovaltine as you start winding down really can help.			
Start relaxing 2 hours before bedtime – a warm bath with candles and smellies; a relaxation or mindfulness technique; soothing music and soft lighting.			
Shut down 1 hour before bedtime – including turning off televisions, radios, computers and even mobile phones.			
Valerian, St John's Wort, Vitamin B6 and other supplements can help – but must not be taken with prescription medication without medical advice.			
Keep a tidy bedroom – used only for sleep.			
Go to bed only when you are sleepy.			
The bedroom should be dark – perhaps blackout blinds?			
The bedroom should be cool, with the bed comfortable and warm.			
Mattresses and pillows need to be supportive and right for you.			
Try orange blossom, rather than lavender.			

and possibly other technical devices. He is likely to be drowsy from the anaesthetic but potentially hyper-aroused by noise and light. Xie et al. (2009) and Van Rompaey et al. (2012) both advocate the use of sound masking, rather than sound-absorbing techniques. Sound masking includes white noise, such as ocean sounds. Xie et al. (2009) found that sound masking improves sleep by 42.7%, while earplugs did so by 25.3%. Hu et al. (2010) used a combination of earplugs to reduce noise exposure and eye masks to reduce light exposure in a laboratory study simulating the ITU and found that the combination resulted in more REM time, shorter REM latency, less arousal and elevated melatonin levels. In the absence of sound-masking devices, earplugs and eye masks are a cost efficient way of promoting sleep in HDUs and reducing the effects of sleep deprivation that may prolong hospital stay. The Alzheimer's Association provide some hints and tips for sleep and sundowning management.

ACTIVITY

Visit the Alzheimer's Association website (http://www.alz.org/care/alzheimers-dementia-sleep-issues-sundowning.asp) and read through their suggested strategies for sleep issues and sundowning. Consider:
- Which of these strategies to improve sleep might you discuss with Violet's husband?
- How do these suggested strategies differ from advice given to people who do not have dementia? (discussed in this chapter)

The strategies to reduce pain and promote comfort, discussed earlier in this chapter, will be important additions to enhance the quality and quantity of sleep. Some of them, such as relaxation techniques, can have a direct impact on sleep by reducing hyper-arousal. Recognising tension is the first step followed by relaxation practice during the daytime until the individual feels competent and confident to try it at night. Imagery relaxation is one example. This approach is about creating pictures, or images, in our minds. These can be based on fantasy, such as being on a beautiful island; on a real event, such as a holiday or on visualising the actual problem and the desired outcome. Imagery can either be guided by another or involve self-visualisation where the individuals make up their own. If the latter approach is adopted, it is worth writing the imagery down so that it can be practised as a prescribed technique. As many of the senses as possible should be involved. In developing one's own imagery, you can experiment with sight, sound, touch, smell and taste. Vividness and clarity can be enhanced by colours, shapes and thoughts. The imagery should be as real and involving as possible. Guided imagery can contain an element of risk if the facilitator creates an image that is unpleasant for the listener. For instance, if the fantasy was based on a walk through a garden and the individual has a poor recollection of pink roses, they may tense up and come out of the imagery. For these reasons, guided imagery can sometimes be generalised, leaving the individual to imagine their favourite flower and perfume.

Pharmacological management of sleep should not be commenced without a detailed sleep assessment and diagnosis. Drugs used for sleep include hypnotics, benzodiazepines, antidepressants, anticonvulsants and beta blockers. Some drugs, such as opioids, can make us drowsy. This may prompt relaxation and aid time taken to get to sleep. Reducing pain during sleep may improve sleep quality. The impact of daytime drowsiness as a consequence of medication side effects may or may not be an issue. For instance, Thomas may be encouraged to nap during his hospital stay, whereas early morning drowsiness for the school run or travel to work is less advisable. Drugs like amitriptyline can leave people feeling drowsy and spaced out in the morning. Conversely, there is evidence that pregabalin has a positive impact on sleep quality as may the SNRIs. These drugs may therefore be useful for Maria whose sleep is disturbed by pain and discomfort.

Poor sleep will enhance perceptions of pain and discomfort, while managing pain and promoting comfort will aid sleep. However, other factors also impact sleep, and a biopsychosocial approach that takes into account individual patterns and behaviours is crucial to managing sleep.

Summary

- Sleep deprivation will affect physical, mental and social health.
- Promoting sleep is a key role of nurses in many different settings and is fundamental to caring.
- Promoting sleep requires an understanding of normal sleep and insight into the individual's usual sleep pattern and any factors that may be contributing to poor sleep.
- A holistic approach to sound sleep hygiene and sleep management is crucial for health.

CHAPTER SUMMARY

Throughout this book, practical nursing skills are contextualised within a philosophy of caring. This final chapter has focused on some fundamental aspects of nursing, managing pain and promoting comfort and sleep and has emphasised a caring approach, including compassion, competence and effective communication. Nurses have an important role in promoting comfort, a role recognised by Florence Nightingale who wrote in 1854:

> The benefits which this Institution [hospital] ought to afford to the sick are perhaps best seen when we are enabled to give comfort in the time of danger and to lessen the agony of death. (quoted in Verney 1970)

Pain management is a huge topic with a developing theoretical base, and this chapter's material aimed to provide a firm basis from which to build your nursing practice. Both pain management and promoting comfort require nurses to integrate a range of skills, with an appropriate attitude and a sound underpinning knowledge base.

ACKNOWLEDGEMENT

The authors thank Dr Ruth Day for her vital assistance and commentary on the pain section.

REFERENCES

Abbey, J., Piller, N., DeBellis, A., et al. 2004. The Abbey Pain Scale: A 1-minute numerical indicator for people with end-stage dementia. *International Journal of Palliative Nursing* 10(1): 6–13.

Al-Samsam, R.H. and Cullen, P. 2005. Sleep and adverse environmental factors in sedated mechanically ventilated pediatric intensive care patients. *Pediatric Critical Care Medicine* 6(5): 562–7.

Alzheimer's and Dementia Caregiver Centre. 2013. Sleep issues and sundowning. Available from: http://www.alz.org/care/alzheimers-dementia-sleep-issues-sundowning.asp (Accessed on 4 March 2013).

Alzheimer's Society. 2012. What is Alzheimer's disease? Available from: http://alzheimers.org.uk/site/scripts/documents_info.php?documentID=100 (Accessed on 4 March 2013).

Alzheimer's Society. 2013. This is me. Available from: http://alzheimers.org.uk/site/scripts/download_info.php?downloadID=399 (Accessed on 4 March 2013).

Ambrogetti, A. 2006. Neuroanatomy and pharmacology of sleep: Clinical implications. In: Ambrogetti, A., Hensley, M.J. and Olson, L.G. (eds.) *Sleep Disorders: A Clinical Textbook*. Chapter 7. London: Quay Books, 211–76.

Arman, M. and Rehnsfeldt, A. 2007. The 'little extra' that alleviates suffering. *Nursing Ethics* 14: 372–86.

Bartlett, D. and Ambrogetti, A. 2006. Insomnia. In: Ambrogetti, A., Hensley, M.J. and Olson, L.G. (eds.) *Sleep Disorders: A Clinical Textbook*. Chapter 7. London: Quay Books, 211–76.

Beacroft, M. and Dodd, K. 2010. 'I feel pain' – Audit of communication skills and understanding of pain and health needs with people with learning disabilities. *British Journal of Learning Disabilities* 39: 139–47.

Bennett, M.I., Bagnall, A.M. and Closs, S.J. 2009. How effective are patient-based educational interventions in the management of cancer pain? Systematic review and meta-analysis. *Pain* 143(3): 192–9.

Bennett, M.I., Hughes, N. and Johnson, M.I. 2011. Methodological quality in randomised controlled trials of transcutaneous electric nerve stimulation for pain: Low fidelity may explain negative findings. *Pain* 152(6): 1226–32.

Berglund, B., Lindvall, T. and Schwela, D.H. 1999. *Guidelines for Community Noise*. Geneva: World Health Organization.

Berr, C., Jaussent, I., Bouyer, J., et al. 2012. Sleep and cognitive decline in the elderly: The French Three-City Cohort. *Alzheimer's & Dementia* 8(4): 233–4.

Bjordal, J., Johnson, M.I. and Ljunggreen, A.E. 2003. Transcutaneous electrical nerve stimulation (TENS) can reduce postoperative analgesic consumption. A meta-analysis with assessment of optimal treatment parameters for postoperative pain. *European Journal of Pain* 7(2): 181–8.

Bland, M. 2007. Betwixt and between: A critical ethnography of comfort in New Zealand residential aged care. *Journal of Clinical Nursing* 16: 937–44.

Breivik, H., Collett, B., Ventafridda, V., et al. 2006. Survey of chronic pain in Europe: Prevalence, impact on daily life, and treatment. *European Journal of Pain* 10(4): 287–333.

Bridges, S. 2012. Chronic pain. In: *Health Survey for England-2011*. 1(9). The Health and Social Care Information Centre. Available from: http://catalogue.ic.nhs.uk/publications/public-health/surveys/heal-surv-eng-2011/HSE2011-Ch9-Chronic-Pain.pdf (Accessed on 31 December 2012).

British Pain Society. 2010. *Opioids for Persistent Pain: Good Practice*. London: The British Pain Society.

Bruce, J. and Quinlan, J. 2011. Chronic post surgical pain. *Reviews in Pain* 5(3): 23–9.

Bundgaard, K. and Nielsen, L.B. 2011. The art of holding hand: A fieldwork study outlining the significance of physical touch in facilities for short-term stay. *International Journal for Human Caring* 15(3): 34–41.

Burrows, D. 2000. *Engaging Patients in Their Own Pain Management: An Action Research Study*. Unpublished PhD thesis. Brunel University.

Burrows, D. 2010. Development of nurse led pain management programmes; meeting a community need. In: Carr, E., Andrews, C. and Layzell, M. (eds.) *Advanced Nursing Practice in Pain Management*. Oxford: Wiley, 143–60.

Burrows, D. and Taylor, E. 2009. The role of personal coping strategies in the management of postoperative pain. In: Cox, F. (ed.) *Perioperative Pain Management*. Oxford: Wiley-Blackwell, 81–94.

Cantrell, M.A. and Matula, C. 2009. The meaning of comfort for pediatric patients with cancer. *Oncology Nursing Forum* 36(6): E303–9.

Castronovo, V. 2006. Basic concepts of polysomnography. In: Ambrogetti, A., Hensley, M.J. and Olson, L.G. (eds.) *Sleep Disorders: A Clinical Textbook*. Chapter 7. London: Quay Books, 211–76.

Chronic Pain Policy Coalition. 2007. Our campaign. Available from: http://www.policyconnect.org.uk/cppc/our-campaign (Accessed on 4 March 2013).

Clarke, H., Bonin, R.P., Orser, B.A., et al. 2012. The prevention of chronic postsurgical pain using Gabapentin and Pregabalin: A combined systematic review and meta-analysis. *Anesthesia & Analgesia* 115(2): 428–42.

Closs, S.J. 2007. Assessment of pain, mood and quality of life. In: Crome, P., Main C.J. and Lally, F. (eds.) *Pain in Older People*. Oxford: Oxford University Press, 11–19.

Closs, S.J., Barr, B., Briggs, M., et al. 2003. Evaluating pain in care home residents with dementia. *Nursing and Residential Care* 5(1): 32–3.

Demir, Y. and Khorshid, L. 2010. The effect of cold application in combination with standard analgesic administration on pain and anxiety during chest tube removal: A single-blinded, randomized, double-controlled study. *Pain Management Nursing* 11(3): 186–96.

Department for Transport. 2005. *Road Safety Research Report No. 58: An In-Depth Study of Work-Related Road Traffic Accidents*. Norwich: HMSO.

Devore, E., Grodstein, F. and Schernhammer, E. 2012. Sleep duration and cognitive function: The nurses' health study. *Alzheimer's & Dementia* 8(4): 233.

Doghramji, K. and Choufani, D. 2011. Taking a sleep history. In: Winkelman, J. and Plante, D. (eds.) *Foundations of Psychiatric Sleep Medicine*. Cambridge, MA: Cambridge University Press, 95–110.

Doghramji, K. and Deane, K. 2010. Nonrestorative sleep in fibromyalgia: From assessment to therapy—Focus on features of fibromyalgia-associated nonrestorative sleep. *Medscape Education Rheumatology*. Available from: http://www.medscape.org/viewarticle/734747 (Accessed on 31 December 2012).

Donaldson, L. 2009. *Pain: Breaking Through the Barrier. 150 Years of the Annual Report of the Chief Medical Officer: On the State of Public Health 2008*. London: DH. Available from http://webarchive.nationalarchives.gov.uk/20130107105354/http://www.dh.gov.uk/en/Publicationsandstatistics/Publications/AnnualReports/DH_096206

Dubinsky, R. and Miyasaki, J. 2010. Assessment: Efficacy of transcutaneous electric nerve stimulation in the treatment of pain in neurologic disorders (an evidence based review). Report of the Therapeutics and Technology Assessment Subcommittee of the American Academy of Neurology. *Neurology* 74(2): 173–6.

Ferrell, B.R., McCaffery, M. and Rhiner, M. 1992. Pain and addiction: An urgent need for change in nursing education. *Journal of Pain and Symptom Management* 7: 117–24.

Ferrie, J.E., Shipley, M.J., Cappuccio, F.P., et al. 2007. A prospective study of change in sleep duration; associations with mortality in the Whitehall II cohort. *Sleep* 30(12): 1659–66.

Fridh, I., Forsberg, A. and Bergbom, I. 2009. Doing one's utmost: Nurses' descriptions of caring for dying patients in an intensive care environment. *Intensive and Critical Care Nursing* 25: 233–41.

Gleeson, M. and Higgins, A. 2009. Touch in mental health nursing: An exploratory study of nurses' views and perceptions. *Journal of Psychiatric and Mental Health Nursing* 16: 382–9.

Hawley, M.P. 2000. Nurse comforting strategies: Perceptions of emergency department patients. *Clinical Nursing Research* 9: 441–59.

Hu, R.F., Jiang, X.Y., Zeng, Y., et al. 2010. Effects of earplugs and eye masks on nocturnal sleep, melatonin and cortisol in a simulated intensive care unit environment. *Critical Care* 14(2): R66.

Hudacek, S.S. 2008. Dimensions of caring: A qualitative analysis of nurses' stories. *Journal of Nursing Education* 47(3): 124–9.

Huizanga, M.M. and Peltier, A. 2007. Painful diabetic neuropathy: A management centred review. *Clinical Diabetes* 25(1): 6–15.

Iber, C., Ancoli-Israel, S., Chesson, A., et al. 2007. *The AASM Manual for the Scoring of Sleep and Associated Events: Rules, Terminology and Technical Specifications*. Westchester, NY: American Academy of Sleep Medicine.

International Association for the Study of Pain Subcommittee on Taxonomy. 1979. Pain terms: A list with definitions and notes on usage. *Pain* 6: 249–52.

Kings College, London. 2012. *Intentional Rounding: What Is the Evidence?* Policy +. London: KCL.

Kingston, K. and Bailey, C. 2009. Assessing the pain of people with learning disability. *British Journal of Nursing* 18(7): 420–3.

Kolkaba, K.Y. 1995. Comfort as process and product, merged in holistic art. *Journal of Holistic Nursing* 13: 117–31.

Kolkaba, K.Y. 2003. *Comfort Theory and Practice: A Vision for Holistic Health Care and Research*. New York: Springer.

Kovach, C.R., Griffie, J. and Muchka, S. 1999. Assessment and treatment of discomfort for people with late-stage dementia. *Journal of Pain and Symptom Management* 18: 412–19.

Kwekkeboom, K.L. and Gretarsdottir, E. 2006. Systematic review of relaxation interventions for pain. *Journal of Nursing Scholarship* 38(3): 269–77.

Lee, O.K., Chung, Y.F., Chan, M.F., et al. 2005. Music and its effect on the physiological responses and anxiety levels of patients receiving mechanical ventilation: A pilot study. *Journal of Clinical Nursing* 14: 609–20.

Leow, Q.H.M., Drury, V.B., Poon, W.H. 2010. A qualitative exploration of patients' experiences of music therapy in an inpatient hospice in Singapore. *International Journal of Palliative Nursing* 16(7): 344–50.

Liu, J.Y.W., Briggs, M. and Closs, S.J. 2010. The psychometric qualities of four observational pain tools (OPTs) for the assessment of pain in elderly people with osteoarthritic pain. *Journal of Pain and Symptom Management* 40(4): 582–98.

Lovering, S. 2006. Cultural attitudes and beliefs about pain. *Journal of Transcultural Nursing* 17(4): 389–95.

Ludlow, C. 2008. One couple's extraordinary story of how they both survived the same cancer. *The Observer*, 27 January: 26–32.

MacIntyre, P.E., Schug, S.A., Scott, D.A., et al. 2010. *Acute Pain Management: Scientific Evidence,* 3rd edn. Melbourne: ANZCA & FPM.

Mann, E. and Carr, E. 2006. *Pain Management: Essential Clinical Skills for Nurses.* Oxford: Blackwell.

McGettigan, P. and Henry, D. 2013. Use of non-steroidal anti-inflammatory drugs that can elevate cardiovascular risk: An examination of sales and essential medicine lists in low-, middle-, and high-income countries. *PLoS Medicine.* DOI: 10.1371/journal.pmed.1001388.

McKay, M. and Clarke, S. 2012. Pain assessment tools for the child with severe learning disability. *Nursing Children and Young People* 24(2): 14–25.

McQuay, H. and Moore, A. 1998. *An Evidence-Based Resource for Pain Relief.* Oxford: Oxford University Press.

MedicineNet.com. 2012. Diabetes mellitus. Available from: http://www.medicinenet.com/diabetes_mellitus/article.htm (Accessed on 18 July 2012).

Melzack, R. 1987. The short-form McGill pain questionnaire. *Pain* 30(2): 191–7.

Melzack, R. 2005. Evolution of the neuromatrix theory of pain. *Pain Practice* 5(2): 85–94.

Melzack, R. and Wall, P. 1996. *Challenge of Pain.* Harmondsworth: Penguin.

Middleton, C. 2006. *Epidural Analgesia in Acute Pain Management.* Chichester: John Wiley.

Morone, N.E. and Greco, C.M. 2007. Mind–body interventions for chronic pain in older adults: A structured review. *Pain Medicine* 8(4): 359–75.

Morse, J.M. and Proctor, A. 1998. Maintaining patient endurance: The comfort work of trauma nurses. *Clinical Nursing Research* 7: 250–74.

Moskow, S.B. 1987. *Human Hand and Other Ailments.* Boston, MA: Little, Brown.

Mottram, A. 2009. Therapeutic relationships in day surgery: A grounded theory study. *Journal of Clinical Nursing* 18: 2830–7.

Multiple Sclerosis Trust. 2007. *Multiple Sclerosis: Information for Health and Social Care Professionals.* Letchworth: Multiple Sclerosis Trust.

Narang, I., Manlhiot, C., Davies-Shaw, J., et al. 2012. Sleep disturbance and cardiovascular risk in adolescents. *CMAJ* 184(17): E913–20.

National Sleep Foundation. Available from: http://www.sleepfoundation.org/article/sleep-topics/dementia-and-sleep (Accesed on 31 December 2012).

Nishimori, M., Ballantyne, J.C. and Low, J.H.S. 2007. Epidural pain relief versus systemic opioid-based pain relief for abdominal aortic surgery. *Cochrane Database of Systematic Reviews* (7). Art. No.: CD005059. DOI: 10.1002/14651858.CD005059.pub3.

Patel, S.R., Ayas, N.T., Malhotra, M.R., et al. 2004. A prospective study of sleep duration and mortality risk in women. *Sleep* 27(3): 440–4.

Patel, S.R., Malhotra, A., Gottlieb, D.J., et al. 2006. Correlates of long sleep duration. *Sleep* 29(7): 881–9.

Patient.co.uk. 2011. Insomnia (poor sleep). Available from: http://www.patient.co.uk/doctor/patient-health-questionnaire-phq-9 (Accessed on 14 September 2012).

Patients Association. 2007. *Pain in Older People – A Hidden Problem.* Available from: http://www.patients-association.com/Portals/0/Public/Files/Research%20Publications/Pain%20in%20Older%20People%20-%20a%20hidden%20problem.pdf (Accessed on 31 December 2012).

Picco, E, Santoro, R. and Garrino, L. 2010. Dealing with the patient's body in nursing: Nurses' ambiguous experience in clinical practice. *Nursing Inquiry* 17(1): 38–45.

Proctor, A., Morse, J.M. and Khonsari, S. 1996. Sounds of comfort in the trauma center: How nurses talk to patients in pain. *Social Science Medicine* 42: 1669–80.

Rasin, J. and Kautz, D.D. 2007. Knowing the resident with dementia: Perspectives of assisted facility caregivers. *Journal of Gerontological Nursing* 33(9): 30–6.

Roche-Fahy, V. and Dowling, M. 2009. Providing comfort to patients in their palliative care trajectory: Experiences of female nurses working in an acute setting. *International Journal of Palliative Nursing* 15(3): 134–41.

Royal College of Psychiatrists (RCP). 2011. Sleeping well. Available from: http://www.rcpsych.ac.uk/mentalhealthinfoforall/problems/sleepproblems/sleepingwell.aspx (Accessed on 4 March 2013).

Sanderson, T. and Cole, F. 2011. *An Audit of the Value of the Pain Toolkit in Facilitating Self-Care: The Patient's Perspective.* Poster Presentation. Bath Pain Management Programmes Conference, Bath.

Sofaer, B. 1998. *Pain Principles, Practice and Patients,* 3rd edn. Cheltenham: Stanley Thornes.

Speigel, K., Knutson, K., Leproult, R., et al. 2005. Sleep loss: A novel risk factor for insulin resistance and type 2 diabetes. *Journal of Applied Physiology* 99(5): 2008–19.

Tutton, E. and Seers, K. 2004. Comfort on a ward for older people. *Journal of Advanced Nursing* 46(4): 380–9.

USA National Sleep Foundation. 2011. Dementia and sleep. Available from: http://www.sleepfoundation.org/article/sleep-topics/dementia-and-sleep (Accessed on 4 March 2013).

Van Rompaey, B., Elseviers, M.M., Van Drom, W., et al. 2012. The effect of earplugs during the night on the onset of delirium and sleep perception: A randomized controlled trial in intensive care. *Critical Care* 16(R73): 1–10.

Verney, H. 1970. *Florence Nightingale at Harley Street: Her Reports to the Governors of Her Nursing Home 1853–4.* London: J.M. Dent.

Walsh, D.M., Howe, T.E., Johnson, M.I., et al. 2009. Transcutaneous electrical nerve stimulation for acute pain. *Cochrane Database of Systematic Reviews* (2). Art. No.: CD006142. DOI: 10.1002/14651858.CD006142.pub2

Werawatganon, T. and Charuluxanun, S. 2007. Patient controlled intravenous opioid analgesia versus continuous epidural analgesia for pain after intra-abdominal surgery. *Cochrane Database of Systematic Reviews* (4). Art. No.: CD004088. DOI: 10.1002/14651858.CD004088.pub3.

Wilby, M.L. 2005. Cancer patients' descriptions of comforting and discomforting nursing actions. *International Journal for Human Caring* 9(4): 59–63.

Williams, A.M., Davies, A. and Griffiths, G. 2009. Facilitating comfort for hospitalized patients using non-pharmacological measures: Preliminary development of clinical practice guidelines. *International Journal of Nursing Practice* 15: 145–55.

Williams, A.M., Dawson, S. and Kristjanson, L.J. 2008. Exploring the relationship between personal control and the hospital environment. *Journal of Clinical Nursing* 17: 1601–9.

Williams, A.M. and Irurita, V. 2004. Therapeutic and non-therapeutic interpersonal interactions: The patient's perspective. *Journal of Clinical Nursing* 13: 806–15.

Williams, A.M. and Irurita, V.F. 2006. Emotional comfort: The patient's perspective of a therapeutic context. *International Journal of Nursing Studies* 43: 405–15.

Wood, S. 2008. Assessment of pain. Available from: http://www.nursingtimes.net/nursing-practice-clinical-research/assessment-of-pain/1861174.article (Accessed on 14 September 2012).

World Health Organization (WHO). 1996. *Cancer Pain Relief,* 2nd edn. Geneva: WHO.

Wright, A. 2012. Exploring the evidence for using TENS to relieve pain. *Nursing Times* 108(11): 20–3.

Xie, H., Kang, J. and Mills, G.H. 2009. Clinical review: The impact of noise on patients' sleep and the effectiveness of noise reduction strategies in intensive care units. *Critical Care* 13(2): 208.

Yilidrim, N., Ulusoy, F. and Bodur, H. 2010. The effect of heat application on pain, stiffness, physical function and quality of life in patients with knee osteoarthritis. *Journal of Clinical Nursing* 19(7–8): 1113–20.

Zanocchi, M., Maero, B., Nicola, E., et al. 2008. Chronic pain in a sample of nursing home residents: Prevalence, characteristics, influence on quality of life (QoL). *Archives of Gerontology and Geriatrics* 47(1): 121–8.

Zerwekh, J.V. 1997. The practice of presencing. *Seminars in Oncology Nursing* 13(4): 260–2.

WEBSITES

http://alzheimers.org.uk/ Accessed 18th July 2012

www.britishpainsociety.org/book_pain_older_people.pdf Accessed 14th September 2012

http://www.medicinenet.com/diabetes_mellitus/article.htm Accessed 18th July 2012

http://www.paincommunitycentre.org Accessed 14th September 2012

http://www.paintoolkit.org/Accessed 14th September 2012

www.patient.co.uk/doctor/Patient-Health-Qusetionnaire-(PHQ-9).htm Accessed 14th September 2012

http://prc.coh.org/PainNOA/DS-DAT_Tool.pdf Accessed 14th September 2012

http://wps.prenhall.com/wps/media/objects/3103/3178396/tools/flacc.pdf

http://www.rcgp.org.uk Accessed 21st August 2012

http://www.wellcome.ac.uk/en/pain/microsite/science4.html Accessed 14th September 2012

Index

Note: Page numbers followed by *b* represent boxes, by *f* represent figures, and *t* represent tables.